# PRACTICAL
# ORTHOPEDICS

FIFTH EDITION

# PRACTICAL ORTHOPEDICS

## LONNIE R. MERCIER, M.D.

Clinical Instructor
Department of Orthopedic Surgery
Creighton University School of Medicine
Omaha, Nebraska

## CONTRIBUTORS
## FRED J. PETTID, M.D.

Associate Professor of Family Practice
Department of Family Practice
Creighton University School of Medicine
Omaha, Nebraska

## DEAN F. TAMISIEA, M.D.

Department of Radiology
Midlands Community Hospital
Papillion, Nebraska

## JOHN J. HEIECK, M.D.

Assistant Clinical Professor
Department of Surgery
Creighton University School of Medicine
Omaha, Nebraska

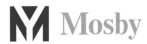

*A Harcourt Health Sciences Company*

St. Louis   London   Philadelphia   Sydney   Toronto

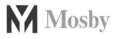

A Harcourt Health Sciences Company

*Acquisitions Editor:* Liz Fathman
*Developmental Editor:* Kathy Falk
*Project Manager:* Deborah Vogel
*Production Editor:* Ed Alderman
*Designer:* Bill Drone

**FIFTH EDITION**

**NOTICE**

Pharmacology is an ever-changing field. Standard safety precautions must be followed, but as new research and clinical experience broaden our knowledge, changes in treatment and drug therapy may become necessary or appropriate. Readers are advised to check the most current product information provided by the manufacturer of each drug to be administered to verify the recommended dose, the method and duration of administration, and contraindications. It is the responsibility of the treating appropriately licensed health care provider, relying on experience and knowledge of the patient, to determine dosages and the best treatment for each individual patient. Neither the publisher nor the editor assumes any liability for any injury and/or damage to persons or property arising from this publication.

Mosby, Inc.
*A Harcourt Health Sciences Company*
11830 Westline Industrial Drive
St. Louis, Missouri 63146

Printed in United States of America

**Library of Congress Cataloging in Publication Data**

Mercier, Lonnie R.
Practical orthopedics / Lonnie R. Mercier; contributors, Fred J. Pettid,
Dean F. Tamisiea, John J. Heieck. —5th ed.
p. cm.
Includes bibliographical references and index.
ISBN 0-323-00827-5 (alk. paper : softcover)
1. Orthopedics. I. Title.
[DNLM: Orthopedics. WE 168 M555p 2000]
RD731 .M43 2000
616.7—dc 21

99-089409

00  01  02  03  04  GW/KPT  9  8  7  6  5  4  3  2  1

*To my wife, Lorraine, and my son, Mark.*

*To my parents, who always encouraged higher education.*

*L.M.*

# Preface to the Fifth Edition

Publication of this edition of Practical Orthopedics reflects the positive responses to the first four editions. The book is based in great part on the author's 25 years of experience in teaching general orthopedics to family physicians and residents. The basic format of the text has been retained, dividing the text into two general sections. The first section deals with musculoskeletal disorders organized by anatomic region and the second discusses the arthritides, infection, roentgenographic diagnosis, and other areas of interest.

As in previous revisions, all material has been updated and additional conditions are discussed. A con-siderable number of new illustrations have been added and older ones revised for clarity. Every effort has been made to identify conditions that are controversial in nature and to explain them in that context.

We would again like to thank the many people who helped in the preparation of the manuscript and illustrations, as well as those who contributed roentgenograms and advice. We hope this edition continues to meet its goals for primary care physicians, residents, and students.

**Lonnie Mercier, M.D.**

# Preface to the First Edition

The stimulus to write this book was our participation in the orthopedic training of students and residents whose primary fields of interest are those other than orthopedic surgery. We were frequently asked to recommend an appropriate text for them to study but we found that none was available that met their needs. Most orthopedic surgery books are either too detailed or not complete enough to have any practical value in general medicine. We discovered, also, that no book existed that could be used as a current, practical guide and clinical reference by practicing physicians in the daily care of their patients. This book was undertaken to meet these needs.

In presenting a useful overview of orthopedic disorders, we have tried to discuss, in some depth, those conditions that are encountered frequently in daily practice. By emphasizing certain common features of these disorders, it is hoped that the fundamental concepts can be applied in the diagnosis and treatment of other musculoskeletal conditions.

The text is divided into two general sections. The first deals with musculoskeletal disorders by anatomic region. The later chapters discuss the arthritides, infection, injuries, and other common problems of interest, including a particularly useful chapter on radiologic aspects of orthopedic disease. The reader interested in sports medicine is directed to the index, where he will find references to discussions throughout the text on treatment of patients with athletic injuries.

The practice of orthopedics is, in a sense, rehabilitative medicine. It has as its goals improvement in the level of function of the patient and the diminution of pain. We hope you will find this book helpful in meeting these goals.

**Lonnie R. Mercier, M.D.**
**Fred J. Pettid, M.D.**

# Contents

*Reproduced from Ferri FF, editor: Ferri's Patient Teaching Guides. In Ferri FF, editor: *Ferri's Clinical Advisor 2000 CD-ROM,* St Louis, 2000, Mosby.

# CHAPTER 1

# Physical Examination

The diagnosis of disorders of the musculoskeletal system begins with compiling a complete history and performing a physical examination. The history is of special significance because physical findings are often minimal. Its importance cannot be overemphasized. It should be possible to diagnose most musculoskeletal conditions by history and physical examination alone. Other additional early testing is usually unnecessary in the analysis of most orthopedic conditions.

## HISTORY

### Birth History

The history of the pediatric patient should include several important points. It should first be determined whether fetal movements were experienced by the mother during pregnancy. Absence or weakness of these movements by the fourth or fifth month of gestation may indicate neuromuscular disease in the newborn. Any maternal diabetes, toxemia, drug ingestion, fetal distress, or prematurity is noted.

The type of delivery should also be determined. This is important because certain disorders such as congenital hip dysplasia are more common after breech delivery.

The condition of the child at birth and immediately after delivery should be ascertained. It should be noted if the hospital stay of the baby was unusually prolonged. The presence of any jaundice, cyanosis, or difficulty with the delivery that might predispose the infant to brain damage is also recorded.

The physical and mental development of the child is then determined, and any deviation from normal progress is noted (Table 1-1).

For accuracy, the ages of all children should be listed by years plus months.

### Family History

A review of the family history is important not only for certain visible musculoskeletal problems such as polydactyly but also for those disorders that may not be so obvious, such as scoliosis, osteoporosis, neuromuscular disease, and tuberculosis. Other family members may even need to be interviewed or examined.

### Past History

The general health of the patient is recorded, as well as any recent weight loss or gain. The patient's exact occupation should be determined and any relevant military history noted, especially if a disability rating resulted from time spent in the service. Impairment ratings from other sources are also recorded. All chronic renal, metabolic, pulmonary, and previous orthopedic disorders should be assessed in view of the initial complaint. Any drug or alcohol use is recorded. The smoking history is especially important because a positive history may adversely affect multiple musculoskeletal conditions including osteoporosis, fracture healing, and low back pain.

The menstrual history, especially the date of onset, is noted when assessing scoliosis and menopause (at which time osteoporosis should always be discussed, even though the present illness may be unrelated).

### Present Illness

The nature of the onset of symptoms, whether gradual or sudden, should be established. If an injury is involved, the exact date and place of the injury are recorded. This is often an important fact in determining injury liability. If the problem seems job related, other information regarding the work history may be helpful:

**TABLE 1–1.**

Normal Milestones*

| Age (mo) | Milestone |
| --- | --- |
| 1-2 | Holds up chin |
| 6-8 | Sits alone |
| 8-10 | Stands with support |
| 10-12 | Walks with support |
| 14 | Walks without support |
| 24 | Ascends stairs one foot at a time |

*Note: There is commonly a wide variation in physical development, but if a child cannot walk unsupported by 18 months of age, a neuromuscular disorder should be suspected. A wide-based gait is often the first noticeable abnormality when neuromuscular disease is present in the child.

(1) whether the symptoms may have been caused by the work or simply developed while the patient was working, (2) if the patient missed any work as a result of the problem, (3) if the patient has ever been on light duty as a result of the disorder, and (4) if a report of the injury was filed at work. The chief complaint should also be evaluated in relation to any previous similar symptoms or other musculoskeletal complaints. In addition, it should be noted whether the patient has had any other recent, seemingly unrelated illness or symptoms, such as fever or chills. The results of any prior treatment or tests should also be ascertained.

The exact location and nature of any *pain* should be determined. In addition, the following important facts are noted: (1) the relationship of the pain to normal daily activities, (2) whether the pain is worse in the morning or late in the day, (3) whether coughing, sneezing, or other similar activities aggravate the pain, (4) whether the pain improves or worsens with rest, and (5) whether the pain remains well localized or is referred or radicular in nature. If the pain is radicular, it should be determined whether the radiation follows any dermatome or peripheral nerve pattern. The effect of any home remedies on the pain should also be assessed.

*Weakness* and *numbness* may be extremely subjective. (Weakness is more often a result of pain than actual motor loss.) An attempt should be made to document these symptoms, however. The following information should be ascertained: (1) whether the weakness is generalized or involves specific muscles or muscle groups, (2) whether there is any loss of sphincter control, and (3) whether the numbness follows a dermatome, peripheral nerve, or stocking/glove pattern. The pain and numbness that follow specific dermatome nerve patterns are often diagnostic, but the numbness that follows a stocking or glove type of distribution is non-anatomic and often indicates symptom magnification. It should also be determined whether the symptoms are worse at night or during the day. The discomfort from carpal tunnel syndrome, for example, is characteristically most severe at night, as is pain from a spinal cord tumor.

When *deformity* is the initial complaint, the following information should be obtained: (1) how long it has been present, (2) whether the patient or someone else first noticed the deformity, (3) whether it is increasing or decreasing, and (4) whether it is associated with any recent injury, joint swelling, or stiffness. The amount of actual disability, if any, that the deformity causes the patient is also of considerable importance.

The assessment of *crepitation* is often difficult. It is commonly an inconsistent finding. Some noise is considered normal in certain joints, especially in the absence of other symptoms such as pain. In other cases, synovial hypertrophy (joint or tendon sheath) or a significantly irregular joint surface may cause crepitus (and pain) with certain movements. By itself, crepitus is not considered pathologic, but its exact etiology may be difficult to explain.

(It should also be recorded whether or not the patient will be released to work and, if so, on what date. Discussing this clearly with the patient and recording it in the chart will simplify future correspondence with the employer or insurance companies.)

## EXAMINATION

Valuable information can often be gained merely by observing the gait, general posture, and stance of the patient. This is especially helpful in the child who may otherwise be difficult to examine. The height and weight of the patient are recorded, and all examinations are performed with the affected area completely exposed (Fig. 1-1). The patient should always be viewed in profile as well as from the front and back. In addition, certain areas may lend themselves to a different view. For example, subtle swelling of the metacarpophalangeal joints and dorsal intermetacarpal soft tissue can be visualized clearly by viewing and comparing the patient's clenched fists pointed toward the examiner. Posterior ankle and heel cord swelling can also be assessed by asking the patient to kneel on a chair and then viewing the swollen areas from behind the patient.

The affected area is then inspected, and any swelling, discoloration, or areas of tenderness are noted. Palpation should be gentle but persistent. In the child it is sometimes easier to start at a distance from the injured or painful site and work slowly toward the area in question. Every attempt should be made to describe affected areas according to their exact anatomic location. Movements or maneuvers that exacerbate the pain are recorded as well as nonorganic behavior or pain magnification during the examination. Any muscle atrophy is noted and compared

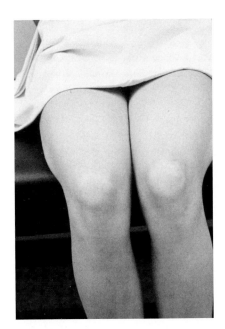

**Fig. 1–1.**
Proper attire for knee examination. Both lower extremities are completely exposed. The patient always needs to be undressed so that the injured area can be well visualized (and compared with an opposite normal extremity, if indicated). Remember: "Much more is missed by not looking than by not knowing" (Osler). To best appreciate increased warmth (synovitis) in a superficial joint such as the knee, place one hand on each knee and then switch hands back and forth.

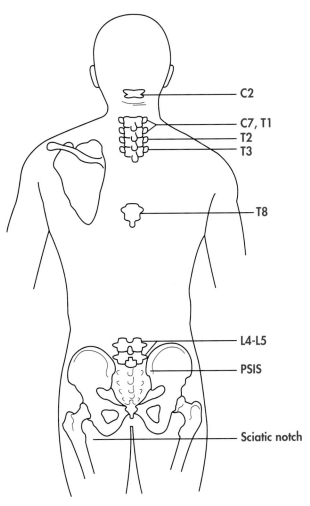

**Fig. 1–2.**
Bony landmarks from the back. C2 is the first palpable cervical spinous process. C7 and T1 are the first prominent spinous processes. (The fat pad over this area is sometimes mistaken for a "mass." It may enlarge with chronic steroid use.) T2 marks the level of the upper tip of the scapula. T3 marks the flattened triangular area of the spine of the scapula. The inferior angle of the scapula is at the level of T8. The iliac crest is at the level of L4-L5. A prominent fat pad over the sacrum may also be misinterpreted as a mass when pain is referred to this area.

with measurements of the opposite extremity. Muscle power is tested in a similar manner. Alterations in skin temperature or perspiration are also noted, especially in the lower extremity. Any signs of circulatory disturbance (edema, dependent rubor, or distal hair loss) should also be recorded. References to known anatomic landmarks are used whenever possible (Fig. 1-2).

Active and passive ranges of joint motion are carefully measured, and the patient is observed for any crepitus or resistance to movement. During the examination, adjacent joints may need to be stabilized to properly measure the affected joint (Fig. 1-3).

Measurements of limb length and circumference are also made when indicated, and a complete neurologic examination is performed if neuromuscular disease is suspected.

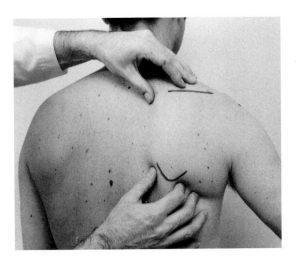

**Fig. 1–3.**
True glenohumeral motion is measured by first stabilizing the scapula to prevent scapulothoracic motion. This is accomplished by prohibiting movement of the palpable spine and inferior angle.

## ORTHOPEDIC TERMINOLOGY

### General

*Ankylosis*:   restriction of motion in a joint (synostosis)

*Antalgic gait*:   gait pattern in which the weight is quickly removed from the affected extremity as a result of pain

*Arthrodesis*:   surgical stiffening of a joint (fusion), usually to relieve pain

*Arthroplasty*:   surgery to restore motion and function to a joint

*Coxa*:   hip bone or joint (os coxae)

*Cubitus*:   elbow

*Diaphysis*:   the shaft of a bone

*Effusion*:   escape of fluid into a cavity

*Extensor*:   the dorsal or posterior surface

*Functional*:   nonorganic, not as a result of a structural defect

*Genu*:   knee or knee joint

*Hallux*:   great toe

*Metaphysis*:   the broad, vascular part of a bone near a joint

*Orthopedic*:   "straight child"

*Osteonecrosis*:   death of bone (aseptic necrosis, avascular necrosis)

*Palmar*:   the anterior surface of the hand (volar)

*Paresthesia*:   abnormal sensation, such as burning or tingling

*Pes*:   foot

*Plantar*:   the sole or flexor surface of the foot

*Pollex (pollicis)*:   thumb

*Radicular*:   spinal nerve involvement

*Spondylitis*:   inflammation involving the spinal column

*Spondylolisthesis*:   slipping of a vertebra, usually as a result of spondylolysis

*Spondylolysis*:   dissolution or loosening of a vertebra

*Spondylosis*:   disease, usually degenerative, of a vertebra

*Sprain*:   injury to joint ligament or capsule

*Strain*:   injury to muscle or tendon

*Subluxation*:   incomplete dislocation

*Synovitis*:   inflammation of the synovial membrane of a joint, usually the result of trauma or an arthritic process and commonly accompanied by fluid production and mild local warmth

*Talipes*:   talus (ankle) plus pes (foot)

*Tenosynovium*:   the synovial sheath in which tendons move, usually at joint levels.

**Note**: When referring to fingers, it is best to use a name (thumb, index, long, ring, and small) rather than a number

### Motion

*Abduction*:   movement away from the middle line (in the hand, the long finger is the middle line)

*Adduction*:   movement toward the middle line

*Eversion*:   turning outward (in the foot, valgus, eversion, and pronation are commonly synonymous)

*Extension*:   straightening of a joint

*Flexion*:   bending of a joint

*Inversion*:   turning inward (in the foot, varus, inversion, and supination are commonly synonymous)

*Pronation*:   to rotate the forearm in such a way that the palm looks backward when the arm is in the anatomic position

*Supination*:   to rotate the forearm in such a way that the palm looks forward when the arm is in the anatomic position

### Deformity

*Calcaneus*:   dorsiflexion of the foot

*Cavus*:   hollow; abnormally high arch

*Equinus*:   plantar flexion of the foot

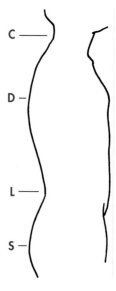

**Fig. 1–4.**
A mild kyphosis is normally present in the dorsal (D) and sacral (S) spine. Lordosis is normally present in the cervical (C) and lumbar (L) spine.

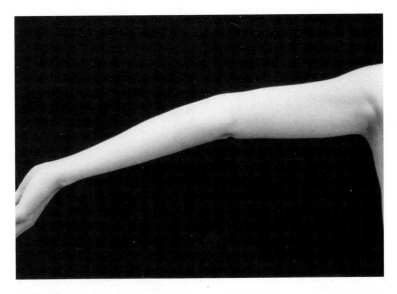

**Fig. 1–5.**
Recurvatum of the elbow.

*Kyphosis*:  curvature of the spine with posterior convexity (Fig. 1-4)

*Lordosis*:  curvature of the spine with anterior convexity

*Planus*:  flat; abnormally low arch

*Recurvatum*:  backward bending or hyperextension (Fig. 1-5)

*Scoliosis*:  abnormal lateral curvature of the spine

*Valgus*:  the distal part angulates away from the midline of the body (Fig. 1-6)

*Varus*:  the distal part angulates toward the midline of the body

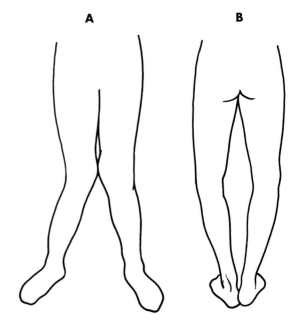

**Fig. 1–6.**
**A**, Genu valgum. **B**, Genu varum.

# Fractures: General Management

Most fractures are easily recognized both clinically and roentgenographically (Fig. 2-1). A satisfactory end result in the treatment of these injuries will depend not only on reduction of the fracture and maintenance of that reduction but also on restoration of the function of the injured extremity. These goals are reached by appreciating both the bony and soft tissue structures involved.

## TERMINOLOGY

*Fracture:* a break in the continuity of a bone

*Avulsion ("chip"):* small fracture near a joint that usually has a ligament or tendon attached

*Closed ("simple"):* fracture that does not have an open wound in the skin

*Comminuted:* fracture with multiple fragments (Fig. 2-2)

*Displaced:* fracture whose ends are separated

*Epiphyseal:* fracture of the growth plate, usually in a long bone

*Greenstick:* incomplete fracture that usually occurs in children

*Impacted:* fracture whose ends are driven into each other

*Intraarticular:* fracture that involves the joint surface of a bone

*Occult:* clinical condition that suggests a fracture. Roentgenograms 2 to 3 weeks later may show the fracture line or new bone formation

*Open ("compound"):* fracture in which there is an open wound of the skin and soft parts that leads into the fracture

*Pathologic:* fracture that occurs because the bone is weakened by some abnormal condition (often tumor)

*Stress:* fracture that occurs when weak bone is stressed normally (insufficiency fracture) or when normal bone is stressed excessively (fatigue fracture). Usually seen only in weight-bearing bones

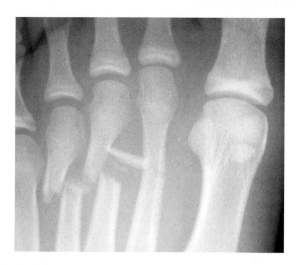

**Fig. 2–1.**
Fractures of the metatarsal necks and a bipartite tibial (medial) sesamoid of the great toe. The fracture is distinguished from the bipartite sesamoid or accessory bone by its sharp, pointed edges and irregular margin.

*Torus:* "buckle" fracture caused by compression of the cortex, most common in the distal portion of the radius of the child

*Alignment:* rotational or angular position

*Apposition:* amount of end-to-end contact of the fracture (Fig. 2-3)

*Delayed union:* fracture healing that is slower than normal

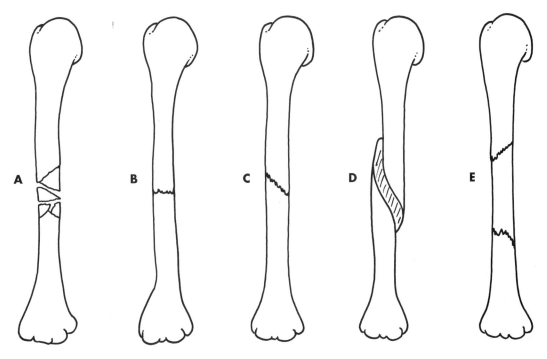

**Fig. 2–2.**
Midshaft fractures of the humerus. **A**, Comminuted. **B**, Transverse, undisplaced. **C**, Oblique, undisplaced. **D**, Spiral.
**E**, Segmental.

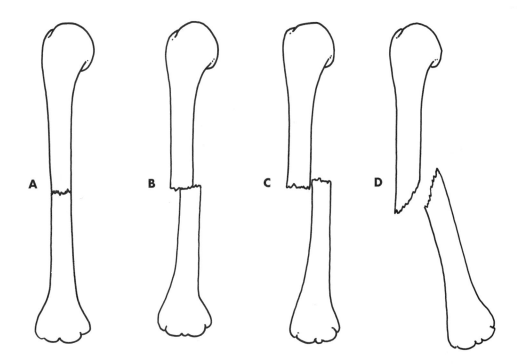

**Fig. 2–3.**
Apposition and alignment of midshaft fractures of the humerus, anteroposterior (AP) view. **A**, Perfect
end-to-end apposition, perfect alignment. **B**, 50% end-to-end apposition, perfect alignment. **C**, Side-
to-side (bayonet) apposition, slight shortening, perfect alignment. **D**, No apposition, approximately
30-degree angulation.

*Dislocation (luxation)*: disruption in the continuity of a joint

*Fracture-dislocation*: dislocation that occurs in conjunction with a fracture of the joint. If incomplete, it is called a fracture-subluxation (Fig. 2-4)

*Malunion*: healing in an unsatisfactory position

*Nonunion*: failure of bony healing

*Pseudarthrosis*: failure of bone healing which produces a "false joint" consisting of soft tissue

*Subluxation*: partial disruption in the continuity of a joint (an incomplete dislocation)

**Note**: Fractures do not dislocate, they *displace* (shorten, angulate, etc.). They are thus described according to the type, place in the bone, amount of displacement, and angulation (Fig. 2-5). Rotation (torsion) is often difficult to visualize roentgenographically but relatively easy to visualize clinically. Rotation is usually described in reference to the distal fragment, as is angulation.

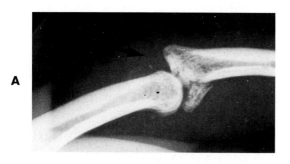
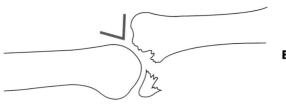

**Fig. 2–4.**
**A**, A fracture-subluxation of the proximal interphalangeal joint with the middle phalanx subluxed dorsally. Remember, each articular surface must match up perfectly with another apposing joint surface. Otherwise, subluxation or dislocation may be present. **B**, Mismatched joint surfaces may only be apparent when the surfaces are no longer parallel and create a "V" appearance.

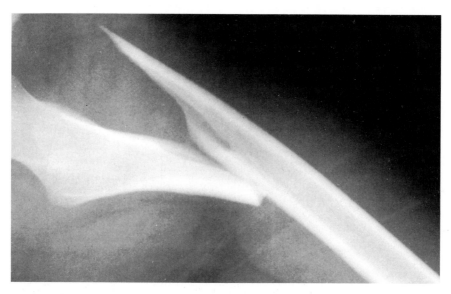

**Fig. 2–5.**
A lateral view of a fracture of the upper portion of the femur. The fracture is closed. It is described as a closed, displaced spiral fracture of the proximal third of the femur with 20- to 30-degree angulation, apex anterior, and shortening of 1 to 2 cm.

# GENERAL CONSIDERATIONS

## Initial Care

All major long-bone fractures should be splinted before the patient is transported. Careless handling of the extremity may further damage the soft tissue and should be avoided, but it is wise to correct any significant rotational or angular malalignment before applying a splinting device. This is done by gentle traction in the long axis of the limb. However, do not pull the protruding bone ends of an open fracture back into the wound.

A variety of splinting devices are available that make transfer of the patient to the hospital more comfortable (Fig. 2-6). Their use should be only temporary, however, until the diagnosis is confirmed roentgenographically. If definitive treatment of the fracture is to be delayed, a well-padded plaster splint or soft dressing such as the "Robert Jones" dressing should be applied. This dressing is made by applying several layers of cast padding or cotton roll to the extremity. Plaster splints are added, and the entire dressing is wrapped with elastic bandage.

The extremity is then elevated above the level of the heart, and ice is applied to control swelling. The neurologic and circulatory status of the extremity distal to the injury should always be checked and recorded (Table 2-1). A complete neurologic examination is usually unnecessary. If the patient can extend the thumb, and flex and spread the fingers, the major nerves (radial, median, and ulnar) of the upper extremity are functioning; if the patient can flex and extend the toes, the major nerves (posterior tibial and peroneal) to the lower extremity are intact. If a neurologic or vascular impairment is present, it is often relieved by reduction of the fracture or dislocation. If a *neurologic* impairment persists after the reduction, it is usually treated by

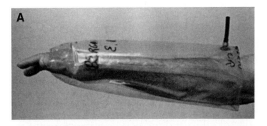
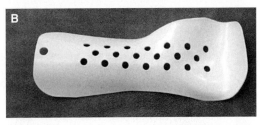
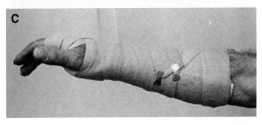

**Fig. 2–6.**
**A** and **B**, Temporary splints used for transfer. These devices should not be used for more than a few hours. They become very uncomfortable in a short time. **C**, Well-padded bulky dressing reinforced with plaster splints that should be applied as soon as possible. An elastic bandage alone should never be used. It does not immobilize, nor does it reduce swelling. In fact, it may do more harm by further compressing the already compromised lymphatic and venous drainage systems. Short arm splints should be well padded around the wrist. Otherwise, the wrist and hand may hang over the edge of the plaster and pain may result.

**TABLE 2–1.**
Occasional Neurovascular Complication of Common Injuries

| Bony Injury | Lesion | Prominent Early Findings |
|---|---|---|
| Anterior shoulder dislocation | Circumflex axillary nerve injury | Mid-deltoid numbness |
| Spiral fracture of humerus | Radial nerve injury | Wrist drop |
| Avulsion fracture of medial epicondyle | Ulnar nerve injury | Numbness of small finger, weak finger abduction, adduction |
| Severe elbow fracture | Brachial artery injury | Severe pain, pain on passive finger extension |
| Fractured distal radius, ulna | Median or ulnar nerve injury | Numbness, motor loss |
| Posterior dislocation of hip | Sciatic nerve injury (usually peroneal portion) | Foot drop, weak extensor hallucis longus, numbness on dorsum of foot or great toe |
| Fracture of upper fibula | Peroneal nerve injury | Same |
| Fracture of upper tibia | Compartment syndrome | Severe pain, pain on passive stretch of involved compartment muscles |

simple observation and exercises to prevent contractures. The prognosis is generally good for complete recovery. *Circulatory* impairment that persists requires immediate vascular evaluation. The initial neurologic examination is particularly important because if a deficit is discovered only *after* treatment, it may not be possible to determine whether it was present before or occurred as a result of treatment.

## DEFINITIVE FRACTURE CARE

Fracture healing is mainly a local event and is influenced little by generalized disease (except smoking) or advanced age. When a fracture occurs, the periosteum and other soft tissues are damaged and there is an outpouring of blood and exudate. The fibrin from this hematoma helps form a mesh that holds all of the elements of the fracture together. Cellular differentiation and tissue organization occur and lead to the formation of a soft, stabilizing callus that encompasses the fracture ends. Eventually, this callus matures into mineralized bone.

To encourage this sequence of healing, the bone ends must be kept in apposition, sufficient blood supply must be maintained, and the bone fragments must be adequately immobilized. Otherwise, fibrous tissue may form instead of callus and lead to nonunion and formation of a pseudarthrosis. Whereas healing bone does have some ability to bridge a gap (especially in the young, whose callus-generating periosteum is so active), distraction of the bone ends is to be avoided. Conversely, compression of the fractured bone ends tends to stimulate fracture healing in many cases. Also, bones such as the clavicle and tibia, which are subcutaneous and have less surrounding soft tissue and blood supply, tend to heal more slowly, whereas fractures in the vascular metaphysis of any bone heal more rapidly. Open fractures or those with soft-tissue interposition will also heal more slowly because these factors compromise the local environment. Another element that influences healing is the type of fracture. Spiral shaft fractures, for example, tend to heal much more readily than do transverse shaft fractures because of the large amount of bone surface and hematoma available in the spiral fracture.

It is with consideration of these various local factors that decisions regarding the treatment of all fractures are made. These decisions are based on the goals of fracture treatment: (1) alignment of the bones in both the angular and rotational planes, (2) restoration of proper length, (3) restoration of apposition of the bone ends, and (4) adequate immobilization.

Some fractures require no treatment or, at most, simple restriction of activity with a sling or crutches (Table 2-2). Many other fractures are treatable by cast immobilization. Fractures that require reduction are usually treated by one of four general methods: (1) open or closed reduction with internal fixation, (2) continuous traction usually followed by cast immobilization, (3) closed reduction with external skeletal fixation, or (4) closed reduction followed by cast immobilization.

**Open or Closed Reduction with Internal Fixation.** Closed treatment, which avoids stripping the soft tissue and periosteum and devascularizing the bone ends, is usually preferred over open treatment for most fractures. Closed treatment also decreases the chance of infection. There are several fractures, however, in which accurate anatomic positioning of the fragments and rigid internal fixation are beneficial: (1) displaced joint fractures, especially the weight-bearing joints; (2) fractures that cannot be reduced or held by closed methods; (3) fractures of the lower extremity in the elderly to allow early activity; (4) certain epiphyseal fractures that could result in a growth disturbance if not accurately reduced; and (5) joint fractures in which early motion would be helpful to prevent stiffness.

**Continuous Traction.** Traction is a means of aligning the bone ends and maintaining the reduction, especially if the fracture is comminuted or unstable. It is usually applied by a skeletal traction pin because prolonged skin traction may cause blisters. Skin traction is sufficient in the very young because their fractures stabilize sooner and require less time in traction. After enough healing has occurred to maintain length and alignment, a cast is applied.

**External Fixation.** External skeletal fixation is a means of fracture treatment that utilizes multiple pins, usually placed above and below the fracture site. The fracture is then reduced and the pins are incorporated into an outrigger or cast. This method is useful in compound fractures with soft tissue damage that requires

**TABLE 2–2.**

Common Fractures Not Requiring Cast Immobilization*

| Fracture | Treatment |
| --- | --- |
| Impacted surgical neck of humerus | Shoulder immobilizer |
| Undisplaced radial head fracture | Sling |
| Undisplaced olecranon | Sling |
| Undisplaced patella | Knee immobilizer |
| Shaft of fibula | Crutches |
| Base of fifth metatarsal | Hard sandal |
| Stress fracture | Avoid offending activity |
| Toe phalanges (undisplaced) | Tape to adjacent toe |
| Undisplaced calcaneus | Crutches |

*These fractures are stable and should not displace if the extremity is moved. A soft compression dressing for the first 2 to 3 days may be helpful in some cases.

exposure of the fracture site. It is particularly helpful in Colles' fractures that are losing position.

## The Elements of Closed Reduction

Most common fractures can be treated by manual reduction and immobilization, but for this procedure to be successful, certain mechanical aspects of the fracture should be understood. When a bone is broken and the fractured ends separate the soft tissue (mainly periosteum) on the side opposite the direction of displace-

ment ruptures, allowing the fracture to angulate and rotate (Fig. 2-7). The tissue on the side to which the displacement occurs remains intact, although it may be stripped off of the bone. This intact soft tissue forms a "hinge" that can be used in the treatment of many fractures to help guide the displaced distal fragment or fragments into place and to help maintain that position.

There are many methods used to place bones back into their original position. Most of these require that the distal fragment be placed into apposition to the proximal one. Some fractures require only a "push" back into place (Fig. 2-8). Others need a more complicated maneuver that incorporates traction and manipulation of the fragments (Fig. 2-9). The nature of the fracture and its displacement will determine which of these is necessary.

Before any reduction is attempted, each fracture should be thoroughly studied and a complete mental plan developed. This should include every detail in the

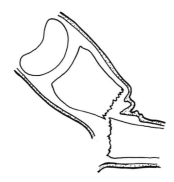

**Fig. 2–7.**
A typical fracture with an intact "periosteal hinge" on the concave side.

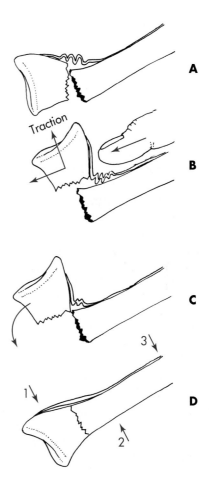

**Fig. 2–9.**
**A,** Typical Colles' fracture. **B,** The distal fragment is disimpacted, and the deformity is increased. Thumb pressure and traction are applied. **C,** The distal fragment is pushed distally to reduce the dorsal cortex. **D,** The reduction is completed by volar pressure and held with three-point cast molding *(arrows)* to keep the soft-tissue hinge tight.

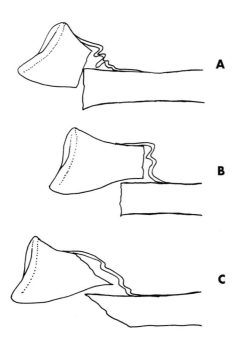

**Fig. 2–8.**
**A,** An epiphyseal fracture that simply requires that the distal fragment be gently pushed back into place. **B,** A transverse fracture that may be reduced by simple traction. **C,** An oblique "toggle" type of fracture that will require a more complicated manipulation. Even though the fracture fragments are not shortened, they must be angulated to accomplish the reduction. Simple traction would only tighten the soft-tissue hinge and prevent reduction of this fracture.

manipulation, including where the operator will be positioned, how the extremity will be grasped and held, and where the assistant should be positioned. In general, most reductions are accomplished as follows. (1) A variable amount of traction is applied to the distal fragment with countertraction on the proximal fragment. (2) The deformity is increased if necessary (reproduce the injury) and rotational malalignment is then corrected. (3) The distal fragment is then reduced and the angular deformity corrected. The periosteal hinge will usually prevent overreduction. A cast is then applied to hold the position. The cast should be properly molded to keep tension on the soft tissue hinge and prevent recurrence of the deformity in the cast (see Fig. 2-9, *D*). Even casts that are applied to undisplaced fractures should be molded to avoid the loss of position, which occasionally occurs in spite of protection (Fig. 2-10).

Utilization of this manipulative method and the soft-tissue hinge applies only to transverse or short oblique fractures that are stable after their irregular bone ends are engaged. It does not work with long oblique or spiral fractures or with markedly comminuted ones because their ends cannot be engaged to prevent shortening.

Questions often arise as to what constitutes an adequate reduction. In general, the following principles are valid:

1. Rotational deformity should always be completely corrected at any age.
2. In adults, angular deformity should also be completely corrected, especially in fractures of the fingers, forearm, and lower extremities.
3. In children, some angular deformity (15 to 20 degrees) that is close to a joint and in the same plane of motion as that joint will correct itself if sufficient growth remains.
4. Perfect apposition is not always necessary for normal healing.
5. Fractures involving the weight-bearing joints require exact reduction.
6. Slight shortening in the upper extremity is often acceptable, but proper length in the lower extremity is preferable.

## Anesthesia

Adequate anesthesia can usually be obtained by direct infiltration of the fracture hematoma on the extensor side under sterile conditions with 5 to 10 mL of a local anesthetic. If a local anesthetic is to be used, the procedure should be undertaken soon after the injury. Otherwise, the hematoma may clot, and the anesthetic will

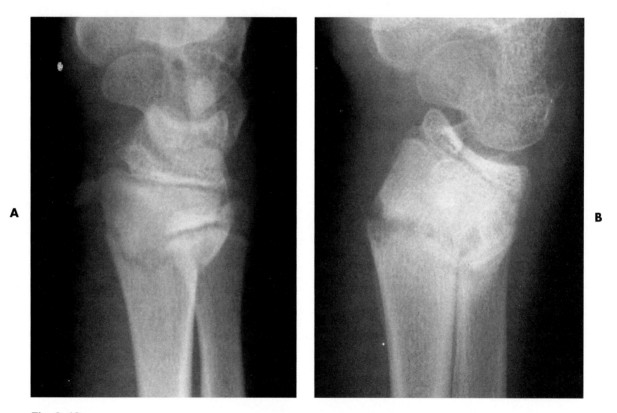

**Fig. 2–10.**
**A**, An undisplaced fracture of the distal radius treated with a loosely fitted cast. **B**, Marked posterior angulation present at the time of cast removal. (Fortunately, the deformity was expected to correct with growth.)

not spread through the fracture as well. Regional anesthetics are also helpful because they eliminate the need to add more volume of fluid to an already swollen area. Digital or metacarpal blocks work well for finger fractures. General anesthesia is often necessary, especially in children.

The intravenous or Bier block is useful in forearm and wrist fractures, although the movement of the extremity required to perform the block is sometimes uncomfortable. An intravenous line is always established in the other upper extremity in the event of a complication. Light sedation is administered. A small needle is then inserted into an appropriate distal vein on the injured extremity, and a double tourniquet is applied to the upper portion of the limb. The extremity is then exsanguinated up to the tourniquet with an elastic wrap or, if this is painful, simply elevated for 3 minutes to empty the venous system. The proximal tourniquet is then inflated above the systolic blood pressure, and any elastic wrap is removed. The venous system is then filled, depending on the size of the patient, with 30 to 50 mL of a 0.5% solution of lidocaine mixed with nonbacteriostatic normal saline. The needle is then removed from the involved extremity. After a few minutes, the fracture will be able to be manipulated. If the proximal tourniquet becomes painful, it can be released after the lower one has been inflated because the lower tourniquet is now in an area that has adequate anesthesia.

After the procedure has been completed, the tourniquet is slowly and intermittently released to avoid the undesirable central nervous system (CNS) and cardiovascular side effects that occasionally occur when the anesthetic enters the general circulation. These are early CNS irritability followed by sedation. Rarely, seizures, tremors, and bradycardia have even been reported. Both tourniquets should not be released until at least 20 minutes after the lidocaine injection, even if the procedure takes less time.

## External Immobilization

Casts are applied for three reasons: (1) to immobilize the ends of a fracture, (2) to allow ambulation, and (3) to hold the position of reduction. A cast never completely immobilizes a fracture. If properly applied, however, it provides enough relative immobilization to allow the fracture to heal.

A variety of materials are available for casting. Plaster of Paris is easy to work with, has a long shelf life, and is relatively low in cost. Synthetic casting materials are becoming increasingly popular because of their light weight and strength. Also, less material is usually needed than for a plaster cast. However, a disadvantage for the generalist using these materials is that they have a relatively short shelf life (2 to 3 months in some cases)

and are also more expensive. When storing lightcast materials, be certain to turn the packages occasionally so that the material does not become dry. Commonly used sizes are 2-, 3-, and 4-inch stockinettes; 3- and 4-inch cast paddings; and 2-, 3-, 4-, and 5-inch plaster or lightcast rolls.

Some physicians occasionally prefer bivalved splints (usually anterior and posterior) to circular casts as primary care to avoid possible circulatory and swelling complications. These splints are sometimes called "sugar tongs" if the units are continuous. The splint system, shaped like an elongated U, is held in position by gauze or an elastic bandage. It can be easily loosened or tightened if needed.

Whenever a cast is used, the extremity should be held in the position of function while the cast is being applied, unless the extremity must be positioned otherwise, such as for maintenance of fracture position (Fig. 2-11). Casts are always applied in the same orderly sequence. The assistant holds the extremity in the proper position, and a single layer of stockinette, although not always necessary, may be applied (Fig. 2-12). Cast padding is then applied, beginning at one end and proceeding to the other, creating a double thickness by overlapping the roll 50% on each turn. Do not overpad because the cast will be loose, but do place "donut" pads over bony prominences or other areas of concern (peroneal nerve at the fibular neck, ulnar styloid, both malleoli, and the olecranon process).

The plaster roll is then placed in lukewarm water and left until the bubbling ceases. Plaster sets more slowly in cold water, thus allowing more time to work; warmer water causes plaster to set more quickly. Never use hot water. After removal from the water, the ends of the plaster are pinched together, and the roll is gently twisted. This removes some of the water but not the plaster. The plaster roll is then applied to the limb in the same manner as the cotton, that is, starting at one end and going up and down the extremity while overlapping by 50% each turn. Moderate tension is used during the application, with greater tension being used on the proximal fleshy part of the extremity. Tucks or pleats are commonly taken to allow the plaster to be smooth and even on parts of the extremity that taper. This also avoids ridges or transverse creases. The roll is applied by pushing it with the thenar eminence and should be kept close to or on the extremity at all times.

The cast should be of uniform thickness, about 0.6 cm. No two turns should be made at the same spot, except at the ends of the cast. Thus the plaster is applied evenly end to end and will not be any thicker at the fracture site than elsewhere. Each layer should be applied moist to allow each turn to bond to the next layer. If this does not occur, a cast results that is several individual layers thick rather than one single thickness.

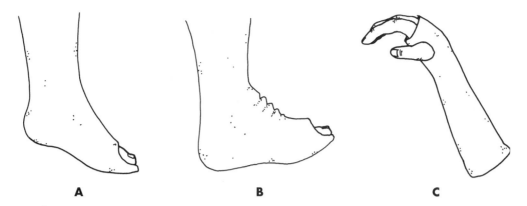

**Fig. 2–11.**
Proper joint positions for casting. **A**, The ankle is in too much equinus. **B**, If the position is changed to the proper position of 90 degrees after the padding or plaster has been applied, a painful cast ridge may develop. **C**, Proper position and length of the short arm cast. Note that the metacarpophalangeal joints should be able to be completely flexed to a right angle and the cast should not extend beyond the distal palmar crease or too far down on the small finger. The patient should also be able to fan the fingers. If they are included in the cast the elbow joint is usually casted at 90 degrees and the knee at 30 degrees. All short leg walking casts should be long enough to include the plantar aspect of the metatarsal heads.

The plaster should be worked and smoothed during the application of each layer.

While the plaster is setting, it is contoured and molded with the flat of the palm or thenar eminence to apply the proper three-point fixation. Overzealous rubbing in the late drying phase may cause the plaster to crumble while it is setting.

Lightcast is easier to apply, because tucks and reinforcing splints are not necessary. Always wear gloves because the bonding material adheres to the skin and is difficult to remove. Use *cool* water for lightcast.

As a general rule, a cast should immobilize one joint above and below the fracture, although short arm casts are often used for wrist fractures and short leg casts for ankle fractures. Two rolls of 4-inch plaster or 2-inch lightcast are sufficient for a short arm cast. Three rolls of 6-inch plaster or 4-inch lightcast are adequate for a short leg cast.

If the fracture is inherently stable, the cast merely acts as a splinting device. Fractures that require reduction or those that are unstable use the cast to hold the position by maintaining three-point tension on the soft tissue hinge, two of the points being the operator's hands that mold the cast into a flat appearance. The third point is a wide area of the proximal portion of the cast. It is unnecessary to apply direct pressure there.

There is an effective *waterproof cast liner* available; it comes in rolls and allows the lightcast to be submerged in water. The liner is applied instead of the stockinette and cast padding. It is rolled on in the same manner as cast padding, overlapping 50% to have a double thickness. Lightcast is then applied in the usual fashion. The liner works best with short arm casts. When used with short leg casts, the material sometimes rolls up at the heel, making walking uncomfortable. After the patient swims or bathes, the water drains out as a result of gravity. Most casts will be dry in 30 to 60 minutes. If the cast has been in salt water or chlorinated water, it should probably be rinsed and then be allowed to dry. Some skin changes do occur because of moisture, but they are usually minor. The cast may be slightly more difficult to remove over the liner because it doesn't "pop" apart quite as easily. Overall, patients are pleased with the liner, especially the younger and more active ones.

## Aftercare

After cast application, the extremity is elevated above the horizontal level of the heart, and ice is applied for 48 to 72 hours. The patient is closely observed for signs and symptoms of circulatory obstruction or acute compartment syndrome. (Excessive pain may be the only early clue.) Hospitalization may even be necessary in some cases. The cast must be split and spread at the earliest sign of circulatory embarrassment. If discomfort secondary to swelling is the only problem, spreading the plaster alone is usually sufficient, but if there is concern for the circulatory status of the extremity, the entire cast, cotton, and every bit of stockinette should be split completely down to the skin and spread apart. If the problem persists, the entire cast should be removed, although this is usually unnecessary.

Plaster splits more easily to relieve swelling than lightcast does. It needs to be cut on only one side and spread. The opposite side will usually crack and keep the split open. Fiberglass must be cut slightly on the opposite side. Otherwise, it springs back.

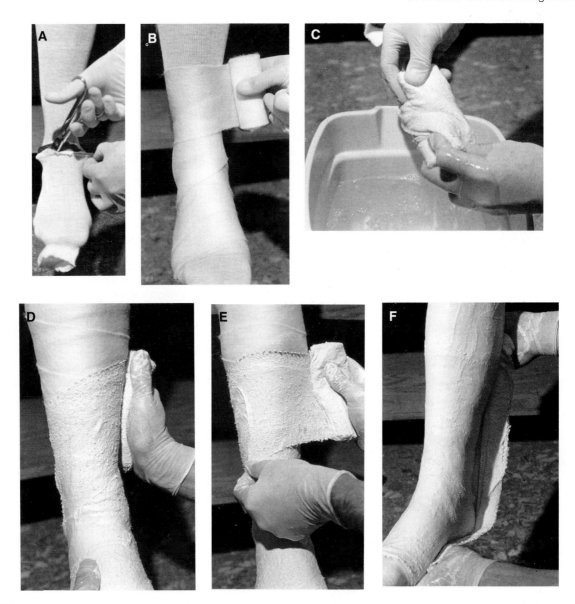

**Fig. 2–12.**
The cast. **A**, A stockinette may be applied first. Any folds in front should be trimmed. **B**, Beginning at one end, cast padding is added while overlapping each turn by half. **C**, The plaster roll is removed from the water after the bubbles cease. The ends are pinched shut, and the roll is gently squeezed to expel excess water. Less water or excess wringing causes faster drying. Using the larger sizes may help avoid premature drying of the roll. Wet plaster makes a smoother cast. **D**, Beginning at one end, the plaster is pushed onto the extremity by using gentle pressure from the thenar eminence against the middle of the roll. The roll should remain in contact with the limb and is usually not lifted from it. Additional rolls are started where the previous one ends. The roll is applied so that the opening side faces the operator and not the extremity. Rolling is continuous, and each layer is rubbed so that all layers fuse together. The short leg cast (SLC) should always extend under the metatarsal heads for support. **E**, Tucks or pleats are taken as often as necessary to guide the roll and to accommodate any tapering of the limb. The stockinette is folded back and incorporated into the cast. **F**, Reinforcing splints five to ten layers thick applied to the sides or back add a great deal of strength without adding much weight. They are particularly useful at the ankle, where the cast is weakest and breakage is most common.                                                                    *Continued.*

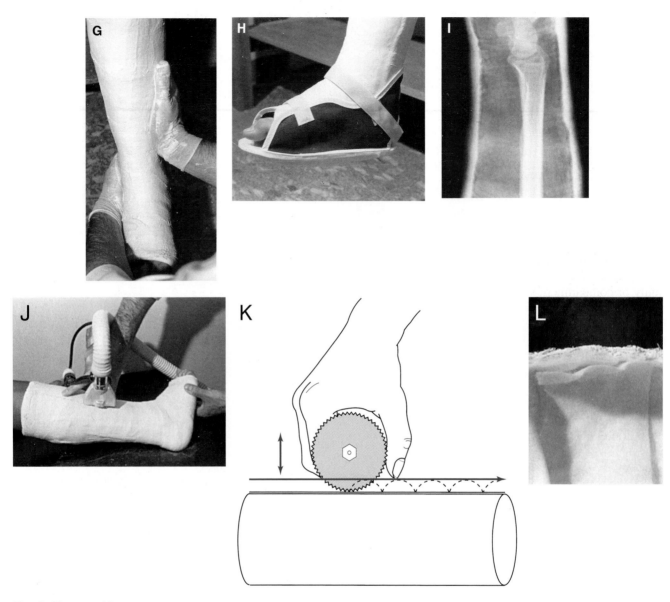

**Fig. 2–12.—cont'd**
**G**, The cast is molded with the flat surface of the hands, if necessary, and trimmed, especially at the small toe. **H**, Cast boots function better than walking heels; there are fewer repairs and a better gait. Wait 48 hours for the cast to cure before allowing weight bearing on plaster (1 hour for lightcast). **I**, Roentgenogram of a portion of a short arm cast (SAC) showing a cast of even thickness without excessive padding between the cast and the skin. **J** and **K**, Casts are removed with the cast saw and spreader. The cast is removed by cutting down through both sides. Do not saw back and forth with the blade. It is better to pick the blade up and move it every time the plaster is cut through. Counterpressure with the thumb and/or index finger on the cast will prevent the blade from injuring the underlying skin. Cut the cast at right angles to the material. Sharp blades cut easier with less force and therefore less potential for skin injury. A hot blade may mean a dull blade. While cutting, the cast may be pulled or pushed away from the skin to give more room. Edema that holds the limb against the cast or the presence of soft rheumatoid skin may increase the chance of the cast saw abrading the skin. **L**, The sectioned cast showing even, fused plaster that is properly contoured and molded. It is as thick at the end as it is in the middle. The use of wider rolls will result in a more even cast than will the use of many small rolls. Two 4-inch rolls of plaster (or two 2-inch rolls of lightcast) will suffice for an adult short arm cast. Three 6-inch rolls of plaster (or three 4-inch rolls of lightcast) are necessary for an adult SAC.

It is often difficult to differentiate among fracture pain, acute compartment syndrome, arterial injury, and nerve palsy, especially in an anxious patient. Peripheral nerve testing will usually rule out nerve palsy, and if peripheral pulses are present, arterial injury is unlikely. The acute compartment syndrome is a condition that develops when perfusion of nerve and muscle decreases to the point where it is unable to sustain viability. Pressure inside the natural fascial compartments of the arm or leg may rise, usually as a result of fracture bleeding, which then obstructs venous outflow. This leads to a further increase in tissue pressure and necrosis, sometimes within a few hours. A compartment syndrome should be suspected if there is (1) pain on passive stretching of the muscles of the affected compartment, (2) sensory loss, and (3) tenseness of the involved compartment. Paralysis may also occur. Arterial injury or compartment syndrome secondary to swelling in a tight cast could lead to Volkmann's ischemic contracture if untreated (Fig. 2-13). This is a rare complication and most often occurs after severe elbow injuries, high tibial fractures, and metatarsal fractures. It is considered a surgical emergency.

Movement of all joints that are not immobilized is encouraged as soon as possible. Fewer vasomotor disturbances, less swelling, and a faster recovery will result. Painful pressure sores may develop rapidly under a cast. *Remember*: the pain will subside when tissue necrosis has occurred. These pressure areas, although rare in a properly padded cast, should be treated or at least evaluated before skin necrosis occurs. If a "window" must be cut in a cast to evaluate the skin or the cast must be split, the window or padding should always be replaced to prevent edema of the soft tissue from swelling through the hole or the split section. If a cast has been properly applied, it should not require changing during the course of treatment, even after swelling subsides. If the cast "telescopes," however, and there is danger of losing the position of the fracture, it should be changed.

Itching beneath the cast is common. It can sometimes be controlled by ice or over-the-counter antihistamines or by blowing warm air into the cast with a hair dryer. The use of any instrument, such as a coat hanger, to scratch the area should be avoided. The cast can be covered with a stockinette to keep it from snagging clothing. It can be kept dry during a shower by wrapping it with a plastic trash bag and avoiding the main flow of the water. If the cast becomes slightly wet, it can be dried with a hair dryer. If the cast becomes too wet, it will need to be changed.

Ecchymosis, which may alarm the patient, may become visible in a few days either distal or proximal to the site of injury. This is a result of the migration of

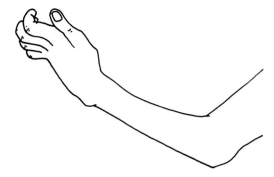

**Fig. 2–13.**
Drawing of a typical Volkmann's ischemic contracture. Contractures and severe muscle loss are the usual end result. The deformity will often persist in spite of prolonged attempts at reconstructive surgery and therapy.

blood by dependent drainage through the tissue planes. Commonly, the toes become bruised in appearance with ankle fractures and the fingers do the same with wrist fractures.

Roentgenograms are repeated weekly for 2 to 3 weeks mainly to assess the position of the fracture. Healing changes may not be visible for some time. The length of time required for complete healing varies with the age of the patient, the nature and site of the fracture, and the specific bone involved. As a rule, fractures in children and fractures near the ends of the bone (metaphysis) heal more rapidly than do those in the relatively avascular midshaft (diaphysis).

The determination as to when a cast may be removed is not made on the basis of the roentgenogram alone. Roentgenographic evidence of complete healing may lag several weeks behind true clinical union. In general, the cast may be removed when sufficient time has passed for the particular bone under treatment to heal. This varies with each bone. Clinical and roentgenographic assessments are made after the cast has been removed, and if the fracture has no motion and is not tender to palpation, pressure, or stress, then sufficient healing has probably occurred to allow the cast to be left off. If any doubt exists, a removable protective splint may be applied for another 2 to 3 weeks, and gradual resumption of limited activity is allowed. If motion, tenderness, or swelling is present, suggesting a slow or delayed union, another circular cast is applied and the fracture is reassessed in 2 to 3 weeks.

## Rehabilitation

It is important that the patient be kept informed of the entire treatment plan from start to finish. This should include what to expect after the cast has been removed:

stiffness for several weeks, swelling, callous bumps, increased hair on the arms and legs in youngsters, or a temporary limp. These usually subside in a few weeks. It is equally important not to let the patient become active too quickly after the cast has been removed. Allow some time for the bone to regain its strength (4 to 6 weeks).

Rehabilitation actually is begun at the time of the injury. By controlling excessive soft-tissue swelling, scar formation is diminished and earlier normal function (once the fracture has healed) is the end result. Early movement is encouraged, and after the initial pain and swelling have subsided, the patient is instructed to use any joints not immobilized by the cast and perform some meaningful tasks at home or work.

After cast removal, active mobilization of joints that were immobilized is begun. A repetitive exercise that the patient may perform at home is preferable to most forms of physical therapy. Exercise in a swimming pool is an excellent method of restoring strength, mobility, and confidence after many kinds of injuries. Most of the motion and strength in extremities can usually be regained within 4 to 6 weeks after the cast has been removed, but it is not uncommon for some stiffness, weakness, and swelling to persist. Formal physical therapy is usually unnecessary.

Discourage the patient from excessive scratching of skin immediately after cast removal. The skin can be somewhat tender at this time. Gentle bathing and the application of a mild skin lotion help restore the skin to normal. Some temporary increase in lower extremity swelling commonly occurs after short leg cast removal because of the loss of the soft tissue compression effect of the cast. A support hose may be needed temporarily.

A bone scan may remain positive up to 2 years after cast removal and signify ongoing fracture remodeling and strengthening. Wait at least 2 months after cast removal before allowing most sports activities.

## Additional Principles

1. Always obtain comparison roentgenograms of the opposite extremity whenever a questionable fracture is present, especially in a child.
2. Always obtain roentgenograms in at least two planes at right angles to each other and include a joint above and below the area of injury. Obtain oblique views whenever necessary.
3. When one bone of a two-bone set (forearm, lower part of the leg) is fractured and becomes shortened or angulated, always look for injury to the other bone or a dislocation.
4. Be certain to correct both rotational and angular malalignment in the reduction.
5. Take stress roentgenograms whenever necessary.
6. Don't be satisfied with one diagnosis (always look for a second injury).
7. Reduce the fracture as soon as possible. There is little to be gained by "waiting for the swelling to go down." The swelling will probably only increase because of the deformity.
8. Avulsion fractures near a joint should always be carefully evaluated for instability and tendon function.
9. The measure of success is the usefulness of the extremity and not just the roentgenographic appearance.
10. Irreducibility may signify soft tissue interposition between the fracture ends, which could require surgery.

## FRACTURES IN CHILDREN

Fractures in children differ from those in adults in many respects. These fractures are usually less complicated and, with a few exceptions, are always treated with closed methods. Nonunion is rare because of the active periosteum and abundant blood supply surrounding the bone of the growing child. The principles of treatment are similar to those in adults. However, the fact that in children the bone continues to grow after the fracture has healed will allow for some correction and realignment of minor deformities.

### Principles of Treatment

1. Mild angular deformities will often correct themselves with growth. The amount of correction depends on the amount of angulation, the age of the child, and the distance of the fracture from the end of the bone. The closer the fracture is to the end of the bone and the younger the patient, the greater the amount of angulation that is acceptable (Fig. 2-14). Correction is also more complete if the angulation is in the same plane of motion as the nearest joint. There is wide variation in the amount of deformity that will realign. The distal radius may correct as much as 10 to 15 degrees per year. Angular deformities that are not in the same plane of motion as the nearest joint will persist, however.
2. Rotational malalignment does not correct itself.
3. Fractures of the midshaft of the bone will not realign.

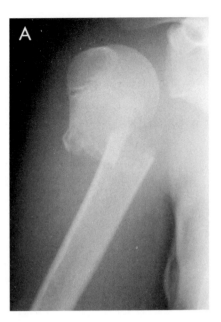
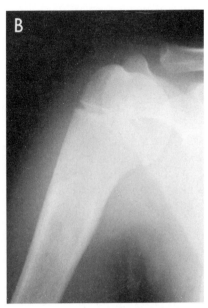

**Fig. 2–14.**
**A**, Fracture of the upper portion of the humerus in a patient aged 6 years. An attempt was made to reduce the fracture, but the position could not be improved and was accepted. **B**, The same patient approximately 10 months later. Although the two roentgenograms are not in the same rotation, the remodeling is obvious.

4. Apposition and mild shortening are of little importance in the young child. Bayonet (side-to-side) apposition is perfectly acceptable in long bone fractures in boys under 12 years of age and girls under 10 years. Slight shortening with reduction may actually be desirable in the leg because acceleration of growth occurs after a displaced fracture. The tibia and femur may overgrow up to 1 cm after a displaced fracture. Thus, some slight overlapping of these bones is occasionally desirable.

5. Physical therapy after the fracture has healed is usually unnecessary and may even be unwise in the child. Forceful manipulation of the extremity will only cause more swelling and stiffness.

6. A tender growth plate after an injury usually means that a fracture is present. Therefore the injury should be treated as a fracture. "Sprains" are rare in children.

7. Nonunion is almost impossible in children.

8. Malposition may not be correctable after 7 to 10 days. Attempts to manipulate the fracture after that may damage the growth plate.

**Note**: *Remodeling* is the process of smoothing off of the sharp bone ends. It occurs in adults as well as children. Only children who have growth left, however, have the ability to straighten or *realign* mild fracture deformities.

## The Epiphyseal Plate

Two types of epiphyses exist in growing bones: the pressure epiphysis and the traction epiphysis (apophysis). Pressure epiphyses occur at the ends of long bones and contribute to the longitudinal growth of the bone. Traction apophyses, such as the iliac crest and trochanters of the hip, contribute primarily to the contour of the bone and little to actual longitudinal growth. They are present at the origin of major muscles and respond to traction rather than to pressure.

The epiphyseal plate itself consists of several zones or layers (Fig. 2-15). The zone nearest the joint is the germinal cell layer. Moving away from the joint are the zone of proliferation, the zone of hypertrophic cartilage, and the zone of provisional calcification. Epiphyseal fractures may be categorized according to the type of injury, the relationship of the fracture line to the germinal cell layer, and the prognosis. Salter's classification is commonly used.

Most epiphyseal fractures occur irregularly through the weakest zone, the zone of hypertrophic cartilage. They are usually transverse and do not travel vertically across the germinal cell layer. These fractures are classified by Salter as type I or type II fractures, and the prognosis for normal healing is good (Fig. 2-16). Manipulative reduction is usually successful. Attempts

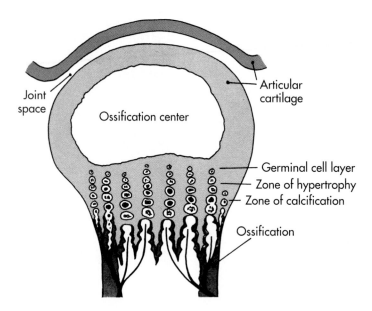

**Fig. 2–15.**
The epiphyseal plate. Most epiphyseal fractures occur through the zone of hypertrophic cartilage.

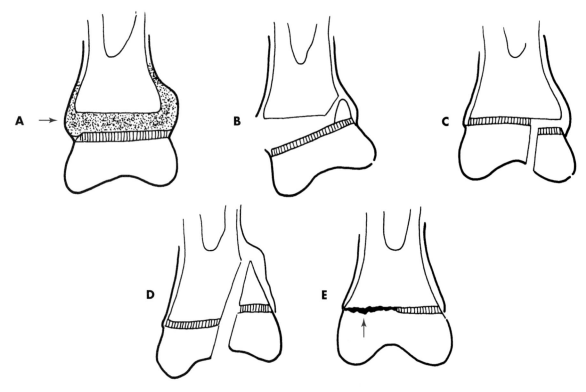

**Fig. 2–16.**
Epiphyseal fractures. **A**, Type I. **B**, Type II. **C**, Type III. **D**, Type IV. **E**, Type V crushing fracture.

to correct persistent minor deformities during the reduction should not be overzealous because these mild deformities will usually correct themselves with growth. Overaggressive treatment may cause further damage to the growth plate.

Fractures that do traverse the growth plate vertically (type III, type IV) may disturb the growth so that angular deformity will result. Cross-union may occur across the epiphyseal plate. These fractures often are also intraarticular, and accurate reduction is mandatory to prevent growth disturbance from occurring and to restore the joint surface. Surgery is usually necessary to accomplish these goals. Type V fractures are crush injuries that have a poor prognosis (Fig. 2-17). Often no definite fracture line is visible.

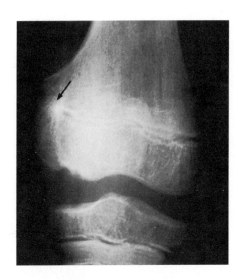

**Fig. 2–17.** Salter type V crush fracture that resulted in a complete bony bridge *(arrow)* being formed in the medial aspect of the lower femoral epiphysis.

## FRACTURES REQUIRING SPECIAL CARE

Most of the fractures described throughout this text can be safely managed by the generalist using nonoperative means. The majority of undisplaced fractures fall into this category. There are, however, several common injuries that are fraught with complications even when treated by one familiar with them. Some fractures will also require surgical intervention or specialized closed treatment. These should always be referred to a surgeon trained in their treatment. Some of the more common of these injuries include the following:

1. All open fractures. These need meticulous cleaning and debridement to prevent osteomyelitis and gas gangrene.

2. Displaced intraarticular fractures. These often require accurate reduction to prevent the onset of traumatic arthritis.
3. All femur fractures. Many of these will require prolonged traction, special casting, or surgery.
4. Most fractures of both bones of the lower leg in adults. In addition, there are several specific fractures in children and adults that should probably be treated only by an orthopedic surgeon (Table 2-3).

**TABLE 2–3.**
Common Fractures and Their Complications

| Fracture | Complication |
| --- | --- |
| **In Children** | |
| Supracondylar fracture of the humerus (displaced) | Volkmann's contracture, malunion |
| Lateral condylar fracture of the humerus | Nonunion, cubitus valgus, late ulnar nerve paralysis |
| Epiphyseal fractures III, IV, V | Growth disturbance |
| Radial neck and head fracture | Growth disturbance |
| **In Adults** | |
| Fracture of both bones of the forearm (displaced) or displaced single forearm bone | Malunion, nonunion, restricted forearm rotation |
| Displaced bimalleolar fracture | Nonunion, traumatic arthritis |
| Supracondylar, intercondylar fracture of the humerus | Traumatic arthritis, joint stiffness |
| Displaced olecranon fracture | Nonunion |
| Displaced radial head fracture | Traumatic arthritis, joint stiffness |
| Fractured upper tibia | Acute compartment syndrome |

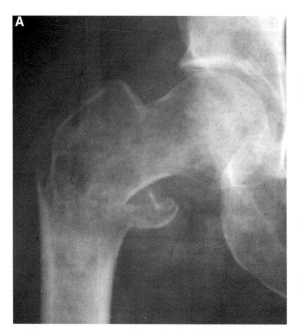
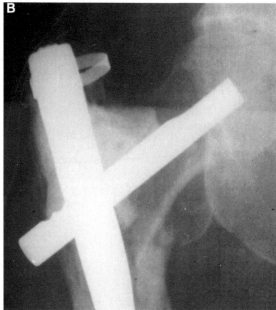

**Fig. 2–18.**
**A**, Pathologic fracture of the intertrochanteric area of the femur as a result of metastatic breast cancer. **B**, After open reduction and internal fixation, pain-free ambulation was possible.

## PATHOLOGIC FRACTURES

Pathologic fractures develop because of some abnormal local condition that causes the bone to become weakened. The most common causes are tumors that metastasize to bone. Other causes are infection, cystic lesions of bone, and Paget's disease. With the increase in the survival rate of cancer victims, there has also been an increase in the incidence of pathologic features. To maintain the highest possible level of function in patients, aggressive management of these fractures is often indicated.

The treatment is usually surgical (Fig. 2-18). Operative procedures are especially indicated in the lower extremities to encourage ambulatory activities. Although radiation therapy may relieve the pain, it can actually impede fracture healing. By stabilizing the fracture surgically, immediate use of the extremity is often possible. This is accomplished by curetting the tumor, filling the resultant cavity with methyl-methacrylate cement, and adding the appropriate internal fixation device. The procedure is often performed on a prophylactic basis.

## FRACTURES OF THE BATTERED CHILD

The term *battered child* refers to a young child who is the victim of physical abuse inflicted by a person usually responsible for the child's care. As a general rule, these children tend to be young, under 4 years of age.

The diagnosis is often difficult. The history is usually suggestive. The parents are often evasive, or the cause of injury seems implausible. The parents are often quite young and seem poorly adjusted. A history of previous injuries should make the physician suspicious. Multiple bruises or signs of other soft tissue trauma may be present. The child may seem malnourished or in poor general health.

The injuries may be visceral, cranial, or musculoskeletal. The characteristic musculoskeletal lesions are

(1) multiple bony lesions, often epiphyseal fractures, in various stages of healing and (2) excessive periosteal reaction indicative of recent trauma with or without fracture (Fig. 2-19).

A complete skeletal survey is indicated in the workup. A bone scan may also be helpful to delineate other fractures. An attempt should also be made to rule out other possible causes of multiple fractures, especially osteogenesis imperfecta.

The treatment of these fractures is no different from that described in the sections on fractures of specific bones. In addition, it is the responsibility of the physician who suspects this condition to report it to the appropriate social service agency to protect the child from further mistreatment.

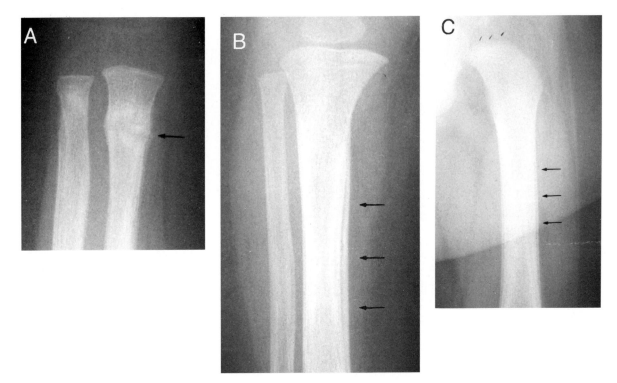

**Fig. 2–19.**
Roentgenograms of a battered child. The child had multiple rib fractures as well as a fractured forearm. **A**, Note the periosteal reaction in the lower extremities, **B** and **C**.

## STRESS FRACTURES

Stress fractures are incomplete fractures. They are often described as either insufficiency or fatigue fractures. Insufficiency fractures may occur when normal stress is applied to weak bone (see Chapters 9 and 10). Fatigue fractures may develop when excess stress is applied to normal bone. Either type may occur in any weight-bearing bone but are most common in the metatarsal ("march" fracture), neck of the femur, calcaneus, tibia, fibula, and pelvis. Osteoporosis is the most common cause of insufficiency fractures.

Fatigue fractures typically occur in unconditioned athletes. They are also common in military personnel subjected to long hikes or marching as part of their physical training program.

Clinically, a history of unusual stress with subsequent pain over a bone is common in a fatigue fracture. Local tenderness and swelling over the affected bone are usually present.

The roentgenogram is usually normal early in the disorder, although a bone scan would be positive. If this condition is suspected, treatment is instituted and roentgenograms are repeated at 2-week intervals (Fig. 2-20). An obvious fracture line is not usually apparent. A healing stress line is generally seen in 2 to 4 weeks. Exuberant periosteal bone formation may even simulate malignancy. Stress fractures in *cancellous* bone usually produce only a sclerotic transverse line without periosteal reaction. In *cortical* bone, however, there is generally considerable formation of periosteal new bone.

Treatment of fatigue injuries consists of protecting the bone from stress. Elimination of the offending activity is usually curative, although occasionally crutches are necessary. Gradual resumption of normal activity is allowed after the pain and tenderness subsides.

## ELECTRICAL STIMULATION OF BONE HEALING

In the early 1950s it was demonstrated that when bone is placed under stress, it exhibits a separation of charge. The side of the bone under compression becomes elec-tronegative, and the side under tension becomes electropositive, thus creating an electrical potential. This is known as the piezoelectric effect. As a result of the

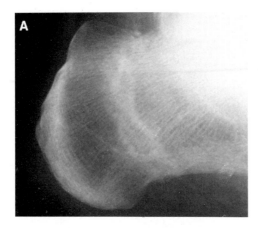 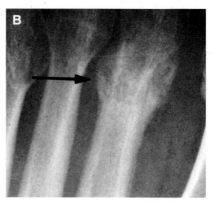

**Fig. 2–20.**
A, Fatigue fracture of the calcaneus with a sclerotic transverse line but no periosteal reaction.
B, "March" fracture of the second metatarsal neck with abundant periosteal callus.

findings, researchers began studying the effects of electricity on bone and cartilage. It was found that delivery of the proper amount of voltage and current by electrodes can stimulate osteogenesis.

A number of bone-stimulating devices are now available: (1) a semi-invasive percutaneous cathode system, (2) an invasive implant system, and (3) a noninvasive external inductive coupling device. These devices are used in conjunction with traditional fracture management (good reduction, adequate immobilization). At this time, they are only used in cases of delayed union or nonunion. The "success" rate varies from 60% to 75%. The indications for the use of these devices remain to be clearly defined.

## BIBLIOGRAPHY

Bassett CA: The development and application of pulsed electromagnetic fields (PEMFs) for ununited fractures and arthrodeses, *Orthop Clin North Am* 15:61, 1984.

Blount WP: *Fractures in children*, Baltimore, 1955, Williams & Wilkins.

Carty HML: Fractures caused by child abuse, *J Bone Joint Surg Br* 75:849-857, 1993.

Charnley J: *The closed treatment of common fractures*, ed 3, Edinburgh, 1970, Churchill Livingstone.

Compere EL, Banks SW, Compere CL: *Pictorial handbook of fracture treatment*, ed 5, Chicago, 1963, Year Book Medical Publishers Inc.

Connolly JF: *Fracture complications*, Chicago, 1988, Year Book Medical Publishers Inc.

Eilsele SA, Sammarco GJ: Fatigue fractures of the foot and ankle in the athlete, *J Bone Joint Surg Am* 75:290-298, 1993.

Flatt AE: *The care of minor hand injuries*, ed 3, St Louis, 1972, CV Mosby Co.

Furia JP, Alioto RJ, Marquardt JD: The efficacy and safety of the hematoma block for fracture reduction in closed, isolated fractures, *Orthopedics* 20:423-426, 1997.

Gitelis S et al: The role of prophylactic surgery in the management of metastatic hip disease, *Orthopedics* 5:1004, 1982.

Harrington KD et al: The use of methylmethacrylate as an adjunct in the internal fixation of malignant neoplastic fractures, *J Bone Joint Surg Am* 54:1665, 1972.

Haverstock BC, Mandracchia VJ: Cigarette smoking and bone healing: implications in foot and ankle surgery, *J Foot Ankle Surg* 37:69-74, 1998.

Holmes CM: Intravenous regional analgesia: useful method of producing analgesia of the limbs, *Lancet* 1:245, 1963.

Howard PW, Makin GS: Lower limb fractures with associated vascular injury, *J Bone Joint Surg Br* 72:116, 1990.

Hunter JM, Cowen NJ: Fifth metacarpal fractures in a compensation clinic population: a report on 133 cases, *J Bone Joint Surg Am* 52:1159, 1970.

Lavine LS, Grodzinsky AJ: Current concepts review: electrical stimulation of repair of bone, *J Bone Joint Surg Am* 69:626, 1987.

Marcove RC, Yang DJ: Survival times after treatment of pathologic fractures, *Cancer* 20:2154, 1967.

McLaughlin HL: *Trauma*, Philadelphia, 1959, WB Saunders.

Milgram C et al: Youth as a risk factor for stress fracture, *J Bone Joint Surg Br* 76:20-22, 1994.

Pool C: Colles' fracture, *J Bone Joint Surg Br* 55:540, 1973.

Rang M: *Children's fractures*, ed 2, Philadelphia, 1983, JB Lippincott.

Rockwood CA, Green DP: *Fractures in adults*, ed 2, Philadelphia, 1984, JB Lippincott.

Ryan JR, Rowe DE, Salciccioli GG: Prophylactic internal fixation of the femur in neoplastic lesions, *J Bone Joint Surg Am* 58:1071, 1976.

Silverman FN: The roentgen manifestations of unrecognized skeletal trauma in infants, *AJR* 69:413, 1953.

Sim FH: Metastatic bone disease: philosophy of treatment, *Orthopedics* 15:541-544, 1992.

Thompson RC: Impending fractures associated with bone destruction, *Orthopedics* 15:547-557, 1992.

Whiteside TE, Heckman MM. Acute compartment syndrome: update on diagnosis and treatment, *J Am Acac Orthop Surg* 4;209-218,1996.

# CHAPTER 3

# The Cervical Spine

The number of patients affected by cervical spine conditions causing pain or dysfunction is exceeded only by the number of those with lumbar spine conditions. Cervical spine disorders vary from those that are annoying to those that may be functionally disabling. The diagnosis and treatment of these disorders is a major part of orthopedics.

## ANATOMY

Seven cervical vertebrae make up the bony elements of the cervical spine. A typical cervical vertebra is similar to other vertebrae in that it is composed of a body and a neural arch (Fig. 3-1). The neural arch is composed of two pedicles that form the sides and two laminae that meet in the midline to form the roof. Projecting dorsally where the laminae meet is the spinous process. On each side, projecting laterally from the junction of the pedicle and lamina, is a transverse process. Also on each side, two articular processes, the superior and inferior, project upward and downward, respectively, from the junction of the pedicle and laminae. These articulate with similar processes on adjacent vertebrae to form the zygapophyseal or facet joints.

The first two cervical vertebrae are atypical in that C1, the atlas, has no body (Fig. 3-2). Its body is attached to C2, the axis, and forms the dens, or odontoid process. This arrangement allows for most of the rotation in the cervical spine. Strong ligaments, the most important of which is the transverse ligament, bind C1 to C2. The seventh cervical vertebra, vertebra prominens, is also somewhat atypical in that it has a long spinous process that is easily palpable beneath the skin. (Patients sometimes misinterpret this bony prominence and its overlying soft tissue as a "mass.")

Several major ligaments stabilize the cervical spine (Fig. 3-3). The anterior and posterior longitudinal ligaments are applied to the respective surfaces of the vertebral bodies. Where the posterior longitudinal ligament crosses the disc, it tends to be somewhat weak laterally, thus forming a point where disc herniation may occur. Some gliding motion is allowed to occur between vertebrae by relatively weak capsular ligaments that bind together each articular joint. The ligamentum flavum, or yellow ligament, is situated between adjacent laminae, and in the cervical spine, extremely strong ligaments— the nuchal ligament and interspinous ligaments—provide posterior support.

The vertebrae are separated from each other by the intervertebral discs, which constitute approximately one fourth of the length of the vertebral column. Each disc is composed of an inner nucleus pulposus, which is mainly gelatinous, and an outer layer, the anulus fibrosus, which is mainly fibrous. The discs function to distribute stress over a wide area of the vertebrae, to absorb shock, and to allow mobility. The nucleus pulposus has a high water content in early life, but with age this tends to diminish. With this loss of water, abnormal pressures begin to be exerted on the anulus, which may lead to herniation and/or disc degeneration. Pathologic changes in adjacent structures (facet joint arthritis, osteophyte formation) may eventually develop as well.

Eight pairs of nerve roots arise from the cervical spinal cord. Each nerve exits above the vertebra of the same number. Thus the sixth nerve root exits at the C5 C6 disc space. Each nerve except the first two pairs leaves the spinal column by passing through an intervertebral foramen (Fig. 3-4). Each foramen has as its superior and inferior boundaries the pedicles of the adjacent vertebrae. Each foramen is bounded posterolaterally by the apophyseal joint and anteromedially by the so-called joint of Luschka. In the cervical spine, this foramen is quite small and is almost entirely occupied by the nerve root. Thus anything that compromises this space, such as disc degeneration with spur formation, could cause pressure on the nerve root.

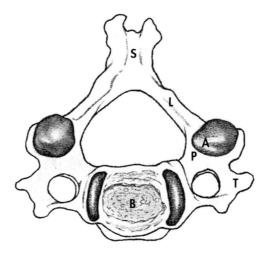

**Fig. 3–1.**
A typical cervical vertebra: *S* = spinous process; *L* = lamina; *A* = articular facet; *P* = pedicle; *T* = transverse process; *B* = body.

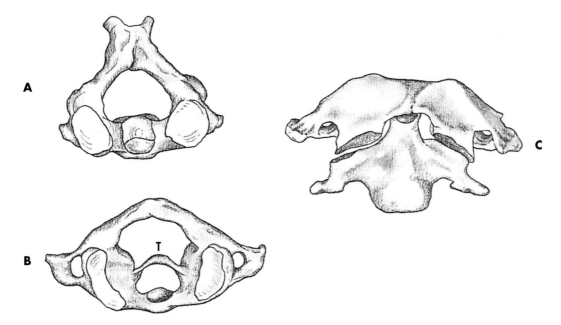

**Fig. 3–2.**
**A**, The axis. **B**, The atlas and transverse ligament *(T)*. **C**, The articulation of the atlas and the axis.

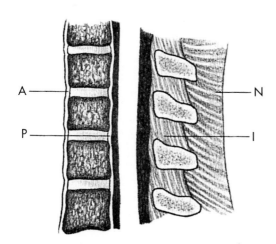

**Fig. 3–3.**
Ligaments of the cervical spine: anterior longitudinal ligament (*A*); posterior longitudinal ligament (*P*); nuchal ligament (*N*); interspinous ligament (*I*).

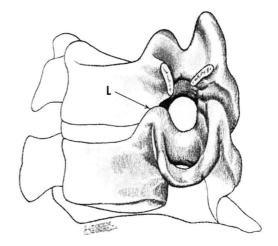

**Fig. 3–4.**
The intervertebral foramen. Note the proximity of the joint of Luschka (*L*).

## EXAMINATION

Examination of the neck begins with observation of the posture of the head and neck in relation to the torso. Any decrease in the normal cervical lordosis is noted. The neck is gently palpated for tender areas and trigger points. The range of motion of the cervical spine is then measured and any movement that reproduces pain is noted. Flexion, extension, right and left bending, and right and left rotation are all recorded. A complete neurologic examination, including muscle strength testing, is always performed. The peripheral nerves are percussed for tenderness and tested for function. In addition, the shoulders and elbows are always carefully examined, particularly if there is any radiation of the pain or numbness and tingling.

## ROENTGENOGRAPHIC ANATOMY

The examination of all neck disorders should include a standard roentgenographic evaluation. The roentgenographic features of the cervical spine are well visualized by the following: (1) anteroposterior view (Fig. 3-5), (2) lateral views in flexion and extension, (3) oblique views in both directions to visualize the intervertebral foramen (Fig. 3-6), and (4) an open-mouth odontoid view to visualize the odontoid process and the relationship between C1 and C2.

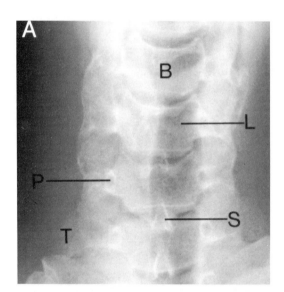

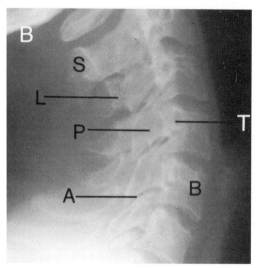

**Fig. 3–5.**
Anteroposterior (**A**) and lateral (**B**) views of the cervical spine: *S* = spinous process; *T* = transverse process; *B* = body; *A* = articular (zygapophyseal) facet joint; *P* = pedicle; *L* = lamina. Note the slight lordosis and even spacing of the vertebrae and discs.

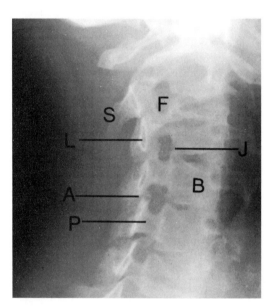

**Fig. 3–6.**
Oblique view: *S* = spinous process; *F* = intervertebral foramen; *J* = joint of Luschka; *L* = lamina; *P* = pedicle; *A* = articular facet joint; *B* = body.

## CERVICAL DISC SYNDROMES

Disease of the cervical spine as a result of disorders of the disc will affect 50% of the population at some time, usually between the ages of 30 and 60. More than 90% of disc lesions in the cervical spine occur at the C5 and C6 levels, those being the most mobile segments. As disc degeneration occurs, two types of lesions produce similar symptoms. The first of these is the soft disc protrusion or nuclear herniation. With this lesion, a mass of nucleus pulposus begins to bulge outward, usually *posterolaterally*, at the area of the greatest weakness in the anulus fibrosus (Fig. 3-7). Complete extrusion of this disc material may even occur. This lesion is more common in the younger patient. With acute rupture of a cervical disc, immediate compression of the nerve root often occurs and results in nerve root symptoms and radicular pain.

The second, more common lesion results from chronic disc degeneration with subsequent settling or narrowing of the disc space and alterations in the surrounding structures. This is the so-called *hard* disc lesion, or cervical spondylosis, and occurs primarily in the older age group. As narrowing and collapse of the disc proceeds, the vertebrae become more closely approximated, which leads to spur formation along the disc edges and at the joints of Luschka. Mild subluxation of the facet joint may also occur. All of these changes decrease the size of the intervertebral foramen, which may result in pressure on the nerve root. Mild inflammation and swelling are usually present in conjunction with osteophyte formation, all of which further contribute to the narrowing of the foramen and nerve root compression.

Rarely, large posterior osteophytes may cause pressure on the anterior portion of the spinal cord and produce mixed symptoms of upper extremity nerve root pain and lower extremity weakness. This is commonly termed *cervical spondylosis with myelopathy*. In many of these cases, the lower extremity symptoms are much more disabling than the neck symptoms, a situation that can cause some difficulty in determining their etiology.

### Clinical Features

Pain associated with cervical disc disease usually develops gradually. Degeneration or slow herniation may initially cause only neck and referred pain, which often begins in the interscapular area and may be mistaken for "shoulder" pain. Patients often complain of a tightness or stiffness in the neck that is made worse with activity. Morning stiffness is common, and certain movements, especially extension, exacerbate the pain. Anterior chest or breast pain may even be the presenting complaint in rare cases. Coughing, sneezing, and straining can accentuate the pain. If nerve root irritation or compression develops, pain may radiate into the shoulder and arm and along the radial aspect of the forearm (Fig. 3-8). Numbness and tingling are often noted in these same areas,

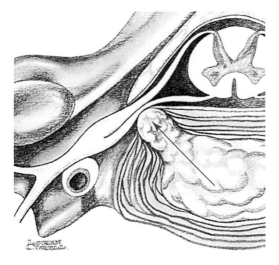

**Fig. 3–7.**
Disc herniation *(arrow)* causing nerve root compression. Spur formation may occur in the same area.

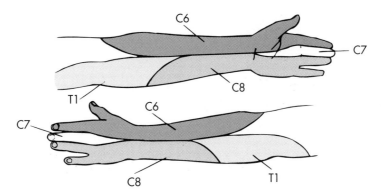

**Fig. 3–8.**
Volar and dorsal dermatome pattern of the forearm and hand. Pain and paresthesias may radiate into these areas when the affected nerve root is compressed. Note: Extremity symptoms as a result of disc disease are almost always unilateral.

and referred pain, which does not follow a dermatome pattern, is common along the medial border of the scapula. Headaches are not uncommon, and dysphagia has even been reported secondary to large anterior osteophytes. Headache or jaw pain may be present with high lesions.

Examination often reveals a decreased range of motion. Pain on hyperextension and local tenderness in the cervical spine are often observed. Trigger point tenderness is commonly noted in the area of referred pain in the interscapular region. (This pain is often reproduced by specific neck movements, usually extension with rotation to the involved side.) Pressure against the top of the head also may reproduce the pain in the arm (Fig. 3-9). Some sensory changes are occasionally present along the specific dermatome, but the sensory examination is often not helpful. Motor weakness and reflex changes may be noted (Table 3-1).

Spondylosis in the cervical spine may occasionally produce symptoms referable to the lower extremities (cervical spondylotic myelopathy). These symptoms result from pressure of posterior osteophytes on the anterior portion of the cervical spinal cord. The symptom

complex appears as a combination of cervical *root* and *cord* symptoms. The patient may have a typical disc syndrome in the upper extremities, but in addition, gait difficulties, weakness, and spasticity may be present in the lower extremities. The lower extremity symptoms have a gradual onset at about 50 years of age and may progress slowly. They are often more disabling than the neck symptoms, which are usually mild.

### Special Studies

In most cases, the diagnosis is clear without further testing. Neck, interscapular, and/or arm pain that is aggravated by neck motion is typical. Eventually, however, the following studies may be needed:

1. Plain roentgenograms are usually performed first, within the first few weeks. Anteroposterior (AP) and lateral views are sufficient. They are usually normal in soft disc rupture. With chronic degenerative disc disease, however, loss of the height of the disc space, anterior and posterior osteophyte formation, and encroachment on the intervertebral foramen by osteophytes are noted on routine films (Fig. 3-10).

2. Myelography, sometimes followed by computed tomography (CT), remains important for the evaluation of cervical radiculopathy. It is helpful in localizing the lesion but is not without some morbidity and is indicated only under the following two circumstances: (1) if surgical intervention is contemplated or (2) if other serious spinal abnormality is suspected. Loss of the normal root "sleeve" and indentation of the dural sac are often seen (Fig. 3-11). Spinal fluid analysis performed at the time of myelography may show a slight increase in protein content.

3. Magnetic resonance imaging is also valuable in the assessment of the cervical spine and may eventually replace myelography. It is attractive partly because it is noninvasive and uses no ionizing radiation. It should be used selectively because of its high cost. Many patients are excluded from this modality for reasons such as obesity, the presence of pacemakers, internal fixation devices, and claustrophobia (although newer models cause less

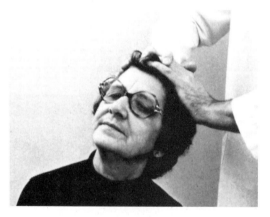

**Fig. 3–9.**
Vertex compression test. Extension and tilting the head to the affected side may narrow the neural foramen and reproduce neck and/or arm pain when disc herniation or spondylosis is present.

**TABLE 3–1.**

Clinical Features of Common Cervical Disc Syndromes

| Disc | Pain | Sensory Change | Motor Weakness, Atrophy | Reflex Change |
|------|------|----------------|-------------------------|---------------|
| C4-5 (C5 root) | Base of neck, shoulder, anterolateral aspect of arm | Numbness in deltoid region | Deltoid, biceps | Biceps |
| C5-6 (C6 root) | Neck, shoulder, medial border of scapula, lateral aspect of arm, dorsum of forearm | Dorsolateral aspect of thumb and index finger | Biceps, extensor pollicis longus | Biceps, brachioradialis |
| C6-7 (C7 root) | Neck, shoulder, medial border of scapula, lateral aspect of arm, dorsum of forearm | Index, middle fingers, dorsum of hand | Triceps | Triceps |

claustrophobia). The examination time is also quite lengthy. Indications for its use are generally the same as those for myelography. Like myelography, it is usually indicated late in the disorder, after several weeks have passed without recovery.

CT scanning, although less expensive, is not as helpful in evaluating degenerative disc disease in the cervical spine as it is in the assessment of traumatic conditions of the neck.

4. Electromyography can confirm the diagnosis in some cases if the disorder has caused nerve root

compression long enough. Nerve conduction studies help rule out peripheral nerve disorders. Discography is also occasionally performed in the evaluation of cervical disc disease, but the diagnosis can usually be well established on the basis of the history, physical examination, and plain films alone.

5. Thermography is mentioned only for completeness. Its validity is uncertain, and it is not commonly used.

**Note**: Roentgenographic studies are not always conclusive. False-negative and false-positive results

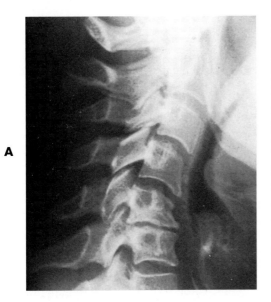
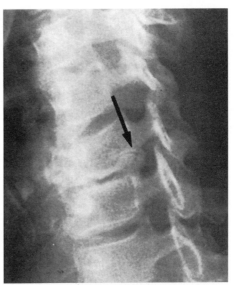

**Fig. 3–10.**
Lateral (**A**) and oblique (**B**) roentgenograms showing degenerative disc disease at the C5-C6 level. Note the osteophyte formation and narrowing of the intervertebral foramen (*arrow*).

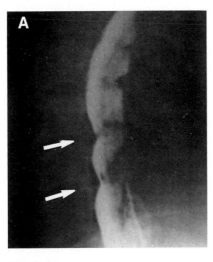
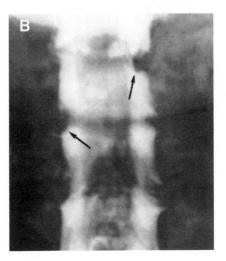

**Fig. 3–11.**
Myelographic findings in cervical disc disease. Note the filling defects from osteophyte formation on the lateral view (**A**) and absence of the normal root sleeve (*arrows*) on the AP view (**B**).

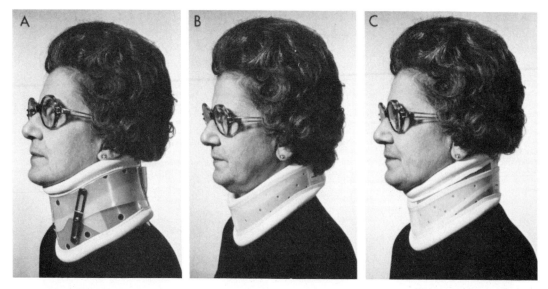

**Fig. 3–12.**
Proper usage of the cervical collar. **A,** A collar too high places the neck in too much extension. **B,** A collar too short does not immobilize and allows too much flexion. **C,** Proper height of the collar maintains the head in a slightly flexed or neutral position.

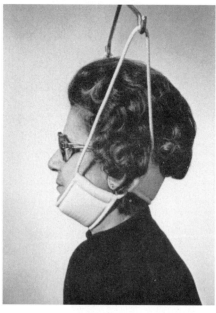

**Fig. 3–13.**
Proper usage of cervical traction. The direction of pull should be neutral; 4 to 6 lb of weight should be used for 20 to 30 minutes. It should be repeated three or four times daily, depending on the response. The pressure should be equally distributed between the chin and the occiput.

are fairly common. These studies should be performed only as an adjunct to, not instead of, a good history and clinical examination. When the results are uncertain, it is best to reexamine the patient. If the symptoms do not correlate well with the roentgenographic findings, it is best to continue to treat the symptoms and not the roentgenogram. Remember that "abnormal" roentgenographic findings in the spine are present in up to 35% of *asymptomatic* adults.

### Treatment

1. Rest is the cornerstone of therapy for cervical disc disease. In acute disc protrusion, it permits the healing of soft parts to occur. (What happens to the disc material is unknown. One theory is that the disc may act as a foreign body and become absorbed or transformed into scar tissue.) In chronic disc disease, rest allows the inflammatory reaction to subside. Rest is accomplished by various means, but absolute bed rest is the most beneficial. Various soft collars that restrict motion and give support are also helpful (Fig. 3-12).

2. Moist heat applied to the affected area will help relieve tenderness and muscle pain. Massage may also give temporary relief of the trigger point soft-tissue pain. Home cervical traction may also help (Fig. 3-13), although it is unlikely that the neck can actually be "stretched." Formal physical therapy such as diathermy or ultrasound, massage, or traction may also provide temporary improvement. (Although most forms of physical therapy are of an unproven value, some patients do respond to these treatments. Pain relief with physical therapy, however, seems short-lived, and any overall improvement usually parallels what would have probably occurred naturally.)

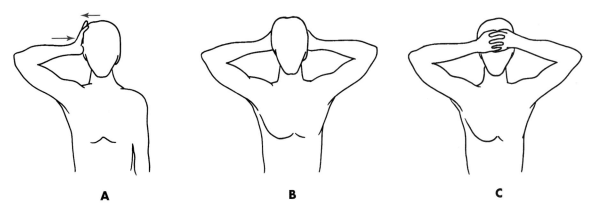

**Fig. 3–14.**
Isometric neck exercises. **A**, The hand is placed against the side of the head slightly above the ear, and pressure is gradually increased while resisting with the neck muscles and keeping the head in the same position. The position is held 5 seconds, relaxed, and repeated five times. **B**, The exercise is performed on the other side and then **C**, from the back and front. The exercise should be performed three or four times daily.

3. NSAIDs may be helpful, especially for degenerative disc disease. Muscle "relaxers" are rarely effective (see Chapter 18) especially if there are signs of nerve compression. The problem is not caused by muscle tissue, nor can "spasm" ever be truly demonstrated. The pain is simply referred to the surrounding soft parts. These medications probably are only effective via their tranquilizing effect. They may be helpful when given at night to allow the patient to rest, but many patients are bothered by their sedative side effects during the day. Mild narcotic analgesics are often necessary to control pain.
4. Epidural pain blocks may be valuable when radicular pain is present.
5. After the acute pain subsides, a program of gentle, graded isometric exercises is recommended (Fig. 3-14). Recurrences are prevented by avoiding fatigue and poor postural habits, especially hyperextension (Fig. 3-15). A pillow approximately 7.5 to 10 cm thick should be used for sleeping and should be placed under the neck rather than under the head. An overly thick pillow may place the head in too much flexion, whereas a thin one may allow too much extension to occur. Most patients may continue a reasonable daily work schedule unless the pain is particularly intense (Fig. 3-16).

### *Prognosis*

Most patients will improve with time, and fewer than 5% will require surgery. Patience is important. The time required for improvement varies considerably among patients. Several weeks may be needed before full recovery occurs. Patients may be advised, how-

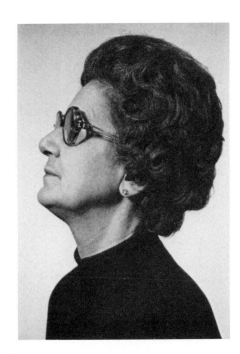

**Fig. 3–15.**
The hyperextended "spectator" attitude that often causes neck strain and aggravates disc disease. The head and neck should be maintained in a neutral position at all times. Positions that produce sharp angulation or rotation of the head, such as sleeping on the abdomen or resting on a couch with the armrest as a "pillow," should also be avoided.

ever, that there is generally no danger in waiting and continuing conservative treatment. Recurrences occur occasionally and are treated in the same manner. Surgery is reserved for those patients in whom the pain and level of disability become intolerable, or in

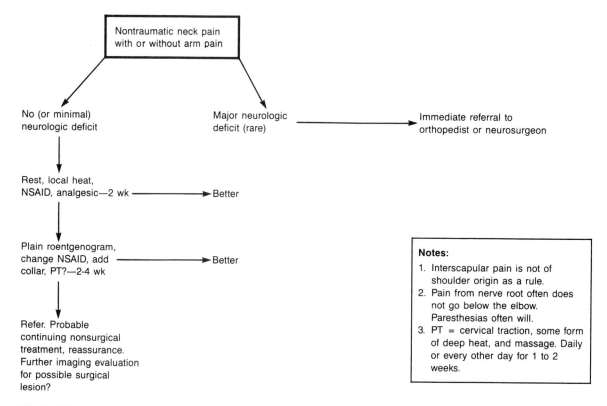

**Fig. 3–16.**
Algorithm for suspected cervical disc syndrome.

Notes:
1. Interscapular pain is not of shoulder origin as a rule.
2. Pain from nerve root often does not go below the elbow. Paresthesias often will.
3. PT = cervical traction, some form of deep heat, and massage. Daily or every other day for 1 to 2 weeks.

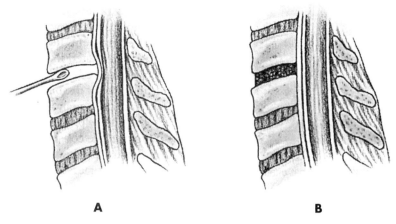

**A**          **B**

**Fig. 3–17.**
Arthrodesis of the cervical spine. The disc is removed and replaced with a bone graft.

whom a major neurologic deficit has developed. Surgery is not as helpful for neck pain as for arm pain. The procedure consists of removal of the affected disc, usually followed by arthrodesis of the two adjacent vertebrae with a bone graft (Fig. 3-17). Some soft disc protrusions are occasionally removed without fusion. The arm pain usually subsides immediately after surgery and osteophytes that have formed in the foramen and adjacent structures are usually absorbed within 9 to 18 months.

# CERVICAL SPRAIN

Most soft-tissue injuries of the cervical spine are the result of a hyperextension force. Although a variety of injuries can produce a cervical sprain, the condition has become virtually synonymous with the disorder called "whiplash" that develops after a rear-end automobile collision. Rarely is there any osseous injury. Most of the force is absorbed by ligaments, muscles, and disc. Acute disc protrusion is not common, but disc "injury" may occur and serial roentgenograms taken later may show significant progressive degenerative changes.

Any soft structures, including muscle, anterior longitudinal ligament, esophagus, and trachea, may be stretched. Dysphagia and hoarseness are sometimes seen shortly after the injury. Hemorrhage and edema may be present in the prevertebral area, and the sympathetic nerve chains, which are located near the vertebral bodies, are occasionally stretched. This may produce somewhat unusual symptoms such as nausea, tinnitus, blurred vision, and dizziness.

Chronic pain that continues for weeks or months is not uncommon. Degenerative changes may eventually result from the injury at one or more levels in a previously normal cervical spine, and this may lead to prolonged disability. Similarly, patients with previously asymptomatic degenerative disc disease may develop their first symptoms of a cervical disc syndrome after a hyperextension injury.

## Clinical Features

Often there are few symptoms immediately after the injury. A few hours later, however, the patient may begin to notice stiffness in the neck followed by pain and an inability to move the neck normally. The pain is generalized to the neck region and may radiate to the occiput along the path of the greater occipital nerve. Shoulder and interscapular discomfort may be noted, and there may even be pain in the anterior chest wall. Radicular pain, suggestive of nerve root involvement, is rare. Symptoms such as nausea, tinnitus, blurred vision, and occipital headaches are not uncommon.

Examination may reveal generalized tenderness in the anterior and posterior neck musculature. Motion may be greatly limited, and extension of the spine is often quite painful. Mild torticollis may be present. The results of the neurologic examination are usually normal. The examination rarely reveals any objective abnormality.

## Special Studies

After the initial examination, if there is any reason to suspect a significant cervical spine injury, a full lateral roentgenogram of the cervical spine should be taken without moving the patient. This view should always include the body of the seventh cervical vertebra; if it

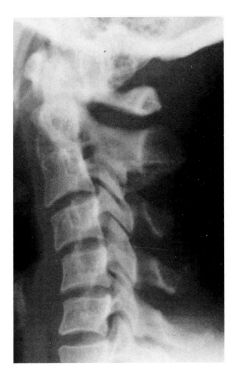

**Fig. 3–18.**
Lateral roentgenogram showing reversal of the cervical lordosis. (This abnormal curvature can become permanent in whiplash injury.)

does not, the vertebra is probably being obscured by the shoulder soft tissue shadow. In this case, the shoulders should be pulled down manually and the roentgenogram repeated. If a satisfactory view of C7 still has not been obtained, then a "swimmer's" view may be performed. If no significant injury is seen on this view, then the remaining cervical spine films are obtained.

Usually, results of the initial roentgenographic examination are normal, but with the passage of time, reversal of the normal cervical lordosis may rarely be observed (Fig. 3-18). This finding is often seen in patients with prolonged disability. Late degenerative changes may even occur. "Loss of the normal cervical lordosis," often quoted on early roentgenograms, is probably not significant. Any degenerative changes present in the cervical spine at the time of the initial injury should also be noted for both medical and medicolegal purposes. Further roentgenographic studies are usually not indicated. CT and bone scanning may be helpful to rule out fracture, however. MRI is usually not helpful and is not generally indicated.

## Treatment

1. Rest is an important treatment modality in acute cervical strain. It should consist primarily of bed

rest for the first few days if the injury is very painful. A soft cervical collar holding the neck in slight flexion is worn day and night for approximately 1 to 2 weeks, depending upon response.

2. Analgesics are given in amounts sufficient to relieve pain. Antiinflammatory drugs given soon after the injury may be helpful, especially in the patient who has preexisting degenerative disc disease of the cervical spine.

3. Cold should be used initially. Heat should be avoided soon after the injury because it may increase swelling. It may be helpful later in the course of care.

4. When the acute pain begins to subside, isometric and gentle range-of-motion exercises are started, and wearing of the collar is gradually discontinued. The patient is encouraged to return to normal activities as soon as possible. General measures—including a proper pillow and the avoidance of stress—should be instituted. If symptoms persist after 4 to 6 weeks, physical therapy may be beneficial (Fig. 3-19).

### Prognosis

Most patients will improve in 4 to 6 weeks unless there is significant underlying degenerative disc disease. Less long-term disability and anxiety on the part of the patient will result if aggressive, conservative treatment is instituted, especially in the initial stage of the injury.

This disorder is well known for its chronicity, especially when associated with motor vehicle accidents. Recovery in these cases is often delayed, taking 6 to 12 months. Surgery is rarely indicated, and the results are often unrewarding. Part of the reason for this is that it is often difficult to localize the exact source of the pain.

Eventually, some patients develop a "chronic benign pain syndrome." Daily exercise, resuming a normal lifestyle, and avoiding excessive *passive* treatment may help these individuals. Reassurance, understanding, and explanation at all stages of care are important. Whether a cervical sprain can ever cause symptoms later in life is impossible to prove because of the common development of disc disease in the general population.

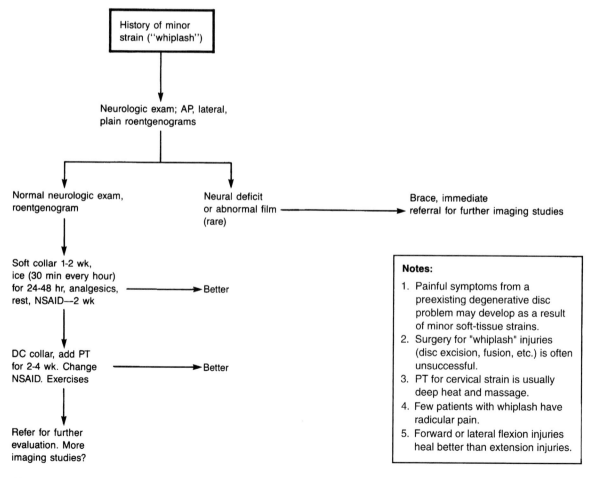

**Fig. 3–19.**
Algorithm for cervical strain.

## Tension Strain

Neck and upper dorsal pain seem to occasionally develop from tension and strain. The common settings are those in which the individual is required to sit at a desk, typing or studying for long periods. Positional strain, sometimes combined with tension and stress, often leads to muscular pain in the upper dorsal and cervical spine. The neck pain may radiate to the occiput.

The examination usually has negative results except for local tenderness and occasional limitation of neck movement. Treatment usually involves changes in work activities and work or study positions and taking frequent breaks from activities for gentle stretching exercises.

# DISC CALCIFICATION

Calcification of the intervertebral disc is not uncommon. It often occurs in the dorsal spine of adults in the anulus fibrosus and is probably secondary to a degenerative process. Multiple disc calcifications also occur with ochronosis. Disc calcification is usually an incidental roentgenographic finding and generally does not produce symptoms.

In children, however, disc calcification occurs more commonly in the cervical spine, and in this age group it appears to be a definite clinical entity with symptoms. The cause is unknown but it may represent a nonspecific inflammatory reaction. It is probably not infectious in nature. In contrast to the adult, it is the nucleus pulposus that calcifies.

### Clinical Features

The disorder has its onset about the age of 7 years and usually begins with neck pain and stiffness. Localized tenderness and a decrease in the range of motion of the cervical spine are usually present. A mild torticollis may be noted. There is usually an elevation of the temperature, sedimentation rate, and white blood cell (WBC) count.

Roentgenograms reveal the disease to primarily affect the lower discs in the cervical spine (Fig. 3-20). Multiple discs may be affected, and the calcification usually begins to regress with the onset of symptoms.

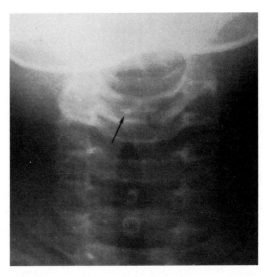

**Fig. 3–20.**
Disc space calcification *(arrow)*.

### Treatment

Treatment is conservative and consists of a soft collar, cervical traction, and analgesics as necessary. Antibiotics are not indicated as a rule. Patients usually become asymptomatic in 1 to 2 weeks without any sequelae.

# TORTICOLLIS

Torticollis is contraction or contracture of the muscles of the neck that causes the head to be tilted to one side. It is usually accompanied by rotation of the chin to the opposite side with flexion, and is usually a *symptom* of some underlying disorder. Often the term is used incorrectly in cases when the torticollis may simply be positional. The condition has been attributed to over 50 causes. It may be present on a congenital basis or acquired as a result of trauma or disease.

## Congenital Muscular Torticollis

This deformity is usually noted at birth and is much more common after breech deliveries. It results from a unilateral contracture of the sternocleidomastoid muscle. The cause is unknown, but fibrosis of the muscle occurs, possibly secondary to a vascular disturbance in the muscle. A "tumor" consisting of dense fibrous tissue is often found in the muscle shortly after birth. This mass gradually subsides over the ensuing weeks to leave a shortened and contracted sternocleidomastoid muscle. If untreated, secondary changes appear in the cervical vertebrae, and marked asymmetry of the face becomes apparent. These changes often persist in spite of later treatment.

### Clinical Features

The diagnosis generally can be made shortly after birth. The "mass" is usually palpable, and the head is characteristically tilted toward the side of the mass and rotated

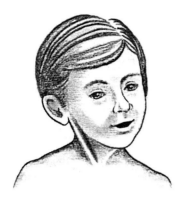

**Fig. 3–21.**
Congenital muscular torticollis.

in the opposite direction (Fig. 3-21). Roentgenograms of the cervical spine are usually performed to rule out injury and congenital osseous disorders of the cervical spine.

### Treatment

Conservative treatment, if instituted early, will usually result in a cure. No improvement can be expected without treatment. In mild deformities, gentle stretching exercises carried out by the mother will usually correct the problem. The exercises should be repeated several times daily. The crib should be placed so that the child must turn toward the corrected position when someone enters the room.

Surgery is reserved for late cases or for those who fail to respond to conservative treatment. The procedure consists of the release of the sternocleidomastoid muscle followed by traction or casting and exercises. The results are usually good.

### Torticollis Secondary to Inflammation

Torticollis may be seen in the 5- to 10-year-old age group after an upper respiratory tract infection or cervical lymphadenitis. A few days after onset of the infection, spontaneous subluxation of the atlas or unilateral subluxation of C2 on C3 occurs. There may be a history of a minor neck injury. Typically, there is no sternocleidomastoid tightness or spasm; if any is present, it is on the long side of the neck rather than on the short side as seen in myositis and congenital muscular torticollis. Examination may reveal tenderness of the spin-

ous process of C2 and an obvious tilting of the head. Treatment consists of cervical traction and warm, moist packs. The subluxation will usually improve, and a collar is worn afterward until all symptoms subside.

A condition sometimes referred to as "myositis" often causes tenderness of the cervical musculature. The cause is unknown, but the disorder is said to follow exposure to cold air or a draft. Clinically, there is tenderness in the musculature of the cervical spine, and the head is held toward the side of the tenderness. This entity is treated with rest, moist heat, and a soft collar until symptoms subside.

### Idiopathic Spasmodic Torticollis

This term refers to a disease entity consisting of the spontaneous onset of painful contractions of various muscles about the cervical spine, including the sternocleidomastoid muscle. The cause is unknown, although some consider it to be a variant or isolated form of dystonia musculorum deformans. It has a gradual onset in adulthood. "Spasms" may occur in the cervical musculature, and they may be bilateral. These spasms tend to hold the head toward the affected side and are uncontrollable.

These patients have strong psychoneurotic tendencies, and there is little likelihood of spontaneous recovery. The disease is usually resistant to ordinary conservative treatment including physical therapy, braces, psychotherapy, and various medications including injection with botulinum toxin. Surgical treatment is sometimes performed and consists of sectioning the spinal accessory nerves and upper cervical rhizotomies. The surgical results are only mediocre. No medical or surgical treatment seems very satisfactory for the majority of patients.

### Miscellaneous Causes of Torticollis

Spinal cord tumor, trauma, drug reactions (phenothiazines), neuritis of the spinal accessory nerve, cervical spine anomalies, and rheumatoid arthritis will all occasionally produce torticollis. Ocular disturbances may produce the same symptoms, and any child who has gradually increasing torticollis should have a complete eye examination. Fracture or unilateral rotatory subluxation may also cause torticollis and should always be ruled out by an adequate roentgenographic examination.

## BIBLIOGRAPHY

Adson AW, Young HH, Ghormley RK: Spasmodic torticollis, *J Bone Joint Surg* 28:299, 1946.

Bernhardt M et al: Cervical spondylotic myelopathy, *J Bone Joint Surg Am* 75:119-129, 1993.

Bohlman HH: Cervical spondylosis with moderate to severe myelopathy, *Spine* 2:151, 1977.

Canale ST, Griffin DW, Hubbard CN: Congenital muscular torticollis: a long-term follow-up, *J Bone Joint Surg Am* 64:810, 1982.

Clark E, Robinson PK: Cervical myelopathy: a complication of cervical spondylosis, *Brain* 79:483, 1956.

Copley LA, Dormans JP: Cervical spine disorders in infancy and childhood, *J Am Acac Orthop Surg* 6:204-214, 1998.

Coventry MB, Harris LE: Congenital muscular torticollis in infancy, *J Bone Joint Surg Am* 41:815, 1959.

Deans GT et al: Neck sprain: a major cause of disability following car accidents, *Injury* 18:10, 1987.

DePalma AF, Rothman RH: *The intervertebral disc*, Philadelphia, 1970, WB Saunders.

Dubousset J: Torticollis in children caused by congenital anomalies of the atlas, *J Bone Joint Surg Am* 68:178, 1986.

Eyring EJ, Peterson CA, Bjornson DR: Intervertebral-disc calcification in childhood: a distinct clinical syndrome, *J Bone Joint Surg Am* 46:1432, 1964.

Ferke RD et al: Muscular torticollis: a modified surgical approach, *J Bone Joint Surg Am* 65:894, 1983.

Gorgan MF, Bannister GC: Long-term prognosis of soft tissue injuries of the neck, *J Bone Joint Surg Br* 72:901-903, 1990.

Helliwell PS, Evans PF, Wright V: The straight cervical spine: does it indicate muscle spasm? *J Bone Joint Surg Br* 76:103-106, 1994.

Hohl M: Soft tissue injuries of the neck in automobile accidents, *J Bone Joint Surg Am* 56:1675, 1974.

Law MD, Bernhardt M, White AA: Evaluation and management of cervical spondylotic myelopathy: instructional course lectures, *J Bone Joint Surg Am* 76:1420-1433, 1994.

Levine MJ, Albert TJ, Smith MD: Cervical radiculopathy: diagnosis and treatment, *J Am Acad Orthop Surg* 4:305-316, 1996.

Miller GM, Forbes GS, Onofrio BM: Magnetic resonance imaging of the spine, *Mayo Clin Proc* 64:986, 1989.

Norris SH, Watt I: The prognosis of neck injuries resulting from rear-end vehicle collisions, *J Bone Joint Surg Br* 65:608, 1983.

Pennie BH, Agambar LJ: Whiplash injuries, *J Bone Joint Surg Br* 72:277, 1990.

Pettersson K, Hildingsson C, Toolanen G, et al: Disc pathology after whiplash injury: a prospective magnetic resonance imaging and clinical investigation, *Spine* 22:283-287, 1997.

Robinson RA: The results of anterior interbody fusion, *J Bone Joint Surg Am* 44:1569, 1962.

Robinson RA et al: Cervical spondylotic myelopathy: etiology and treatment concepts, *Spine* 2:89, 1977.

Robinson RA, Smith GW: Anterolateral cervical disc syndrome, *Bull Johns Hopkins Hosp* 96:223, 1955.

Ruge D, Wiltse LL: *Spinal disorders: diagnosis and treatment*, Philadelphia, 1977, Lea & Febiger.

Scoville WB: Types of cervical disc lesion and their surgical approaches, *JAMA* 196:105, 1966.

Sherman WD et al: Calcified cervical intervertebral discs in children, *Spine* 1:55, 1976.

Sonnabend DH, Taylor TKF, Chapman GK: Intervertebral disc calcification syndromes in children, *J Bone Joint Surg Br* 64:25, 1982.

Tachdjian MO: *Pediatric orthopedics*, Philadelphia, 1972, WB Saunders.

Tamura T: Cranial symptoms after cervical injuries: aetiology and treatment of Barre-Lieou syndrome, *J Bone Joint Surg Br* 71:283, 1989.

# CHAPTER 4

# The Cervicobrachial Region

Disorders of the brachial plexus are usually the result of either compression or injury. The resultant symptoms and signs are often confusing, but these conditions should always be considered in the differential diagnosis of neuropathies of the upper extremity.

## ANATOMY

The brachial plexus is formed by the anterior rami of the last four cervical nerves and the first thoracic nerve (Fig. 4-1). In general, the upper portion of the plexus innervates the shoulder abductors and external rotators and the elbow flexors. It also provides sensation to the shoulder and radial side of the arm. The lower portion of the plexus primarily innervates the forearm and hand muscles and provides sensation to the ulnar side of the arm, forearm, and hand. The first thoracic ramus also communicates with the first thoracic ganglion, through which sympathetic fibers are carried to the face from the spinal cord. Thus involvement of the lower portion of the plexus by disease or injury may produce Horner's syndrome (ptosis, miosis, enophthalmos, and anhidrosis).

The plexus passes distally between the middle and anterior scalene muscles, which attach to the first rib (Fig. 4-2). Beneath the clavicle, it is joined by the subclavian artery. The subclavian vein passes anterior to the scalenus anticus muscle. Artery, vein, and plexus then enter the axilla beneath the pectoralis minor muscle, with the lower trunk of the plexus (C8, T1) lying on the first rib.

## THORACIC OUTLET SYNDROMES

*Thoracic outlet syndrome* is a term used to describe a controversial condition thought to produce upper extremity symptoms as a result of neurovascular compression at the base of the neck. The thoracic outlet is the space through which pass the brachial plexus, subclavian artery and vein on their way into the arm. Three types of syndromes have been described based on the point of compression: (1) the cervical rib and scalenus anticus syndromes, in which a cervical rib or abnormal scalene muscle insertions may cause compression; (2) the costoclavicular syndrome, in which compression may occur under the clavicle; and (3) the hyperabduction syndrome, in which compression may develop in the subcoracoid region. These disorders all have similar clinical features and it is often impossible to differentiate among them on this basis alone. The symptoms and signs are related to the degree of involvement of each of the various structures at the level of the first rib. Primary neural involvement may lead to pain and numbness. Arterial involvement usually causes the extremity to feel "asleep." This symptom may have a glove type of distribution and is occasionally associated with paresis. Venous involvement, such as that seen with acute thrombosis of the subclavian vein (effort thrombosis), may produce swelling. True arterial or venous compression or thrombosis is quite rare. The diagnosis of thoracic outlet syndrome is most often used in the consideration of *pain* affecting the arm.

### Cervical Rib Syndrome

The cervical rib usually arises from the seventh cervical vertebra and is the most common cause of neurovascular compression at the base of the neck (Fig. 4-3). The condition may be bilateral. The rib or its fibrous extension narrows the interval between the anterior and middle scalene muscles and produces a higher barrier that the neurovascular structures must arch over on their way into the arm. In older patients or those with muscular weakness, the shoulder may also sag more than

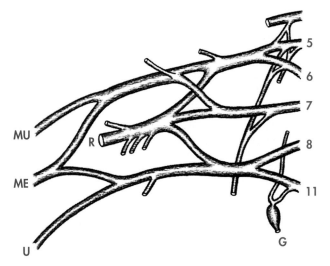

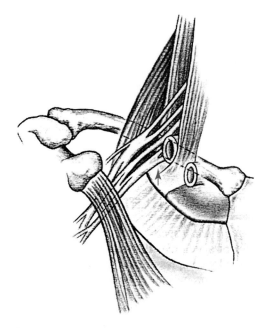

**Fig. 4–1.**
The brachial plexus. Five rami normally combine to form three trunks, which divide to form three cords. The lower trunk *(C8, T1)* lies on the first rib and is most commonly involved in thoracic outlet syndromes. The posterior cord continues as the radial nerve *(R)*. The medial cord contributes half of the median nerve and continues as the ulnar nerve *(U)*. The lateral cord continues as the musculocutaneous *(MU)* nerve after contributing the other half of the median nerve *(ME)*. *G* is the ganglion.

**Fig. 4–2.**
Anatomy of the cervicobrachial region. Note that the lower trunk of the brachial plexus (C8, T1) lies on the first rib *(arrow)*.

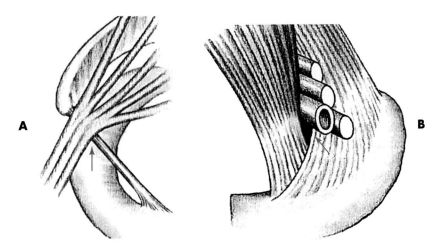

**Fig. 4–3.**
**A,** Compression caused by a cervical rib *(arrow)*. **B,** Abnormal scalene muscles that may cause compression at the cervicobrachial region *(arrow)*.

normal, further increasing the tension on the neurovascular structures. The compression is also increased by carrying a heavy object in the hand.

In the absence of a cervical rib, compression can occur between the middle and anterior scalene muscles because of abnormal insertions or the presence of additional muscle slips in the interscalene interval (scalenus anticus syndrome).

The lowest components (C8, T1) of the plexus are most commonly involved because of their position against the rib. The symptoms therefore tend to be most noticeable in the hand and inner aspect of the forearm. Pain and paresthesias are often produced along the distribution of the ulnar nerve. Weakness, numbness, and clumsiness in use of the hand are common complaints. Coldness, Raynaud's phenomenon, or even gangrene may be the initial symptom.

Clinically, the cervical rib may be palpable, and the brachial plexus is often tender. Weakness and atrophy of the muscles supplied by the lower trunk (interosseous, hypothenar muscles) is occasionally seen. Sensation may be diminished over the ulnar aspect of the forearm,

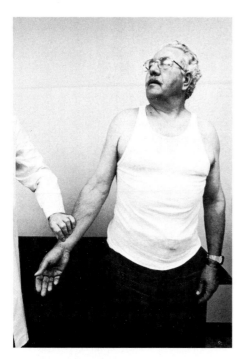

**Fig. 4–4.**
Adson's test.

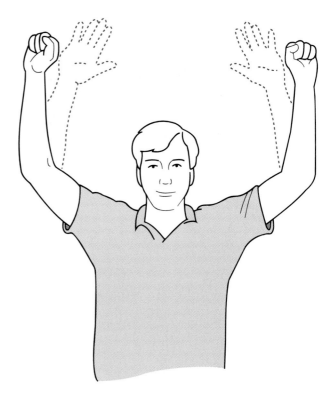

**Fig 4-5.**
Elevated arm stress test. With the arms held overhead, the hands are opened and closed. A positive test is pain and fatigue within 30 seconds.

arm, and the ulnar 1½ fingers. Swelling, coldness, cyanosis, trophic skin changes, and other signs of circulatory insufficiency are occasionally observed.

Provocative positioning tests are often described in the assessment of thoracic outlet syndromes. Adson's test may be positive in cervical rib and scalenus anticus syndromes (Fig. 4-4). This test takes advantage of the fact that when the scalene muscles are tensed, the interval between them is decreased and any existing compression of the subclavian artery is increased. The test is performed by having the patient breathe deeply, extend the neck, and turn the chin toward the affected side. When the test is positive, a decrease in the radial pulse is noted and pain is reproduced. If the test is negative, it is repeated with the chin turned to the opposite side. Although a positive test is suggestive of compression in the interscalene region, it is often positive in the normal population and is not necessarily diagnostic of cervical rib or scalenus anticus syndrome. Symptoms can also be reproduced occasionally by exercising the fingers with the arms elevated (Fig. 4-5).

Roentgenographic examination may reveal an extra rib extending from the transverse process of the seventh cervical vertebra (Fig. 4-6). The rib may be fully developed or rudimentary, and it is often bilateral. Its presence does not necessarily imply that it is symptomatic, however, because it is often present in asymptomatic individuals.

Electromyography and nerve conduction studies are not useful in the diagnosis of any of the thoracic outlet syndromes. Vascular studies are occasionally helpful if diminished pulsations and reproduction of the neurologic and/or vascular symptoms occur during one of the various maneuvers.

## Costoclavicular Syndrome

The space between the clavicle and the first rib may be narrowed by downward and backward pressure on the shoulders for a prolonged period. Abnormalities of the clavicle, such as malunion or nonunion after fracture, may contribute to the narrowing.

The syndrome is occasionally seen in individuals who are required to carry heavy packs on their shoulders. Intermittent numbness and pain in the hand and arm are the most common symptoms. They may be reproduced by the costoclavicular maneuver (Fig. 4-7). In this test, the shoulders are drawn downward and backward, and any change in the radial pulse or reproduction of symptoms is noted.

## Hyperabduction Syndrome

Neurovascular symptoms may also follow prolonged assumption of the position of shoulder hyperabduction. This position is often assumed during sleep and in certain occupations such as overhead painting. The neurovascular structures are compressed as they pass under the cora-

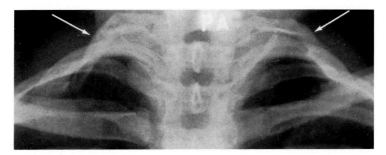

**Fig. 4–6.**
Bilateral cervical ribs *(arrows).*

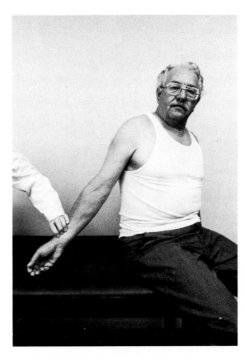

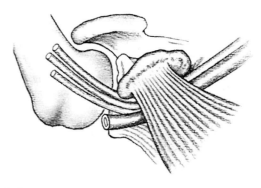

**Fig. 4–8.**
Hyperabduction of the upper extremity that may produce neurovascular compression.

**Fig. 4–7.**
The costoclavicular maneuver. The radial pulse may be diminished in many normal individuals.

coid process and pectoralis minor muscle with the arm in hyperabduction (Fig. 4-8). Numbness and paresthesias are common, but the pain tends to be less severe than that seen in the other compression syndromes. Wright's test (diminution of pulse or reproduction of symptoms on hyperabduction of the arm) may be positive (Fig. 4-9).

### Treatment

The initial treatment is conservative in all thoracic outlet syndromes except those rare cases with vascular complications. Symptomatic relief may be obtained by resting the elbow of the affected side on the arm of the chair, thereby elevating the shoulder. A sling may serve the same purpose. Specific strengthening and stretching exercises for the shoulder girdle muscles, taught by a knowledgeable physical therapist, can help (Fig. 4-10). Faulty posture and poor body

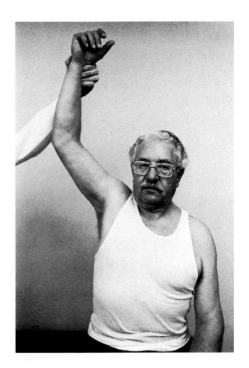

**Fig. 4–9.**
Wright's test.

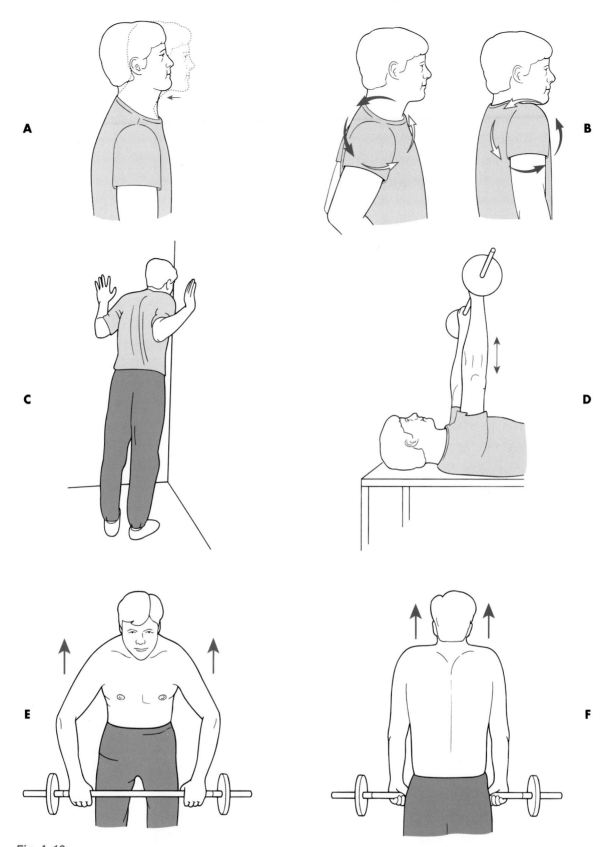

**Fig. 4–10.**

Shoulder exercises for thoracic outlet syndrome. **A,** Neck retraction. The head is pulled straight back keeping the jaw level. The position is held for 5 to 10 seconds. **B,** Shoulder rolls are performed by shrugging up, back, and down in a circular motion. **C,** Corner stretch. With the hands at shoulder height, the patient stands and leans into a corner until a gentle stretch is felt. This is held for 5 to 10 seconds. **D,** To strengthen the serrati, the weight is pushed upward so that the shoulders are lifted off the table. **E** and **F,** The trapezius is strengthened by raising the shoulders and drawing them backward to bring the scapulae upward and together.

mechanics should be corrected, and positions that aggravate the condition should be avoided. General health factors should be addressed as well, especially deconditioning and obesity. If symptoms are worsened by certain work activities, a minor alteration in the position of the arms while working could help.

For the hyperabduction syndrome, avoidance of the hyperabducted position is usually the only treatment necessary. A gauze strip tied to the wrist and attached to the foot of the bed to prevent hyperabduction at night may be temporarily necessary for those patients whose symptoms occur primarily at night.

The rare emergency is a case of acute vascular involvement. Otherwise, operative treatment is considered only when conservative measures fail to obtain significant relief after 4 to 6 months. Removal of the first dorsal and cervical ribs, combined with release of any abnormal scalene muscle insertions, is performed. These procedures are all combined with vascular repair when indicated.

**Note**: Although its actual incidence is difficult to assess, thoracic outlet syndrome is probably quite uncommon. Unfortunately, the diagnosis is often used in an attempt to explain symptoms difficult to correlate with known neuroanatomical pathways. The standard physical tests (Adson's, etc.) are of somewhat questionable value, and except for those rare cases with vascular involvement, there are no good special studies that can be used to confirm the diagnosis. The results from surgery are also quite variable and surgery is associated with a significant complication rate.

## BIRTH PALSY

Paralysis of the upper extremity at birth occurs in approximately 0.1% of live births. It usually follows a difficult and prolonged delivery. Injury to the upper plexus may occur as a result of lateral flexion of the neck against either a fixed head or a fixed shoulder. The lower plexus may be damaged by an injury that forces the arm upward. The damage may vary from simple stretching to complete avulsion of nerve roots.

Clinically, the involved extremity is noted to remain motionless at the side with the elbow extended. The Moro reflex is also absent on the affected side. There may be swelling above the clavicle because of hemorrhage. Tenderness to palpation is often present from a traumatic neuritis. Fractures of the clavicle or upper portion of the humerus may be present and cause a "pseudoparalysis." They should always be ruled out in cases of birth palsy. Horner's syndrome may be observed if the injury involves the thoracic root.

Recovery may occur within a few days or may take 3 to 6 months. No improvement can be expected after the age of 2 years. In older patients, underdevelopment of the entire upper extremity is often seen, and the humerus is often markedly shortened. Contractures and disuse atrophy are also observed. Unawareness of the extremity, despite satisfactory motor and sensory recovery, may also be noted in late cases.

Three types of paralysis are seen, depending on the area of the injury: Erb-Duchenne, or upper-arm paralysis; whole-arm paralysis; and Klumpke's, or lower-arm paralysis.

### Erb-Duchenne Paralysis

This is the most common type of obstetric paralysis. Damage to the upper roots (C5 and C6) leads to paralysis of the deltoid muscle, the external rotators of the shoulder, the elbow flexors, and the supinators of the forearm. Residual weakness of these muscles leads to the characteristic "waiter's-tip" position in which the arm is held adducted and internally rotated and the forearm is pronated (Fig. 4-11). Wrist and finger function is usually normal.

### Whole-Arm Paralysis

The limb is often completely flaccid and without motor function in this uncommon type of birth palsy. The hand tends to be dry and atrophic, and extensive sensory loss is often present.

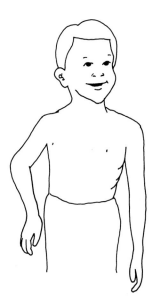

**Fig. 4–11.**
The "waiter's-tip" position. After partial upper arm paralysis, the upper extremity is often shortened and slightly smaller, and the palm often faces backward at rest.

## Klumpke's Paralysis

Klumpke's paralysis is quite rare. In this condition, the lower cervical and first thoracic roots are involved. The finger and wrist flexors are denervated along with the intrinsic muscles. A clawhand deformity often results. Horner's syndrome may also be present. Sensory loss involves the affected dermatomes of the lower plexus. The upper part of the arm is often uninvolved.

### *Treatment and Prognosis*

Treatment is designed to prevent fixed soft tissue contractures from developing so that any muscles that regain function will have a flexible joint on which to act. Gentle, repetitive, meticulous range-of-motion exercises to the shoulder and elbow are instituted as soon as the tenderness disappears (usually about 2 weeks). Supportive splints for the wrist and fingers are helpful when used in conjunction with a good exercise program. Casts are not recommended because they may lead to overimmobilization and contractures.

Reconstructive surgery is often beneficial for late deformities. Muscle transfers and osteotomies are utilized to restore motor function and correct malposition.

The overall prognosis for Erb's palsy is relatively good when compared with those for Klumpke's and whole-arm paralyses. More than 50% to 80% of upper-arm paralyses show fair to good recovery of arm function, usually within 3 to 6 months. Only about one in ten patients, however, will have complete return of normal use of the extremity.

## BRACHIAL PLEXUS INJURIES

Injuries of the brachial plexus are uncommon and often severe. They are usually caused by motorcycle accidents. Both traction and compression of the plexus may occur anywhere along its course.

The diagnosis is sometimes delayed because the patient commonly has other serious injuries, often to the head and chest. Eventually it is noted that the arm is completely paralyzed and hangs loosely from the shoulder. It may be completely anesthetic except for the small area on the inner aspect of the upper portion of the arm that is innervated by T2. Severe pain is common. If the site of injury is close to the spinal cord, Horner's syndrome may be present. This usually implies a poor prognosis.

The initial treatment is always conservative for the first several weeks. Range-of-motion exercises are begun to prevent joint stiffness. During this time the patient is observed for spontaneous recovery. If this occurs, the prognosis is often favorable. If it does not occur, the patient should be evaluated to determine whether a reparable lesion is present. Myelography and electromyography can be helpful in this regard. If the myelogram shows the presence of several traction meningoceles or dye pockets, this indicates that the nerve roots have been avulsed from the cord. This suggests that the injury is probably complete and not reparable and that the prognosis is poor. This status is also suggested by the absence of any appropriate electromyographic activity.

If results of the myelogram are normal and there is some potential for recovery suggested, early surgery with microscopic assistance may be beneficial. Neurolysis and nerve repair may then be performed. Some improvement can be expected after the surgery.

The patient with irreversible lesions is faced with a difficult decision. The extremity is now anesthetic, flail, often painful, and frequently in the way during normal activities. Amputation above the elbow is usually recommended about 1 year after the injury. Prostheses may be tried, but these are often discarded. Amputation should not be expected to relieve pain, however. Most patients are able to adapt to being one-handed.

## BIBLIOGRAPHY

Aston JW: Brachial plexus palsy, *Orthopedics* 2:594, 1979.

Britt LP: Nonoperative treatment of thoracic outlet syndrome symptoms, *Clin Orthop* 51:45, 1967.

Burge P, Rushworth G, Watson N: Patterns of injury to the terminal branches of the brachial plexus: the place for early exploration, *J Bone Joint Surg Br* 67:630, 1985.

Derkash RS et al: The results of first rib resection in thoracic outlet syndrome, *Orthopedics* 4:1025, 1981.

Dunkerton MC: Posterior dislocation of the shoulder associated with obstetric brachial palsy, *J Bone Joint Surg Br* 71:764, 1989.

Eng GD: Brachial plexus palsy in newborn infants, *Pediatrics* 48:18, 1971.

Fechter JD, Kuschner SH: The thoracic outlet syndrome, *Orthopedics* 16:1243-1251, 1993.

Ferguson AB Jr: *Orthopaedic surgery in infancy and childhood*, ed 3, Baltimore, 1968, Williams & Wilkins.

Grant JCB: *A method of anatomy*, ed 6, Baltimore, 1958, Williams & Wilkins.

Hardy AE: Birth injuries of the brachial plexus: incidence and prognosis, *J Bone Joint Surg Br* 63:98, 1981.

Jackson ST, Hoffer MM, Parish N: Brachial plexus palsy in the newborn, *J Bone Joint Surg Am* 70:1217, 1989.

Leffert RD: Thoracic outlet syndrome, *J Am Acad Orthop Surg* 2:317-325, 1994.

Michelow BJ et al: The natural history of obstetrical brachial plexus palsy, *Plast Reconstr Surg* 93:675-681, 1994.

Nichols HM: Anatomic structures of the thoracic outlet, *Clin Orthop* 51:17, 1967.

Oates SD, Daley RA: Thoracic outlet syndrome, *Hand Clin* 12:705-718, 1996.

Omer GE Jr, Spinner M: *Management of peripheral nerve problems*, Philadelphia, 1980, WB Saunders.

Ransford AO, Hughes SPF: Complete brachial plexus injuries: a ten-year follow-up of twenty cases, *J Bone Joint Surg Br* 59:417, 1977.

Roos DB: The thoracic outlet syndrome is underrated, *Arch Neurol* 47:327-328, 1990.

Roos DB: Thoracic outlet syndromes: update 1987, *Am J Surg* 154:568-573, 1987.

Rorabeck CH, Harris WR: Factors affecting the prognosis of brachial plexus injuries, *J Bone Joint Surg Br* 63:404, 1981.

Sedal L: The results of surgical repair of brachial plexus injuries, *J Bone Joint Surg Br* 64:54, 1982.

Tachdjian MO: *Pediatric orthopedics*, Philadelphia, 1972, WB Saunders.

Telford ED, Mottershead S: Pressure at the cervicobrachial junction: an operative and anatomical study, *J Bone Joint Surg Br* 30:249, 1948.

Travlos J, Goldberg I, Boome RS: Brachial plexus lesions associated with dislocated shoulders, *J Bone Joint Surg Br* 72:68, 1990.

Waters PW: Obstetric brachial plexus injuries: evaluation and management, *J Am Acad Orthop Surg* 5:205-214, 1997.

Wickstrom J: Birth injuries of the brachial plexus: treatment of defects of the shoulder, *Clin Orthop* 23:187, 1962.

Wilburn AJ: The thoracic outlet syndrome is overdiagnosed, *Arch Neurol* 47:328-330, 1990.

# CHAPTER 5

# The Shoulder

The shoulder is a complex series of joints that provides an extraordinary range of motion. This extreme mobility is accomplished at the expense of some stability, however. This lack of stability, combined with its relatively exposed position, makes the shoulder vulnerable to injury and degenerative processes.

## ANATOMY

The shoulder is composed of three bones: the scapula, the clavicle, and the humerus. The scapula is a thin bone that articulates widely and closely with the posterior chest wall. It also articulates with the humerus by way of a small, shallow glenoid cavity and with the clavicle at the acromion process. The clavicle and scapula are suspended from the cervical and thoracic vertebrae by the trapezium, levator scapulae, and rhomboid muscles.

Four articulations constitute the shoulder joint: the glenohumeral, scapulothoracic, acromioclavicular, and sternoclavicular joints. The stability of these joints is provided by a series of ligaments and muscles (Fig. 5-1).

Motion of the arm results from the coordinated efforts of several muscles. With the initiation of shoulder motion, the scapula is first stabilized. The muscles of the rotator (musculotendinous) cuff then steady the humeral head in the glenoid cavity and cause it to descend (Fig. 5-2). Elevation of the arm results from a combination of scapulothoracic and glenohumeral joint movements. One third of total shoulder abduction is provided by forward and lateral movement of the scapula. The remaining two thirds occurs at the glenohumeral joint through progressively increasing activity of the deltoid and supraspinatus muscles. Thus even in the complete absence of glenohumeral motion, scapulothoracic movement can still abduct the arm approximately 60 to 70 degrees.

The muscles of the rotator cuff (supraspinatus, teres minor, infraspinatus, and subscapularis) are separated from the overlying "coracoacromial arch" by two bursae, the subdeltoid and the subcoracoid (Fig. 5-3). These bursae often communicate and are affected by lesions of the musculotendinous cuff, acromioclavicular joint, and adjacent structures. They are often referred to as the subacromial bursae. Primary diseases of this bursa are rare, although secondary involvement is quite common.

## EXAMINATION

The examination is performed with both shoulders widely exposed (Fig. 5-4). The general contour of the shoulder is noted, as well as any atrophy or swelling. The shoulder is thoroughly palpated, and any areas of tenderness are determined. These are often located over the acromioclavicular joint and the rotator cuff.

Active and passive ranges of motion are tested and compared with those of the opposite arm. The examiner should determine whether the scapula and humerus move together or independently. Any crepitus during the examination is also noted. Active motion is measured in abduction, forward flexion, and extension. External and internal rotation can be measured by instructing the patient to reach behind the head and then backward behind the shoulder blades. Involvement of the acromioclavicular joint is tested by directing the patient to adduct the arm across the front of the chest and touch the opposite shoulder (Fig. 5-5). Pain with this test suggests acromioclavicular or sternoclavicular disease. The strength of the shoulder, especially at 90 degrees of forward flexion and then at 90 degrees of abduction, is tested and compared with the opposite arm.

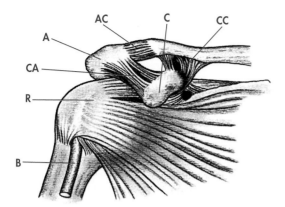

**Fig. 5–1.**
Bones and ligaments of the shoulder. *R* = rotator cuff; *B* = long head of the biceps; *AC* = acromioclavicular joint capsule; *CC* = coracoclavicular ligaments; *A* = acromion; *C* = coracoid process; *CA* = coracoacromial ligaments.

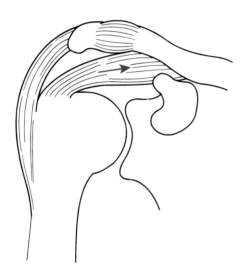

**Fig. 5–2.**
Abduction of the shoulder. By stabilizing the humeral head in the glenoid *(arrow)*, the superior portion of the rotator cuff prevents it from being forced into the acromion by the deltoid muscle.

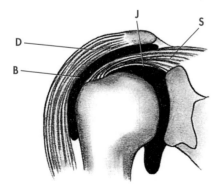

**Fig. 5–3.**
The subacromial bursa *(B)* is shown between the deltoid *(D)* and supraspinatus *(S)* muscles. Deep to the rotator cuff is the glenohumeral joint cavity *(J)*.

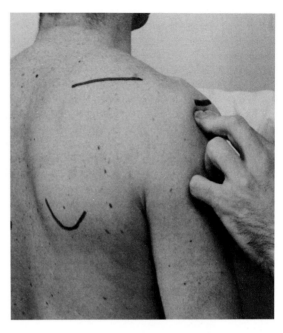

**Fig. 5–4.**
Superficial landmarks of the shoulder. The spine of the scapula lies at the level of the third dorsal vertebra. The inferior angle lies at the level of the seventh rib and eighth dorsal vertebra. The rotator cuff is palpated just distal to the acromion process.

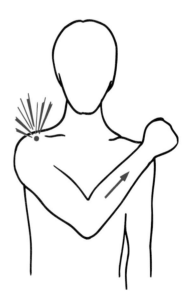

**Fig. 5–5.**
The crossover maneuver. Testing for acromioclavicular pain by having the patient touch behind the opposite shoulder *(arrow)*. Local AC tenderness may also be present.

## ROENTGENOGRAPHIC ANATOMY

The shoulder is routinely examined by anteroposterior views with the arm rotated externally and internally (Fig. 5-6). A lateral view may be obtained by utilizing a transaxillary or transthoracic exposure. The scapular "Y"

view is helpful in evaluating abnormalities of the acromion that could be associated with rotator cuff conditions. It is also valuable in determining if the humeral head is dislocated or not.

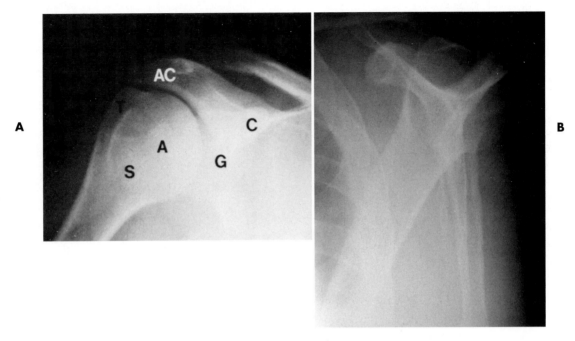

**Fig. 5–6.**
Roentgenographic anatomy of the shoulder: **A,** The AP view. *S* = surgical neck of the humerus; *A* = anatomic neck of the humerus; *T* = greater tuberosity; *C* = coracoid process; *AC* = acromion process; *G* = glenoid fossa. **B,** The scapular Y view. The humeral head should be centered at the intersection of the coracoid, spine, and body.

## DISORDERS OF THE ROTATOR CUFF

The tendons of the rotator cuff muscles fuse together near their insertions into the tuberosities of the humerus to form a musculotendinous cuff. Degeneration of these tendons probably is the result of many factors. Repetitive microtrauma, impairment in cuff vascularity as a result of age, shoulder instability with secondary overload of the cuff and an abnormally downward shaped acromion all may play a role. Degeneration is most severe near the tendon insertion. The supraspinatus is affected most. Secondary changes in the form of thickening and chronic inflammation often develop in the overlying bursa. With abduction, the tendon and bursa may impinge against the coracoacromial arch, causing further irritation. Many authors agree that the rotator cuff is the source of the majority of all shoulder pain and that the throwing motion or "overhead" work is often the cause. (Overhead work is work performed above shoulder height.)

A spectrum of disorders may affect the rotator cuff, and some difficulty may be encountered in diagnosing them. Tendinitis, complete and incomplete rotator cuff ruptures, and calcific deposits are all capable of producing similar signs and symptoms. A variety of terms have been developed to describe these diseases: supraspinatus syndrome, chronic impingement syndrome, painful arc syndrome, and internal derangement of the subacromial joint. The treatment for all of these lesions tends to be similar except that for complete rupture of the capsular rotator muscles, which causes loss of motor function. Surgical repair is sometimes necessary for this lesion.

### Tendinitis

At any age, a chronic irritation of the musculotendinous unit may develop. Repetitive use may even produce small tears in the rotator cuff of the young athlete or laborer. Scarring and thickening of the involved area of tendon occurs with secondary inflammation of the overlying bursa. Thickening of all of these tissues decreases the distance between the cuff and the overlying coracoacromial arch. Pain and crepitus ("impingement") may be noted when motions of the arm (especially abduction) squeeze and pinch these tissues between the humerus and the overlying arch. Impingement may also develop because the cuff doesn't function effectively and the humeral head is pulled upward with deltoid contraction even if the cuff is intact.

### Clinical Features

The major clinical manifestations are pain, especially at night; tenderness; and, occasionally, atrophy. The patient is often unable to lie on the affected shoulder, and may feel a locking sensation with certain motions (especially abduction). The pain is often referred to the deltoid region. When abducting the shoulder, the patient will often automatically turn the palm up, thereby externally rotating the shoulder. This maneuver gives the rotator cuff more room beneath the coracoacromial arch. Active, palm-down abduction is often painful. Forced passive elevation of the arm may cause the supraspinatus to impinge against the acromion, producing pain. Pain may also be reproduced by internal rotation and forward flexion (Fig. 5-7).

Maximum tenderness is usually noted over the supraspinatus insertion because this is the most common area of involvement. The acromioclavicular joint may also be tender because of degenerative arthritis, which is often present as well. There is usually little loss of muscle power. The pain and crepitus are most severe in the arc of motion between 60 and 120 degrees of abduction. This is where the traumatized soft tissues are maximally compressed between the tuberosity and the overlying arch. The roentgenogram is usually normal, but some sclerosis may be present in the tuberosity secondary to long-standing local inflammation.

### Treatment

1. Relief of pain and restoration of function are the therapeutic goals. An important part of the treatment program is rest. This allows the inflammatory process to subside, relieves pain, and restores function. Rest should not be complete, however, because stiffness is prone to develop in the shoulder joint, especially in the older patient. Simply avoiding excessive use of the arm may constitute sufficient rest, but occasionally a sling is needed temporarily. The patient should avoid all "overhead" work until pain-free.
2. Antiinflammatory medication is usually helpful.
3. Moist heat or other counterirritants are used several times each day.
4. Local steroid injections often dramatically relieve pain and swelling but should be used with caution, especially in the young patient: 1 to 2 mL of steroid mixed with 2 to 3 mL of lidocaine is injected, under sterile conditions, into the subacromial space (Fig. 5-8). The injection may be repeated two or three times every 3 weeks.
5. Function is restored by a careful, gentle exercise program directed at preserving muscle tone and preventing stiffness (Fig. 5-9). Pendulum exercises are begun early but are performed only within the limits of pain. As pain subsides, the exercises are increased, and further range-of-motion exercises are added. Work

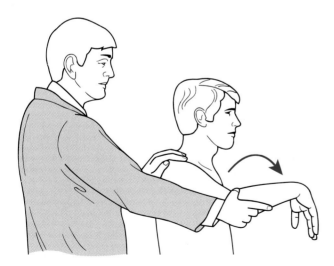

**Fig. 5–7.**
The impingement sign. Forced internal rotation of the abducted, slightly flexed arm may impinge the supraspinatus tendon against the coracoacromial ligament.

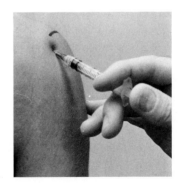

**Fig. 5–8.**
Injection of the rotator cuff and bursa. A slightly posterior approach is often best because there is more room. The needle is angled slightly upward and placed in the sulcus between the head of the humerus and the acromion *(marked)*. It should be able to be inserted completely, and, if the needle tip is properly positioned, the fluid should flow easily without resistance. If not, the needle should be repositioned.

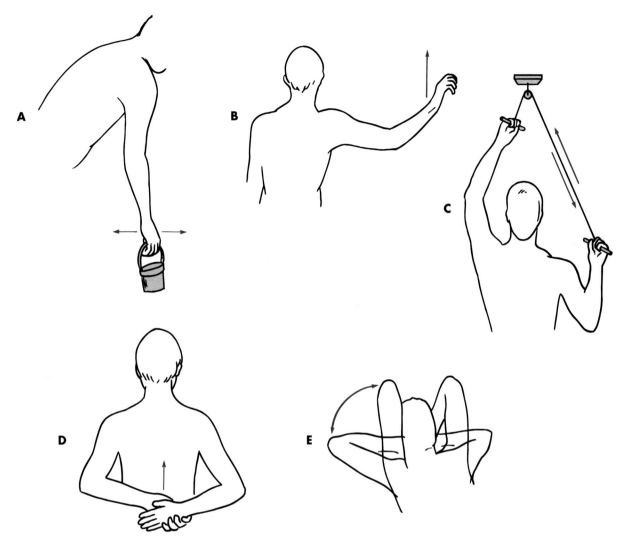

**Fig. 5–9.**
Shoulder stretching exercises. **A,** Pendulum exercises. **B,** Wall-climbing exercise. **C,** Rope and pulley exercises. The normal arm assists in the elevation of the stiffened arm. **D,** Exercise for restoring internal rotation. **E,** Exercise for restoring external rotation. Each exercise should be performed hourly or at least four times a day. Applying moist heat before the exercise may be helpful. In addition, activities that aggravate the pain, such as overhead work, should be avoided. For sitting work, a chair that supports the arms and shoulders should be used, and the patient should sit as close to the working surface as possible.

habits and other activities that cause compression and pinching of the inflamed tissue should be avoided. If needed, a sling may initially be worn between the exercises to rest the shoulder, but this is gradually discontinued as the exercise is increased.

Improvement is usually seen within 3 to 5 weeks (Fig. 5-10). If it is not, a more serious cuff lesion such as a rupture should be suspected. Surgery is reserved for those cases that fail to respond to conservative treatment. It consists of partial excision of the acromion to provide more space and remove osteophytes, release of obstructing soft tissue, and repair of any rotator cuff tears.

## Ruptures of the Rotator Cuff

Ruptures of the rotator cuff result from continued deterioration and degeneration (Fig. 5-11). The tear may be partial or complete. Ruptures are uncommon before the age of 40 years, although they may occur in the young athlete.

### Clinical Features

Obtaining a history sometimes reveals a fall on the outstretched hand or an attempt at lifting a heavy object, but usually there is no obvious injury. The pain may become progressively worse and the patient will note an inability to abduct or flex the shoulder, depending on

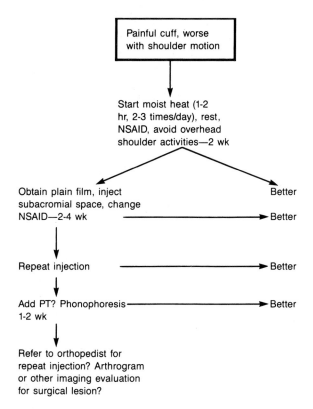

Painful cuff, worse
with shoulder motion

↓

Start moist heat (1-2
hr, 2-3 times/day), rest,
NSAID, avoid overhead
shoulder activities—2 wk

Obtain plain film, inject
subacromial space, change
NSAID—2-4 wk ————————————→ Better

Better

Repeat injection ————————————→ Better

↓

Add PT? Phonophoresis————————→ Better
1-2 wk

↓

Refer to orthopedist for
repeat injection? Arthrogram
or other imaging evaluation
for surgical lesion?

**Fig. 5–10.**
Algorithm for rotator cuff inflammation.

**Notes:**
1. Night pain is common with cuff tendinitis.
2. No trauma—always consider METS.
3. Bone scans are often abnormal in tendinitis and reflect the local increased bone circulation caused by the adjacent soft-tissue inflammation.

the area of the tear. The pain is often referred down the deltoid muscle. Occasionally the patient may have had previous impingement pain, and the diagnosis is often considered when the patient fails to respond to the usual treatment for tendinitis.

If the rupture is partial, the clinical findings are similar to those seen in chronic tendinitis. Even with complete rupture, the shoulder may have a full range of motion because of continued function of the other rotator muscles. With both partial and complete ruptures, however, there is usually at least some weakness in abduction or flexion. The weakness is usually most severe in abduction because the muscle most commonly torn is the supraspinatus. If the tear is more anterior into the subscapularis, forward flexion will be weak. It may be impossible to actively abduct the arm more than 45 to 50 degrees, after which further abduction is obtained by scapulothoracic motion. A painful "catch" may be noted on passive motion between 50 and 100 degrees, where compression of the swollen tissues between the tuberosity and the overlying arch occurs. Tenderness at the site of the tear is a common finding, and with complete ruptures a defect in the cuff may be palpated through the deltoid muscle. Passive range of motion is often normal in the pain-free shoulder although there is usually a positive impingement sign. With some com-

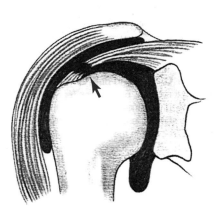

**Fig. 5–11.**
Rupture of the rotator cuff *(arrow)*. Full thickness rupture allows joint fluid to escape from the glenohumeral joint into the subacromial region. This is often an MRI clue to a full thickness tear.

plete tears, the patient can only "shrug" the shoulder and may have to use the opposite hand to raise the arm any further.

Atrophy of the cuff muscles is often present, and the "drop-arm" test may be positive. In this test, the arm is passively abducted to 90 degrees with the thumb pointing down, and then released. If the shoulder can maintain abduction, slight downward pressure is applied to

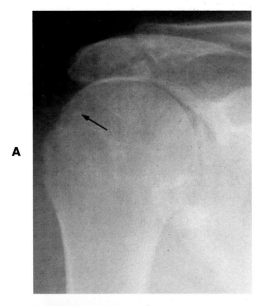

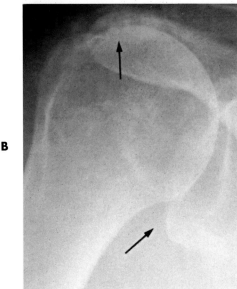

**Fig. 5–12.**
**A,** Cystic changes and sclerosis *(arrow)* often seen in the humeral head in chronic rotator cuff disorders. **B,** Proximal migration of the humeral head is occasionally seen in rotator cuff tears *(arrows)*. This occurs because the cuff can no longer stabilize the head in the glenoid. The deltoid, acting alone in abduction, pulls the head proximally. Some limited abduction can then be achieved by a fulcrum effect with the head stabilized against the underneath side of the acromion. After the head migrates upward, subacromial injection is more difficult because little space remains for needle insertion.

the forearm, and the strength of the affected shoulder is compared with the normal shoulder. If pain is severe during the examination, lidocaine infiltration of the tender area can relieve the pain. The strength is then measured again. Inability to maintain shoulder abduction with this test is suggestive of a rotator cuff tear.

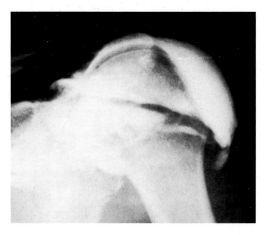

**Fig. 5–13.**
Arthrography of the shoulder reveals dye leakage through the rotator cuff into the subacromial bursa; this indicates a complete rupture.

Acute hemarthrosis and prominent ecchymosis down the arm may occasionally accompany long-standing rotator cuff tears, especially those with cuff-tear arthropathy (a term used to describe end stage rotator cuff disease as a result of a large defect with additional humeral head roughening and glenohumeral joint changes). This is probably the result of further rupture with bleeding of remaining rotator cuff musculature.

Chronic subdeltoid swelling usually means synovial fluid has escaped from the glenohumeral joint to the subacromial space and indicates a large rotator cuff rupture. The entire deltoid may appear grossly enlarged as a result of the underlying swelling.

### Special Studies

In patients who have shoulder pain that clearly originates in the shoulder, it may be difficult to differentiate tendinitis from partial or complete rotator cuff tears on a clinical basis.

Roentgenographic evaluation may be of assistance:

1. Plain films should be obtained within the first few weeks of symptoms although they may not be necessary on the first visit. They are often indicated simply because of the nonspecific nature of rotator cuff symptoms and to rule out other obvious causes of shoulder pain. The examination may reveal chronic changes in the tuberosity of the humerus or calcific deposits (Fig. 5-12). Degenerative arthritis may also be present in the acromioclavicular or glenohumeral joint.

2. Arthrography of the shoulder may help distinguish between complete and incomplete tears (Fig. 5-13). Its main drawback is its invasive nature. It should probably only be performed if there has been serious discussion regarding surgery.

3. Ultrasonography has some popularity in the evaluation of the rotator cuff. It is safe and noninvasive and is most accurate in large and moderately large tears.
4. Magnetic resonance imaging (MRI) now plays a major role in diagnosing rotator cuff disease. It can diagnose if a tear is present, and may help determine whether the tear is reparable or not reparable because of the amount of separation and atrophy.

### Treatment

Partial tears or small, complete tears may respond to the conservative treatment program outlined for chronic tendinitis. Occasionally it is necessary to surgically repair the rupture and remove any impinging structures beneath the coracoacromial arch.

Complete tears may also need repair if they are sufficiently disabling. Occasionally, however, there is little loss of function and minimal pain. Operative intervention is probably not justified in these patients, especially if they are relatively inactive.

## Calcific Deposits in the Rotator Cuff

Calcium deposits in the rotator cuff tendon may be associated with pain and stiffness in the shoulder. These deposits probably result from degenerative changes in the same area where ruptures take place and are most often found in the supraspinatus tendon. Most of them remain small and deep in the tendon, and pain may be absent. Others produce an inflammatory reaction and swelling, perhaps as the process of resorption takes place. Impingement of these swollen tissues on the overlying coracoacromial arch may increase the inflammation and pain.

### Clinical Features

Symptoms may have gradual or acute onset, and are similar to simple tendinitis. The pain is characteristically severe and accentuated by the slightest motion. Night pain and an inability to sleep on the shoulder are common complaints. The pain may radiate to the deltoid and even down the arm and forearm.

Examination in the acute stage reveals markedly limited motion and exquisite tenderness over the bursa and calcific deposit.

The symptoms and signs in chronic cases are less pronounced. Shoulder motion is often normal. However, symptoms of intermittent impingement and tenderness of the rotator cuff may be present.

Roentgenographic examination in internal and external rotation will usually reveal the deposit (Fig. 5-14). If the deposit is either anterior in the subscapularis mus-

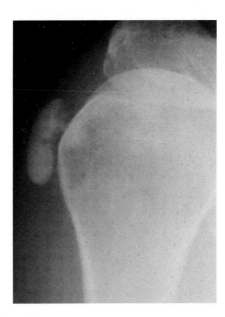

**Fig. 5–14.**
Large calcific deposit in the rotator cuff.

cle, or posterior, a transaxillary view may be necessary to demonstrate it.

### Treatment

Treatment is directed at relief of the inflammation. A subacromial injection of 1 mL of steroid mixed with 4 to 5 mL of lidocaine will often give dramatic relief. If the deposit appears soft, fluffy, and irregular on roentgenographic examination, aspiration and needling of the deposit may also be indicated. However, if the deposit is dense, round, and well circumscribed, this procedure is less helpful.

Aspiration and needling are performed under local anesthesia. A syringe with an 18-gauge needle is partially filled with lidocaine and inserted directly into the deposit. Multiple areas are then injected and aspirated. A fine, flaky material may be withdrawn. The aspiration and needling are repeated over several areas until all accessible material is withdrawn. A second large needle placed in the calcific mass can be used for aspiration while the first needle is used for injection. At the end of the procedure, 2 mL of steroid is left in the bursa.

Analgesics and NSAIDs are given as necessary. Warm, moist packs are applied to the shoulder. The arm is allowed to hang in a sling until the acute pain subsides, and pendulum exercises are then initiated within the limits of pain. Motion progresses as it can be tolerated.

Surgical excision of the calcific deposit is reserved for those rare cases that fail to respond to conservative treatment. The calcific material often resorbs on it own, however, and the tendon reconstitutes itself.

# DISORDERS OF THE BICEPS TENDON

## Tenosynovitis

Tenosynovitis of the long head of the biceps is a common cause of shoulder pain in adults over 40 years old. It may also occur in the young athlete from repeated strains, such as those caused by the throwing motion. The basic lesion is an inflammation in the tendon and its sheath in the bicipital groove. The disorder may be primary or secondary to disease of the overlying rotator cuff. It may be difficult to differentiate from rotator cuff inflammation.

### Clinical Features

The most common symptom is pain over the anterolateral aspect of the shoulder that may be referred down the anterior aspect of the arm. The most constant physical finding is tenderness to palpation over the bicipital groove. Active and passive shoulder motions are often restricted because of pain. Maneuvers that stretch the biceps tendon or cause it to glide in the groove may reproduce the pain. Forceful external rotation with abduction or backward flexion with the elbow extended is often painful. Supination against resistance with the elbow flexed is also commonly uncomfortable (Fig. 5-15). The roentgenograms are usually normal.

### Treatment

In the acute stage, treatment consists of rest, moist heat, and gentle range-of-motion exercises. All motions that stretch the biceps tendon should be avoided. A sling may be used temporarily. NSAIDs may be helpful, and local steroid injections into the tendon sheath are often beneficial (Fig. 5-16). The majority of cases respond well to conservative treatment. Surgery is recommended for those cases that fail to improve.

## Rupture of the Biceps Tendon

The long head of the biceps tendon may rupture as a result of advanced degeneration from chronic tendinitis. The rupture is usually complete and may follow a forceful contraction of the biceps muscle.

### Clinical Features

The onset is usually sudden. A sharp snap may be felt by the patient, followed by pain and weakness of the arm. The diagnosis is easily made by the observation of an abnormally large mass in the arm that represents the retracted muscle belly of the long head of the biceps (Fig. 5-17). There may be some loss of elbow flexion power.

### Treatment

No treatment is necessary in most cases. There is only minimal loss of function and usually little pain associated with rupture. Often, if the patient has had chronic anterior shoulder pain consistent with biceps tendinitis,

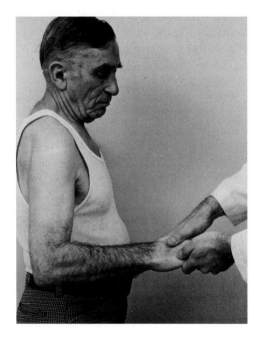

**Fig. 5–15.**
Yergason's test. The patient supinates the forearm against resistance. Pain in the region of the bicipital groove is suggestive of bicipital tenosynovitis.

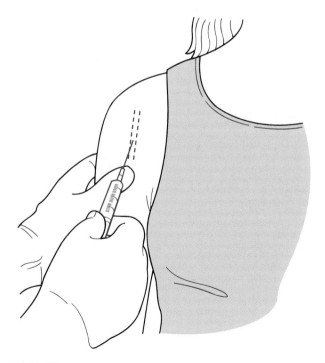

**Fig. 5–16.**
Injecting the bicipital groove. The elbow rests in the flexed position with the upper arm in neutral rotation. The biceps groove faces forward. The area of point tenderness is injected.

the pain may actually be relieved by the rupture. In the young patient, however, surgical repair of the rupture may be indicated.

## Subluxing Biceps Tendon

The biceps tendon may occasionally dislocate from the bicipital groove. The usual cause is a tear in the overlying subscapularis tendon as the result of degenerative changes, but the condition may result from a congenitally shallow groove. The disorder may also occur in the young patient on forceful external rotation and abduction of the shoulder. Recurrences are common and may

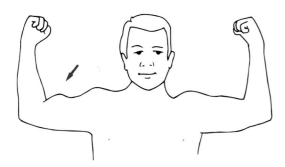

**Fig. 5–17.**
Rupture of the long head of the biceps. A localized bulge *(arrow)* that is more prominent when the elbow is flexed against resistance is present in the distal part of the biceps.

be reproducible by the patient (Fig. 5-18). Tenosynovitis often develops and leads to pain and stiffness.

The only cure for this lesion is anchoring the tendon in the bicipital groove surgically. The results are uniformly good.

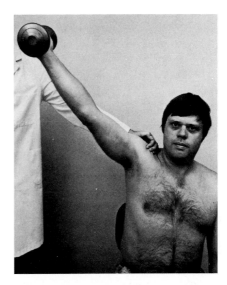

**Fig. 5–18.**
Test for a subluxing biceps tendon. With a weight in the hand, the arm is elevated and externally rotated. As the arm is slowly adducted from this position, a snap may be heard or felt in the bicipital groove.

# FROZEN SHOULDER (ADHESIVE CAPSULITIS)

Frozen shoulder is a disorder characterized by the insidious onset of pain and restriction of motion. The disease tends to be chronic, and full recovery may take several months. It is more common in women and diabetic patients, and it is also more recalcitrant in diabetic patients. The cause is unknown, but bicipital tenosynovitis, rotator cuff tendinitis, and reflex sympathetic dystrophy have all been blamed. It is often found in association with ischemic heart disease, thyroid disease, and lung disease. The term capsulitis is probably a misnomer because inflammation is not a constant finding.

### Clinical Features

The onset is usually gradual and begins in the fifth decade. The disorder may develop during a period of inactivity in the use of the extremity or after a relatively minor injury to the shoulder, but usually there is no precipitating event. Pain is a constant symptom but often does not occur until much of the shoulder motion has already been lost. It is usually well localized in the region of the rotator cuff and may radiate down the deltoid and anterior aspect of the arm. It often interferes with sleep, especially when the patient attempts to lie on the affected shoulder.

Examination reveals an apprehensive patient who holds the arm protectively at the side. Varying degrees of deltoid and spinatus atrophy may be noted. Generalized tenderness is present around the rotator cuff and biceps tendon. Active and passive shoulder motion is restricted to varying degrees, depending on the stage of the disease. The signs of reflex sympathetic dystrophy may be present in the involved extremity (edema of the hand, coolness, and discoloration).

Roentgenograms should always be performed. Although their findings are usually normal, a missed *posterior shoulder dislocation* should always be ruled out.

The course of the disease is variable. Some patients recover relatively early in the disorder, but in many cases the condition is progressive over several months. In these patients, shoulder motion gradually decreases and the pain subsides. As soon as the pain diminishes, the shoulder begins to regain its motion. Recovery is slow, and complete recovery in less than 6 months is rare. Most patients will eventually regain full motion of their shoulder, although some mild loss of motion and discomfort may persist for years.

### Treatment

The most important facet of treatment is prevention. Every attempt should be made to maintain motion in the shoulder during those periods when the patient may be inactive because of disease or injury. Once the disease process has begun, treatment is directed at the relief of pain, and restoration of motion. Moist heat, sedation, and analgesics are prescribed as necessary. A local injection of a steroid/lidocaine mixture into the subacromial space may also prove beneficial. Pendulum and overhead pulley exercises are begun as soon as possible and initially performed on an *hourly* basis.

The initial stage of pain followed by stiffness may last several months. The recovery, or "thawing" phase, may also last several months. Complete recovery is usually the case. Recurrence in the same shoulder is rare although the opposite limb may develop the same symptoms, sometimes months to years later. Most patients will eventually respond to a well-supervised program of physical therapy. Some will have mild permanent residual loss of motion but without any significant functional impairment. Those patients who fail to respond may benefit from careful manipulation of the shoulder under general anesthesia followed by aggressive range-of-motion exercises. Surgical intervention is rarely indicated.

## SNAPPING SCAPULA

Snapping scapula is an uncommon disorder in which an audible grating sound occurs with motion of the scapulothoracic joint. Normally, the serratus anterior and subscapularis muscles cushion the scapula from the underlying rib cage. The scapula is poorly protected at its medial border and at its superior and inferior angles, however. Abnormal angulations at these locations may cause pain and snapping sensations. Tumors of the scapula or ribs, bursae between these bones, and poor posture with sagging of the shoulder joint are other causes of crepitus in this area. Often no cause is found.

### Clinical Features

The onset is usually gradual, but the process is often precipitated by a traumatic event. The snapping is often palpable and painful. The origin of these noises can often be well localized by the patient to a specific area in the scapulothoracic articulation. Roentgenograms of the scapula, including oblique views, are obtained to discover such lesions as exostoses and tumors when they are present (Fig. 5-19).

### Treatment

If the roentgenograms are normal, physical therapy, rest, and local steroid injections will often relieve the pain. An exercise program is important. Correction of poor posture is also often beneficial. If the snapping is secondary to tumor or exostosis, and the pain and disability are sufficient to justify surgery, the involved area of the scapula is removed surgically.

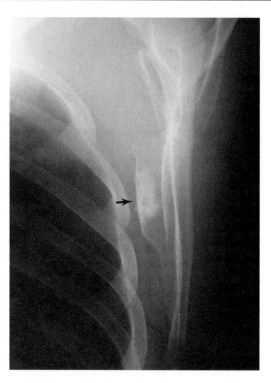

**Fig. 5–19.**
A "Y" view of the scapula revealing an osteochondroma *(arrow)* of the inner wall.

## DISTAL CLAVICLE OSTEOLYSIS

In this disorder, pain and tenderness develop at the AC joint, often in individuals who are weightlifters. The etiology is unknown but the condition may be related to microfractures that cause hyperemia, a destructive synovitis, and localized osteopenia.

Plain roentgenographic evaluation reveals loss of bone detail of the distal tip of the clavicle as a result of osteopenia (Fig. 5-20). Bone scanning is abnormal although the test is usually not required to establish the diagnosis.

Treatment is symptomatic. NSAIDs and heat are helpful. Weightlifting activities should be discontinued. Steroid injection into the AC joint is often helpful. Rarely, excision of the tip of the clavicle may be required.

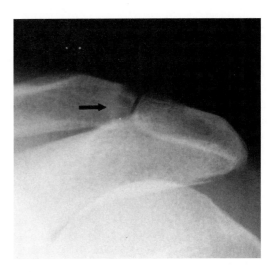

**Fig. 5–20.**
Distal clavicle osteolysis *(arrow)*.

## SERRATUS ANTERIOR PARALYSIS

The serratus anterior pulls the scapula forward, stabilizing it when pushing. Paralysis of the long thoracic nerve can lead to the characteristic winging, which is most obvious when the patient does a push-up against a wall (Fig. 5-21). The etiology may be direct trauma, but usually no cause is found.

Treatment is usually by observation and an exercise program to maintain strength. Many cases recover spontaneously, but full return of function may take 6 months to a year.

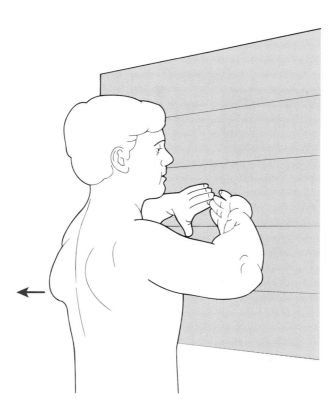

**Fig. 5–21.**
Winging of the scapula. Paralysis of the serratus anterior is most prominent when the patient pushes against the wall.

# GLENOHUMERAL DISLOCATION

Dislocations of the shoulder are most commonly *anterior* and usually result from a fall on the externally rotated, abducted arm (Fig. 5-22). This force levers the humerus out of the glenoid cavity into its anterior position.

*Posterior* dislocations are less common and may result from a force directed against the internally rotated arm. Many posterior dislocations occur at the time of a seizure in patients with convulsive disorders. Some individuals can reproduce a posterior dislocation *voluntarily* and use this maneuver to attract attention.

*Multidirectional instability* is a condition in which glenohumeral dislocation or subluxation can occur in multiple directions. The main abnormality is generalized excessive laxity of the joint capsule.

### Clinical Features

The diagnosis of dislocation is usually not difficult. Clinically, the acromion is much more prominent than normal, and there is an absence of the normal fullness of the humeral head beneath the deltoid and acromion process. Little movement of the shoulder is possible without severe pain. With anterior dislocations, the arm is held externally rotated, the anterior shoulder is full, and internal rotation is painful. In posterior dislocations, the arm is held in internal rotation with the forearm resting on the abdomen, the anterior portion of the shoulder is flat, and external rotation is painful (the arm is locked in internal rotation). The integrity of the neu-

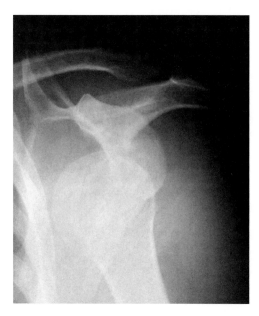

**Fig. 5–22.**
Anterior dislocation of the shoulder.

rovascular structures of the arm, especially the axillary nerve, should always be assessed. Numbness in the middle of the deltoid may be present.

The diagnosis of multidirectional instability may be difficult if dislocation has not occurred. The sulcus test is helpful. This test assesses inferior movement of the humeral head. With the patient standing and the arms hanging, the arms are pulled inferiorly. A sulcus will form between the acromion and humeral head in cases of multidirectional instability.

Roentgenographic evaluation is mandatory, but interpretation is sometimes difficult with *posterior* dislocations (Fig. 5-23). A "true" anteroposterior (AP) view of the shoulder may be helpful, and a lateral view of the glenohumeral joint is essential. A variety of lateral views may be performed (transscapular Y, transthoracic, transaxillary). Perhaps the easiest to perform and interpret is the *transaxillary* (Fig. 5-24).

### Treatment and Prognosis

Shoulder dislocations are usually reducible without general anesthesia if good muscular relaxation can be obtained. Intravenous sedation or analgesia is often helpful. Gentle, straight traction on the arm is usually sufficient to reduce both the anterior and posterior dislocation (Fig. 5-25). If straight traction does not reduce the dislocation, Stimson's method may be used for the anterior dislocation. The patient is placed in a prone position with the affected arm hanging over the side of the table. A 5- to 10-kg weight is tied to the wrist for traction. As the shoulder muscles relax, spontaneous reduction often occurs. If the shoulder remains dislocated, reduction under a general anesthetic is usually necessary. Open reduction is rarely required.

Primary dislocations in either direction in patients under the age of 30 years have a high rate of recurrence, often with little trauma. It had been theorized that prolonged immobilization for 3 to 4 weeks would encourage better capsular healing and prevent recurrent dislocation. It now appears that extended protection offers no benefit against recurrence and that the likelihood of recurrence is determined primarily by the age of the patient at the time of the injury, regardless of treatment. Patients under the age of 30 have a 50% recurrence rate irrespective of the type or length of immobilization after reduction. Thus after reduction, the arm is rested in a sling for 1 to 2 weeks and motion is gradually allowed as symptoms subside after the injury. Rehabilitative exercises are often helpful (Fig. 5-26). The patient is educated to avoid positions of known instability (usually external rotation and abduction with the common anterior dislocation). Recurrent dislocations in either direction usually require corrective surgery, and there is an almost 100% recurrence after the third dislocation.

Primary dislocations in patients over the age of 40 years are not generally complicated by recurrence but often result in shoulder joint stiffness. In this age group, light immobilization with a sling for a few days is all the treatment that is necessary. Active motion is then encouraged to prevent stiffness.

Occasionally, an old anterior dislocation is seen in the elderly patient. The length of time the shoulder has been dislocated may be impossible to determine.

Closed reduction may be attempted, but if the injury is more than 2 to 3 weeks old, enough soft-tissue healing will probably have occurred to make the procedure unsuccessful. If it fails, accepting the disability and working to improve motion may be the most logical treatment in this age group. In the young, open reduction or even arthroplasty will be needed.

Multidirectional instabilities can be difficult to diagnose, especially when only subluxation occurs. These instabilities are usually treated nonsurgically with strengthening exercises. Voluntary dislocators are always treated nonsurgically.

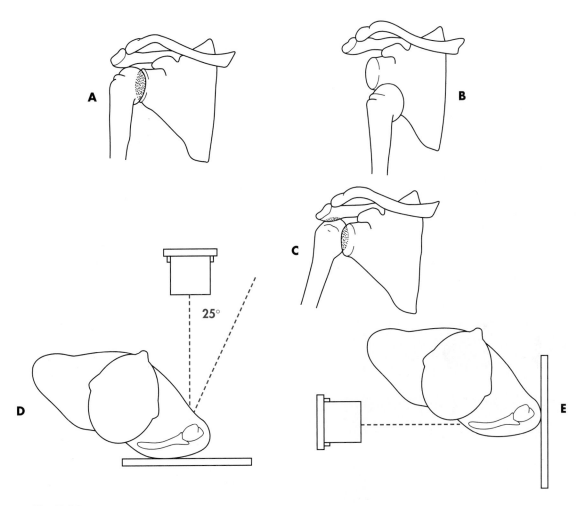

**Fig. 5–23.**
**A,** The "normal" AP roentgenographic anatomy of the glenohumeral joint. There is normally a 50% elliptical overlap or "half moon" of increased density where the humeral head overlaps the posterior glenoid rim. The anterior edge of the glenoid should parallel the medial border of the humeral head, and the distance between these two lines should not exceed 6 mm. **B,** Anterior dislocation, which is usually not a problem in diagnosis. **C,** Posterior dislocation. Up to 50% of these are missed initially. The humeral head barely overlaps the glenoid and may be higher or lower than normal. The greater tuberosity is usually internally rotated, and the area of overlap is abnormal. **D,** The "true" AP view of the glenohumeral joint is taken 25 degrees toward the midline. **E,** A true lateral (the scapular Y) view may be taken at a right angle to this film. (The Y is formed at the glenoid fossa where the bases of the coracoid and spine of the scapula join the distally projecting body.) The humeral head should be present at the intersection.

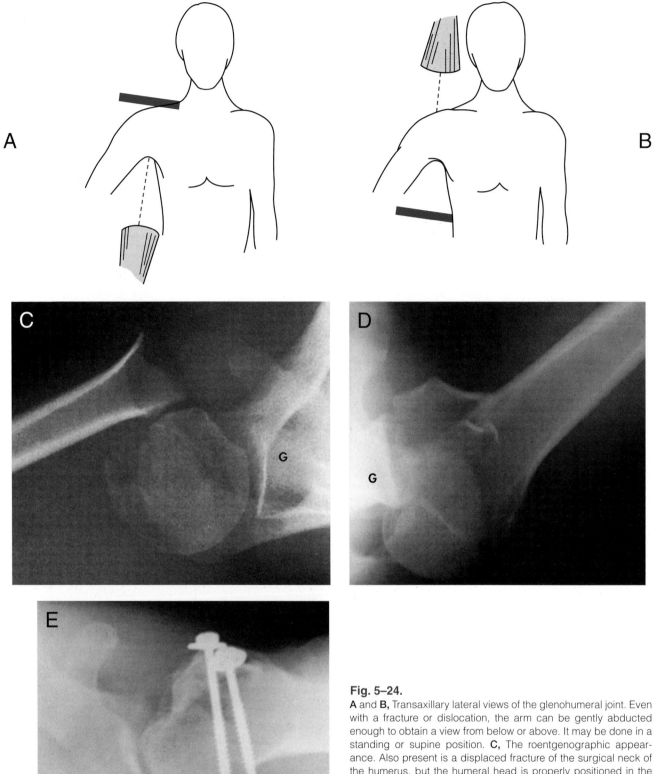

**Fig. 5–24.**
**A** and **B,** Transaxillary lateral views of the glenohumeral joint. Even with a fracture or dislocation, the arm can be gently abducted enough to obtain a view from below or above. It may be done in a standing or supine position. **C,** The roentgenographic appearance. Also present is a displaced fracture of the surgical neck of the humerus, but the humeral head is properly positioned in the glenoid *(G)*. **D,** A posterior fracture-dislocation. **E,** The injury in D is reduced and the fracture has been internally fixed.

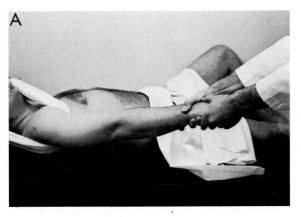

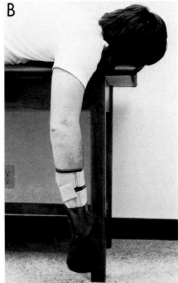

**Fig. 5–25.**
Reduction of shoulder dislocation. **A,** Straight traction is applied to the wrist with countertraction to the axilla. If straight traction fails, try pulling upward. **B,** Stimson's method for anterior dislocations. Kocher's maneuver is usually not necessary. Relaxation, explanation, and reassurance often help more than high doses of narcotics.

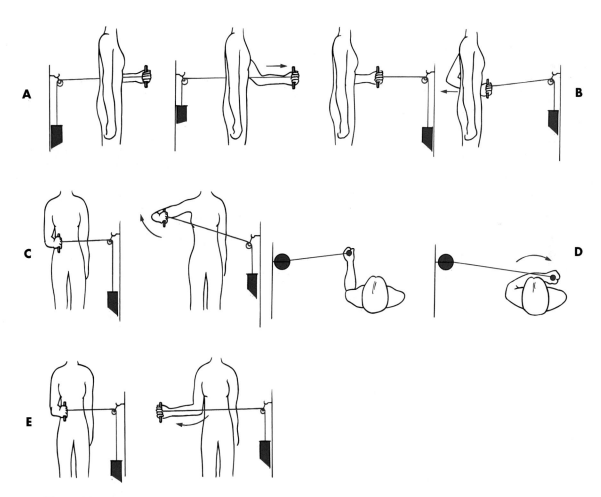

**Fig. 5–26.**
Exercises for shoulder strengthening after dislocations. These should be performed with the arm below shoulder level. A simple rope and pulley system is all that is needed, with the pulley being attached to the wall or stud with an eye bolt. Exercises are performed two or three times a day, and each is repeated 15 to 30 times beginning with a 2-kg weight and progressing to 10 kg. **A,** Flexion. **B,** Extension. **C,** Abduction. **D,** Internal rotation. **E,** External rotation.

# ACROMIOCLAVICULAR DISLOCATION

Acromioclavicular (AC) dislocations and "separations" usually occur as a result of a fall on the shoulder or a direct blow to the top of the shoulder. The acromion is driven away from the clavicle. They are graded I through V. Grade I is a simple AC contusion or strain. In grade II, there is rupture of the AC ligaments. Grade III includes the additional rupture of the coracoclavicular ligaments. The uncommon, severe grades IV and V involve more significant displacement, often with penetration through the overlying muscle. Grades I and II are sometimes called *incomplete*, and grades III through V called *complete* (Fig. 5-27).

### Clinical Features

These injuries are characterized by tenderness and swelling over the acromioclavicular joint. The outer clavicle is usually elevated in both complete and incomplete dislocations (Fig. 5-28). Downward traction on the arm may increase the deformity.

Complete dislocations may be differentiated from incomplete dislocations by an AP roentgenogram taken while the patient has a 10-kg weight hanging from each arm. (The patient should not *hold* the weights.) If complete rupture of the coracoclavicular ligaments has occurred, widening between the coracoid process and the clavicle will be present on the affected side (Fig. 5-29).

### Treatment

Usually no treatment is necessary for incomplete separations. A sling is used for a few days to minimize the pain, and active shoulder motion is begun when it can be tolerated. The outer end of the clavicle will remain prominent, but this is usually painless and does not interfere with function. If it does, the tip of the clavicle may be surgically removed at a later date. Complete acromioclavicular dislocations sometimes require surgical intervention with reduction of the dislocation and repair of the ruptured ligaments. But except for the rare grade IV and above, even these are not usually treated surgically.

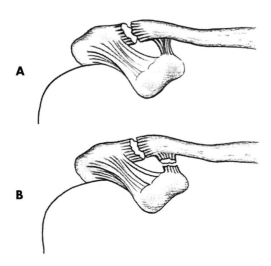

**Fig. 5-27.**
**A,** Incomplete dislocation of the acromioclavicular joint. The coracoclavicular ligaments are intact. **B,** Complete dislocation.

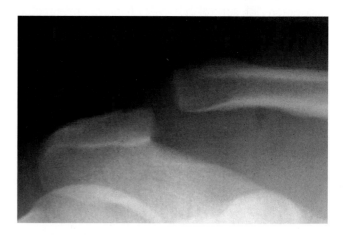

**Fig. 5–29.**
Complete acromioclavicular dislocation.

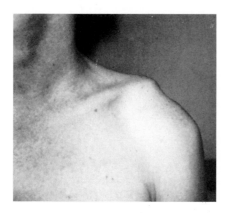

**Fig. 5–28.**
Clinical deformity with acromioclavicular dislocation.

## STERNOCLAVICULAR DISLOCATION

Sternoclavicular dislocations are uncommon injuries that occur as the result of a fall on the shoulder. The anterior dislocation is more common than the posterior dislocation. The rare posterior dislocation may cause pressure on the anterior structures of the neck and lead to dyspnea and vascular compression that may require immediate reduction.

The injury usually produces a tender, visible prominence at the sternoclavicular joint. Some discomfort with shoulder motion is usually present.

This is an area that is difficult to visualize roentgenographically. A view angled upward including the uninjured side may give some information. MRI may be required.

Anterior dislocations can be reduced by traction and manipulation, but the reduction is difficult to maintain. Recurrence after the reduction is common, but except for minor cosmetic deformity, no function is lost. Surgical intervention, therefore, is rarely justified in the acute case, and most injuries are simply treated with a sling.

*Spontaneous anterior sternoclavicular (SC) dislocation* may occasionally occur without any clear history of trauma. The patient may present with a relatively painless "mass," the enlargement being the sternal end of the clavicle. This is most commonly seen in the older adult. Reassurance is usually the only treatment, after routine examination and plain films.

In the child, an *epiphyseal fracture* can also occur in this area, sometimes causing confusion with an SC dislocation. Reduction may be obtained by manipulation but is difficult to maintain. Fortunately, some remodeling eventually occurs that will diminish the size of the fracture bump. Surgery would be required to keep the fracture reduced, but an unsightly scar usually results. As with SC dislocations, only nonsurgical management is needed.

## DEGENERATIVE ARTHRITIS

Degenerative arthritis of the glenohumeral joint is relatively uncommon. It is usually the end stage of chronic rheumatoid arthritis, avascular necrosis, or long-standing chronic rotator cuff disease (cuff-tear arthropathy) (Fig. 5-30). It may also result from recurrent shoulder dislocations or severe fractures of the shoulder joint. Chronic pain and limited shoulder motion are common, and atrophy and crepitus are often present.

Treatment is usually directed at providing symptomatic relief by injections, antiinflammatory medication, and stretching exercises. The surgical options are fusion, resection of the humeral head, and total joint replacement, but the search continues for the ideal surgical intervention.

The AC joint is a common site of osteoarthritis. Local tenderness is usually present, and the crossover maneuver is painful. Symptomatic treatment with NSAIDs and local injections of cortisone into the joint are helpful (Fig. 5-31). Distal clavicle resection is the surgical treatment of choice and offers a high success rate with low morbidity.

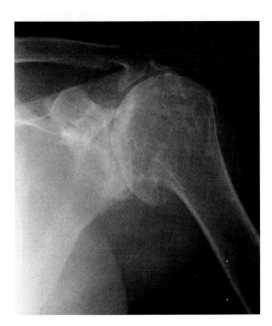

**Fig. 5–30.**
Osteoarthritis of the glenohumeral joint.

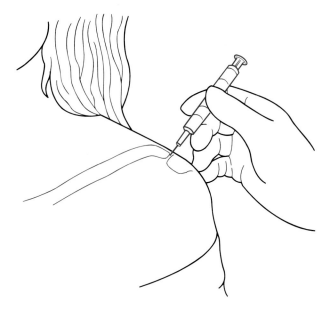

**Fig. 5–31.**
AC joint injection.

# FRACTURES OF THE SHOULDER REGION

## Fractures of the Clavicle

The clavicle is the only rigid, bony connection between the shoulder and the chest, and it functions to hold the shoulder upward and backward. It may be injured by a fall against the shoulder or on the outstretched hand (Fig. 5-32). Examination usually reveals a tender deformity. Some tenting of the skin may be present but the skin is rarely penetrated.

Historically, treatment has been directed at reduction with immobilization using either a canvas or plaster

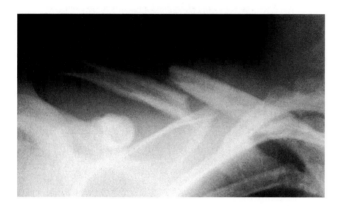

**Fig. 5–32.**
Fracture of the clavicle.

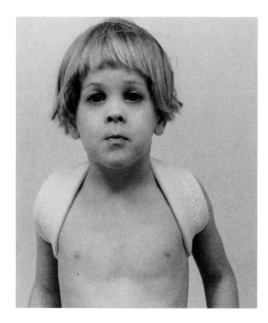

**Fig. 5–33.**
The clavicle fracture is immobilized by a figure-8 dressing. The dressing should remain snug and may have to be tightened.

figure-8 strapping system (Fig. 5-33). Reduction can sometimes be obtained by manipulation, but it is difficult to maintain and some element of overriding and overlap seem inevitable in most cases in spite of reduction. Pressure problems in the axilla sometimes occur with figure-8 bandages (discomfort, venous congestion, skin pressure, nerve dysfunction), which require frequent readjustment. As a result, the use of a simple sling has been studied as a treatment method and appears to be a safe and simple alternative treatment. If the figure-8 bandage is used, discomfort can be relieved by having the patient lie down and temporarily abduct the arms. The addition of a sling may also be helpful.

The fracture should be protected for 4 to 5 weeks in the child and 6 to 8 weeks in the adult. A prominence at the fracture site will often persist in the adult, but usually disappears in the child a few months after remodeling of the bone has occurred. Open reduction is never indicated in the child and only rarely in the adult (usually when fragments are markedly displaced). Nonunion is rare regardless of age. Fractures distal to the coracoclavicular ligament may be managed by a sling alone.

## Fractures of the Scapula

Fractures of the scapula usually result from a direct blow or fall (Fig. 5-34). Fractures that do not involve the articular surface of the glenoid cavity require little treatment. A sling or shoulder immobilizer may be used for 1 to 2 weeks until the pain subsides. Gentle motion of the shoulder is encouraged as soon as possible, and the results are usually excellent. The rare fracture that involves the shoulder articulation may require more extensive surgical treatment.

**Note**: A sling worn *under* a snug undershirt (to keep the arm against the body) is often more comfortable than the shoulder immobilizer.

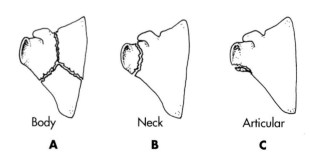

**Fig. 5–34.**
Various fractures of the scapula.

## Fractures of the Upper Portion of the Humerus

Minimally displaced or impacted fractures of the surgical neck of the humerus are common in elderly patients (Fig. 5-35). Slight degrees of malalignment should be accepted in this age group. Treatment consists of wearing a sling for 4 weeks. Pendulum exercises are performed in the sling after 2 weeks. All immobilization is discontinued after 4 weeks, and exercises are increased. A hanging cast should not be used in these fractures because it may disimpact the bony fragments. The disability in this injury results not from the fracture itself, which usually heals readily, but from the secondary stiffness that develops in the shoulder, especially in elderly patients. It is not uncommon for some permanent loss of abduction to result from this injury, and full range of motion may take several months to return.

Displaced fractures of the surgical neck may require manipulative reduction and a hanging long arm cast. If closed methods fail, open reduction is occasionally indicated.

Fractures of the tuberosities of the upper humerus may occur from a fall or in association with a shoulder dislocation (Fig. 5-36). Undisplaced fractures require only a sling for 7 to 10 days, followed by early range-of-motion exercises. Fractures that are displaced over 5 to 10 mm often require open reduction and internal fixation. If this is not performed, a bony impingement to abduction could result.

## Fractures of the Shaft of the Humerus

Fractures of the shaft of the humerus usually heal well with nonoperative treatment. The function of the radial nerve should always be evaluated because it may be injured in its course around the humeral shaft.

Manipulative reduction under local anesthesia may be required, but distraction of the fracture fragments should be avoided. With the patient sitting on a stool and leaning forward, the weight of the arm will often reduce the fracture (Fig. 5-37). The wrist is supported to overcome apprehension, but the elbow should hang free. Gentle traction and countertraction are applied, and the fracture fragments are manipulated to correct any angulation. End-to-end apposition is tested by upward pressure on the elbow. If no "telescoping" of the fracture fragments occurs, apposition is usually secure.

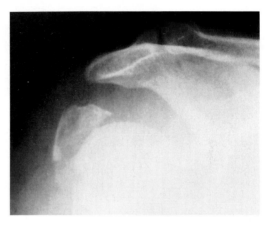

**Fig. 5–36.**
Displaced fracture of the greater tuberosity of the humerus.

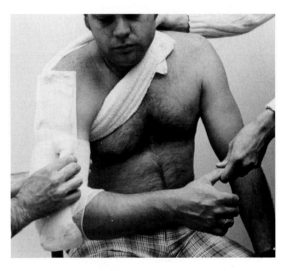

**Fig. 5–37.**
Fracture of the humerus reduced by downward traction and countertraction. A "sugar-tong" or U-shaped splint is then applied and wrapped with gauze or elastic bandage. The splint begins in the axilla and ends over the shoulder. It may have to be tightened at intervals. A collar and cuff or sling is added.

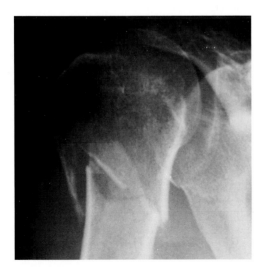

**Fig. 5–35.**
Fracture of the surgical neck of the humerus.

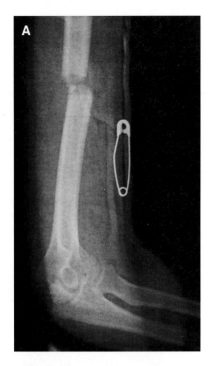
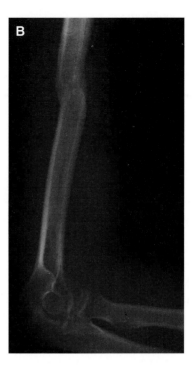

**Fig. 5–38.**
**A,** Transverse fracture of the humerus immobilized in a U-shaped splint. **B,** The end result.

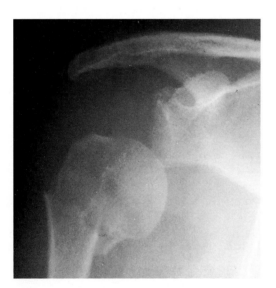

**Fig. 5–39.**
Inferior "subluxation" of the humeral head after a fracture of the upper humerus.

The fracture is immobilized by a cast brace or by the application of a U-shaped plaster splint (Fig. 5-38). Additional fixation may be obtained by strapping the humerus to the chest wall. Healing is usually complete by 8 to 10 weeks. (This form of fracture care requires frequent reevaluation and readjustment of the brace system.)

## Inferior Subluxation of the Humeral Head

Inferior displacement of the head of the humerus may occur as a result of the following: (1) fractures about the shoulder area (Fig. 5-39), (2) local neurogenic impairment such as brachial neuritis, and (3) strokes or other central nervous system (CNS) disorders.

The most common cause is "hypotonicity," which may develop in conjunction with fractures of the upper humerus or dislocations of the glenohumeral joint. When the musculoskeletal injury heals, muscle tone usually returns to normal, and the abnormal increase in acromiohumeral distance disappears. Simple strengthening and range-of-motion exercises after the injury has healed are the only necessary treatment.

If the subluxation is atraumatic, electromyography may be needed to determine whether a neurogenic disorder has developed.

## MEDICAL CAUSES OF SHOULDER PAIN

Shoulder pain may develop not only from primary disease of the neck and shoulder but also by referral from disorders of thoracic or abdominal origin. Care should be taken not to assume the patient's description of shoulder pain is from "arthritis." Visceral disorders must be borne in mind, especially when other causes of pain are not apparent.

### Abdominal Causes

Pain may be referred to the shoulder via the phrenic nerve. This pain may refer to any part of the shoulder but is most commonly on top of the shoulder, in the supraspinous fossa, or over the acromion or clavicle, that is, in the region of distribution of the cutaneous branches of the fourth cervical nerve. Lesions affecting a certain portion of the diaphragm may cause pain over the corresponding part of the shoulder on the same side of the body. In general, pain on top of both shoulders indicates a median diaphragmatic irritation. When the diaphragm is irritated by a neighboring lesion, such as blood from a ruptured spleen, tenderness may even be elicited by pressure on the corresponding phrenic nerve in the neck.

When a gastric or intestinal ulcer perforates, the escaping fluid may impinge on the lower surface of the diaphragm. This may irritate the terminations of the phrenic nerve on one or both sides and cause pain on top of one or both shoulders. Pain felt on top of both shoulders at the onset of the attack suggests that the perforation has occurred in the anterior portion of the stomach, causing irritation of the median portion of the diaphragm. In the case of pyloric duodenal ulcer, the shoulder pain is usually felt in the right supraspinous fossa or on the corresponding side.

Referred shoulder pain may also develop in cases of subphrenic abscess, diaphragmatic pleurisy, acute pancreatitis, gallstones, ruptured spleen, and appendicitis with peritonitis. It may be the only signal with a liver abscess that is threatening to perforate the diaphragm. Pelvic inflammatory disease with perihepatic inflammation (so-called Fitz-Hugh-Curtis syndrome) is also an occasional cause of shoulder pain.

In addition, a history of shoulder pain should be sought in all patients who have had serious abdominal trauma. Injury to solid viscera such as liver, spleen, pancreas, and kidney may result in hemorrhage, which in turn may cause diaphragmatic irritation and shoulder pain.

**Note**: In summary, although most shoulder pain is musculoskeletal in origin, it is important to be suspicious of abdominal causes of the pain. This is especially true if the pain is not aggravated by neck or shoulder movement and the patient has a history of gastrointestinal symptoms. In these cases, further studies and referral to a gastroenterologist may be indicated.

### Thoracic Causes

Although most disorders of intrathoracic origin will cause chest pain, shoulder discomfort is not uncommon and may be the main presenting complaint. Diseases of *cardiac* origin (such as pericarditis) commonly cause left arm and shoulder pain. Cardiac pain may also be referred to the neck, lower jaw, and interscapular area. The pain associated with ischemic disease is usually exertional but may occur at rest and cause more confusion. Clinically, there is usually no tenderness or aggravation of the pain by neck or shoulder motion.

*Pulmonary* diseases (such as carcinoma, pneumonia, and abscess) may also result in shoulder pain. Of special interest are tumors of the superior sulcus of the lung (Pancoast). This tumor produces a syndrome by virtue of its growth in the thoracic inlet. This region is bounded roughly by the first rib, the first costal cartilage, the manubrium, and the body of T1. The apex of the lung occupies most of the area. The superior pulmonary sulcus is a groove in the lung tissue made by the subclavian artery as it crosses the apex of the lung, and because the majority of apical lung tumors occur in relation to this sulcus, they are often called superior sulcus tumors. The structures in this area are the internal jugular and subclavian veins; the vagus, phrenic, and recurrent laryngeal nerves; the subclavian and common carotid arteries; the eighth cervical and first thoracic nerves; and the stellate ganglion and sympathetic chain. Any of these structures may be involved, and therefore the symptoms may be variable and complex. Pain is the most common initial complaint. Its distribution is often wide and unusual, commonly being present throughout the shoulder, scapular or infrascapular area, upper anterior portion of the chest, arm, neck, and axilla. Other components of this syndrome include Horner's syndrome, weakness and sensory disturbances on the involved side (possibly because of involvement of the lower portion of the brachial plexus), supraclavicular fullness, venous distension, and edema of the extremity. A superior sulcus tumor should always be kept in mind in patients with neck or shoulder pain, especially if there is a history of cigarette smoking. Shoulder roentgenograms may reveal the lesion, but usually a more complete roentgenographic examination is needed (Fig. 5-40).

Other diseases of thoracic origin that may cause shoulder pain are disorders of the mediastinum, aorta, and esophagus. The pain of hiatus hernia, in particular, can radiate to the top of both shoulders and down the arms.

## Miscellaneous Causes

*Malignant tumor*, either primary, locally spread, or metastatic from a distant origin, may also be the cause of shoulder pain. The diagnosis may be obvious in the patient with a known history of malignancy. The major sources are tumors of thyroid, prostate, breast, lung, and kidney, and Hodgkin's disease. The most common primary tumor that metastasizes to bone is multiple myeloma. The shoulder is less commonly involved than the ribs, spine, and pelvis. Pathologic fractures may occur but are uncommon in the upper extremity. Plain roentgenograms may be normal because more than 50% bone destruction is needed before destructive changes become apparent. Bone scanning is usually helpful, but myeloma and some aggressive sarcomas may destroy bone so fast that repair cannot occur, resulting in a false-negative study.

*Paget's disease* may also cause localized bone pain (see Chapter 18). As a result of periosteal bone formation impinging on cranial and spinal nerves, impairment of nerve function may even occur. Most patients with Paget's disease have minimal or no symptoms. The onset of increased pain in an area of Paget's disease should suggest sarcomatous degeneration.

*Shoulder-hand syndrome*, a form of reflex neurovascular dystrophy, is a poorly understood disorder (see Chapter 18). The disease is probably caused by reflex sympathetic stimulation analogous to that proposed for causalgia. The patients are usually above the age of 50 years and often have had a recent acute illness, often a myocardial infarction, cerebrovascular accident (CVA), pulmonary disorder, or minor musculoskeletal trauma. The patient develops pain, stiffness in the shoulder, and swelling and vasomotor phenom-

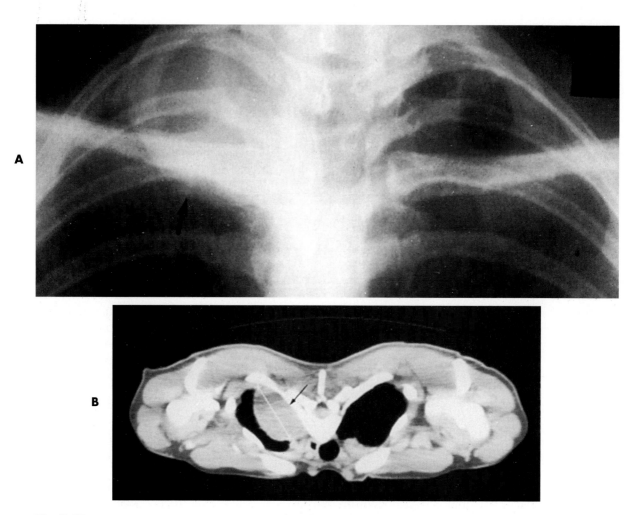

**Fig. 5–40.**
Pancoast tumor *(arrows)*. **A,** Plain film. **B,** Computed tomographic (CT) appearance.

ena in the involved extremity. There is a marked variability in the intensity of the pain, duration of acute symptoms, and extent of dystrophic change. A common complication is frozen shoulder. Treatment is nonspecific and includes: (1) an active exercise program facilitated by analgesics, (2) physical therapy, (3) a trial of a corticosteroid (prednisone, 10 to 20 mg/day) for a short time, and (4) stellate ganglion blocks if all other forms of medical management are unsuccessful. The condition will usually resolve on its own in the course of several months.

*Herpes zoster* ("shingles") is an acute viral infection that produces an inflammatory reaction in a segmental nerve. Initially, fever with unilateral pain and paresthesias may be present. In a few days, an erythematous rash appears that becomes vesicular. Early, before the rash develops, its symptoms may be confused with other painful disorders.

*Brachial neuritis* is an unusual disorder of unknown cause that can also be confused with other causes of shoulder pain or weakness, especially rotator cuff disease. Many terms have been used to describe this syndrome: shoulder-girdle syndrome of Parsonage and Turner, acute brachial radiculitis, neuralgic amyotrophy, and brachial plexus neuropathy. The cause is unknown, but a viral or allergic reaction is suspected. It is characterized by acute severe pain, usually in the shoulder but often in the arm and neck. The pain is often worse at night. Shoulder weakness follows the pain, usually within 1 month and sometimes as soon as 1 day. The pain is typically of short duration. The deltoid, rotator cuff, biceps, and triceps are commonly involved, and electromyography usually demonstrates changes of neurogenic atrophy. The prognosis is usually good, although recovery may take 2 to 3 years. Treatment is symptomatic.

*Carpal tunnel syndrome* (see Chapter 7) is a common cause of shoulder pain. Whereas the predominant symptoms occur in the hand, they are often accompanied by arm and shoulder pain. Carpal tunnel syndrome and cervical disc syndrome with radiculopathy also occasionally occur at the same time and involve the same extremity. This situation is called the "double-crush" syndrome. Under this circumstance, there may be two causes of shoulder pain, neither of which has its origin in the shoulder itself.

## DIFFERENTIAL DIAGNOSIS (TABLE 5-1)

**TABLE 5–1.**

Differential Diagnosis of Common Causes of Neck and/or Arm Pain* (see Fig. 5-41)

| Disorder | Most Common Pain Location or Radiation | Findings Present | Findings Absent |
|---|---|---|---|
| Cervical disc syndrome | Posterior neck, usually unilateral, intrascapular and trapezius pain. May radiate down one shoulder (if nerve root pressure), lateral arm, dorsoradial forearm to thumb, index, or long finger (see Fig. 5-41) | Pain aggravated by neck movement. Weak biceps or triceps. Paresthesias in forearm, hand. Trigger point in interscapular area | Symptoms not aggravated by shoulder motion. Usually no radicular symptoms on ulnar aspect of arm or hand |
| Rotator cuff syndrome | Acromion down to deltoid insertion (often worse at night) | Painful shoulder motion especially abduction, external rotation. Mild limitation of shoulder motion. Crepitus. Tender rotator cuff. Mild weakness | No interscapular pain or pain with neck motion. No paresthesias. Usually no symptoms below elbow |
| Bicipital tendinitis | Bicipital groove down anterior arm | Tender bicipital groove, pain on shoulder extension. Positive Yergason's test | No symptoms below elbow, no pain with neck motion, no neurologic symptoms |
| Pancoast tumor | Variable symptoms. Shoulder, plexus pain into arm | Supraclavicular tenderness. Horner's syndrome? Palpable mass. Pain with shoulder motion | Pain not increased with neck movement |
| Thoracic outlet syndrome | Shoulder, medial arm, forearm, and hand symptoms (C8, T1) | Ulnar (medial) paresthesias; signs of vascular compression? | No neck findings. Full, pain-free shoulder motion |

**\*Notes:** (1) Symptoms of *cervical strain* are usually bilateral and involve the neck and occiput. The symptoms are often diffuse, and the areas of soft-tissue tenderness often change. (2) *Acromioclavicular arthritis* has localized acromioclavicular pain and tenderness. (3) *Glenohumeral arthritis* presents with generalized shoulder pain and considerable loss of shoulder movement. (4) *Carpal tunnel syndrome* may cause shoulder aching, but the symptoms are mainly in the hand and forearm.

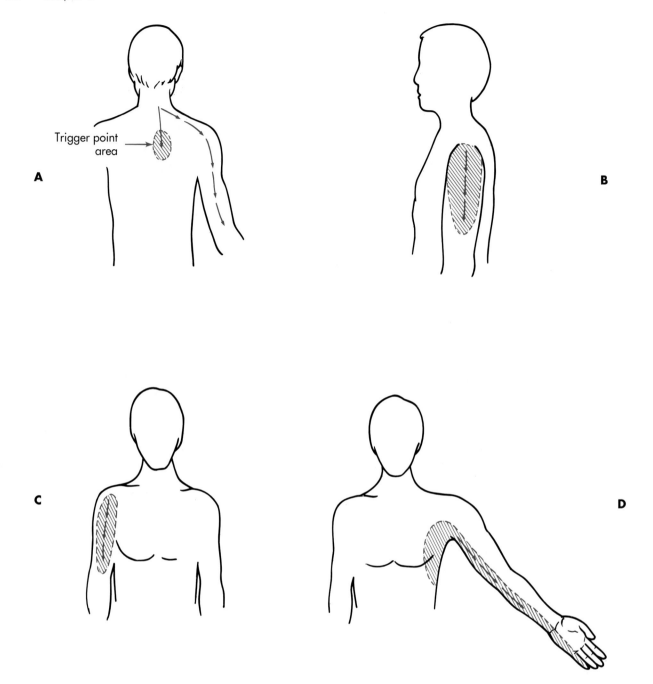

**Fig. 5–41.**
General pain distribution of common neck and arm disorders. **A,** Cervical disc syndrome. **B,** Rotator cuff syndrome. **C,** Bicipital tendinitis. **D,** Disorders involving the lower portion of the brachial plexus (Pancoast tumor, thoracic outlet syndrome). When the shoulder pain has a visceral origin, the patient sometimes recognizes it as "deep" and perhaps not arising in the exact region where it is felt.

## BIBLIOGRAPHY

Almekinders LC: Tendinitis and other chronic tendinopathies, *J Am Acad Orthop Surg* 6:157-164, 1998.

Andersen K, Jensen PO, Lauritzen J: Treatment of clavicular fractures: figure-8 bandages versus a simple sling, *Acta Orthop Scand* 57:71, 1987.

Arendt EA: Multidirectional shoulder instability, *Orthopedics* 11:113, 1988.

Balich SM, Sheley RC, Brown TR, et al: MR imaging of the rotator cuff, tendon: interobserver agreement and analysis of interpretive errors, *Radiology* 204(1):191-194, 1997.

Bacevich BB: Paralytic brachial neuritis. A case report, *J Bone Joint Surg Am* 58:262, 1976.

Bannister GC et al: The management of acute acromioclavicular dislocation, *J Bone Joint Surg Br* 71:848, 1989.

Bateman JE: The diagnosis and treatment of ruptures of the rotator cuff, *Surg Clin North Am* 43:1523, 1963.

Baxter MP, Wiley JJ: Fractures of the proximal humeral epiphysis. Their influence on humeral growth, *J Bone Joint Surg Br* 68:570, 1986.

Bergenudd H, et al: Shoulder pain in middle age: a study of prevalence and relation to occupational workload and psychosocial factors, *Clin Orthop* 231:234, 1988.

Buckerfield CT, Castle ME: Acute traumatic retrosternal dislocation of the clavicle, *J Bone Joint Surg Am* 66:379, 1984.

Bush LH: The torn shoulder capsule, *J Bone Joint Surg Am* 57:256, 1975.

Cofield RH: Rotator cuff disease of the shoulder, *J Bone Joint Surg Am* 67:974, 1985.

Cope Z: *The early diagnosis of the acute abdomen*, ed 12, Oxford, England, 1963, Oxford University Press.

Cox JS: Current treatment of acromioclavicular joint dislocation, *Orthopedics* 15:1041-1051, 1992.

Crass JR, Craig EV: Noninvasive imaging of the rotator cuff, *Orthopedics* 11:57, 1988.

DeDeuxchaisnes CN, Krone SM: Paget's disease of bone: clinical and metabolic observation, *Medicine* (Baltimore) 43:233, 1964.

de Laat EAT et al: Nerve lesions in primary shoulder dislocation and humeral neck fractures, *J Bone Joint Surg Br* 76:381-383, 1994.

DePalma AF: *Surgery of the shoulder*, ed 2, Philadelphia, 1973, JB Lippincott.

Dillin L, Hoaglund FT, Scheck M: Brachial neuritis, *J Bone Joint Surg Am* 67:878, 1985.

Fery A, Sommelet S: Dislocation of the sternoclavicular joint: a review of 49 cases, *Int Orthop* 12:187, 1988.

Fronek J et al: Posterior subluxation of the glenohumeral joint, *J Bone Joint Surg Am* 71:205, 1989.

Gerber C, Garz R: Clinical assessment of instability of the shoulder, *J Bone Joint Surg Br* 66:551, 1984.

Gore DR et al: Shoulder-muscle strength and range of motion following surgical repair of full-thickness rotator-cuff tears, *J Bone Joint Surg Am* 68:266, 1986.

Goss TP: Anterior glenohumeral instability, *Orthopedics* 11:87, 1988.

Goss TP: Scapular fractures and dislocations: diagnosis and treatment, *J Am Acad Orthop Surg* 3:22-33, 1995.

Grant JC: *A method of anatomy*, ed 6, Baltimore, 1958, Williams & Wilkins.

Hammond G: Complete acromionectomy in the treatment of chronic tendinitis of the shoulder, *J Bone Joint Surg Am* 53:173, 1971.

Hawkins RJ, McCormack RG: Posterior shoulder instability, *Orthopedics* 11:101, 1988.

Howell SM et al: Normal and abnormal mechanics of the glenohumeral joint in the horizontal plane, *J Bone Joint Surg Am* 70:227, 1988.

Jupiter JB, Leffert RD: Non-union of the clavicle. Associated complications and surgical management, *J Bone Joint Surg Am* 69:753, 1987.

Kessel L, Watson M: The painful arc syndrome: clinical classification as a guide to management, *J Bone Joint Surg Br* 59:166, 1977.

Kozin F et al: The reflex sympathetic dystrophy syndrome: I. Clinical and histologic studies: evidence for bilaterality, response to corticosteroids, and articular involvement, *Am J Med* 60:321, 1976.

Kuhn JE, Planchy KD, Hawkins RJ: Symptomatic scapulothoracic crepitus and bursitis, *J Am Acad Orthop Surg* 6:267-273, 1998.

Laskin RS, Schreiber S: Inferior subluxation of the humeral head: the drooping shoulder, *Radiology* 98:585, 1971.

Lyons AR, Tomlinson JE: Clinical diagnosis of tears of the rotator cuff, *J Bone Joint Surg Br* 74:414-416, 1992.

Marans HJ, Angel KR, Schemitsh EH, Wedge JH: The fate of traumatic anterior dislocation in children, *J Bone Joint Surg Am* 74:1242-1244, 1992.

McConville OR, Iannotti JP: Partial-thickness tears of the rotator cuff: evaluation and management, *J Am Acad Orthop Surg* 7:32-43, 1997.

McLaughlin HL: The "frozen" shoulder, *Clin Orthop* 20:126, 1961.

Miller MD, Wirth MA, Rockwood CA: Thawing the frozen shoulder: the "patient" patient, *Orthopedics* 19:849-853, 1996.

Miniaci A, Froese WG: Magnetic imaging evaluation of the rotator cuff tendons in the asymptomatic shoulder, *Am J Sports Med* 23:142-145, 1995.

Moseley HF: *Ruptures of the rotator cuff*, Springfield, Ill, 1952, Charles C Thomas Publisher.

Neer CS: Anterior acromioplasty for the chronic impingement syndrome in the shoulder, *J Bone Joint Surg Am* 54:41, 1972.

Neer CS, Craig EV, Fukuda H: Cuff-tear arthropathy, *J Bone Joint Surg Am* 65:1232, 1983.

Nuber GW, Bowen MK: Acromioclavicular joint injuries and distal clavicle fractures, *J Am Acad Orthop Surg* 5:11-18, 1997.

Parker RD et al: Frozen shoulder, *Orthopedics* 12:869, 1989.

Parsons TA: The snapping scapula and subscapular exostosis, *J Bone Joint Surg Br* 55:345, 1973.

Percy EC, Birbragen D, Pitt MJ: Snapping scapula: a review of the literature and presentation of 14 patients, *Can J Surg* 31:248, 1988.

Pollock RG, Duralde XA, Flatow EL, Bigliani LU: The use of arthroscopy in the treatment of resistant frozen shoulder, *Clin Orthop Related Res* 304:30-36, 1994.

Quigley TB: The nonoperative treatment of symptomatic calcareous deposits in the shoulder, *Surg Clin North Am* 43:1495, 1963.

Rockwood CA, Lyons FR: Shoulder impingement syndrome: diagnosis, radiographic evaluation and treatment with a modified Neer acromioplasty, *J Bone Joint Surg Am* 75:409-424, 1993.

Rockwood CA, Odor JM: Spontaneous atraumatic anterior subluxation of the sternoclavicular joint, *J Bone Joint Surg Am* 71:1280, 1989.

Rowe CR, Zarins B, Ciullo JV: Recurrent anterior dislocation of the shoulder after surgical repair: apparent causes of failure and treatment, *J Bone Joint Surg Am* 66:159, 1984.

Samelson RL, Prieto V: Dislocation arthropathy of the shoulder, *J Bone Joint Surg Am* 65:456, 1983.

Shaffer B, Tibone JE, Kerlan RK: Frozen shoulder: a long-term follow-up, *J Bone Joint Surg Am* 5:738-746, 1992.

Shaffer BS: Painful conditions of the acromioclavicular joint, *J Am Acad Orthop Surg* 7:176-188, 1999.

Schenk TJ, Brems JJ: Multidirectional instability of the shoulder: pathophysiology, diagnosis and management, *J Am Acad Orthop Surg* 6:65-72, 1998.

Sher JS, Uribe JW, Posada A, et al: Abnormal findings on magnetic resonance images of asymptomatic shoulders, *J Bone Joint Surg Am* 77:10-15, 1995.

Silferskiold JP, Straehley DJ, Jones WW: Roentgenographic evaluation of suspected shoulder dislocation: a prospective study comparing the axillary view and the scapular "Y" view, *Orthopedics* 13:63, 1990.

Spengler DW, Kirsh MM, Kaufer H: Orthopedic aspects and early diagnosis of superior sulcus tumor of lung (Pancoast), *J Bone Joint Surg Am* 55:1645, 1973.

Steinbrocher O: The painful shoulder. In Hollander JL, McCarty D Jr, editors: *Arthritis and allied conditions*, ed 8, Philadelphia, 1972, Lea & Febiger.

Taft TN, Wilson FC, Oglesby JW: Dislocation of the acromioclavicular joint: an end-result study, *J Bone Joint Surg Am* 69:1045, 1987.

Tsairis P, Dyck PJ, Mulder DW: Natural history of brachial plexus neuropathy, *Arch Neurol* 27:109, 1972.

Uhthoff HK, Loehr JW: Calcific tenopathy of the rotator cuff: pathogenesis, diagnosis and management, *J Am Acad Orthop Surg* 5:183-191, 1997.

Warner JJ: Frozen shoulder: diagnosis and management, *J Am Acad Orthop Surg* 3:130-140, 1997.

Watson M: Major ruptures of the rotator cuff: the results of surgical repairs in 89 patients, *J Bone Joint Surg Br* 67:618, 1985.

Young TB, Wallace WA: Conservative treatment of fractures and fracture-dislocations of the upper end of the humerus, *J Bone Joint Surg Br* 67:373, 1985.

Zeman CA et al: The rotator cuff-deficient arthritic shoulder: diagnosis and surgical management, *J Am Acad Orthop Surg* 6:337-348, 1998.

# CHAPTER 6

# The Elbow

The elbow is a strong hinge joint that allows flexion and rotation of the forearm. It also provides the bony origin for most of the extrinsic muscles of the wrist and hand. It is often affected by inflammatory and traumatic conditions that seriously alter its function. Osteoarthritis is rare, however.

## ANATOMY

The elbow joint is formed by the articulation between the humerus and the radius and ulna (Fig. 6-1). The humerus widens distally to form the lateral and medial condyles. The capitellum of the lateral condyle articulates with the radial head, and the trochlea articulates with the ulna. The head of the radius also articulates with the lateral aspect of the ulna and is held in position by the orbicular ligament. Medial and lateral collateral ligaments provide additional stability.

Adjacent to each condyle are the epicondyles, which are the bony attachments for many forearm muscles. The flexor-pronator muscle group takes its origin from a common tendon that attaches to the medial epi-condyle, and the extensor-supinator group arises in a similar manner from the lateral epicondyle. Posteriorly, the triceps attaches to the olecranon; anteriorly, the biceps and brachialis attach to the radius and ulna, respectively.

Three major nerves cross the elbow joint on their way into the forearm. The median nerve passes deep in the antecubital fossa medial to the biceps and brachialis, and the radial nerve passes lateral to them. The ulnar nerve reaches the forearm by coursing posteriorly in a groove between the medial epicondyle and the olecranon process, where it is easily palpated. It is also vulnerable to injury in this superficial location.

## EXAMINATION

The tip of the olecranon process and the epicondyles form useful bony landmarks (Fig. 6-2). When the elbow is fully extended and viewed from behind, these points form a straight, transverse line. With the elbow flexed, they form an isosceles triangle. Just distal to the lateral epicondyle lies the radial head. These two points, along with the olecranon process, form another triangle on the posterolateral aspect of the joint. This triangle is occupied by the anconeus muscle. This area usually bulges when the joint is distended by fluid and is an excellent site for joint aspiration.

With the forearm in the supinated position, an angle is formed with the arm at the elbow joint. This is referred to as the "carrying angle" and normally measures 15 to 20 degrees. Alterations in this angle may occur after injury or infection, especially in the young, and may lead to excessive cubitus valgus or even varus (Fig. 6-3).

## ROENTGENOGRAPHIC ANATOMY

The roentgenographic features of the elbow are well visualized by standard anteroposterior and 90-degree flexion lateral views (Fig. 6-4). Comparison views of the opposite elbow should be obtained whenever necessary.

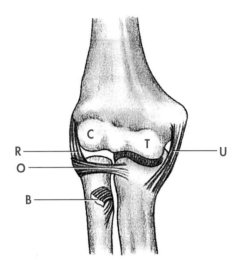

**Fig. 6–1.**
Bony and ligamentous anatomy of the elbow: *R* = radial collateral ligament; *O* = orbicular ligament; *B* = biceps insertion; *U* = ulnar collateral ligament; *C* = capitellum; *T* = trochlea.

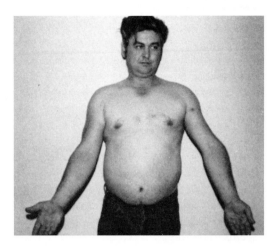

**Fig. 6–3.**
Gunstock deformity (cubitus varus) of the left elbow with reversal of the carrying angle because of an old fracture with malunion.

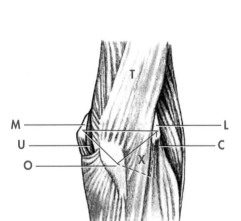

**Fig. 6–2.**
The flexed elbow from behind: *T* = triceps; *M* = medial epicondyle; *U* = ulnar nerve; *L* = lateral epicondyle; *C* = common extensor tendon; *X* = the posterolateral triangle. The isosceles triangle between the epicondyles and the olecranon *(O)* is altered in most fractures and dislocations of the elbow except the supracondylar fracture, where all three points move together.

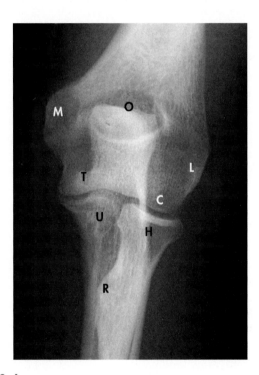

**Fig. 6–4.**
Roentgenographic anatomy of the elbow: *M* = medial epicondyle; *O* = olecranon fossa; *L* = lateral epicondyle; *T* = trochlea; *C* = capitellum; *U* = coronoid process of the ulna; *H* = radial head; *R* = radial tuberosity. Regardless of the position of the elbow, the long axis of the radius always passes through the capitellum.

# EPICONDYLITIS

Epicondylitis is one of a large group of musculoskeletal disorders commonly termed "overuse syndromes." Although it is often called an inflammatory condition, degeneration (tendinosis) is usually present instead. The condition is characterized by pain at the origin of the flexor muscles at the medial epicondyle or the extensor muscles at the lateral epicondyle. Some cases may start with a direct blow, but usually the cause is unknown. Minor tears in the tendinous attachments of these muscles are often present. The disorder is common in those individuals whose activities require repeated use of the extensor or flexor mechanism of the forearm. The lateral side ("tennis elbow") is more commonly involved. In tennis players, the backhand swing seems to be the main offender. Involvement of the medial epicondyle is often called "golfer's elbow."

## Clinical Features

The onset is usually gradual. A dull ache appears over the affected epicondyle, and it worsens with use of the involved muscles. Palm down lifting is painful. Activities that require rotation and grasping, such as opening a jar, increase the pain. The pain often radiates into the forearm. Extension or flexion of the hand against resistance will reproduce the pain at the affected epicondyle. The point of maximum tenderness can usually be well localized by digital pressure applied to the epicondyle. The roentgenograms are usually normal, although a traction spur or calcification may be present.

## Treatment

Treatment is similar to that for other "musculotendinous overuse syndromes." Rest is important and can often be obtained merely by avoiding the offending activity. Applying ice after exercise can help. An exercise program is begun after pain subsides (Fig. 6-5). NSAIDs are given as necessary. Local infiltration of the affected area with 1 to 2 mL of a steroid/lidocaine mixture will often

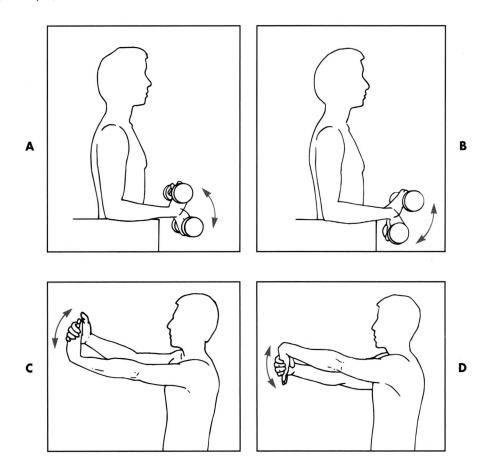

**Fig. 6–5.**
Exercise program for tennis elbow. It should be performed daily only after pain has subsided. **A** and **B**, Wrist curls and reverse curls are performed with light weights, lifting quickly and releasing slowly. Twenty repetitions are done each time, starting with 6 ounces and progressing to 2 pounds. **C** and **D**, Stretching exercises are performed with the elbow extended. Each position is held for 5 seconds and is repeated five times. Ice is applied for 1 to 2 minutes after the exercise program.

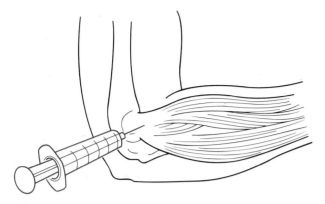

**Fig. 6–6.**
Soft tissue injection for lateral epicondylitis. The patient is supine and the elbow is flexed 90 degrees. A 25-gauge needle is used to inject the tender spot, which is usually about 1 cm. distal to the bony epicondyle.

give permanent relief (Fig. 6-6). The injection is placed in the area of maximum local tenderness and may be repeated two or three times. A tennis elbow counter-force strap may also be tried. Theoretically, this works by dampening the force transmitted to the elbow from the hand and wrist (see Chapter 15). If these modalities are not effective, the elbow and wrist may be immobilized in a long arm cast. The cast is applied so that the wrist is immobilized in a position that maintains relaxation of the affected muscles. For the more common lateral epicondylitis, the cast is applied with the elbow flexed 90 degrees, the forearm supinated, and the wrist slightly dorsiflexed.

The disease is usually self-limited, but symptoms may persist for several months before full recovery occurs. Conservative treatment is effective in most cases. Surgery is reserved for resistant cases.

# OSTEOCHONDRITIS DISSECANS

Osteochondritis dissecans is a condition in which a portion of subchondral bone undergoes avascular necrosis. This segment of bone, with its overlying articular cartilage, may partially or completely separate from the adjacent bone and even extrude into the joint to form a loose body (Fig. 6-7). The disorder is most commonly seen in the knee joint, but a similar condition also occurs in the elbow, ankle, and hip joints. The cause is unknown, but it is probably traumatic in origin. Repetitive compression of the lateral elbow joint may be responsible. The condition is sometimes a cause of "Little League elbow."

### Clinical Features
In the elbow, the disorder is most common during adolescence, and males are usually affected. The onset of symptoms is gradual, and a history of trauma may be elicited. The patient will often complain of a dull, aching pain that is often associated with stiffness. Occasionally, episodes of locking will occur if the fragment has become extruded into the joint. The physical findings consist of limitation of motion, local tenderness, and joint effusion. Roentgenographically, the capitellum is the most common site of involvement.

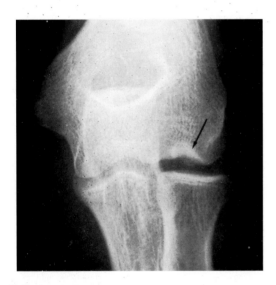

**Fig. 6–7.**
Osteochondritis dissecans of the elbow. Sclerosis, rarefaction, and a small loose body are present *(arrow)*.

### Treatment
The treatment in early cases consists of rest. This may require the use of a sling. All throwing activities are discontinued. Surgery is indicated for removal of any loose bodies. The prognosis is usually good in patients under age 10 (Panner's disease). When the condition develops later, some residual stiffness may occur and late osteoarthritis may even develop.

# PULLED ELBOW

Pulled elbow, or "nursemaid's elbow," is a disorder in which the head of the radius becomes subluxed beneath the orbicular ligament (Fig. 6-8). This occurs as a result of longitudinal traction on the hand with the elbow extended and the forearm in a pronated position. A common situation in which this occurs is when a child is lifted up by the wrist or hand.

### Clinical Features

The disorder is most common between the ages of 1 and 3 years and is rare after the age of 6. Clinically, an audible snap may be heard when the radial head subluxes. The arm is then held motionless at the side in slight flexion and pronation. The radial head is tender. Roentgenographic findings are usually normal.

### Treatment

Reduction is easily accomplished by supinating and flexing the forearm while applying manual pressure over the radial head (Fig. 6-9). A palpable click can be noted as reduction occurs, and the pain is immediately relieved. Reduction sometimes occurs in the radiology department when the technician places the forearm and the elbow in the flexed and supinated position to obtain a lateral view of the elbow. After reduction, a sling is worn for 5 to 7 days, if needed. Recurrences occasionally take place and are treated in a similar manner.

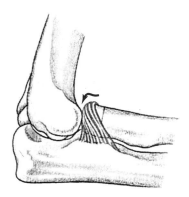

**Fig. 6–8.**
The radial head is pulled beneath the orbicular ligament.

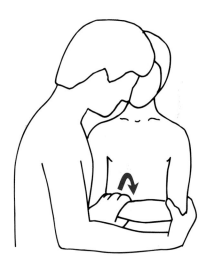

**Fig. 6–9.**
Reduction of a "pulled elbow."

## OLECRANON BURSITIS

The olecranon bursa overlies the olecranon process and is extremely vulnerable to direct trauma and repeated irritation. After an *acute* traumatic episode, usually a contusion, a tender, painful swelling may develop over the tip of the olecranon. The bursa sac fills with blood or clear fluid. At this stage, aspiration of the fluid (with culture if the fluid is suspicious for infection) and application of a compression dressing and ice may prevent reformation of the fluid and recurrence. Many acute lesions will spontaneously subside, however. Roentgenograms should be obtained to rule out fracture of the olecranon if trauma is involved.

With repetitive trauma, a *chronic* inflammatory reaction may occur that results in the formation of a thickened, rubbery bursa (Fig. 6-10). This bursa is usually not painful, in contrast to the swelling that occurs after an acute injury. Palpation may reveal multiple, small, hard nodules that feel like loose bodies. These usually are not chips of bone but instead represent villous thickenings of the bursa. Aspiration of the bursa may be attempted but the fluid often recurs. Incision is not rec-

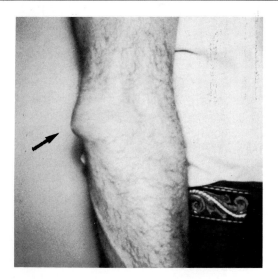

**Fig. 6–10.**
Chronic olecranon bursitis *(arrow).*

ommended, because a chronic draining sinus infection often results. If the bursa is chronically painful, excision is recommended. The bursa will eventually "dry up" on its own, however. Elbow pads or other forms of protection may be helpful.

Occasionally, sometimes following trauma, the bursa is the site of an acute infection. The treatment is the same as for any infection and consists of antibiotics, moist heat, and splinting, with repeated aspirations or incision and drainage when necessary.

## DISTAL RUPTURE OF THE BICEPS TENDON

The distal end of the biceps tendon may rupture as the result of degenerative changes near its insertion into the radial tuberosity. The distal end of the biceps tendon undergoes the same attritional changes that occur in the long head at the shoulder. Sudden, forceful flexion of the elbow against resistance may then cause it to rupture at its insertion into the radius.

A painful snap is felt at the elbow, followed by swelling and tenderness. Flexion of the elbow and supination of the forearm are weakened. The overlying deep fascia of the antecubital fossa may remain intact, thus preventing a significant loss of elbow flexion power. On flexion of the elbow, the belly of the biceps retracts to produce a bulbous swelling in the upper arm similar to that seen with proximal rupture of the long head.

Surgical repair of the ruptured tendon is usually indicated if a significant amount of motor power is lost. If the strength is satisfactory, surgical repair then becomes elective.

## DISLOCATION OF THE ELBOW

Dislocation of the elbow is a common injury and is usually posterior in direction (Fig. 6-11). It is generally the result of a fall on the outstretched hand with the elbow extended. Examination will reveal obvious deformity that must be differentiated from a supracondylar fracture. Avulsion fractures of the medial epicondyle and fractures of the radial head occasionally occur at the same time and may require surgical intervention.

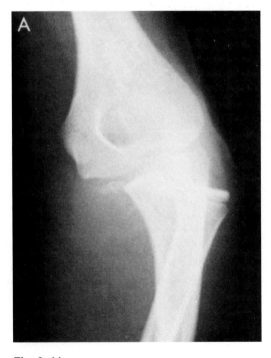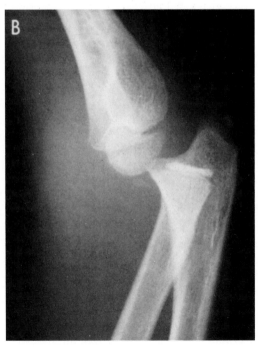

**Fig. 6–11.**
Posterior dislocation of the elbow. A line drawn through the center of the radius no longer passes through the capitellum. **A,** AP view. **B,** Lateral view.

Reduction is performed as soon as possible. It can usually be accomplished by gentle, steady traction on the wrist with countertraction on the shoulder (Fig. 6-12). A general anesthetic is usually unnecessary. Extension of the elbow to unlock the olecranon may be necessary. After reduction, the elbow is tested for stability, and post-reduction roentgenograms are always obtained. Lack of full motion after reduction suggests the possibility of an intraarticular fracture fragment. If the elbow is stable after reduction, it is immobilized in a molded posterior plaster splint for 1 to 2 weeks in a position of 90 degrees of flex-

ion. If instability is present, immobilization is continued for a total of 3 weeks to allow ligamentous and capsular healing. The splint is then removed and gentle range-of-motion exercises are instituted. Temporary stiffness is common, and full recovery of elbow motion may take several months. Motion should never be forced. The patient should be allowed to progress as tolerated. Forced passive motion only encourages more swelling, which leads to more stiffness. Some residual restriction of motion is not uncommon, but it is usually of such a minor degree that it does not interfere with function.

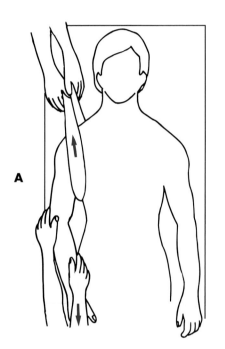
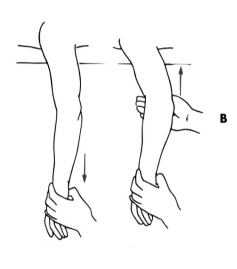

**Fig. 6–12.**
**A,** Reduction of an elbow dislocation by straight traction. **B,** Parvin's method. With the patient prone, gentle downward traction is applied to the wrist. A few minutes later, the arm is gently lifted upward, often reducing the dislocation.

## DISLOCATION OF THE RADIAL HEAD IN CHILDREN

This is a disorder that is usually traumatic but may occasionally be congenital or developmental in nature. Most of the traumatic cases dislocate anteriorly (Fig. 6-13). The mechanism of injury is usually a fall on the outstretched pronated arm, and the injury is often missed. Some cases may be associated with a "bent" ulna suggesting a Monteggia type of injury.

*Congenital* dislocations are usually posterior and are often bilateral. They may be associated with other congenital anomalies such as Ehlers-Danlos syndrome. *Developmental* dislocations are usually the result of cere-

bral palsy or neurologic injury and are commonly posterolateral. These two types of radial head dislocations usually have no pain and little functional impairment. No treatment is required unless symptoms are present.

*Traumatic* dislocations, however, need early reduction to prevent stiffness and pain. Old neglected dislocations may benefit from surgery.

Recognition is important. *Remember*: a line drawn through the long axis of the radius should always pass through the capitellum in any view, and all articular surfaces should match.

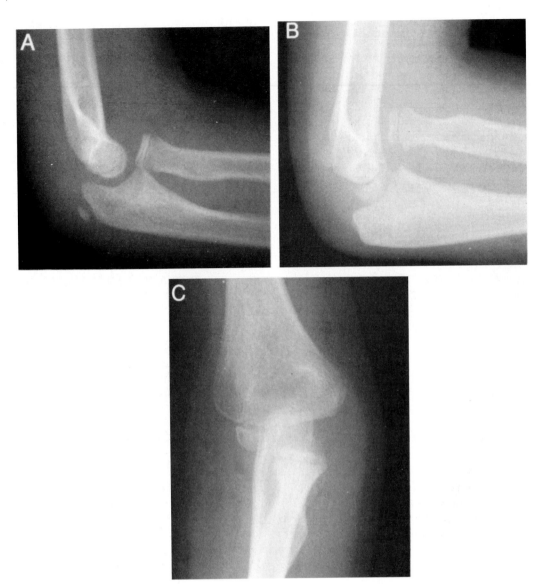

**Fig. 6–13.**
Anterior radial head dislocation. **A,** Lateral view showing subtle anterior dislocation. **B,** A more obvious dislocation. **C,** Anteroposterior view.

## FRACTURES OF THE ELBOW REGION

### Fractures of the Head and Neck of the Radius

Fractures of the radial head and neck result from a fall on the outstretched hand with the elbow extended (Fig. 6-14). All are characterized by tenderness over the radial head, local swelling, and pain on rotation or flexion of the forearm.

Undisplaced or minimally displaced fractures in adults and children are treated conservatively. If the swelling is extremely painful, the joint may be aspirated through the posterolateral triangle. A sling alone may be used or a light posterior splint may be added with the elbow flexed 90 degrees. Protection beyond 7 to 10 days is usually not required and early motion is encouraged. (Undisplaced radial head fractures can be missed on initial roentgenograms. If there is a clinical suspicion of fracture, treatment is indicated.)

Significantly comminuted fractures in adults are usually treated by early excision of the entire radial head. Otherwise, permanent restriction of joint motion and traumatic arthritis may result. Early removal is especially indicated in grossly comminuted and displaced fractures because the fracture fragments may act as a nidus for soft tissue calcification and lead to myositis ossifi-

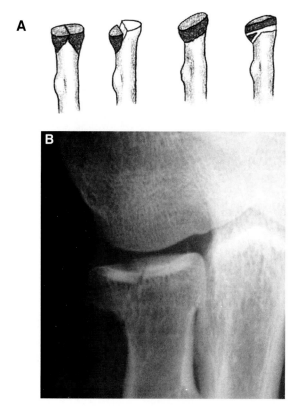

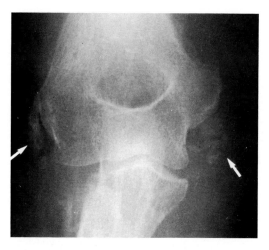

**Fig. 6–15.**
Roentgenogram of the elbow after a comminuted radial head fracture shows multiple areas of ossification (myositis ossificans) in the adjacent soft tissue *(arrows)*.

**Fig. 6–14.**
**A,** Various types of fractures of the radial head or neck that may be treated nonsurgically. **B,** Typical head fracture in which full, pain-free motion was restored after conservative treatment.

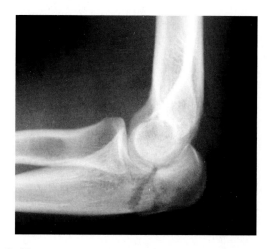

**Fig. 6–16.**
Fracture of the olecranon.

cans in the anterior elbow region (Fig. 6-15). Open reduction may be considered in fractures with a single large displaced fragment.

Children's fractures with less than 15 to 30 degrees of angulation are treated as undisplaced fractures, with a long arm splint applied for 3 weeks. Displaced fractures, or fractures that are angulated greater than 15 to 30 degrees, are treated by closed or open reduction. However, the radial head is never removed in the growing child because removal of the epiphysis will result in unequal growth of the forearm bones.

Regardless of the method of treatment, some loss of extension of the elbow is not uncommon. However, little functional impairment usually results.

## Fractures of the Olecranon

Fractures of the olecranon usually result from falls on the tip of the elbow (Fig. 6-16). They are either displaced or undisplaced. The extensor mechanism is intact in undisplaced fractures, and further displacement is unlikely. These fractures are easily treated with ad posterior splint for 2 weeks, followed by a sling and gradually increasing range-of-motion exercises.

Displaced fractures usually require open reduction and internal fixation to restore the bony alignment and repair the triceps insertion.

Displaced fractures in the very elderly or debilitated are often treated with a sling and early motion. Function returns reasonably well in these patients, but some weakness is present.

## The Supracondylar Fracture

This is the most common elbow fracture in children. The distal fragment is usually displaced posteriorly (Fig. 6-17). Neurologic and vascular injuries are not uncommon, but usually present only when the fracture is severely displaced.

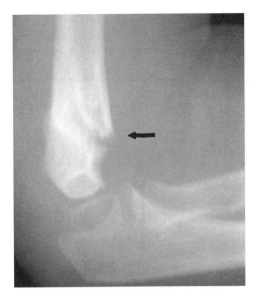

**Fig. 6–17.**
Supracondylar fracture of the humerus with minimal displacement.

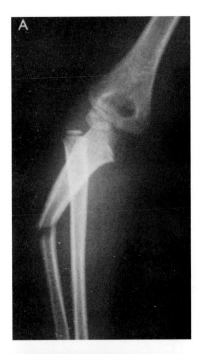

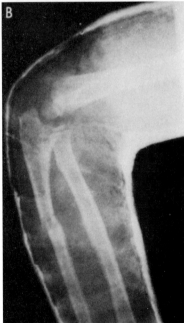

**Fig. 6–19.**
**A**, Monteggia's fracture-dislocation of the elbow. Note the angulation of the ulna. Also, a line drawn through the shaft of the radius no longer passes through the capitellum. **B**, After reduction it is always important to obtain a roentgenogram of the joint above and below any fracture.

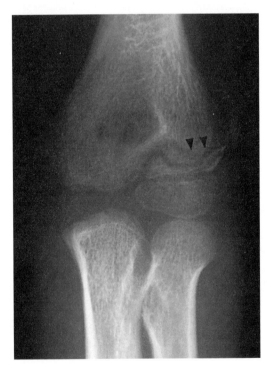

**Fig. 6–18.**
Fracture of the lateral condyle.

Displaced fractures are considered an emergency. Reduction with pinning is performed as soon as possible and the extremity is closely observed for neurovascular complications.

Undisplaced or minimally angulated fractures are treated with a posterior splint for 4 weeks.

## Fracture of the Lateral Humeral Condyle

This is a common fracture in children and is usually a Salter-Harris type IV injury. The fracture is sometimes missed because only a thin line of metaphyseal fragment may be visible, the remainder of the fracture line crossing the cartilaginous trochlea (Fig. 6-18). It is a potentially serious injury because the fracture line often passes through the growth plate and into the joint. Nonunion, malunion and traumatic arthritis are potential complications.

Undisplaced fractures are treated with a posterior splint for 5 weeks. Roentgenograms are repeated at 1 week to be certain that displacement has not occurred.

Fractures displaced over 2 mm usually need open reduction with pinning.

## Monteggia's Fracture-Dislocation

This injury consists of a fracture of the proximal third of the ulna and a dislocation of the radial head (Fig. 6-19).

Closed treatment may suffice in the child, but open reduction with internal fixation is often necessary in the adult.

Occasionally, especially in children, the fracture of the ulna may not be obvious, or the ulna fracture may be greenstick in nature and the radial head dislocation overlooked. Remember: always obtain roentgenograms of the joint above and below any fracture, especially if there is any shortening or angulation.

## BIBLIOGRAPHY

Ackerman G, Jupiter JB: Nonunion of fractures of the distal end of the humerus, *J Bone Joint Surg Am* 70:57, 1988.

Adams JE: Bone injuries in very young athletes, *Clin Orthop* 58:129, 1968.

Baker BE, Bierwagen D: Rupture of the distal tendon of the biceps brachii: operative versus non-operative treatment, *J Bone Joint Surg Am* 67:414, 1985.

Blount WP: *Fractures in children*, Baltimore, 1955, Williams & Wilkins.

Boyd HB, McLeod AC: Tennis elbow, *J Bone Joint Surg Am* 55:1183, 1973.

Broberg MA, Morrey BF: Results of delayed excision of the radial head after fracture, *J Bone Joint Surg Am* 68:669, 1986.

Cohen MS, Hastings H: Acute elbow dislocation: evaluation and treatment, *J Am Acad Orthop Surg* 6:15-23, 1998.

Dobbie RP: Avulsion of the lower biceps brachii tendon: analysis of 51 previously unreported cases, *Am J Surg* 51:662, 1941.

Galloway M, DeMais M, Mangine R: Rehabilitation techniques in the treatment of medial and lateral epicondylitis, *Orthopedics* 15:1089-1099, 1992.

Garden RS: Tennis elbow, *J Bone Joint Surg Br* 43:100, 1961.

Goldberg I et al: Late results of excision of the radial head for an isolated closed fracture, *J Bone Joint Surg Am* 68:675, 1986.

Hotchkiss RN: Displaced fractures of the radial head: internal fixation or excision? *J Am Acad Orthop Surg* 5:1-10, 1997.

Hudson DA, DeBeer JD: Isolated traumatic dislocation of the radial head in children, *J Bone Joint Surg Br* 68:378, 1986.

Jobe FW, Giccotti MG: Lateral and medial epicondylitis of the elbow, *J Am Acad Orthop Surg* 2:1-8, 1994.

Letts M, Locht R, Wiens J: Monteggia fracture-dislocations in children, *J Bone Joint Surg Br* 67:724, 1985.

Lloyd-Roberts GC, Bucknell TM: Anterior dislocation of the radial head in children: aetiology, natural history and management, *J Bone Joint Surg Br* 59:402-407, 1977.

March HC: Osteochondritis of the capitellum (Panner's disease), *AJR* 51:682, 1944B.

Mehlhoff TL et al: Simple dislocation of the elbow in the adult: results after closed treatment, *J Bone Joint Surg Br* 70:244, 1988.

Morrey B: Current concepts in the treatment of fractures of the radial head, the olecranon, and the coronoid process, *J Bone Joint Surg Am* 77:316-327, 1995.

O'Donoghue DH: *Treatment of injuries to athletes*, ed 3, Philadelphia, 1976, WB Saunders.

Otsuka NY, Kasser JR: Supracondylar fractures of the humerus in children, *J Am Acad Orthop Surg* 5:19-26, 1997.

Pirone AM, Krajbich JE: Management of displaced extension-type supracondylar fracture of the humerus in children, *J Bone Joint Surg Am* 70:641, 1988.

Ramsey ML: Distal biceps tendon injuries: diagnosis and treatment, *J Am Acad Orthop Surg* 7:199-207, 1999.

Reckling FW: Unstable fracture-dislocations of the forearm (Monteggia and Galeazzi lesions), *J Bone Joint Surg Am* 64:857, 1982.

Ring DR. Jupiter JB, Waters PW: Monteggia fractures in children and adults, *J Amer Acad Orthop Surg* 6:215-224, 1998.

Roberts N, Hughes R: Osteochondritis dissecans of the elbow joint, *J Bone Joint Surg Br* 32:348, 1950.

Salter RB: *Disorders and injuries of the musculoskeletal system*, Baltimore, 1970, Williams & Wilkins.

Skaggs DL: Elbow fractures in children: diagnosis and management, *J Amer Acad Orthop Surg* 5:303-312, 1997.

Tullos HS, King JW: Lesions of the pitching arm in adolescents, *JAMA* 220:264, 1972.

Woodward A, Bianco A: Osteochondritis dissecans of elbow, ankle, and hip: a comparison survey, *Clin Orthop* 148:245, 1980.

# CHAPTER 7

# The Forearm, Wrist, and Hand

The importance of the wrist and hand is evidenced by the fact that the rest of the upper extremity functions primarily to place the hand in a position where it can operate most effectively. Treatment of the variety of disorders that occur in the hand requires an understanding of its complicated anatomy and functional physiology.

## ANATOMY

### Skin, Fascia, and Nail

The skin on the dorsum of the hand is loose and overlies a subcutaneous space through which pass many veins and most of the lymph vessels of the hand. This abundance of lymph vessels accounts for the dorsal lymphedema that commonly occurs secondary to infection in the palm or fingers.

The palmar skin, however, is firmly attached to the underlying palmar aponeurosis, which is continuous with the palmaris longus tendon (Fig. 7-1). This thick fascia sends extensions into the fingers and protects the important deeper structures of the hand. It may become nodular and shortened in Dupuytren's contracture.

The nail of each finger originates close to the distal interphalangeal joint and is surrounded by thick folds of tissue on the sides and at the base by the eponychium. The nail covers a rich capillary bed that may be tested to determine the circulation of the extremity. The nail should be retained, whenever possible, in fingertip injuries.

### Blood Supply

Most of the blood supply to the hand enters on the palmar aspect through the radial and ulnar arteries. Each of these arteries terminates in a superficial and a deep branch. The superficial branches join to form the superficial palmar arch, which is located at the level of the base of the first web space. The deep palmar arch, located 1 cm proximal to the superficial arch, is formed by the junction of the deep branches. The arches are named for their position relative to the flexor tendons.

Many branches and anastomoses from these arches provide the blood supply to the fingers and hand. In the fingers, digital vessels (and nerves) lie just ventral to the flexor skin crease of the interphalangeal joints (Fig. 7-2).

### Muscles of the Hand

Motions of the wrist and fingers are controlled by groups of muscles that are classified as either intrinsic or extrinsic. Intrinsic muscles arise within the hand and are responsible for the delicate movements of the fingers. Thenar refers to intrinsic muscles of the thumb. Hypothenar refers to those on the ulnar side of the hand. Extrinsic muscles are those that take origin within the forearm.

#### Extrinsic Muscles

Motion at the wrist is accomplished by the various wrist flexors and extensors. In addition to providing wrist motion, these muscles stabilize the wrist in slight dorsiflexion, a position that allows maximum function of the extrinsic flexors.

Nine finger flexors and the median nerve pass into the hand through the carpal tunnel beneath the transverse carpal ligament (Fig. 7-3). Five deep flexors pass to the distal phalanx of each finger and thumb, and four superficial flexors pass to the middle phalanx of each finger. Each of these finger flexors can be tested individually (Fig. 7-4).

The finger flexors pass beneath a series of ligaments between the distal palmar crease and the distal interphalangeal joint. These annular ligaments, or "pulleys,"

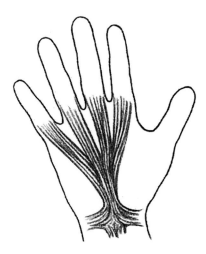

**Fig. 7–1.**
The palmar aponeurosis.

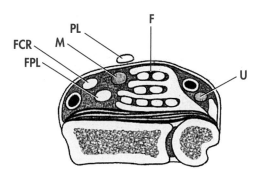

**Fig. 7–3.**
Structures proximal to the wrist joint. The ulnar nerve *(U)* and artery continue distally through the ulnar tunnel of Guyon. The nine finger flexors *(F, FPL)* and median nerve *(M)* pass through the carpal tunnel beneath the transverse carpal ligament. Note the superficial location of the median nerve and the sublimis to the long and ring fingers. *FCR* = flexor carpi radialis; *PL* = palmaris longus.

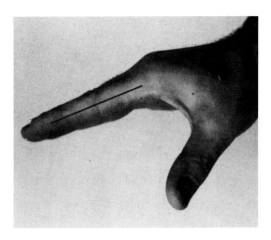

**Fig. 7–2.**
The neurovascular bundle is situated just ventral to the flexor skin crease.

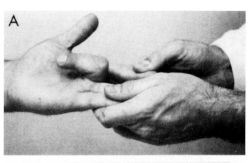

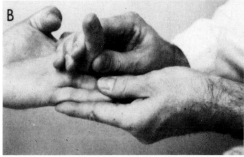

**Fig. 7–4.**
**A,** The sublimis is functioning if the proximal interphalangeal joint can be flexed while the adjacent fingers are held extended. **B,** The profundus is functioning if the distal interphalangeal joint can be flexed while the rest of the finger is stabilized.

prevent the tendon from bowstringing. Tendon repair in this area called "no-man's-land" is often unrewarding because of adhesions that form between the lacerated tendon ends and these ligaments.

The extensor tendons pass dorsally over each finger and thumb and insert into the phalanges. They extend the proximal phalanges and assist the intrinsic muscles in interphalangeal joint extension. The thumb extensors are easily palpated at the anatomic "snuffbox."

## Intrinsic Muscles

The thenar (median nerve) and hypothenar (ulnar) muscles act primarily to position the thumb and small finger for the purpose of pinching. The rest of the intrinsic muscles (interossei and lumbricals) insert into the

proximal phalanges and extensor hoods and assist in flexion of the metacarpophalangeal joints and in extension of the interphalangeal joints.

## Nerve Supply

The ulnar nerve provides the motor supply to all of the intrinsic muscles of the hand except the two radial lumbricals and the thenar muscles. It also provides sensation to the entire ulnar 1½ fingers (Fig. 7-5). Its function is easily evaluated by testing finger abduction and palpating the belly of the first dorsal interosseous muscle (Fig. 7-6).

The thenar muscles and the two radial lumbricals are supplied by the median nerve, which also supplies sensation to the palmar aspect of the radial 3½ fingers as well as the tips of these fingers on their dorsal aspect. Its function is evaluated by testing opposition of the thumb to each finger and observing the thenar muscles for contractions.

The radial nerve has no intrinsic muscle supply but does provide sensation to the dorsum of the hand over the radial 3½ fingers. It supplies motor function to the extrinsic wrist and finger extensors.

## Bones and Ligaments

The carpal bones contribute to the mobility of the hand by allowing flexion, extension, and radial and ulnar deviation to occur. The eight carpal bones are arranged into a distal and proximal row. They are bound together by strong ligaments, one of the strongest being the transverse carpal ligament. At the metacarpophalangeal and interphalangeal joints, strong collateral ligaments provide mediolateral stability.

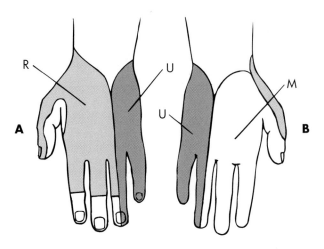

**Fig. 7–5.**
Dorsal (**A**) and palmar (**B**) sensation of the hand: *R* = radial nerve; *U* = ulnar nerve; *M* = median nerve.

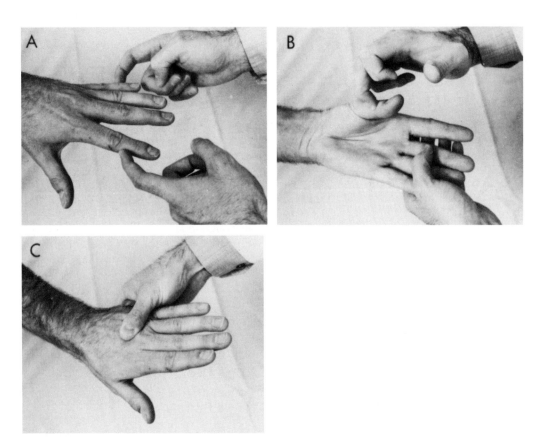

**Fig. 7–6.**
**A**, Testing for ulnar motor function. **B**, Testing for median nerve function by determining thenar muscle strength.
**C**, Testing for radial nerve function by examining wrist extension against resistance.

## ROENTGENOGRAPHIC ANATOMY

The 27 bones of the hand are visualized by anteroposterior, lateral, and oblique roentgenograms when appropriate (Fig. 7-7).

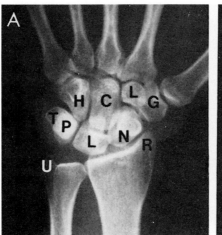
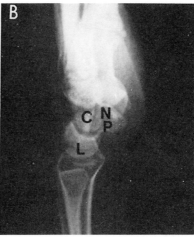

**Fig. 7–7.**
Roentgenographic anatomy of the wrist: *H* = hamate with its prominent hook; *C* = capitate; *L* = lesser multangular (trapezoid); *G* = greater multangular (trapezium); *T* = triquetrum; *P* = pisiform; *L* = lunate; *N* = navicular (scaphoid); *U* = ulnar styloid; *R* = radial styloid. On the lateral view, note that the capitate, lunate, and distal portion of the radius are in a direct line.

## CARPAL TUNNEL SYNDROME

Carpal tunnel syndrome, or compression of the median nerve at the wrist, is the most common entrapment neuropathy in the upper extremity. It usually occurs when vigorous use of the hand results in compression of the nerve between the transverse carpal ligament and the flexor tendons with their inflamed and enlarged synovium. Often no cause is found, but the disorder is also seen in association with hypothyroidism, rheumatoid and gouty arthritis, and aberrant or anomalous muscles in the wrist. A deficiency in vitamin $B_6$ has even been postulated. It is sometimes seen after fractures of the wrist, and is not uncommon in the third trimester of pregnancy. (**Note**: When it does occur late in pregnancy, the symptoms tend to subside after delivery, often quite dramatically within a few days. Thus treatment is strictly symptomatic, and surgery is generally not recommended in these cases. The disorder often recurs in subsequent pregnancies.) The syndrome is bilateral in up to 50% of cases and may occur in the workplace as a result of repetitive hand activities. Whether occupational and job-related overuse is a risk factor remains controversial.

Sometimes, a combination of neck and hand pain occurs, especially in patients who suffer from degenerative cervical disc disease. This is termed the "double-crush syndrome" lesion and results from nerve compression at two separate levels, the neck and the wrist. This suggests that proximal compression may decrease the ability of the nerve to tolerate a second, more distal compression.

### Clinical Features

The onset is usually spontaneous, with gradually increasing night pain being common. The nocturnal pain is often the reason the patient seeks medical attention. It may occur because of a slight increase in swelling at the wrist with inactivity, or perhaps as a result of wrist flexion at night. The pain may radiate into the forearm, arm, and even the shoulder. Numbness and tingling occurs along the median nerve distribution, but the sensory impairment rarely involves all 3½ fingers supplied by the median nerve. Often, only the long and index fingers are involved. A sense of weakness and clumsiness in the use of the hand is common. All of these symptoms may be precipitated by various manual activities such as typing or painting. They commonly subside after shaking and moving the hand or allowing it to hang downward. The patient often describes "poor circulation" and "stiffness," but the hand is usually warm and the motion is full. These symptoms are usually a result of the numbness.

Physical examination may reveal some sensory disturbance along the median nerve. Tinel's sign and Phalen's maneuver are often positive (Fig. 7-8). Atrophy of the thenar muscles is seen in cases of long-standing duration.

Roentgenograms of the wrist are helpful in ruling out local bony abnormality. Nerve conduction studies may be of benefit but are often unnecessary in classic cases. Delayed electrical conduction across the wrist is usually present. Electromyography is generally not required. Some error may exist in electrodiagnostic testing and it should not be the sole guide to diagnosis and treatment.

### Treatment

1. Eliminate the cause. If repetitive trauma is a factor, cessation of that trauma may alleviate the symptoms in some cases. Patients should avoid the extremes of wrist positions. Ergonomic changes in the workplace may be beneficial.
2. Antiinflammatory medication for any tenosynovitis.
3. Splinting. Occupational ("job-specific") splints or braces or night splints may be helpful (Fig. 7-9).
4. Injection of the carpal canal (avoiding the median nerve!) will occasionally provide some relief, although improvement is often only temporary. It can be harmful if improperly performed. Inject on the ulnar side of the palmaris longus tendon.
5. Stretching exercises for the wrist and forearm may be helpful.

### Prognosis

Resolution of symptoms may occur with medical management. If symptoms warrant, or if motor weakness is developing, surgical release of the transverse carpal lig-

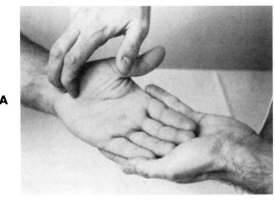
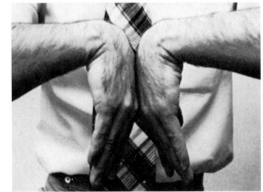
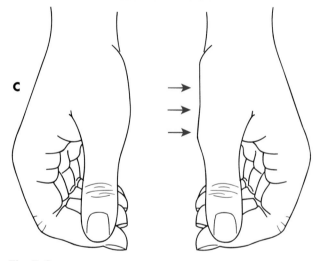

**Fig. 7–8.**
**A,** Tinel's sign. Percussion of the median nerve at the carpal tunnel may reproduce the pain and tingling along the median nerve distribution. **B,** Phalen's maneuver. The symptoms may also be reproduced after 1 minute of gentle, unforced wrist flexion. **C,** Thenar atrophy. Loss of the normal thenar bulk is best seen from the top and is present only in long-standing cases.

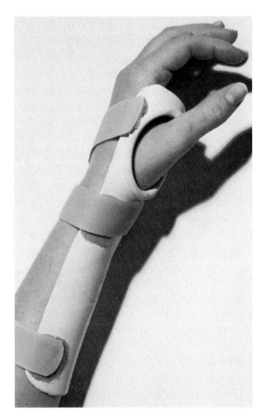

**Fig. 7–9.**
Polypropylene occupational wrist splint.

ament is indicated. This is usually followed by prompt and permanent relief of pain. Improvement of sensory and motor function may take several weeks or months, with motor function returning last. No disability results from sectioning the transverse ligament, and the surgi-

cal results are uniformly good. Some discomfort may persist because of the underlying tenosynovitis, however. The treatment of job-related carpal tunnel disease is much more difficult, and the results are more unpredictable.

## ULNAR TUNNEL SYNDROME

Pain or numbness along the ulnar border of the hand secondary to compression of the ulnar nerve in its "tunnel" at the wrist (Guyon's canal) is much less common than median nerve compression. It may result from pressure on the nerve by soft-tissue tumors, ganglia, constricting bands or muscles, or thrombosis of the ulnar artery. The incidence is high in bike riders. The symptoms and signs are similar to those found with carpal tunnel syndrome except that they are ulnar nerve

in distribution. They are also similar to cubital tunnel syndrome, except that the forearm is not affected and sensation to the dorsum of the hand and dorsal ulnar 1½ fingers is intact. This is because the dorsal sensory branch of the ulnar nerve passes to the back of the hand proximal to the ulnar tunnel at the wrist.

The treatment is the same as that for carpal tunnel syndrome, except cortisone injections are not given. Surgical release of the Guyon's tunnel is sometimes necessary.

## GANGLION

Ganglions are soft tissue lesions that are commonly found in the extremities. They are always found adjacent to a joint or tendon sheath. The cause is unknown, but myxoid degeneration of connective tissue and repetitive trauma with chronic irritation are possible causes. The cyst contains a thick, mucinous material and usually has a stalk that can be traced to a tendon sheath or joint.

The ganglion cyst is the most common soft-tissue mass in the hand. It is usually found on the dorsum of the wrist at the radiocarpal region, but volar cysts radial to the palmaris longus are not rare. Tendon sheath cysts also can develop on the flexor aspect of the hand near the base of the fingers at the MP joint flexion crease. Ganglion cysts are occasionally seen in children but often subside spontaneously in this age group in 2 to 3 years.

### Clinical Features
A history of trauma is rarely elicited. Local pain and a feeling of weakness may be experienced by the patient.

The mass may change in size, and this change is usually related to the level of activity of the patient. Ganglia are most common on the dorsum of the wrist. They are more prominent with the wrist flexed and are usually freely movable (Fig. 7-10).

An "occult" ganglion may be the source of local dorsal wrist pain. Clinically, it is difficult to detect because it is deep to the extensor tendons. Special imaging studies such as MRI may be needed to determine its presence.

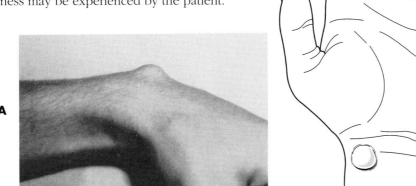

**A**                                                                                          **B**

**Fig. 7–10.**
**A**, Dorsal ganglion cyst. **B**, The volar wrist ganglion and flexor tendon sheath cyst in their usual locations.

### Treatment

Simple observation is recommended if symptoms are minimal. The lesion may subside on its own. A cure may be effected by aspirating or puncturing the cyst in multiple areas and injecting it with a steroid compound.

A large (22-gauge) needle is required to aspirate the thick gel. A compression pad is then applied over the lesion for 48 to 72 hours. Recurrence is common.

If symptoms persist, excision of the cyst may be indicated. The recurrence rate is 5% to 10%.

## DEGENERATIVE ARTHRITIS

Although osteoarthritis of the wrist and hand is much less common than in the lower extremities, it is sometimes more disabling. In the hand, it is 10 times more common in females than males, and the most common area of involvement is the trapeziometacarpal or "base joint" of the thumb (Fig. 7-11). Involvement at the base joint of the

thumb is particularly bothersome because of the tremendous mobility required by this joint in daily use. Sometimes deformity of this joint has the appearance of a "mass" because of osteophyte formation, swelling, and subluxation. Many other joints may also be affected, especially after fractures. When the distal interphalangeal (DIP) joints become involved with arthritis, persistent nodular swellings called *Heberden's nodes* may develop. Similar lesions at the proximal interphalangeal (PIP) joints are termed *Bouchard's nodes*. Occasionally, *mucous cysts* also develop at these interphalangeal (IP) joints.

### Treatment

Treatment is similar to arthritis elsewhere. Antiinflammatory medication, intermittent splinting, moist heat, and occasional local cortisone injections are usually successful in temporarily relieving symptoms (Fig. 7-12). Cystic lesions may be aspirated but should not be drained open. Arthroplasty and arthrodesis are occasionally necessary to control pain.

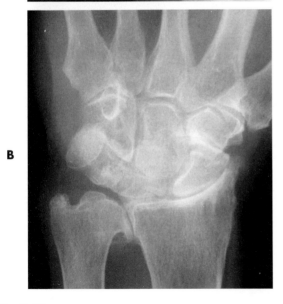

**Fig. 7–11.**
**A**, Osteoarthritis *(arrow)* of the carpometacarpal (CMC) joint of the thumb. Joint space narrowing and subluxation are present. **B**, Generalized osteoarthritis of the wrist.

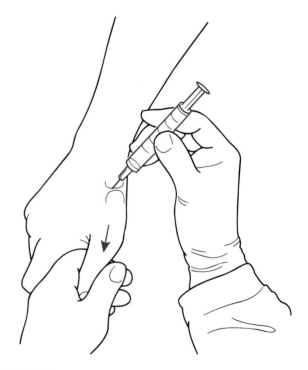

**Fig. 7–12.**
Injection of the CMC joint of the thumb for osteoarthritis. Distal traction on the thumb may open the joint for easier access. One mL of medication is usually sufficient.

# DUPUYTREN'S CONTRACTURE

Dupuytren's contracture is a disease of the palmar fascia in which progressive contractures of the fascia occur and lead to a flexion deformity of the distal portion of the palm and fingers. The cause is unknown, but it is often hereditary and bilateral. Predisposing disorders are diabetes, alcoholism, epilepsy, and liver disease. It is seen more often in Scandinavians, and some northern European populations have a 25% prevalence over age 60. Lesions develop more often and earlier in certain families. It is 10 times more common in males, and 5% of patients develop a similar condition elsewhere, such as Peyronie's disease or Ledderhose disease (involvement of the plantar fascia). Soft tissue "pads" in the knuckles may also be present. Individuals with these additional findings are considered to have Dupuytren's diathesis and their disease is generally more severe and recurrent.

Pathologically, the contracture consists of proliferating vascular fibrous tissue that later develops into mature collagen.

## Clinical Features

The disorder is usually painless. Age of onset is usually between 40 and 60 years. The most common complaints are deformity and interference with the use of the hand from the flexed, contracted fingers. The process usually begins on the ulnar side of the hand, often starting at the ring finger. An isolated nodule may appear in this area that eventually hardens and later dis-

appears. The overlying skin becomes adherent to the fascia, and a strong fibrous cord develops that extends into the finger (Fig. 7-13). In the later stages of the disorder, the cord may begin to contract and pull the finger into flexion. Multiple fingers may be affected.

## Treatment

The treatment is often surgical, although stretching exercises may help prevent contractures in the early stages. Fasciectomy is indicated as soon as joint contracture occurs. If performed early, complete restoration of extension can be anticipated. Nodules without contracture usually require no treatment. Referral is indicated if contracture begins to develop.

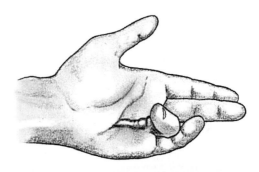

**Fig. 7–13.**
Dupuytren's contracture. A flexion deformity of the finger is present, with nodular thickening of the fascia to the ring finger.

# STENOSING TENOSYNOVITIS

This is a common condition that may result from repetitive overuse or direct trauma. The resultant inflammation and irritation hinder the normal gliding motion of the tendon. Several distinct syndromes can be described, depending on the site of involvement. Many of them occur in the hand and some are associated with rheumatoid arthritis. They are common in the workplace.

## de Quervain's Disease

Tenosynovitis often occurs in the first dorsal extensor compartment of the wrist (Fig. 7-14). The extensor pollicis brevis and abductor pollicis longus occupy this compartment and are involved where they cross over the radial styloid.

## Clinical Features

Pain and tenderness are usually present at the first dorsal compartment, and crepitus with motion of the tendon may be noted. The pain may radiate up the forearm and down into the thumb. Active and passive motion of the thumb aggravates the pain, and local thickening of the tendon

sheath is often present. Characteristically, pain is reproduced by passive stretching of the affected thumb tendons (Finkelstein's test). The overlying radial sensory nerve may become involved because of adjacent inflammation leading to tingling or numbness over the thumb and web space. Long-standing inflammation may even cause a tendon sheath cyst to develop near the radial styloid.

## Treatment

Treatment in mild cases includes NSAIDs, immobilization, avoidance of the offending activity, and steroid injections into the tendon sheath (Fig. 7-15). Braces or other immobilizing devices should always include the thumb and wrist. Moist heat is applied as necessary for comfort.

The symptoms usually subside with conservative treatment, but if they persist, surgical release of the tendon sheath is indicated.

## Trigger Finger and Thumb

If swelling of the flexor tendon and sheath occurs, passage of the tendon through the constricted sheath may become difficult (Fig. 7-16). This may result in snapping or "triggering" of the affected finger at the metacarpophalangeal joint as the swollen, nodular tendon passes through the constricted sheath. The symptoms are often worse after rest and improve with active use of the finger. The triggering effect itself is transmitted to the DIP joint, and the finger may even lock completely in either flexion or extension. If in flexion, manipulation may be required to extend the finger, a maneuver usually accompanied by a palpable snap. A congenital form is occasionally seen in the thumb of children. Examination usually reveals tenderness and a firm swelling at the proximal flexor pulley.

The treatment is the same as that for de Quervain's disease. Sometimes splinting only the DIP joint is needed. Surgical release is often necessary, but many patients, especially children, recover spontaneously.

## Extensor Carpi Radialis Tenosynovitis

Pain and tenderness affecting the radial wrist extensors are occasionally seen in heavy laborers. The symptoms, signs, and treatment are similar to those in de Quervain's disease.

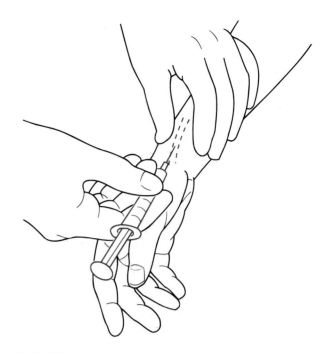

**Fig. 7–15.**
Injecting for de Quervain's tenosynovitis. The synovial compartment is gently grasped between the thumb and index fingers. These fingers can be used as a "sight" with the needle being inserted midway between them. Flow of the fluid up and down the sheath confirms the needle is in the sheath and not the tendon. Resistance to injection indicates incorrect placement and the needle tip should be readjusted.

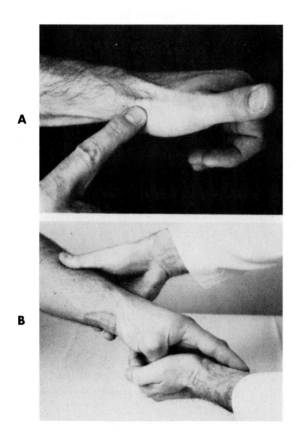

**Fig. 7–14.**
**A**, The first dorsal extensor compartment. **B**, Finkelstein's test. Pain is reproduced in the first dorsal compartment by passively flexing the thumb and adducting the wrist.

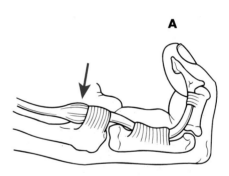

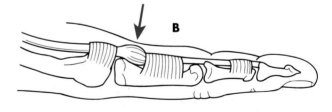

**Fig. 7–16.**
Trigger finger. In (**A**), the nodule is proximal to the first pulley. With extension (**B**), the nodular tendon thickening (along with narrowing of the sheath) prohibits smooth passage of the tendon causing the typical "triggering" effect. The finger may even completely lock in flexion or extension. The nodular thickening is usually palpable and often quite tender.

# REPETITIVE MOTION SYNDROME

This is one of several terms given to a controversial and increasingly common new diagnosis, in which pain develops in the forearm and hand in the course of normal activities in the workplace. Among other names used are *cumulative trauma disorder* and *repetitive strain injury*. A similar chronic pain syndrome may be seen in the neck and shoulder area as well as in the lower part of the back. The disorder has been the subject of much media attention and has even set labor against management in many large industries. It has also been the source of a great deal of litigation, mainly directed at workers' compensation carriers. The condition appears to reflect a complicated mixture of physical and psychosocial factors.

Some of the reasons why it is so controversial are the following:

1. It is not known whether the condition is really an "injury" and therefore compensable under law.
2. It is not known whether the syndrome is simply discomfort or whether any actual harm or damage ever results.
3. Often there is an absence or paucity of objective physical findings to support any clear working diagnosis or explanation for the pain.
4. There is considerable controversy surrounding a number of epidemiologic studies based on data gathered from the workplace.

## Clinical Features

Typically, pain occurs in the forearms after activity. The pain may not even be improved by rest or restricted activities. The syndrome sometimes presents with symptoms consistent with one or more disorders known to cause upper extremity pain. Thus some patients may present with symptoms compatible with tenosynovitis, whereas others may suggest occupational cramps, epicondylitis, reflex sympathetic dystrophy, thoracic outlet syndrome, carpal tunnel syndrome, or even a combination of several disorders. Often the symptoms are vague. The patient often lacks specific objective physical findings, with only diffuse soft-tissue tenderness being present. Occasionally, however, there may be mild generalized hand swelling and tenderness of the median nerve. Electrical studies may even be abnormal in some patients without any symptoms suggestive of nerve compression. This causes difficulty in arriving at a specific diagnosis (and is misleading if surgery is being contemplated).

## Treatment

The usual remedies are tried first: stretching exercises, moist heat, splints, rest, and antiinflammatory medication. The splint should keep the wrist straight, not flexed or cocked, and the patient should avoid extremes of wrist position. Local steroid injections are occasionally useful if the condition is clearly defined. If possible, task modification, frequent breaks, and shortening the exposure time improves the situation, although this is not always possible in most job situations. Occasionally, surgery such as carpal tunnel release is indicated if the diagnosis is clearly established, but surgery often fails to completely resolve the patient's symptoms in this setting in spite of positive nerve conduction studies.

## Prognosis

Occasionally, some permanent "injury" does occur as a result of repetitive motion, but it is not common. There is little doubt that discomfort does occur, however. Many patients continue with symptoms in spite of job changes, with pain occurring even with slight domestic tasks. These patients can usually be allowed to work but will often experience discomfort with any light job. Unfortunately, few jobs are available that do not require upper extremity use to at least some degree. Some patients may even have to completely change occupations.

# ULNAR NERVE ENTRAPMENT (CUBITAL TUNNEL SYNDROME)

Cubital tunnel syndrome is the second most common nerve compression in the upper extremity. It may occur from several causes, but the most common is chronic trauma to the nerve where it passes behind the elbow. The nerve is most superficial at this location and is easily subjected to external pressure. Leaning on the elbow or repeated flexion and extension may also be factors in its onset. Elbow synovitis with synovial enlargement and muscular hypertrophy may also cause localized pressure in the tunnel. A cubitus valgus deformity at the elbow secondary to a growth plate fracture or infection may also cause paralysis ("Tardy Ulnar Palsy") by progressive stretching of the nerve in its groove behind the elbow (Fig. 7-17). The nerve may even sublux in and out of its groove on occasion, thereby giving rise to symptoms.

## Clinical Features

Minimal pressure against the elbow may lead to paresthesias and numbness along the distribution of the ulnar nerve in the forearm and hand, mainly the small finger (Table 7-1). Tinel's sign is often positive. The elbow flexion test may be abnormal. This test is performed by having the patient flex the elbow for 30 to 60 seconds with the wrist extended. This maneuver increases the volume and pressure in the cubital tunnel and may reproduce symptoms. The test is not diagnostic, however, because it is positive in many asymptomatic individuals. In contrast to ulnar tunnel syndrome at the wrist, symptoms are also present on the dorsum of the hand and ulnar forearm. More severe involvement leads to progressive forearm, hypothenar, and intrinsic motor weakness (weak fanning of the fingers) and atrophy, especially the first dorsal interosseous muscle (Fig. 7-18). If the nerve subluxes, the subluxation is usually palpable with elbow flexion and extension. Nerve conduction studies usually reveal delayed conduction at the elbow.

### Treatment

Protecting the nerve from pressure may improve the symptoms in most mild to moderate cases. Elbow pads may be helpful. Keeping the elbow straight at night may be beneficial. A rolled towel wrapped around the elbow may be sufficient for this purpose. Otherwise,

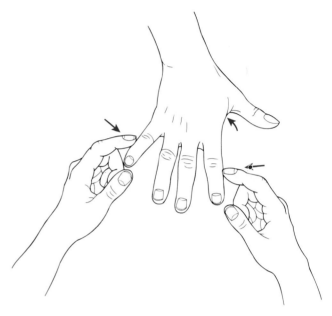

**Fig. 7–18.**
Testing for intrinsic (ulnar) motor weakness. Always look for atrophy of the first dorsal interosseus *(curved arrow)* when ulnar nerve lesions are suspected.

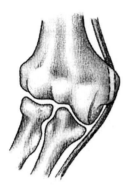

**Fig. 7–17.**
Valgus deformity of the elbow that may stretch the ulnar nerve and lead to paralysis ("Tardy Ulnar Palsy").

**TABLE 7–1.**

Differential Diagnosis of Common Causes of Forearm and Hand Pain*

| Disorder | Findings Present | Findings Absent |
|---|---|---|
| Carpal tunnel syndrome | Painful paresthesias along portions of median nerve (i.e., palm side of hand). Index and long often only fingers involved. May have night pain in long-standing cases. Pain may radiate as high as shoulder. Tinel's sign may be positive at wrist | Pain not worsened by resisted motion or stretching. No symptoms on dorsum of hand. Full range of motion |
| Tenosynovitis | Pain and tenderness usually well localized to site of involvement. Pain may be reproduced by passive stretch or resistance against movement of affected tendon. May be local swelling | Full range of motion. No paresthesias or night pain |
| Tennis elbow (most common lateral) | Pain may radiate from elbow to forearm and hand. Localized tenderness at epicondyle. Pain aggravated by resisted dorsiflexion of wrist (if lateral). Pain with gripping activities | Full range of motion. No paresthesias or night pain |
| Osteoarthritis | Local tenderness, sometimes with swelling of affected joint. Pain with motion. Decreased motion | No paresthesias. Tinel's sign negative |
| Cubital tunnel syndrome | Painful paresthesias along ulnar nerve distribution in forearm and hand. Tinel's sign may be positive behind medial epicondyle | Full range of motion. Pain not worsened by resisted motion. No night pain |

* **Notes**: Treatment and workup:
1. NSAID, moist heat, splint, and modification of activities as indicated for 2 to 4 weeks
2. Roentgenogram, inject (if appropriate), change NSAID for 2 to 4 weeks
3. Nerve conduction studies, referral as indicated

the treatment is usually surgical. The ulnar nerve is usually transferred anterior to the medial epicondyle and any constricting bands are released. The pain is usually relieved immediately, but sensory recovery is often delayed, and motor function may not be completely restored. It is important, therefore, that all compression neuropathies undergo definitive treatment before significant motor weakness develops.

## KIENBÖCK'S DISEASE

Avascular necrosis of the carpal lunate bone is an uncommon disorder that may follow an injury. The cause is unknown, but the condition is considered to represent a circulatory disturbance to the bone. An abnormally short ulna (negative ulnar variance) may be a risk factor. A similar involvement of the navicular is termed *Preiser's disease.*

### Clinical Features

Although it is uncertain if trauma plays a role, a history is sometimes obtained of a single major injury. Multiple minor injuries such as those that occur with certain manual occupations may also lead to symptoms. Chronic pain, tenderness, swelling, and restriction of wrist motion (especially dorsiflexion) are common. The pain may be aggravated by passive dorsiflexion of the long finger in Kienböck's disease or the index finger in Preiser's disease. The initial roentgenogram is usually normal, but eventually the affected bone becomes abnormally dense and white (Fig. 7-19). Later, fragmentation and collapse occur. Often the end result is degenerative arthritis.

### Treatment

In the early stages before collapse has occurred, intermittent immobilization for several months may permit reconstitution of the normal bony architecture. Surgery is often effective if performed before collapse has occurred.

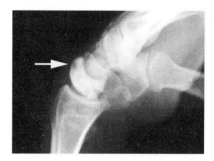

**Fig. 7–19.**
Kienböck's disease. The lunate is dense and sclerotic *(arrow).*

## SOFT-TISSUE INJURIES

### Fingertip Injuries

A variety of fingertip injuries are encountered in daily practice. By definition, these are injuries that occur distal to the distal interphalangeal joint. Bone, skin, and nail may all be involved in varying degrees. Examination and treatment of most of these injuries may be performed under a metacarpal block using 1% lidocaine anesthesia. The anesthesia is instilled into the web space rather than the digit to prevent pressure on the digital vessels (Fig. 7-20). Epinephrine should not be used. A small Penrose drain applied to the base of the finger makes a satisfactory tourniquet. Some general principles in the treatment of these injuries should be followed:

1. Proper healing occurs only in a clean wound. Gentle cleansing and thorough debridement are mandatory.
2. The nail should be retained. It protects the nail bed, acts as a splint for bone and soft tissue, and prevents excessive dorsal scar formation. The partially avulsed nail should be restored to its normal

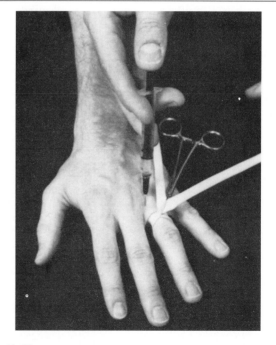

**Fig. 7–20.**
Metacarpal block. The anesthesia should be instilled into the web space. (The tourniquet is added later when the block becomes effective.)

position and held in place with one or two sutures through the nail into the adjacent soft tissue.

3. Repair the nail bed whenever possible. One should use 6-0 chromic or other absorbable suture. Sometimes, this requires elevation or even removal of the nail. After repair, the nail is replaced and attached. Failure to repair the bed can result in scarring and future nail deformity.

4. Working surfaces should be replaced with as near-normal skin as possible.

5. Preserve length, especially the radial three digits (thumb, index, and long fingers).

The treatment of all fingertip injuries is directed toward coverage of the deeper tissue. This may be accomplished by simple closure, free grafts, or flaps. *Major* wounds should not be allowed to heal by the "open" treatment method without closure or coverage. Epithelialization of the wound will eventually occur but may take up to 12 weeks, and the resultant skin coverage is often thin and tender and breaks down easily.

### Simple Closure

Simple closure is effective when skin loss is minimal and sufficient looseness of the surrounding skin and soft tissue is present to permit suturing of the wound without undue tension. A small portion of the distal phalanx may be removed with a rongeur. The scar line should be kept on the dorsal aspect if possible to prevent a tender scar from being present on the volar aspect of the finger. Never trim "dog ears." They will usually disappear with time, and trimming them may compromise healing.

### Epithelialization

Many *minor* soft-tissue amputations of the pulp without bone loss that are less than 1 cm square can be treated by thorough cleansing, debridement, and healing by secondary intention, especially if the amputation is transverse or dorsal oblique (Fig. 7-21). (Even some amputations with minimal exposed bone may be treated in the same fashion if the protruding bone is shortened first.) Dressings are changed in 2 days and then daily, using tube gauze and petroleum jelly. Recovery is usually rapid (2 to 3 weeks). Significant volar pulp loss may

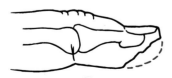

**Fig. 7–21.**
A common type of fingertip amputation easily treated by epithelialization.

be a contraindication to this method of care, where a padded flap graft might be more appropriate. If there is any question, it is always acceptable to temporize on fingertip injuries. The wound may be cleaned and dressed and referred for further care at a later date.

### Free Grafts

Free grafts are usually split thickness or full thickness. The thinner grafts tend to "take" better than do thicker grafts but do not afford the protection of a full-thickness graft. Although they may heal over bone or tendon, secondary revisions are often necessary. Their use should be limited to dorsal wounds or those without exposure of bone or tendon. These thin grafts may be obtained from a number of areas. The donor area often ends up being unsightly after healing, however, and should be chosen carefully. The thigh or lateral aspect of the buttock is a satisfactory donor site.

Full-thickness grafts provide better protection for the volar aspect of the finger but have the same limitations as split-thickness skin grafts when used over bone and tendon. They are less sensitive and may be used on volar injuries. The flexor creases of the wrist and elbow are excellent donor sites. The donor wound is easily closed without undue tension in these areas. The graft should include no subcutaneous tissue. As with all grafting procedures, it is wise to plan backward and be certain that the graft will completely cover the area of the wound. If the patient brings in the amputated fingertip, it may be used as a full-thickness graft if it is in good condition. All fat must be removed prior to application. In children less than 5 years of age, defatting the tip is not necessary. As healing progresses, full-thickness grafts may become dark after a few days. This should not be a cause for alarm because the deeper portion is usually viable in spite of the appearance of the more superficial layers.

### Flap Grafts

Extensive wounds may require local flaps. A variety of flap grafts are available depending on the need. These grafts provide more bulk and protection and are used when subcutaneous tissue is needed, for example, over bone and tendon. They are occasionally used by the experienced surgeon.

## Crush Injuries

These injuries are the result of direct violence to the tip of the finger. A painful subungual hematoma or fracture of the distal phalanx may occur (Fig. 7-22). The treatment of these injuries is directed at the soft tissues. Isolated painful hematomas may be drained by gently drilling a hole into the nail with a No. 11 blade or an 18-gauge needle spun between the fingertips. A heated paper clip may also be used. The hematoma should not be drained, however, when a fracture of the phalanx is present. Minimally displaced fracture fragments are stabilized by the adjacent soft tissue and can usually be ignored. A tube-gauze compression dressing and ice are applied, and the hand is elevated to combat swelling. Warm soaks are started in 48 to 72 hours, and gentle motion is encouraged. Recovery is usually rapid.

## Extensor Tendon Injuries

The extensor mechanism of each finger is a complex system, only a part of which is the extrinsic tendon itself. Restoration of normal function requires accurate diag-

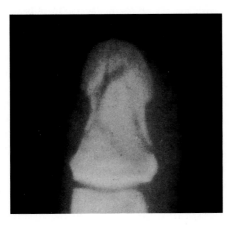

**Fig. 7–22.**
Fracture of the distal phalanx.

nosis and repair. All skin lacerations over the hand should be thoroughly inspected for tendon injury, but special attention should be paid to lacerations over the metacarpophalangeal joint. Extensor tendon lacerations in this area are particularly difficult to diagnose because the injury often occurs with the metacarpophalangeal joint in *flexion*, and the examination is usually carried out with the finger in *extension*. The tendon laceration then lies at a different level than the skin laceration and often goes undetected. With any extensor tendon injury, there is variable loss of active extension of the finger.

Lacerations in the extensor complex must be repaired accurately, and there should be no hesitation to extend the wound proximally or distally to properly visualize the ends of the tendon. Direct end-to-end repair using nonabsorbable suture such as nylon is desirable (Fig. 7-23). The finger and wrist are splinted in extension to remove tension from the suture line. Immobilization is maintained for approximately 4 weeks.

Partial lacerations consisting of greater than one third of the tendon should also be repaired. Small "nicks" can usually be left alone.

*Spontaneous rupture* of extensor tendons can also occur in patients with rheumatoid synovitis or after wrist fractures. When this occurs, it can mimic a peripheral nerve entrapment.

## Flexor Tendon Injuries

Flexor tendon injuries are diagnosed by history and examination. Partial or complete loss of finger flexion will

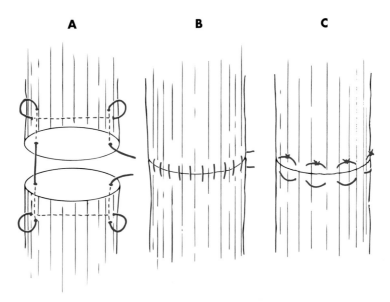

**Fig. 7–23.**
**A**, The Kessler technique for tendon repair: 4-0 nylon is used. A running suture of 6-0 nylon is added (**B**). **C**, Simple horizontal mattress sutures may be used instead of the Kessler technique.

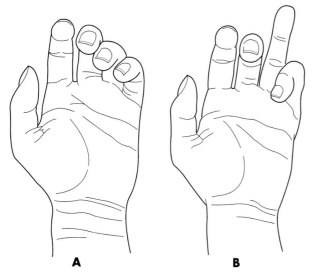

**Fig. 7–24.**
**A,** The position of rest. With the hand lying on a flat surface, the fingers will maintain a position of slight flexion. **B,** When the flexor tendon is lacerated, the affected finger will rest in extension.

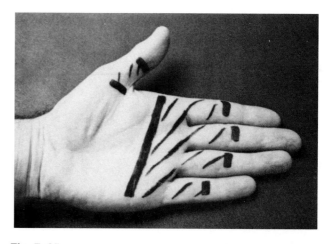

**Fig. 7–25.**
"No-man's-land," the critical area of the annular ligaments.

be accompanied by a typical posture of the finger (Fig. 7-24). There are often associated digital nerve injuries.

Repair of flexor tendon injuries is a complex problem that should be undertaken only in the operating room by an experienced surgeon. Primary repair of these injuries is indicated when the laceration occurs distal to the sublimis insertion or proximal to the distal palmar crease.

Primary tendon repair between these two points, in so-called "no-man's-land," is often unrewarding because adhesions are likely to form between the lacerated tendon ends and the flexor sheath and pulleys (Fig. 7-25). In selected cases of sharp wounds, primary tendon repair may be undertaken in this area. Otherwise, simple closure of the skin laceration followed by secondary tendon grafting in 6 to 8 weeks is often preferable.

Lacerations of the wrist that involve the palmaris longus tendon should always be carefully evaluated for *median nerve injury* because these two structures are close in this area.

## HAND INFECTIONS

### Human Bites

These are common injuries that are often mistaken for innocuous lacerations. Serious complications and disability often result, however, usually from the inoculation of virulent oral bacteria into the wound. A variety of organisms may be involved but the most common are mixed anaerobes and aerobes, streptococci, and *Staphylococcus aureus.*

The usual mechanism of injury is a fistfight in which the clenched fist strikes the opponent's tooth. Most commonly, the metacarpophalangeal (MCP) joint of the index or long finger is involved. The injury may cause penetration of the tendon, MCP joint capsule, and even the metacarpal head. When the finger is extended, the site of injury is often obscured and obliterated. Thus drainage is hindered, and infection is encouraged. (Laceration of the extensor tendon may also occur but is often overlooked because the finger is examined in the extended position.) The stage is set for spread of the infection into the joint and sometimes throughout the entire hand.

### Treatment

Appreciation of the injury is most important so that the initial wound is properly treated. Always assume that puncture wounds on the dorsum of the IP or MP joints are clenched fist injuries unless proven otherwise and examine the hand with the fist clenched. Thorough inspection, cleansing, and debridement are needed. The laceration may need to be enlarged to fully visualize the extent of the wound. Cultures are taken, and the wound is left open. No structures are repaired. A wick may be placed in the wound, and a soft bulky dressing is applied. Tetanus prophylaxis is given.

Antibiotics are administered on an empiric basis. They are initially given intravenously and later followed by the oral route. They are changed as needed, depending on the results of the initial culture and sensitivity.

If a wick is used, it is removed the next day, and daily wound cleansing and dressing changes are begun. The laceration is inspected closely, and if it is not improving, further surgical debridement and intravenous antibiotic therapy may be necessary. If the wound is healing satisfactorily, antibiotic coverage is continued for 2 to 3 weeks. Secondary closure of the wound is usually unnecessary. Complete extensor tendon lacerations may eventually require secondary repair, usually in 5 to 10 days when the wound is clean.

Wounds treated within a few hours can usually be managed on an outpatient basis. Older injuries may require hospitalization because cellulitis and abscess formation are often well established. Roentgenograms are always taken to rule out fracture (or infection in late cases).

## Felon

A felon is an infection of the closed space of the pulp of the distal phalanx (Fig. 7-26). It occurs secondary to a local puncture wound and is characterized by rapidly increasing pressure and pain. Osteomyelitis of the distal phalanx and extension of the infection into the flexor sheath or adjacent joint may result. *S. aureus* is the most common offending organism. Early incision and drainage are indicated. A short 24-hour trial of conservative treatment with antibiotics and hot packs may be attempted, but if symptoms do not rapidly diminish, early drainage is advisable. A metacarpal block is adequate anesthesia. A tourniquet is applied to the base of the finger, and a direct incision is made into the point of maximum tenderness and swelling. The incision does not have to be any longer than 5 to 10 mm. If no specific "point" can be detected, a straight lateral incision, which may be extended around the tip of the finger, is made (Fig. 7-27). The "fish-mouth" incision should not be used. A pack should be inserted and then removed in 2 days. Routine care of the wound after drainage includes dressing changes every 2 to 3 days and maintenance of antibiotic therapy. The wound will usually be healed in 2 weeks.

## Paronychia

Paronychia is an infection of the distal phalanx that occurs along the edge of the nail. The organism, usually *Staphylococcus*, is often introduced by biting the nail or by a rough manicure. Local signs of infection such as redness, swelling, and tenderness are invariably present (Fig. 7-28).

Acute paronychia will usually require drainage, although oral antibiotics and local care will occasionally result in a cure in 3 to 5 days. Once the pus has localized, incision and drainage are indicated. This is easily accomplished by passing a scalpel *between* the nail and the adjacent eponychium with the patient under local anesthesia (Fig. 7-29). If the infection has penetrated under the nail, a small portion of it may have to be excised. Incision and drainage *through* the eponychium should be avoided.

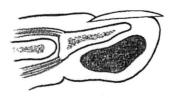

**Fig. 7–26.**
Felon. The pus accumulates in the pulp of the distal phalanx.

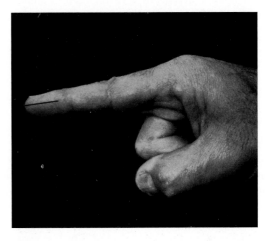

**Fig. 7–27.**
Drainage of a felon. The incision is placed posterior to the neurovascular bundle. Incisions in the thumb and small finger should be on the radial side. In the index, long, and ring fingers, the incision should be on the ulnar side.

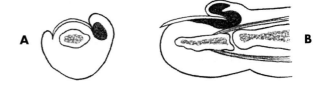

**Fig. 7–28.**
Paronychia. **A**, The abscess is present beneath the eponychium. **B**, The infection has penetrated under the nail and extended proximally.

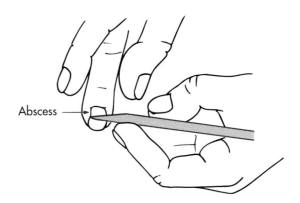

**Fig. 7–29.**
Drainage of acute paronychia. Under digital block, a scalpel blade is passed between the nail fold and the nail. This usually evacuates pus.

Once the infection spreads under the nail, a subungual abscess results. In this case, drainage is only effective if the proximal part of the nail is excised (Fig. 7-30). The nail will usually regrow. Chronic paronychia is treated in a similar manner.

## Tendon Sheath Infections

Infection may occur inside a flexor tendon sheath from extension of a felon or directly from a puncture wound. The rapid increase in pressure because of the accumulation of pus may obliterate the blood supply to the tendon and result in necrosis and complete loss of function of the tendon. The infection may also spread through the rest of the hand. Early diagnosis and treatment are therefore important.

### Clinical Features

The patient with suppurative tenosynovitis is febrile and often in a toxic condition. The disorder can usually be diagnosed by the presence of the four cardinal signs of Kanavel: (1) the finger is uniformly swollen, (2) the finger is held in slight flexion for comfort, (3) intense pain is present on passive extension of the finger, and (4) marked tenderness is present along the course of the inflamed sheath.

### Treatment

Early treatment with high doses of antibiotics, elevation, and splinting may result in a cure. In addition, wide incision and drainage are usually necessary to prevent sloughing of the tendon and further spread of the infection.

*High-pressure injection wounds* of the hand can cause severe infections. These occur when a material such as paint, oil, or grease is accidentally injected into the soft tissues of the hand. The puncture wound may be quite small, but extensive debridement and decompression are necessary to control infection and prevent the need for amputation. Paint appears to be the most toxic substance. Prompt recognition of the problem is important.

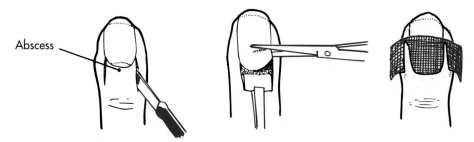

**Fig. 7–30.**
Drainage of paronychia when a subungual abscess is present. Lateral incisions are made through the eponychium, and the base of the nail is removed. Packing is applied, and the eponychium is replaced but not sutured.

# FRACTURES OF THE FOREARM

## Fractures in Adults

Fractures that occur through both bones of the forearm in adults are usually shortened and displaced. Accurate reduction of these injuries by closed methods is difficult, and there is a strong tendency for these unstable fractures to angulate after swelling subsides in spite of a good reduction and cast immobilization. Strong muscular forces acting across the fracture fragments predispose to this loss of correction. Consequently, there is a high rate of nonunion. For these reasons, displaced fractures of both bones of the forearm in the adult are often treated by primary open reduction and internal fixation (Fig. 7-31). Closed treatment may be attempted, but if it is unsuccessful the first time, operative intervention is usually indicated. The length of immobilization is shorter with surgery, and there is a more rapid return of function. Undisplaced fractures of both bones are treated with a long arm cast for 8 to 12 weeks.

Isolated fractures of either the radius or the ulna are treated in a similar manner. If enough angulation is present to interfere with rotation, closed reduction is attempted. If it is unsuccessful, open reduction and internal fixation are indicated. Undisplaced fractures are treated with a long arm cast for 8 to 12 weeks or until healing is complete.

## Fractures in Children

Fractures in children differ from those in adults in that surgery is rarely necessary. Reduction is usually possible by manipulation with the patient under light anesthesia. Angulated fractures are reduced by traction and countertraction, with manual correction of the angulation. It is often necessary to break the opposite cortex of the greenstick fracture to prevent reangulation from occurring in the cast (Fig. 7-32). Displaced fractures are treated by reduction with traction and countertraction (Fig. 7-33). Slight "bayonet" apposition is acceptable in young children if the alignment is satisfactory because subsequent remodeling of growth will correct minor deformities.

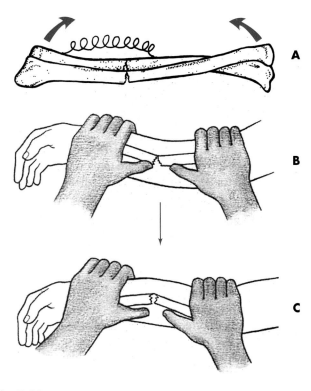

**Fig. 7–32.**
**A**, Greenstick fracture of the forearm. The tension side of an angulated greenstick fracture of both bones of the forearm will often act as a spring and may cause the angulation to recur. **B** and **C**, These fractures should be manually broken through to prevent recurrence. The periosteum on the concave side will remain intact. Reduction is then accomplished by simple traction.

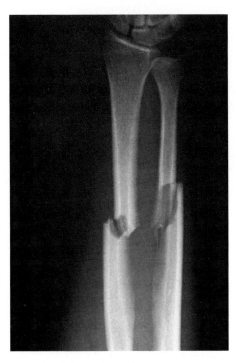

**Fig. 7–31.**
Roentgenogram of a fracture of both bones of the forearm that required primary open reduction with internal fixation.

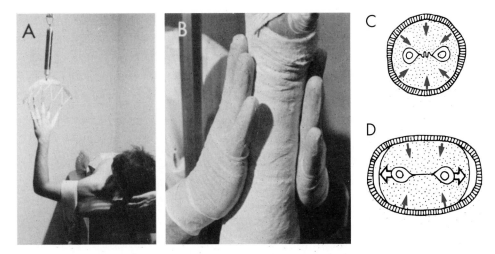

**Fig. 7–33.**
Reduction of a forearm fracture by simple vertical traction and countertraction. **A**, The fingers are incorporated into finger "traps." Countertraction is applied with a weight or water bucket. **B**, A long arm cast is applied with the elbow flexed 90 degrees and molded into an oval shape and straight by placing the hands on the anterior and posterior sides. **C**, An improperly molded circular cast may allow the forearm bones to encroach on the interosseus space, which could limit rotation. **D**, A properly molded elliptical cast will prevent this from occurring.

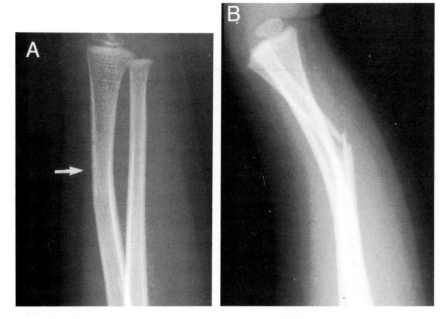

**Fig. 7–34.**
**A,** Traumatic bowing of the radius *(arrow).* **B,** Fracture of the ulna with bowing of the radius.

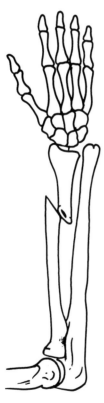

**Fig. 7–35.**
Galeazzi fracture-dislocation. There is a fracture of the distal portion of the radius with shortening. This shortening can only occur if there is injury elsewhere (in this lesion, a radio-ulnar dislocation). On the lateral view, the distal portion of the ulna is usually dislocated dorsally.

Children are examined at weekly intervals for 3 weeks to determine whether any reangulation of the fracture is occurring after the swelling subsides. If angulation does recur before 2 weeks pass, it can usually be corrected manually. However, if more than 2 weeks pass, the healing is so rapid in children that the angulation may be permanent. The cast is worn for 7 to 8 weeks.

All forearm fractures in children and adults are immobilized by a long arm cast with the elbow flexed 90 degrees. The forearm portion is always molded to prevent encroachment on the interosseous space.

## Traumatic Bowing of the Forearm

This is an unusual clinical entity in which "plastic deformation" of the radius and/or ulna occurs in the absence of typical clinical and roentgenographic findings for fracture (Fig. 7-34). The usual cause is a fall on the outstretched hand. There may be a fracture of one bone and bowing of the other or, less commonly, bowing of both bones.

Management of these injuries is controversial. Persistent angulation could limit pronation and supination, although young children (less than 5 years old) will undergo bone remodeling and probably do not need reduction. An angulated fracture of one bone is also difficult to reduce until the bowing of the other bone is corrected. In older children, the angulation should be corrected. The reduction may require significant force, and general anesthesia is usually needed.

## Galeazzi Fracture-Dislocation

This injury is a fracture of the shaft of the radius with a dislocation of the distal radio-ulnar joint (Fig. 7-35). It is rare in children. The disorder is sometimes called the reverse Monteggia fracture. Usually the radius is fractured in its distal third, and the radio-ulnar disruption is often missed. Surgery is usually required for repair.

# FRACTURES OF THE WRIST

Several common injuries occur in the region of the wrist joint: Colles' fracture, fracture of the distal portion of the radius in children, epiphyseal fractures of the distal aspect of the radius, and fractures of the scaphoid. Treatment of all these injuries is similar.

## Colles' Fracture

Colles' fracture is the most common injury of the wrist. It usually results from a fall on the outstretched hand. The force of the fall fractures the distal portion of the radius and displaces it into the typical "silver-fork" position. In addition to the dorsal angulation, there is shortening and radial deviation of the distal fragment. There is usually an associated injury to the ulnar styloid or ulnar collateral ligament of the wrist (Fig. 7-36).

The fracture can usually be reduced under local anesthesia if reduction is performed within a few hours. If more time passes, a general anesthetic may be necessary, because the local anesthetic may not diffuse through the clotted hematoma after several hours have passed. The tip of the ulna should also be injected.

With the assistant grasping the forearm for countertraction, the surgeon grasps the hand of the affected wrist (Fig. 7-37). The thumb of the surgeon's other hand is placed over the distal fragment, and the wrist is hyperextended to break up any impaction. Traction and countertraction are then applied, and by using the thumb for pressure on the distal fragment, the rotation is corrected, and the dorsal cortex of the distal fragment is forced onto the dorsal cortex of the proximal fragment (see Chapter 2). Ulnar and volar pressure over the distal fragment will then correct the radial and dorsal angulation. The radial styloid is palpated to determine whether the length has been restored. With the assistant maintaining volar and ulnar tension on the hand, a well-molded cast is applied with the wrist slightly pronated. The cast is well molded over the dorsal and radial aspects of the distal fragments and the volar aspect of the proximal fragment to keep the dorsal soft tissue tight. A short arm cast is usually sufficient. Excessive volar flexion of the wrist should be avoided and is unnecessary if the cast is properly applied and molded. Excessive flexion of the wrist may cause median nerve compression. The base of the thumb may be included to the interphalangeal joint to help prevent radial collapse.

An alternative method of treatment is to use the method of traction previously described for forearm fractures. After anesthesia has been obtained, the fracture is disimpacted, and the patient's index finger and thumb are placed in the finger traps. A counterweight is placed on the upper part of the arm, and the fracture is manipulated. A properly molded cast is then applied with the forearm in slight pronation. Roentgenograms are then repeated.

If the reduction is satisfactory, the wrist is elevated, and ice is applied for 48 to 72 hours. Active motion of the fingers is encouraged, and the roentgenogram is repeated in 7 to 10 days. The fracture is immobilized for approximately 6 weeks.

After the cast is removed, some temporary stiffness should be expected for several weeks. This usually subsides gradually as the activity level is increased. A temporary splint that is removed several times a day for exercise is often helpful in the transition period between cast removal and full use of the extremity.

Occasionally, some loss of reduction may occur after the swelling subsides. This is particularly true if there is comminution of the dorsal cortex. In the elderly patient, this position should be accepted rather than attempting to remanipulate the fragments to improve the roentgenographic appearance. This would only lead to more swelling, stiffness, and loss of function. Accepting the minor cosmetic deformity caused by the slight malunion is preferable in the older patient. If this occurs in younger patients (especially radial shortening), remanipulation with pinning or the application of an external fixator is indicated.

## Smith's Fracture

This fracture has often been called the reverse Colles' fracture (Fig. 7-38). One form of this fracture may be considered as such. The type that does not involve the articular surface may be treated by traction, manipulation, and casting in supination. Treatment in supination is important. "Cocking up" the wrist (the reverse of the Colles' treatment) will often not hold the reduction.

One type of Smith's fracture has an articular component that results in volar subluxation of the carpal bones. This injury often requires open reduction with internal fixation for satisfactory results.

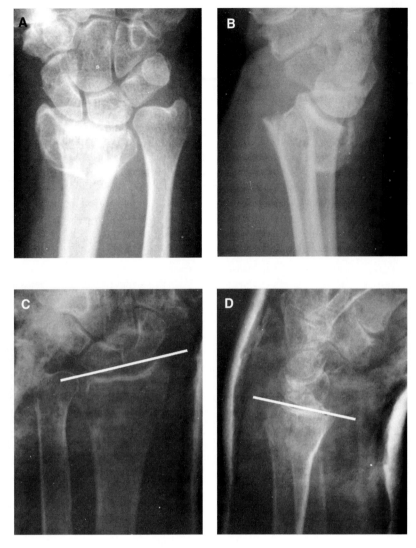

**Fig. 7–36.**
**A** and **B**, Typical Colles' fracture with dorsal and radial displacement. Normally, the tip of the styloid process of the distal portion of the radius extends 1 cm distal to the tip of the ulnar styloid. The articular surface of the lower part of the radius inclines 25 degrees ulnarward and 10 degrees volarward. **C** and **D**, After complete reduction, the length and these angular relationships are restored.

## Barton's Fracture

This is an oblique fracture that is essentially the reverse of the intraarticular Smith's fracture. The injury involves an oblique dorsal rim fracture-dislocation through the articular surface of the distal portion of the radius. Because this fracture involves the joint surface, accurate reduction is necessary, and open reduction is often required.

## Fracture of the Distal Portion of the Radius in Children

In children and adolescents, a fracture may occur through the distal radial epiphysis. If it is displaced or angulated over 15 to 20 degrees, it is reduced in the same manner as Colles' fracture and immobilized in a well molded cast for 5 weeks. Roentgenograms should always be repeated at 7 to 10 days to be certain that loss of position has not occurred. If the fracture is undisplaced, the diagnosis may be difficult. It should be kept in mind, however, that sprains of the wrist are rare in children. This is because the epiphyseal plate is weaker than the surrounding ligamentous structures and trauma will usually produce an epiphyseal fracture rather than a ligamentous sprain. Clinical tenderness over the epiphysis is highly suggestive of a fracture, and a short arm cast should be applied to these injuries for 2 weeks even though the roentgenographic findings

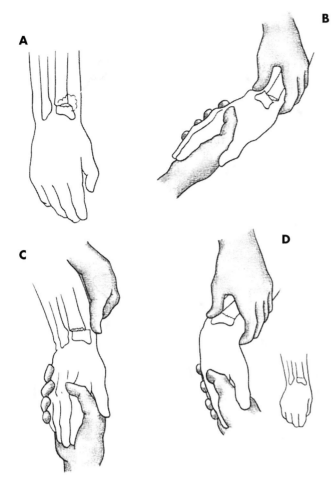

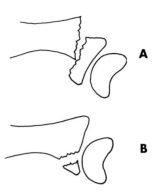

**Fig. 7–38.**
Smith's fracture. Closed reduction is usually successful with the type that does not involve the articular surface (**A**), but surgery is usually necessary for the intraarticular type (**B**).

**Fig. 7–37.**
Reduction of Colles' fracture. **A**, The needle is inserted dorsally into the fracture hematoma, and 5 to 10 mL of local anesthesia is injected. **B**, The distal fragment is disimpacted, and longitudinal traction is applied. Thumb pressure is then applied to the distal fragment to correct the dorsal displacement. **C**, The radial displacement is corrected by further digital pressure and ulnar deviation of the wrist. **D**, Upward pressure on the proximal fragment and tension on the slightly flexed, ulnarly deviated hand will maintain the reduction. A cast is then applied and properly molded. (Adapted from Compere EL, Banks SW, Compere CL: *Pictorial handbook of fracture treatment*, ed 5, Chicago, 1963, Year Book Medical Publishers Inc.)

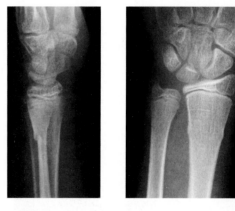

**Fig. 7–39.**
The "buckle" or torus fracture of the distal portion of the radius.

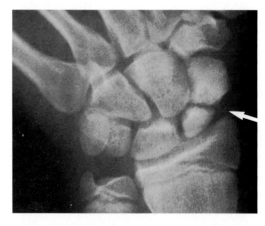

**Fig. 7–40.**
Fractured scaphoid *(arrow)*.

may be normal. If a healing callus is present at the end of 2 weeks, the cast is continued for an additional 2 weeks. If no callus is present, the cast is removed, and the "sprain" has had excellent treatment.

Fractures of the distal portion of the radius also occur in children approximately 2.5 cm above the wrist joint. They are treated in the same manner as Colles' fracture. Undisplaced or so-called *torus* fractures also occur in this area (Fig. 7-39). No displacement occurs with this injury, but it should be immobilized in a short arm cast for 3 weeks.

## Fractures of the Scaphoid

The scaphoid is the carpal bone that is most prone to fracture (Fig. 7-40). This injury also occurs as the result of a fall on the outstretched hand.

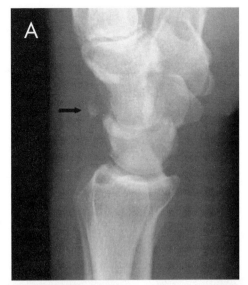

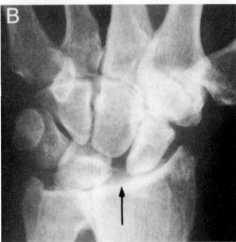

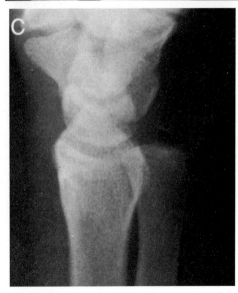

**Fig. 7–41.**
**A**, Avulsion fracture of the triquetrum *(arrow)*. **B**, Scapholunate dissociation *(arrow)*. Note the widening between the scaphoid and lunate. **C**, Dislocation of the distal ulna.

The blood supply to this bone often enters the distal portion. Consequently, fractures that occur through the midportion of the bone may lead to avascular necrosis of the proximal fragment. This complication almost always occurs in more proximal fractures. Nonunion is also more common after this injury.

The diagnosis is sometimes difficult. It should be suspected, however, in any patient with a history of a "sprained wrist" who has persistent swelling and pain in the wrist. Clinically, tenderness and swelling in the anatomic snuffbox are characteristic findings.

Initial roentgenographic findings are often normal because there may be little or no displacement of the fracture fragments. The fracture usually becomes visible in 2 to 4 weeks, however, as decalcification around the fracture line occurs.

Whenever this injury is suspected, even if the roentgenographic findings are normal, a short arm cast including the thumb should be applied. The roentgenogram is repeated in 2 to 3 weeks. If a fracture is present, the immobilization is continued until the fracture has healed, which in this case may take from 2 to 3 months. If pain persists but the roentgenogram remains normal, bone scanning is indicated.

The type and length of immobilization used in the treatment of the acute nondisplaced navicular fracture is controversial but a short arm thumb spica cast for 8 to 12 weeks is usually required. Failure of the fracture line to fill in by this time may indicate the need for surgery.

Displaced fractures may require open reduction and internal fixation and should be referred.

## The Sprained Wrist

Although simple, uncomplicated ligamentous injuries of the wrist do occur, there are a number of conditions that are often misdiagnosed as sprains. Failure to appreciate and properly treat these disorders can lead to permanent disability and chronic pain. Among the more common injuries presenting as "sprains" are the following:

1. Fractures of the navicular (usually as a result of a fall)
2. Undisplaced epiphyseal fractures of the distal portion of the radius in children
3. Fracture of the hook of the hamate (often occurring when a baseball bat handle strikes the palm)
4. Avulsion fractures of the triquetrum, an injury that may signify serious ligamentous disruption (Fig. 7-41)
5. Carpal instability, often manifested by scapholunate dissociation, a separation of lunate from the scaphoid that may require surgery
6. Subluxation of the distal portion of the ulna (usually resulting from complete ligamentous rupture

between the ulna and its attachments to the radius and carpal bones)

Careful clinical examination will usually reveal the site of injury. Routine wrist roentgenograms are always performed, and special views are added as indicated.

The true simple sprain is well treated by light immobilization for 10 to 14 days, followed by re-evaluation and further testing as indicated. Elastic wraps or "light braces" are often inadequate. More serious fractures or ligamentous disruptions should be referred.

## FRACTURES OF THE HAND

The principles of treatment of finger injuries are similar to those for other fractures except that the reduction must be more accurate in the hand. With certain exceptions, manipulation and external immobilization constitute satisfactory treatment. Principles of treatment include the following:

1. Avoid overimmobilization.
2. Be certain to correct *rotational* as well as angular malalignment.
3. Early surgery in the form of open reduction and internal fixation is often more "conservative" than are overzealous manipulation and prolonged, improper splinting.
4. Fingers should be immobilized in the position of moderate flexion. Avoid splinting the finger joints in extension, especially the metacarpophalangeal joint (Fig. 7-42).

5. Displaced intraarticular fractures involving greater than 25% of the joint surface are unstable and usually require open reduction and internal fixation (Fig. 7-43).
6. In the position of grasping, the axes of all flexed fingers point to the navicular bone (Fig. 7-44). Failure to appreciate this fact may result in rotational malunion.
7. "Chip" fractures near joints usually have a tendon or ligament attached. These injuries require careful evaluation (Fig. 7-45).

### Fractures of the Metacarpal

Fractures of the shaft of the finger metacarpal often present with dorsal angulation because of the action of the interosseous muscles (Fig. 7-46). Fractures that are in good alignment and apposition will heal satisfactorily in

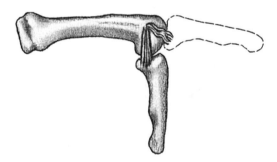

**Fig. 7–42.**
Collateral ligaments of the metacarpophalangeal joint. These ligaments are normally lax in extension and tight in flexion. Prolonged splinting in extension may allow them to shorten slightly, thereby making future flexion difficult.

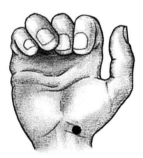

**Fig. 7–44.**
Normally, the axes of the flexed fingers point to the navicular *(dot)*. Malunion with rotation will cause the fingers to overlap when a fist is made. The resultant functional disability may be great.

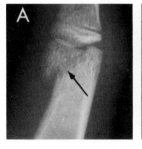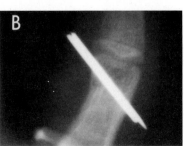

**Fig. 7–43.**
**A,** A displaced intraarticular IP joint fracture *(arrow)*. Open reduction with internal fixation (**B**) was required.

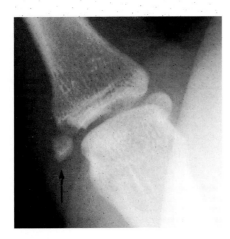

**Fig. 7–45.**
Collateral ligament avulsion fracture, which usually causes instability.

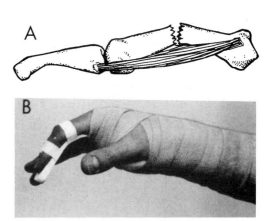

**Fig. 7–46.**
**A,** Fracture of the metacarpal. **B,** Reduction is maintained by a metal splint incorporated in a cast or plaster splint.

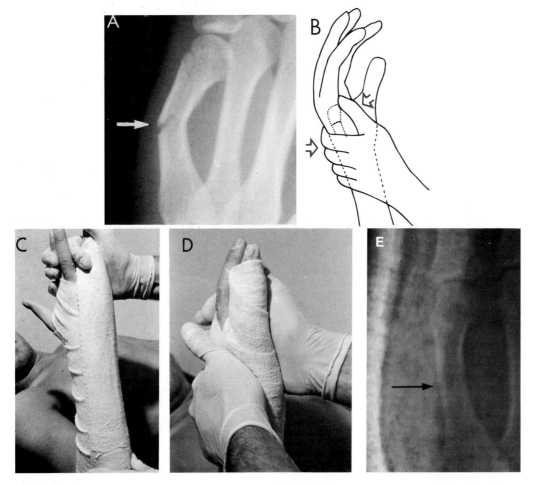

**Fig. 7–47.**
**A,** Fracture of the small finger metacarpal *(arrow).* **B,** Reduction is obtained by digital pressure against the distal fragment with counterpressure on the dorsum of the proximal fragment. **C** and **D,** Applying and molding the ulnar gutter splint. **E,** The end result.

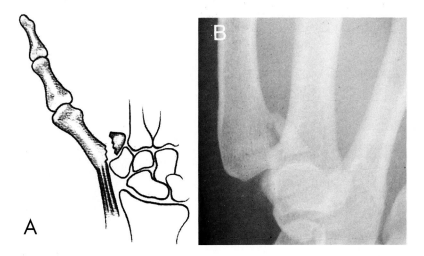

**Fig. 7–48.**
**A**, Bennett's fracture of the base of the thumb metacarpal. **B**, The roentgenographic appearance.

3 to 4 weeks. Slight shortening may be accepted. A short arm ulnar or radial "gutter" splint or a volar splint incorporating an aluminum splint and extending over the finger provides adequate immobilization.

Fractures of the neck of the metacarpal are common in the small finger (Fig. 7-47). These commonly occur in fistfights and are sometimes called "boxer's fractures." Clinically, there is swelling over the fracture site and depression of the "knuckle" of the affected finger. Impacted fractures with minimal angulation are treated with a compression dressing for 1 week followed by gradually increasing active exercises. Fractures with angulation over 25 to 30 degrees should be reduced. If closed reduction is successful, the finger is immobilized in a plaster or fiberglass gutter splint for 4 weeks. In the ring or small fingers, even if fractures of the metacarpal neck heal with a mild amount of angulation, the functional result is usually good as a result of the high mobility of the carpometacarpal joints of these fingers. However, the patient must be warned that the "knuckle" will never be as prominent. The same fracture in a child will usually correct itself with further growth. Open reduction is occasionally indicated in severely angulated fractures. Fractures of the index and long fingers are less forgiving than those of the ring and small fingers and should probably be referred if there is any doubt about the alignment.

*Bennett's fracture* is actually a fracture-dislocation that occurs at the carpometacarpal (CM) joint of the thumb (Fig. 7-48). The metacarpal is usually dislocated proximally because of the pull of the long abductor muscle that inserts at its base. This injury requires exact reduction to avoid disturbing the function of this

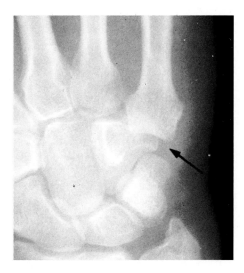

**Fig. 7–49.**
Fracture-dislocation of the small finger CM joint *(arrow),* sometimes called the "reverse Bennett" injury.

important joint. Most of these injuries are displaced and require reduction and internal fixation for the best overall results.

A similar fracture-dislocation occurs at the CM joint of the small finger (Fig. 7-49). Although not as potentially serious as the injury to the thumb, reduction and internal fixation are often required, nonetheless. Failure to recognize and properly treat the injury may lead to a weakness in grip because more power is provided by the ulnar side of the hand than the radial side.

The *Rolando fracture* is a comminuted intraarticular fracture of the base of the thumb metacarpal. It is often difficult to restore normal anatomic alignment to the fracture, even by open reduction. The prognosis for return of normal use of this joint after a Rolando fracture is often poor.

## Fractures of the Phalanges

Fractures of the proximal phalanx usually angulate to the volar aspect of the hand (Fig. 7-50). This angulation is produced by the pull of the intrinsic muscles. Oblique fractures of this bone are the most common cause of rotational deformity of the fingers (Fig. 7-51). Reduction of the transverse fracture is usually possible by traction on the flexed finger toward the tubercle of the scaphoid. Immobilization in moderate flexion with

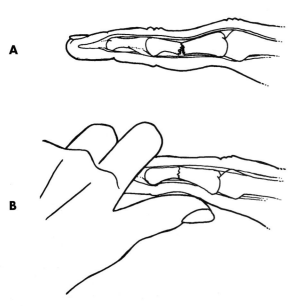

**Fig. 7–50.**
**A**, Fracture of the proximal phalanx. **B**, Reduction by flexion of the distal fragment. The position is maintained by a splint.

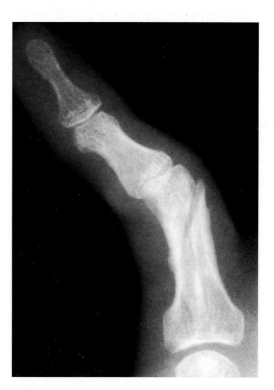

**Fig. 7–51.**
Oblique fracture of the proximal phalanx with malrotation. Always evaluate for proper rotation.

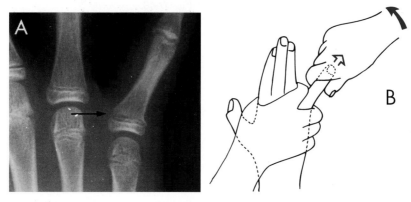

**Fig. 7–52.**
**A**, Epiphyseal fracture of the proximal phalanx of the small finger in the typical position of ulnar deviation. **B**, Reduction by traction and pressure against the finger in the web space.

a splint for 4 weeks is usually sufficient for healing to occur. Unstable displaced fractures usually require open reduction and internal fixation.

The common epiphyseal fracture of the base of the proximal phalanx of the small finger is usually a type II Salter fracture and is usually displaced into abduction (Fig. 7-52). It is reduced under local anesthesia by applying traction with the finger in slight flexion and then adducting the finger against a pencil or the physician's finger, which acts as a fulcrum. It is taped to the ring finger and immobilized with a padded splint for 4 weeks.

Fractures of the middle phalanx may angulate volarward or dorsally (Fig. 7-53). Traction with manipulation of the fracture will usually effect a reduction. The finger is splinted for 4 weeks.

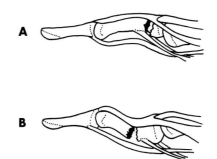

**Fig. 7–53.**
Fracture of the middle phalanx. If the fracture is proximal to the insertion of sublimis tendon, the fracture will tend to angulate into flexion (**A**). This fracture may require treatment in slight extension. Fractures distal to the sublimis insertion (**B**) often angulate into extension, and flexion is therefore required for reduction.

## DISLOCATIONS OF THE FINGERS

Metacarpophalangeal (MP) dislocations may be classified as simple or complex. Simple dislocations may be reduced by traction and manipulation (Fig. 7-54). If the MP joint is stable after reduction, "buddy taping" to the adjacent finger for 2 to 3 weeks is usually sufficient. If it is unstable, referral is indicated.

Complex MP dislocations usually have soft tissue interposed in the joint, or the metacarpal neck is buttonholed through a window in the soft tissue (Fig. 7-55). It is usually impossible to treat them by closed methods. Some improvement may seem apparent after the manipulation, but the joint does not "snap" back into place and does not feel reduced. Reduction of the complex MP dislocation is prevented by the soft tissue. The more traction and pressure applied to the finger, the tighter the soft tissue becomes. Open reduction is usually necessary.

Interphalangeal (IP) joint dislocations are common injuries and occur most often in the athlete (Fig. 7-56).

Distal IP joint dislocations are unusual. Dorsal PIP joint dislocations are the most common. They are usually reduced easily, under digital block if needed, by increasing the angular deformity, applying traction and digital

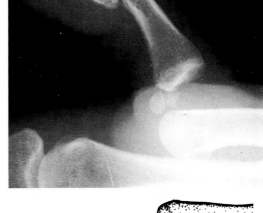

**Fig. 7–55.**
A, Complex MP dislocation. B, Soft-tissue interposition that may prevent reduction. (Remember: Push rather than pull to reduce most dislocations. Otherwise, a simple one may be converted to a complex one.)

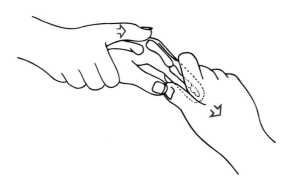

**Fig. 7–54.**
An MP dislocation that may be reduced by simple traction and digital pressure.

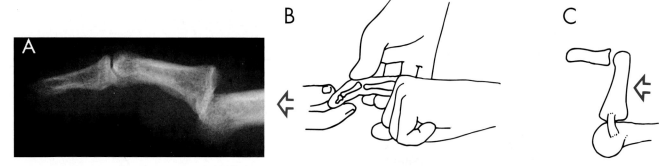

**Fig. 7–56.**
**A**, PIP dislocation. Traction and digital pressure are usually successful for reduction (**B**). Occasionally, the deformity must be increased before reduction can be accomplished (**C**).

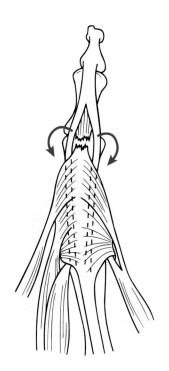

**Fig. 7–57.**
Central slip rupture. If this occurs, the lateral bands may eventually migrate around the condyles of the proximal phalanx past the axis of movement and become flexors of the PIP joint rather than extensors. This is called the boutonnierre deformity.

pressure to the distal portion, and manipulating it into flexion. Roentgenograms are always repeated after the reduction to exclude avulsion fractures. Dorsal PIPJ dislocations sometimes cause disruption of the volar plate although this usually heals and the joint is generally stable immediately after reduction. If the finger is stable after reduction, it may be taped to an adjacent finger for 3 to 4 weeks. If the dislocation is unstable, an avulsion fracture may be present, and the injury may represent a fracture-dislocation or ligament rupture rather than a simple dislocation. Examination may reveal some instability in the volar direction or mediolaterally. Special care of this injury is necessary, and referral is often indicated (see Chapter 15).

The rare volar PIP joint dislocation has the potential for rupture of the central slip and the formation of the boutonniere deformity (Fig. 7-57). This injury should be referred for extended splinting of the PIP joint in extension for 4 to 6 weeks allowing MCP and DIP motion.

## MISCELLANEOUS DISORDERS

### Carpometacarpal Boss

This abnormality is in the same area as the usual dorsal ganglion cyst although slightly distal to where the typical ganglion presents. The deformity is a bony prominence that develops at the base of the index and long finger metacarpals (Fig. 7-58). The etiology is unknown, although repetitive trauma may be a factor. A spur or thickening develops at these CM joints and may be-

come painful. Treatment is usually conservative with splinting and antiinflammatory medication. Surgical removal is occasionally necessary.

### Writer's (Occupational) Cramps

This is a disorder in which the individual develops pain when performing a habitual motor activity. Typically, as the individual begins to write or type, pain develops

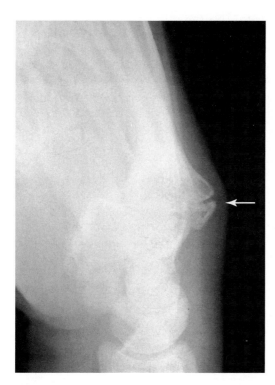

**Fig. 7–58.**
The carpometacarpal boss.

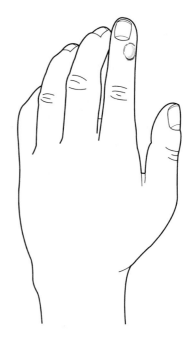

**Fig. 7–59.**
Mucous cyst. The lesion often develops next to an osteophyte at the DIP joint, usually to one side of the extensor tendon insertion. It may cause pressure furrowing of the nail. It may occasionally drain a clear fluid spontaneously and then heal. The cyst may be aspirated but should not be opened. Excision is sometimes required.

that increases in severity with more use. Eventually, the activity becomes impossible. The etiology remains unknown, although a variety of neurologic and psychiatric causes have been suggested. The condition may be similar to "spasmodic" torticollis in the neck. Most attempts at treatment fail, including changing pen sizes, desk angles, and even psychological counseling. Sometimes, the only cure is a complete change in jobs.

## Mucous Cysts

Mucous cysts are benign lesions that are similar to ganglia. They usually develop on the dorsal aspect of the DIP joints of the index or long fingers and are usually associated with osteoarthritis and osteophytes of the joint (Fig. 7-59). Heberden's nodes are also commonly present. Mucous cysts may produce grooving of the nail of the affected digit. They are characteristically located on one side of the extensor tendon. Treatment ranges from needle aspiration followed by massage, to excision, and there is a fairly high recurrence rate regardless of treatment.

## Raynaud's Disease and Raynaud's Phenomenon

*Raynaud's disease* is a benign idiopathic paroxysmal vasospasm that occurs mainly in young women and usually affects the fingers and toes. The term "disease"

is used when no cause can be found. The "attacks" often occur daily and are often precipitated by cold or emotional stress. They are typically symmetric and bilateral and are relieved by warming. Extreme pallor is followed by cyanosis and then by hyperemia. Serious sequelae are rare, although small areas of gangrene occasionally occur if the disorder is of many years' duration. Treatment is directed at avoiding cold situations that trigger vasoconstriction. Reassurance, dressing sensibly (often with gloves), and avoiding sudden temperature changes are important. Stress management and avoiding tobacco products are also necessary. Medication is usually not required.

*Raynaud's phenomenon* (or secondary Raynaud's disease) consists of similar attacks of ischemia of the digits that occur in the course of other diseases, mainly scleroderma and other connective tissue diseases. It is often seen before the characteristic skin changes develop. Early on, however, it may be impossible to differentiate benign Raynaud's disease from scleroderma with Raynaud's phenomenon. (β-Blockers like propranolol may cause a similar peripheral vasospasm, as may ergot preparations, amphetamines, and nitroglycerin.)

## Hypothenar Hammer Syndrome

Occlusion of the ulnar artery at the wrist may produce symptoms similar to those seen with ulnar tunnel

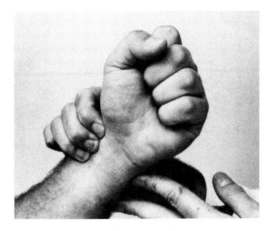

**Fig. 7–60.**
Allen's test. The hand is elevated. The radial and ulnar arteries are occluded, and the patient clenches the fist for 20 seconds. The arteries are released one at a time. Release of either artery will usually allow rapid restoration of the circulation to the hand. If one artery is occluded, however, revascularization of the hand will be delayed or absent.

syndrome. This disorder is usually secondary to some repetitive trauma to the ulnar aspect of the hand, such as what occurs when the hand is used as a mallet. This produces a thrombosis of the ulnar artery and results in ischemic manifestations such as pain, pallor, paresthesias, cold intolerance, and decreased temperature of the affected digits. Local tenderness may be present and a mass may be palpable. Allen's test is often positive (Fig. 7-60).

Treatment is mainly symptomatic and is directed at avoiding the offending practice. The symptoms may resolve in many cases without any further treatment. Vasodilators and sympathetic blocks are often tried. Surgical intervention may be necessary if symptoms fail to respond to conservative treatment.

## BIBLIOGRAPHY

Abrams RA, Botte MJ: Hand infections: treatment recommendations for specific types, *J Am Acad Orthop Surg* 4:219-230, 1996.

Allen MJ: Conservative management of fingertip injuries in adults, *Hand* 12:257, 1980.

Barton NJ: Fractures of the hand, *J Bone Joint Surg Br* 66:159, 1984.

Benson LS, Ptaszek AJ: Injection versus surgery in the treatment of trigger finger, *J Hand Surg Am* 22:138-144, 1997.

Benson LS, Williams CS, Kable M: Dupuytren's contracture, *J Am Acad Orthop Surg* 6:24-35, 1998.

Bishop AT, Beckenbaugh RD: Fracture of the hamate hook, *J Hand Surg Am* 13:135, 1988.

Borden S: Traumatic bowing of the forearm in children, *J Bone Joint Surg Am* 56:611, 1974.

Boswick JA, Kilgore ES, Watson HK, et al: Symposium: Dupuytren's contracture, *Contemp Orthop* 16:71, 1988.

Bowers WH, Hurst LC: Gamekeeper's thumb, *J Bone Joint Surg Am* 59:519, 1977.

Boyes JH: *Bunnell's surgery of the hand*, ed 5, Philadelphia, 1970, JB Lippincott Co.

Carey PJ et al: Both-bone forearm fractures in children, *Orthopedics* 15:1015-1023, 1992.

Clay NR et al: Need the thumb be immobilized in scaphoid fractures? *J Bone Joint Surg Br* 73:828-832, 1991.

Conklin JE, White WL: Stenosing tenosynovitis and its possible relation to the carpal tunnel syndrome, *Surg Clin North Am* 40:531, 1960.

DeOliveira JC: Barton's fractures, *J Bone Joint Surg Am* 55:586, 1973.

Dias JJ et al: Suspected scaphoid fractures, *J Bone Joint Surg Br* 72:98, 1990.

Dinham JM, Meggitt BF: Trigger thumbs in children, *J Bone Joint Surg Br* 56:153, 1974.

Entin MA: Repair of extensor mechanism of the hand, *Surg Clin North Am* 40:275, 1960.

Fassler PR: Fingertip injuries: evaluation and treatment, *J Am Acad Orthop Surg* 4:84-92, 1996.

Fisk GR: The wrist, *J Bone Joint Surg Br* 66:396, 1984.

Flatt AE: *The care of minor hand injuries*, ed 3, St Louis, 1972, CV Mosby Co.

Fuhr JE, Farrow A, Nelson HS: Vitamin $B_6$ levels in patients with carpal tunnel syndrome, *Arch Surg* 124:1329, 1989.

Gebuhr P et al: Isolated ulnar shaft fractures, *J Bone Joint Surg Br* 74:757-760, 1992.

Geilberman RH et al: Current concepts review. Fractures and non-unions of the carpal scaphoid, *J Bone Joint Surg Am* 71:1560, 1989.

Hadley NM: Illness in the workplace: the challenge of musculoskeletal symptoms, *J Hand Surg Am* 10:451, 1985.

Henderson JJ, Arafa MA: Carpometacarpal dislocation. An easily missed diagnosis, *J Bone Joint Surg Br* 69:212, 1987.

Herndon WA, Hershey SL, Lambdin CS: Thrombosis of the ulnar artery in the hand, *J Bone Joint Surg Am* 57:994, 1975.

Hill NA: Dupuytren's contracture: current concepts review, *J Bone Joint Surg Am* 67:1439, 1985.

Jones WA: Beware the sprained wrist. The incidence and diagnosis of scapholunate instability, *J Bone Joint Surg Br* 70:293, 1988.

Kaplan EB: *Functional and surgical anatomy of the hand*, ed 2, Philadelphia, 1965, JB Lippincott.

Koman LA, Urbaniak JR: Ulnar artery insufficiency: a guide to treatment, *J Hand Surg* 6:16, 1981.

Kuschner SH et al: Tinel's sign and Phalen's test in carpal tunnel syndrome, *Orthopedics* 15:1297-1309, 1992.

Leddy JP: Infections of the upper extremity, *J Hand Surg* 11:294, 1986.

Louis DS, Huebner JJ, Hankin FM: Rupture and displacement of the ulnar collateral ligament of the metacarpophalangeal joint of the thumb: preoperative diagnosis, *J Bone Joint Surg Am* 68:1320, 1986.

McKerrell J et al: Boxers fractures: conservative or operative management, *J Trauma* 27:486, 1987.

Milford L: The hand. In Crenshaw AH, editor: *Campbell's operative orthopaedics,* ed 5, St Louis, 1971, CV Mosby Co.

Millender LH, Conlon M: An approach to the work-related disorders of the upper extremity, *J Am Acad Orthop Surg* 4:134-142, 1996.

Muddu BN, Morrias MA, Fahmy NR: The treatment of ganglia, *J Bone Joint Surg Br* 72:147, 1990.

Nelson CL, Sawmiller S, Phalen GS: Ganglions of the wrist and hand, *J Bone Joint Surg Am* 54:1459, 1972.

Osterman AL: The double crush syndrome, *Orthop Clin North Am* 19:147, 1988.

Posner MA. Compressive ulnar neuropathies at the elbow I: etiology and diagnosis, *J Am Acad Orthop Surg* 6:282-288, 1998.

Posner MA: Compressive ulnar neuropathies at the elbow II: treatment, *J Am Acad Orthop Surg* 6:289-297, 1998.

Putzakis MJ, Wilkins J, Bassett RL: Surgical findings in clenched-fist injuries, *Clin Orthop* 220:237, 1987.

Rang MD: *Children's fractures,* ed 2, Philadelphia, 1983, JB Lippincott.

Rayan GM, Flournoy DJ: Chronic paronychia due to multiple pyogenic organisms, *J Hand Surg Am* 13:790, 1988.

Reckling FW: Unstable fracture-dislocations of the forearm (Monteggia and Galeazzi lesions), *J Bone Joint Surg* 64:857, 1982.

Rockwood CA, Green DP: *Fractures in adults,* Philadelphia, 1984, JB Lippincott.

Rodrigo JJ, Kiebauer JJ, Doyle JR: Treatment of Dupuytren's contracture, *J Bone Joint Surg Am* 58:380, 1976.

Roysam GS: The distal radio-ulnar joint in Colles fractures, *J Bone and Joint Surg Br* 75:58-61, 1993.

Sakellarides HT, DeWeese JW: Instability of the metacarpophalangeal joint of the thumb, *J Bone Joint Surg Am* 58:106, 1976.

Scheyer RD, Haas DC: Pyridoxine in carpal tunnel syndrome, *Lancet* 1:42, 1984.

Schwartz RG: Cumulative trauma disorders, *Orthopedics* 15:1051-1057, 1992.

Slater RR, Bynum DK: Diagnosis and treatment of carpal tunnel syndrome, *Orthop Review* 22:1095-1105, 1993.

Smith RJ: Post-traumatic instability of the metacarpophalangeal joint of the thumb, *J Bone Joint Surg Am* 59:14, 1977.

Spinner RJ, Bachman JW, Amadio PC: The many faces of carpal tunnel syndrome, *Mayo Clin Proc* 64:829, 1989.

Stark HH et al: Fracture of the hook of the hamate, *J Bone Joint Surg Am* 71:1202, 1989.

Upton AR, McComas AJ: The double crush in nerve entrapment syndromes, *Lancet* 2:359, 1973.

Villar RN et al: Three years after Colles fracture: a prospective review, *J Bone Joint Surg Br* 69:635, 1987.

Walsh HP, McLaren CA, Owen R: Galeazzi fractures in children, *J Bone Joint Surg Br* 69:730, 1987.

Wehbe MA, Schneider LH: Mallet fractures, *J Bone Joint Surg Am* 66:658, 1984.

Weiss AP, Akelman E, Tabatabai M: Treatment of de Quervain's disease, *J Hand Surg Am* 19:595-598, 1994.

Weiss AP, Sachar K, Gendreau M: Conservative management of carpal tunnel syndrome: a re-examination of steroid injection and splinting, *J Hand Surg Am* 19:410-415, 1994.

Zook EG, Guy RJ, Russell RC: A study of nailbed injuries: causes, treatment and prognosis, *J Hand Surg Am* 9:247, 1984.

# CHAPTER 8

# The Back

Back pain is one of the most common conditions requiring medical treatment. It is also the most expensive ailment for those between the ages of 30 and 60 years and one of the most difficult to treat. Back pain may be the result of a variety of disorders, including gynecologic, genitourinary, and gastrointestinal diseases, but the most common causes are disorders of the lumbar disc.

## ANATOMY

The vertebrae, discs, and ligaments of the dorsal and lumbar spine are similar in most respects to their counterparts in the cervical spine. The lumbar vertebrae are larger and thicker, however, because of their weight-bearing function (Fig. 8-1). Anterior and posterior longitudinal ligaments are applied to the respective surfaces of the vertebral bodies, and posterior stability is aided by supraspinous and interspinous ligaments and the ligamentum flavum. The discs account for over one third of the total height of the lumbar spine and account for most of the normal lordosis.

Spinal nerves exit the canal by passing through intervertebral foramina, each foramen consisting of the inferior aspect of the pedicle above and the superior aspect of the pedicle below the level of exit. In the lumbar spine, disc disease usually affects the nerve root exiting one level below because that is the nerve that actually passes over the disc (Fig. 8-2). Thus a herniated disc between the fourth and fifth lumbar vertebrae commonly affects the fifth nerve root and not the fourth.

## EXAMINATION

Examination of the back is performed with the patient standing, sitting on the examining table, and lying in the supine position. The patient is first observed in the standing position. Any list or excessive kyphosis or lordosis is noted. Next, the chest is measured in full inspiration and expiration. Normal expansion is greater than 5 cm but may be less than 2.5 cm in ankylosing spondylitis. The iliac crests are then palpated to determine whether they are level. If they are not, footboards of varying thicknesses may be placed under the shorter extremity to assess the amount of shoe lift necessary to level the pelvis. (Up to 2 cm difference seems to be well tolerated.) The shoulders are also observed for evenness, although the dominant shoulder is often lower in the normal population. The spine and sacroiliac joints are palpated and percussed for spasm and tenderness. Any varicosities in the lower extremities are also noted.

The range of motion is then slowly tested. With the patient bending forward as far as possible, flexion is measured as the distance between the fingertips and the floor. This calculation represents a combination of lumbar spine mobility and hamstring flexibility. While the patient is flexed forward, the back is viewed from behind to detect any scoliosis and from the side to detect any persistence of the normal lumbar lordosis that might be present secondary to protective muscle spasm. Extension and right and left bending are then measured. Pain on bending *toward* the affected side commonly signifies disc disease, whereas pain on bending *away* from the affected side commonly denotes muscle strain. The gait pattern is then observed, and the ability to walk on the heels (L5 root) and balls of the feet (S1 root) is tested.

With the patient in the sitting position, a complete neurologic examination of the lower extremities is per-

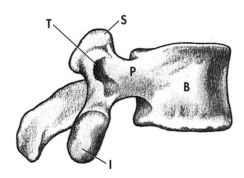

**Fig. 8–1.**
A typical lumbar vertebra: *S* = superior articular facet; *I* = inferior articular facet; *P* = pedicle; *T* = transverse process; *B* = body.

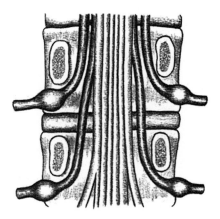

**Fig. 8–2.**
Relationship of nerve roots to discs in the lumbar spine.

**Fig. 8–3.**
The lower extremities are measured between the anterior superior iliac spines and the medial malleoli with the leg in neutral alignment. Discrepancies under 1 cm are probably not significant.

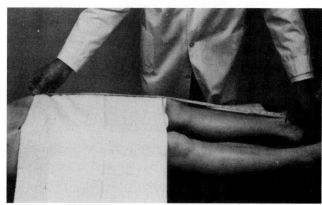

formed. Reflexes, motor strength, and sensation are tested. The thighs and calves are measured to detect any muscular atrophy. Discrepancies of ½ inch in the thigh and ½ inch in the calf are significant. Straight leg raising in the sitting position is also tested and compared with straight leg raising tests that will be performed in the supine position. The peripheral pulses are palpated and any abnormalities in the vascular status of the extremity noted.

With the patient in the supine position, the hip is placed through a full range of motion and thoroughly tested to rule out primary hip abnormality. The straight-leg–raising tests are then performed, and the leg lengths are measured (Fig. 8-3). Next, with the patient on the side, manual pressure is applied to the iliac crest (pelvic compression test). Reproduction of pain in the sacroiliac joints or symphysis pubis with this maneuver may suggest disorders of these areas.

## ROENTGENOGRAPHIC ANATOMY

An evaluation of disorders of the lumbar spine should include a standard roentgenographic examination. The roentgenographic features are well visualized by the following: anteroposterior view (Fig. 8-4, *A*), lateral view (Fig. 8-4, *B*), and oblique views in both directions (Fig. 8-5). In addition, a spot lateral view of the lumbosacral space may be necessary.

## LUMBAR DISC SYNDROMES

The intervertebral disc is probably the source of most back pain, and the pattern of disc deterioration in the lumbar spine is similar to what occurs in the cervical spine. Some 95% of disc lesions in the lumbar spine oc-

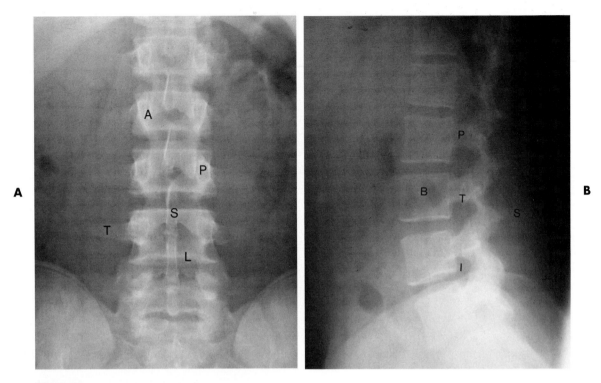

**Fig. 8–4.**
Anteroposterior (**A**) and lateral (**B**) view of the lumbar spine: *S* = spinous process; *P* = pedicle; *T* = transverse process; *L* = lamina; *A* = articular facet joint; *B* = body; *I* = intervertebral foramen.

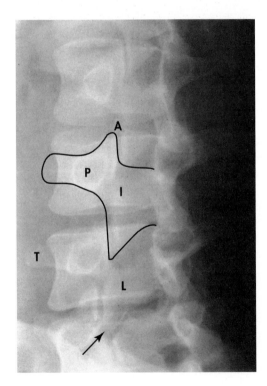

**Fig. 8–5.**
Oblique view: *A* = articular facet joint; *I* = isthmus or pars interarticularis; *T* = transverse process; *L* = lamina; *P* = pedicle. The oblique view visualizes the so-called "Scottie dog." Spondylolysis occurs through the isthmus *(arrow).*

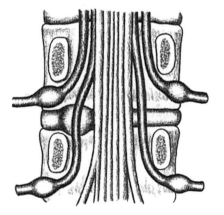

**Fig. 8–6.**
Lumbar disc protrusion. Note that the herniation affects the root that exits one level below.

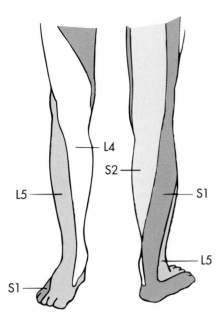

**Fig. 8–7.**
Dermatomes of the lower extremity.

cur at the fourth and fifth spaces, with most of the remainder occurring at the third space. With normal aging and repetitive trauma, progressive degeneration of the nucleus pulposus occurs and may lead to protrusion or complete extrusion of a portion of the disc contents into the neural canal. This usually occurs in the area of greatest weakness at the posterolateral aspect of the disc (Fig. 8-6). Chronic disc deterioration (spondylosis) may also occur and result in spur formation, disc space narrowing, and degenerative changes in the facet joints and between adjacent vertebral bodies. In addition to anatomical causes, biochemical and inflammatory factors may play some role in the development of back and leg pain from disc disease.

Disc herniation is most common in the third and fourth decades and is uncommon before the age of 20 years.

A rare but serious complication of lumbar disc disease is the *cauda equina syndrome*. This results from a massive central disc protrusion and may produce variable degrees of permanent paralysis in the lower extremities. Bladder and bowel function may also be severely impaired. This condition is a true emergency and usually demands immediate surgery.

### Clinical Features

Disc disease may result in several overlapping clinical syndromes: (1) mild herniation without nerve root compression, (2) herniation with nerve root compression, (3) cauda equina syndrome, (4) chronic degenerative disease with or without leg symptoms, and (5) spinal steno-

sis. The onset of symptoms is variable. One specific traumatic episode may produce symptoms, but because of the progressive nature of the disease process in the disc, the symptoms usually occur gradually. The most common complaint is low back pain, which is often deep and aching in nature. The pain is aggravated by activity and relieved by rest. Coughing, sneezing, or other actions that increase the stress on the disc tend to intensify the pain. The back pain is often localized near the disc and may be referred to the iliac crest or buttock. It is probably the result of stretching of the annulus by the expanding, protruding disc. *Radicular* pain occurs when the disc protrudes far enough to press on the adjacent nerve root. Nerve root pain is usually quite intense. Often, if the disc herniates completely (extrudes), the low back pain may be relieved, but the leg pain intensifies.

Low back pain may occur in combination with radiating pain, or the two pain patterns may occur separately. Radicular pain characteristically spreads over the buttock and passes down the posterior or posterolateral aspect of the thigh and calf and may even spread onto the foot. Both types of pain usually improve with bed rest. If little or no relief of pain occurs with rest, inorganic causes should be considered. Relentless pain that is not relieved or may even be aggravated by recumbency suggests a spinal cord tumor.

Paresthesias in the form of numbness and tingling are common and are usually more marked in the distal portion of the extremity. They may follow a specific dermatome pattern (Fig. 8-7).

Examination often reveals restriction of low back motion. Bending toward the affected side commonly exacerbates the pain. Variable degrees of local tenderness and muscle guarding are present. In an attempt to relieve pressure or tension on the nerve root, the patient may list or bend away from the painful side and stand with the affected hip and knee slightly flexed. A characteristic clinical picture may be present, depending on the level of nerve root involvement (Table 8-1). The sensory examination may reveal diminished sensation along the affected dermatome, although the sensory examination is usually not helpful. The various tests measuring sciatic nerve root tension are commonly positive (Fig. 8-8).

### Special Studies

The diagnosis usually becomes apparent on the basis of the history and physical examination. Early disc herniation may be difficult to differentiate from other causes of back pain, however.

1. Plain roentgenograms are not indicated before 2 to 4 weeks. They are usually normal.
2. Electromyography, computed tomography (CT), magnetic resonance imaging (MRI), or myelogra-

**TABLE 8–1.**

Clinical Features of Common Lumbar Disc Syndromes

| Disc | Pain | Sensory Change | Motor Weakness Atrophy | Reflex Change |
|---|---|---|---|---|
| L3-L4 (L4 root) | Low back, posterolateral aspect of thigh, across patella, anteromedial aspect of leg | Anterior aspect of knee, anteromedial aspect of leg | Quadriceps (knee extension) | Knee jerk |
| L4-L5 (L5 root) | Lateral, posterolateral aspect of thigh, leg | Lateral aspect of leg, dorsum of foot, first web space, great toe | Great toe extension, ankle dorsiflexion, heel walking difficult (footdrop may occur) | Minor (posterior tibial jerk depressed) |
| L5-S1 (S1 root) | Posterolateral aspect of thigh, leg, heel | Posterior aspect of calf, heel, lateral aspect of foot (3 toes) | Calf, plantar-flexion of foot, great toe; toe walking weak | Ankle jerk |
| Cauda equina syndrome (massive midline protrusion) | Low back, thigh, legs; often bilateral | Thighs, legs, feet, perineum; often bilateral | Variable; may be bowel, bladder incontinence | Ankle jerk (may be bilateral) |

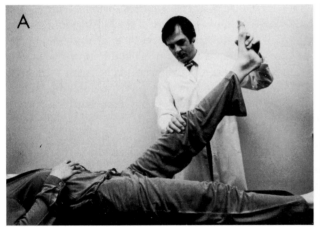 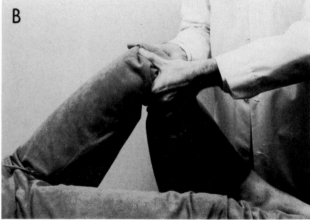

**Fig. 8–8.**

Tests of nerve root tension, the most important examination in herniation of the lumbar intervertebral disc. **A,** The foot is slowly raised, keeping the knee straight, until sciatic pain is produced. A positive test includes the following: (1) pain produced before 70 degrees is reached, (2) aggravation of the pain by dorsiflexion of the ankle, and (3) relief of the pain by flexion of the knee. **B,** The popliteal compression test is then performed by flexing the knee and applying pressure to the popliteal nerve in the fossa. Reproduction of leg pain by this maneuver is further evidence of nerve root irritation. If the patient can extend the leg to 90 degrees while sitting but the same test is impossible in the supine position, pain magnification should be suspected. If raising the leg on the contralateral side reproduces pain in the affected leg, disc herniation should be strongly suspected.

phy are used to confirm the diagnosis (Fig. 8-9). They are not usually indicated for at least 4 to 6 weeks. The myelogram is not a procedure without some morbidity, and all of these tests are costly. They are indicated: (1) if surgical intervention is being contemplated or (2) if other, more serious spinal pathology is suspected. Myelography is gradually being replaced by the other imaging studies. If it is performed, spinal fluid analysis may show a slight increase in protein content.

3. Discography is considered to be of only limited value.

**Note**: The number of symptomatic conditions discovered by special studies but not suspected clinically is very small. These tests should only be adjuncts to the clinical assessment.

### Treatment

The initial treatment is always conservative. Bed rest is indicated for the first 1 to 2 weeks in the treatment of acute disc herniation (mainly if leg pain is present), followed by a careful exercise program. While the patient is in bed, the hips and knees are kept moderately flexed. Lying on the abdomen, which increases the lumbar lordosis, is avoided. Hip flexion and pelvic tilt ex-

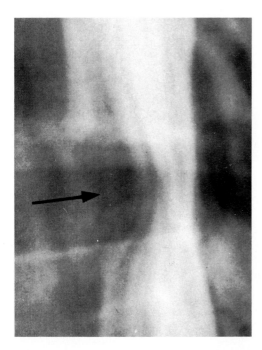

**Fig. 8–9.**
Abnormal lumbar myelogram revealing a large extradural defect *(arrow)* in the dye column that is consistent with disc herniation.

ercises are begun within the limits of pain (Fig. 8-10). NSAIDs, analgesics, and moist heat are used as necessary. If improvement occurs, which it does in the majority of cases, gradual resumption of activity is allowed. A lumbosacral corset may be temporarily used. (There is no evidence that continued use of any brace promotes back weakness, however, especially if the patient adheres to an exercise program.) Recurrences are prevented by a proper exercise program and the avoidance of stress to the lower part of the back (Fig. 8-11).

Caudal or epidural cortisone injections are often used. They may help relieve residual radicular pain. They may have no effect on acute leg pain from ongoing disc pressure. The majority of patients will improve with conservative treatment. What happens to the disc material that has herniated is unknown. It is theorized that it may act as a foreign body and be absorbed or transformed into scar tissue.

Disc removal is reserved for those patients with major or progressing neurologic deficits or those with intractable leg pain who fail to respond to conservative management for at least 6 weeks. There are three general ways of removing disc tissue:

1. *Laminotomy* ("laminectomy"). The disc is removed through a small incision, and the nerve is explored under direct vision. A small portion of the lamina is sometimes removed for better visualization. With a positive history, physical findings, myelography (or similar study) and electromyelography (EMG), there is a 90% to 95% success rate for surgery. In the absence of one or more of these, the cure rate for disc removal by any means declines considerably. Patients must also be cautioned that although their leg pain will usually disappear postoperatively, some mild intermittent low back pain may persist.

    *Microdiscectomy* is the same procedure except that an operating microscope is used and the incision and surgical exposure are minimized. Advocates of this procedure note that there is less postoperative pain and a shorter hospital stay. A disadvantage to the procedure may be the narrower view afforded to the disc, nerve root, and adjacent bony structures.

2. *Automated percutaneous discectomy.* In this procedure, a small suction cutter is used to remove the disc. The instrument is placed through a cannula that has been passed through the flank to the posterolateral aspect of the disc under fluoroscopic control. It is performed through a very small incision, and no dissection or bone removal is needed. The disc is actually removed anterior to the herniation. The procedure's success rate is 70% to 85%. One of the reasons for failure is that portions of the disc extruded or trapped in the spinal canal (or pressing on the nerve root) are never directly removed as they are with posterior surgery (laminectomy, microdiscectomy). An advantage is that the procedure has few side effects and can often be performed under local anesthesia, which makes recovery rapid.

3. *Chemonucleolysis.* In 1964 enzymatic dissolution of the nucleus pulposus was introduced for the treatment of a herniated lumbar disc. The procedure involves injecting the affected disc with chymopapain, a derivative of the papaya plant that digests the disc. It was developed partly because of its "noninvasive" nature and partly because of a relatively high rate of poor results in some series after traditional laminectomy and disc excision. Preliminary reports of its use seemed encouraging, but a double-blind study left its efficacy in doubt, and it was removed from general use in the United States. It continued to be used in other countries and some centers in the United States and has recently been re-released.

    Its main advantages are a shorter hospital stay and a short convalescence. The most common complication from the procedure is a relatively severe anaphylactoid reaction in approximately 1% of the cases. Its main disadvantages are that the pathologic process being treated is never directly

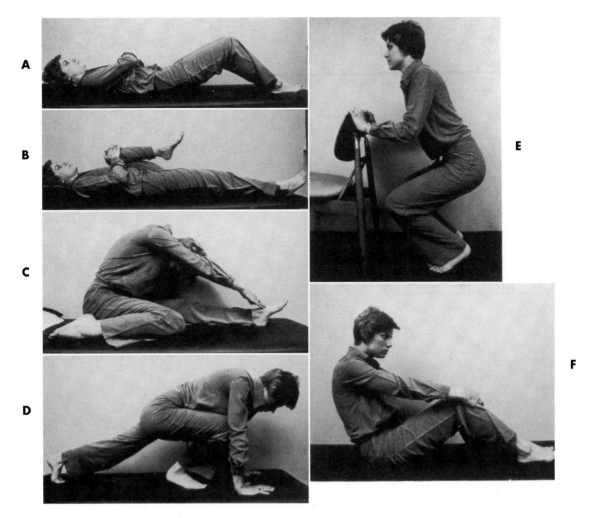

**Fig. 8–10.**
Low back exercises. **A**, Pelvic tilt performed to decrease the lumbar lordosis and raise the anterior aspect of the pelvis. The small of the back is pressed to the floor and the abdominal and buttock muscles are tightened. **B**, Hip flexion, performed to stretch the tight posterior spinal musculature and unload the posterior disc. Each knee is drawn up and pulled firmly to the chest several times and held for 10 to 20 seconds. The exercise is then repeated with both knees. After the acute pain has subsided, the remainder of the exercises are performed: **C**, Hamstring stretching exercises; **D**, Hip flexor stretching exercises; **E**, Quadriceps strengthening and heel cord stretching exercise; and **F**, Abdominal strengthening exercise (sit-ups, which may be partial). All exercises are performed on a carpeted floor and should be repeated in sets of five to ten at least three times daily.

visualized and the patient with extruded disc material will certainly not benefit from its use.

Its success rate is about 75%. Enthusiasm for this procedure is waning, partly because of the complication rate and partly because of the lower success rate. Like percutaneous discectomy, its less invasive nature also carries a greater risk of overuse.

### *Summary*

Surgery is effective in well over 85% of cases but patient selection is the key. When advising treatment, the following well-known facts should always be kept in mind:

1. There is no long-term difference in the outcome of most patients treated conservatively (by nature) and those treated surgically. The major benefit to surgery is that the intense pain in the leg is relieved sooner.
2. Disc removal by any means does not cure back pain, only leg pain.
3. Having sciatic nerve root pain does not assume surgery.
4. Before any procedure is contemplated, *radicular* symptoms should have been present for at least 6 weeks and should have failed to improve

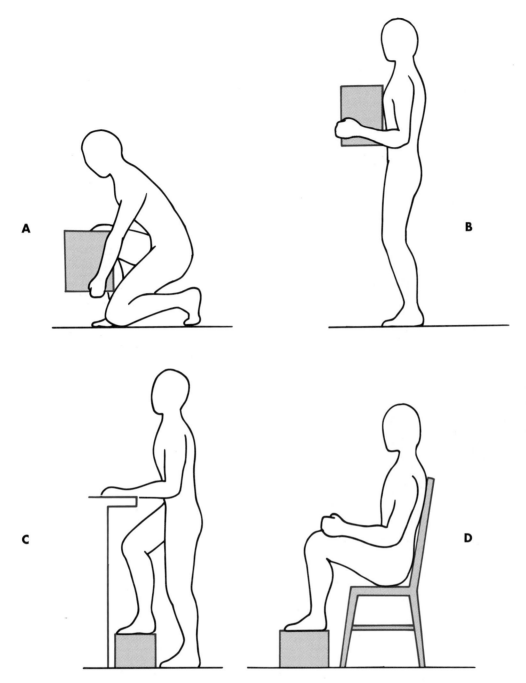

**Fig. 8–11.**
General postural instructions. Patients should be instructed to do the following. **A,** Bend the knees and hips and keep the back straight when lifting. **B,** Hold objects close to the body when carrying. **C,** Place one foot on a stool when standing. **D,** Keep the knees higher than the hips when sitting, and keep the back straight when standing by "tucking in" the abdomen and tightening the buttocks to decrease swayback. In addition, they should avoid high-heeled shoes and sleeping on the abdomen, activities that increase lordosis.

with at least 2 weeks of complete bed rest. If this rule is strictly followed, the majority of patients will get better on their own without surgery.

5. Cauda equina syndrome (back pain, bilateral sciatica, saddle anesthesia, motor weakness sometimes with incontinence) is the only absolute indication for disc removal.

## Chronic Lumbar Disc Disease

A high percentage of adults over the age of 40 years have degenerative disc disease at one or more levels on roentgenographic examination (Fig. 8-12). Significant thinning of the disc accompanied by osteophyte formation is often present. These roentgenographic changes are common in the general population and are present in many asymptomatic individuals. Degenerative changes in the adjacent facet joints and surrounding

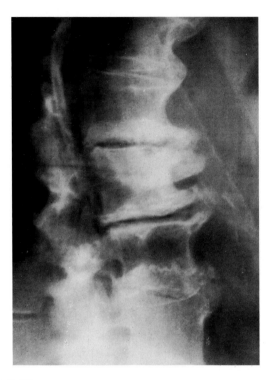

**Fig. 8–12.**
Chronic degenerative disc disease in an adult with only minimal symptoms.

soft tissue inflammation may, however, lead to intermittent low back pain and even nerve root irritation or compression with leg pain.

Pain of this nature will usually respond to conservative management. NSAIDs, rest, moist heat, and the use of a lumbosacral corset may be the only treatment necessary. Exercises, education, and correction of postural problems are important. Risk factors associated with chronic back pain, such as smoking and poor physical conditioning, should be addressed. A physical therapist can be helpful in this regard. When signs of nerve root irritation with radicular pain are present, compression of the root by a small, acute, soft disc herniation or degenerative spur should be suspected. The leg pain often responds well to epidural pain blocks. Surgical intervention is occasionally indicated to relieve nerve pressure. Arthrodesis of the adjacent vertebrae may rarely be indicated to relieve chronic low back pain by stabilizing the degenerated painful disc segment (see Chapter 18). Conservative treatment is usually successful in most cases, however.

## The Facet Syndrome

The small articular facet joints of the spine have occasionally been implicated as a cause of chronic low back pain. They may be affected because of disc thinning and even develop arthritis. The diagnosis is difficult to make, and some doubt its existence. The patient is often one who has a long history of chronic spine pain that has not responded to the traditional methods of management. Clinically, there may be local facet tenderness and pain on side bending.

To alleviate the symptoms, injection and even denervation of these joints has occasionally been performed. The results of these treatments are only modestly successful.

## LUMBAR STRAIN

Muscular or ligamentous injury is a common cause of low back pain. It may follow single or multiple traumatic episodes. Incomplete muscular tears or ligament sprains occur and lead to pain and tenderness over the affected area. The simple acute injury usually heals quickly and responds well to brief rest and symptomatic treatment. When the injury is superimposed on a chronic pattern of low back pain or lumbar disc disease, however, the course is often more protracted. A variety of factors predispose to chronic low back pain. Obesity, poor muscular tone, smoking, faulty work habits, the wearing of high-heeled shoes, and the lack of a daily exercise program are among the contributing factors. The center of gravity of the body may become

shifted forward, which leads to an increase in the lumbar lordosis. This places an added strain on the discs, ligaments, and muscles to maintain an upright posture. The condition is also commonly seen in teenagers who are vigorous weightlifters.

Obesity contributes to chronic low back pain in other ways. First, it is known that intraabdominal pressure aids the erector spinae muscles in keeping the lumbar spine erect and decreases intradiscal pressure. Obese patients have poor abdominal muscular tone. Obese patients also typically have an increase in their lumbar lordosis, which adds further stress to the lower part of the back.

With a daily program of proper postural exercises, weight loss, and a general exercise program, most patients with chronic back pain will be able to rehabilitate the lower part of the back. The use of modalities in physical therapy is discouraged. Full cooperation is necessary.

**Note**: The term *lumbar strain* is often used as a "wastebasket" diagnosis. An exact diagnosis of low back pain in many cases of this nature may be difficult. Muscle strain, ligament sprain, and mild early disc herniation or degeneration may all present with similar clinical findings. Regardless of the cause, the initial treatment is the same. A short (1 to 2 days) period of rest and mild analgesics followed by a gradual return to activities may be all that is needed. Walking or other similar aerobic exercise is started early to prevent generalized cardiovascular and musculoskeletal deterioration. Patients with chronic back pain benefit from postural back exercises and correction of obesity. Relaxation techniques are sometimes helpful. Active participation by the patient is most important. Proper lifting and bending habits are stressed. Only the acute disc herniation benefits from bed rest.

## ISTHMIC SPONDYLOLISTHESIS

Spondylolisthesis is a disorder, usually in the lumbar spine, in which one vertebra gradually slips on another. Several types have been described (congenital, degenerative, pathologic, traumatic, and spondylolytic). However, most spondylolisthesis is secondary to spondylolysis, which represents a fibrous defect in the pars interarticularis or isthmus of the vertebra (Fig. 8-13). A hereditary predisposition to develop this defect is usually manifested by repetitive stresses to the lower part of the back. This causes a fatigue fracture at the isthmus that fails to heal, resulting in a fibrous nonunion. Most common at L5-S1, it develops in the teen years but may not become symptomatic until years later, if at all. The defect is often associated with lumbosacral anomalies such as transitional vertebrae. There is an increased incidence in football players and gymnasts. Spondylolisthesis is classified according to the amount of forward slippage of the affected vertebra (Fig. 8-14).

### Clinical Features

Spondylolysis may be symptomatic even without spondylolisthesis, and both conditions may be associated with lumbar disc herniation. The disorder is often asymptomatic, however, and is commonly discovered incidentally in adults when roentgenograms are taken for other purposes. When it is seen on roentgenograms taken as a part of a routine evaluation for back pain, it is often difficult to determine whether or not it is playing any role in the patient's complaints.

Symptoms from spondylolisthesis may begin gradually in the second or third decade. Low back pain, sometimes radiating into the buttocks, occurs with activity and is relieved by rest. Symptoms of nerve root irritation may also be present, along with radiation of the pain into the extremities. These symptoms often progress in severity, especially in the teenager.

Examination may reveal guarding of the lower part of the back and "spasm" of the paraspinal muscles, especially in the adolescent. With moderate forward slippage, the lumbar lordosis appears increased, and the buttocks may appear more prominent. A palpable "step-

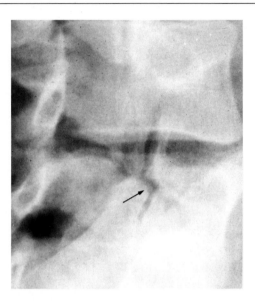

**Fig. 8–13.**
Bony defect *(arrow)* in the isthmus or neck of the "Scottie dog" present in spondylolysis (oblique view).

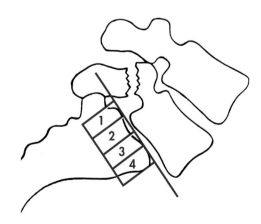

**Fig. 8–14.**
Meyerding's classification of spondylolisthesis. The amount of slippage is graded 1 to 4. Grade 1 represents 25% forward displacement; grade 2, 25% to 50%; grade 3, 50% to 75%; and grade 4, greater than 75%.

off" in the spinous processes of the lumbar spine may be present. There may be tenderness in the affected area and hamstring tightness. Neurologic deficits are rare.

Roentgenograms reveal the typical findings of a defect in the pars interarticularis, which may be accompanied by forward slippage (Fig. 8-15). A bone scan may be positive if the lesion is "acute" in the adolescent.

### Treatment

In the adolescent it is helpful to determine if the lesion is acute or chronic. If the bone scan is "hot" (suggesting an acute lesion) and no slip is present, the patient may benefit from prolonged bracing and restricted activities for several months. This is an attempt to encourage bony healing before fibrous nonunion can develop that could allow slippage to occur. If the scan is "cold," then the lesion probably will not heal and such limitations on the patient's activities would not be helpful. The treatment then is similar to that in the adult.

Management in the adult is usually conservative and consists of rest, a careful exercise program, weight loss, antiinflammatory medication, and the use of a lumbosacral orthosis. A change in occupation or work habits is sometimes indicated. The spondylolisthesis may increase in degree, but this is a gradual process and usually ceases by maturity. Further slippage in adulthood is rare. Progressive symptoms or intractable pain occasionally warrant surgical intervention. Decompression with spinal fusion is usually performed.

## Degenerative Spondylolisthesis

This type of spondylolisthesis results from disc degeneration and narrowing. When the process of "settling" is uneven, spondylolisthesis can develop (Fig. 8-16). The signs and symptoms are those of degenerative disc disease, sometimes accompanied by those of stenosis. Although many patients are pain-free, low back and radicular leg pain may occasionally develop. The treatment is the same as that for degenerative disc disease.

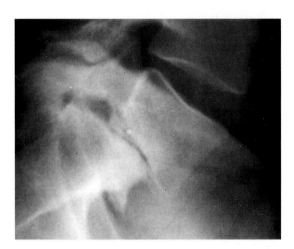

**Fig. 8–15.**
Spondylolisthesis of the lumbosacral junction.

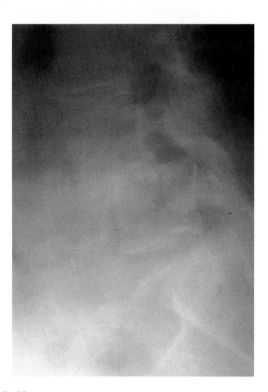

**Fig. 8–16.**
Degenerative spondylolisthesis at L4-L5. The disc is markedly narrowed.

## LUMBAR SPINE STENOSIS

Lumbar spinal stenosis is a syndrome in which narrowing of the spinal canal and nerve root foramina occurs. This may lead to vague and unusual symptoms. The disorder occurs secondary to a combination of disc degeneration, facet joint arthritis, and subluxation; and, occasionally, to a congenitally small spinal canal. These changes can lead to abnormal pressure on spinal nerve roots.

### Clinical Features

The history is highly suggestive. Neurogenic claudication is a hallmark symptom. Low back pain, motor weakness, leg cramping (pseudoclaudication), and a sensation of "poor circulation" in the extremities are typical. The patient is usually more than 40 or 50 years of age. The symptoms are characteristically aggravated by walking and by extension of the lumbar spine.

Improvement usually occurs with rest or flexion of the back. These symptoms are often misinterpreted as being vascular in origin. Sphincter disturbances and muscle atrophy rarely may be present.

Physical findings typical of disc herniation are usually absent. Neurologic findings are also commonly minimal, and results of a straight-leg–raising test are usually normal. Pain on extension of the lumbar spine may be severe. The vascular examination is usually normal but because vascular disease and stenosis occur in similar age groups and can produce similar symptoms, vascular studies may be necessary in some cases to differentiate the two conditions.

Roentgenographic examination of the lumbar spine usually reveals degenerative changes throughout the lower part of the back. Electromyography and myelography may help localize the disorder, and computerized axial tomography is often diagnostic (Fig. 8-17). MRI is also helpful.

### Treatment

Treatment is directed at reducing the lumbar lordosis. A light corset is sometimes beneficial, as is antiinflammatory medication. Hip flexion and abdominal strengthening exercises may also be helpful. Periodic epidural pain blocks can relieve the leg symptoms. Operative treatment consists of wide complete decompression of the involved area. Spinal fusion may also be necessary.

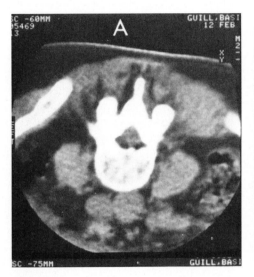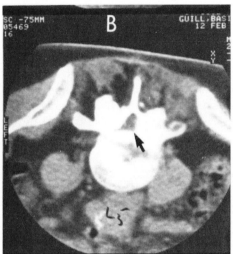

**Fig. 8–17.**
Normal (**A**) and abnormal (**B**) computerized axial tomographic scans of the lumbar spine. Marked narrowing *(arrow)* is present in **B** because of hypertrophic spurring.

## BACK PAIN IN THE WORKPLACE

Work-related low back pain is a growing problem in industrial societies, not only from a medical standpoint but also because of its legal and socioeconomic aspects. Low back pain accounts for as much as 25% to 30% of workers' compensation payments and the majority of long-term disability cases.

A variety of terms have been used to describe this condition, including "chronic benign industrial back pain," "compensation lumbago," and "chronic pain syndrome." This terminology partly reflects the difficulty in assigning a specific diagnosis and cause for the pain. A part of this difficulty, in turn, is a result of the fact that low back pain in general—and especially back pain in the workplace—may be caused by a variety of biomechanical, biochemical, behavioral, socioeconomic, and psychophysiologic disorders.

### Evaluation

An accurate history is especially important to determine whether an "injury" actually occurred or if the pain simply developed during or after a job. The pain may be referred to one or both legs, but it is usually not truly radicular in nature. Commonly, a description of the location and nature of the pain changes slightly from visit to visit.

Physical findings are often nonspecific. There is usually generalized low back tenderness and diminished range of motion. Often, the physical findings are "nonanatomic" in nature. There is usually no neurologic deficit, and sciatic tension tests are generally normal but often difficult to assess.

### Special Studies

Any of the anatomic structures of the lower part of the back (discs, ligaments, facet joints, bone, and muscle) can be the source of pain. The intervertebral disc is thought by many to be the source of most low back pain. Unfortunately, as many as 35% of asymptomatic adults who have myelography, CT, or MRI will have abnormal findings that are usually related to the disc. This makes evaluation of this problem difficult, and it is felt by many that the exact underlying pathology probably cannot be determined in the majority of these patients with work-related injuries.

Initially, a routine roentgenographic examination should be performed in 2 to 4 weeks if the patient does not improve, mainly to rule out any serious disorder. Further studies (EMG, CT, MRI, bone scan, myelography) should be performed only as adjuncts to the physical examination and history. The yield of clinically useful information from these studies is often poor. Subjecting these patients to further extensive testing in a search for the exact etiology of their pain is likely to be futile and is certainly costly. The same can be said for the various forms of instrumented back-testing devices. Diagnosing a spinal disorder solely on the basis of any of these tests should be avoided. It is rare that these special tests clearly demonstrate a source for the pain when it is not suspected clinically. In addition, any treatment (surgery, etc.) based solely on a special study will often fail. In general, myelography and other special studies should be used only under the following circumstances: (1) if surgical disc removal is contemplated for intractable leg pain or a serious neurologic deficit, or (2) if other serious spinal abnormality is suspected.

### Treatment and Prognosis

Considerable controversy exists regarding the treatment of this problem. Historically, the disorder has always been resistant to traditional medical care. Thus there has been a proliferation of rehabilitation services, pain centers, work-hardening programs, surgical procedures, chiropractic care, and physical therapy services. Patients often prefer this type of "hands-on" treatment, but no scientific proof exists that any of these treatments are any better than nature's own. And although orthopedic and neurologic surgeons are commonly called on to assess and treat this condition, in fewer than 1% of these cases is surgery ever indicated (usually for leg pain associated with severe disc herniation), and not for at least 6 to 8 weeks. Surgery may even become a negative factor for returning the patient to work in that it gives "validity" to the injury.

Fortunately, the natural history of most back problems is that they improve, and the end result of conservative management is usually good. Unfortunately, the longer the patient is off of work with benign low back pain, the less likely it is that the patient will ever return to gainful employment. After 6 months of not working, the chances that the patient will return to *any* work are minimal. Thus for a number of reasons, the trend for managing this condition has changed. There has been a deemphasis on the initial rest period and more encouragement for early exercise and returning to work on a limited basis. This trend has developed largely because of the low success rate with prolonged bed rest and the belief that it causes a deterioration of the musculoskeletal and cardiopulmonary systems. It has also been shown in limited studies that patients who begin exercise programs quickly after minor low back injuries have less pain and are disabled for shorter periods. (Only the patient with nerve root impingement because of disc herniation may require more rest.) The following approach may be helpful:

1. Reassurance and education. Instructions should be given regarding proper body mechanics and lifting habits. The patient needs to know that hurt does not mean harm and that returning to work is safe.
2. Bed rest for no more than a few days, and mild analgesics followed by over-the-counter medication.
3. Temporarily avoid bending and lifting, and use a chair with good lumbar support and armrests when sitting.
4. Begin a walking, biking, or swimming program as soon as possible. Back exercises are gradually added as tolerated.
5. Avoid the excessive use of passive treatment (massage, heat, etc.). Encourage active patient involvement, especially with the exercise program. Relaxation techniques may be helpful.
6. Encourage a return to work within the first 2 to 4 weeks (work activities may initially have to be modified). Time off from work is discouraged.

Patients should be made to understand that the pain may recur if they resume light work, but it is usually not as severe as it was initially and does not mean any damage is occurring. It should not require further time off from work. The patient should continue the exercise program and practice good body mechanics. (A formal education program may be necessary.) Active participation by the patient and compliance are extremely important.

If no improvement has occurred in 4 to 6 weeks, referral to a specialist is indicated. Psychosocial factors and work-related conditions may also need investigation. The attitude of the patient about the job and involvement of the employer also play important roles in the length of disability. Workers who like their jobs and employers who promote a good working environment are more likely to have a mutually satisfactory relationship.

# THORACIC DISC DISEASE

Symptomatic disc degeneration in the dorsal spine is uncommon. The cause is often traumatic. The most serious sequela of thoracic disc disease is acute or progressive spinal cord compression from central disc herniation. Progressive paralysis is not uncommon. Unilateral nerve root compression from lateral herniation also occurs.

## Clinical Features

Only dorsal spine pain occurs in most cases. With central herniation, however, gradually increasing motor weakness in the lower extremities becomes apparent. Sphincter control may be lost, and diffuse numbness is common. Examination usually reveals limited motion in the dorsal spine. Major neurologic deficits (spasticity, clonus) may be present in the lower extremities. Roentgenographic examination often reveals calcification, narrowing, and spondylosis in the dorsal spine. Myelography may reveal a complete block in central lesions. MRI is often needed.

## Treatment

Treatment is symptomatic for the typical case with thoracic pain as a result of degenerative disc disease. The treatment is surgical in those with significant neurologic deficits as a result of disc rupture.

# SCOLIOSIS

Scoliosis is a lateral curvature of the spine in the upright position greater than 10 degrees. The lateral curvature is usually accompanied by some rotational deformity and sometimes by kyphosis or lordosis. Scoliosis may be classified as either structural or nonstructural. Structural curves are fixed and nonflexible and fail to correct with side bending. Nonstructural curves, on the other hand, are flexible and readily correct with side bending.

*Nonstructural* scoliosis is often seen as a compensatory mechanism secondary to a leg length discrepancy, local inflammation, or irritation from acute lumbar disc disease. This type of scoliosis tends to disappear when the offending disorder is corrected.

*Structural* scoliosis may occur from a variety of causes. Congenital abnormalities in the spine with anomalous vertebral formation may lead to asymmetric growth and result in scoliosis. Neurofibromatosis and a variety of neurologic and myopathic conditions may also lead to structural scoliosis. The most common type, however, has no known cause and is usually termed "idiopathic."

Idiopathic scoliosis accounts for approximately 90% of all scoliosis. It appears to represent a hereditary disorder, but the exact mechanism of its production is unknown.

## Clinical Features

Genetic or idiopathic scoliosis usually appears clinically between the ages of 10 and 13 years but may be seen at any age. It is six times more common in females, and serious curvatures are also more common in females. Right thoracic curves are the most common. In young people, the disease is usually asymptomatic, and subjective complaints are absent. (Pain should suggest tumor or other disorder.) Many cases are diagnosed by nurses in screening clinics or by other family members.

The diagnosis is usually made on routine physical examination. Attention should be focused on the problem in all children, but especially in those between 10 and 14 years, the ages when spinal growth is most rapid. For the examination, the patient should be undressed to the waist or wear a bathing suit, and a routine should be followed. The shoulders and iliac crests are inspected to determine whether they are level. The scapulae, rib cage, and flanks are then observed for symmetry. The spinous processes are palpated to determine their alignment. The patient is then asked to bend symmetrically forward at the waist with the arms hanging free (Fig. 8-18). Observation from the back or front will detect the spinal rotation in the form of a rib hump or abnormal paraspinal muscular prominence.

The diagnosis is confirmed and the degree of curvature is measured by a *standing* roentgenogram of the spine (Fig. 8-19). There is no other method of determining the severity of the curve, and a patient should never leave the office without an accurate roentgenographic measurement of the curvature. The roentgenogram may have to be repeated at intervals to determine whether or not the curve is progressive. Breasts and gonads should be shielded when films are done.

MRI is usually not indicated unless there is: (1) pain, (2) a neurologic deficit, or (3) a left thoracic curve (which is often associated with an underlying spinal disorder).

## Natural History

Although it is impossible to accurately predict the outcome of most curves, the following facts are known about scoliosis:

1. Curves under 20 degrees will improve spontaneously more than 50% of the time.
2. There is no accurate method of predicting which curves will get better and which will get worse.

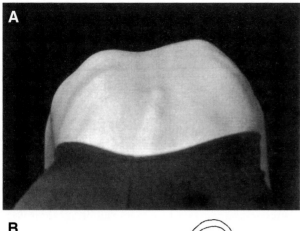

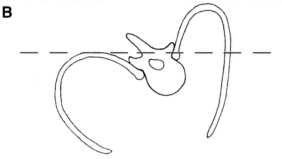

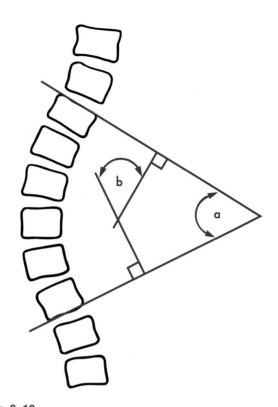

**Fig. 8–18.**
**A,** Scoliosis with rib prominence resulting from vertebral rotation is best exhibited on forward bending (the Adams position). **B,** Cross section of the chest showing rib distortion as a result of vertebral rotation.

**Fig. 8–19.**
Cobb method of measuring the severity of a curve. The upper and lower end vertebrae are identified. The upper end vertebra is the highest one whose superior border converges toward the concavity of the curve, and the lower end vertebra is the one whose inferior border converges toward the concavity. Lines are drawn along these borders, and the curve is measured directly *(a)* or geometrically *(b)*.

3. Twenty percent of curves under 30 degrees will progress.
4. Progression is more common in young children who are beginning their growth spurt.
5. The larger the curve at detection, the greater the chance of progression.
6. Curves in females are more likely to progress.

### *Treatment*

The most important aspect in treatment is early detection. A curve that is obviously present when the patient is standing is often already approaching 30 to 40 degrees. Detecting a curve before it reaches 20 degrees is important because curves over 20 degrees tend to progress. Prompt referral of all scoliosis patients to a specialist is mandatory. Regular reexaminations are essential while the child is at an age where progression is common. The failure to diagnose or treat this problem early may result in progressive deformity, pain, cardiopulmonary compromise, and disability. Early discovery and treatment can prevent this progression.

The treatment depends on the age of the patient and the severity of the curve (Fig. 8-20). In the immature patient, regular observation is necessary until the curve reaches 20 degrees. Curvatures over 20 to 25 degrees usually require treatment. The curve can be stabilized and, in many cases, improved by spinal bracing; but full, permanent correction is not possible or necessary. The Milwaukee brace or a thoracolumbosacral orthotic (TLSO) is commonly used for this purpose (Fig. 8-21). Young patients more easily accept the newer underarm orthotics as a result of their low profile design. Treatment in the brace is continuous for 23 hours a day, and the brace may have to be worn for 2 years or longer. Exercises are performed in the brace to improve the cosmetic appearance and decrease the curvature. Exercises alone will effect no change in the curvature, nor will they prevent any progression without the brace. Excellent results are obtained with proper use of the brace in curvatures between 20 and 40 degrees. The brace will not fully correct the curve, but it will usually prevent progression to the stage where spinal surgery is necessary.

Surgery is generally reserved for those cases in which the curvature is more than 45 to 50 degrees. Correction of the curvature by intraoperative instrumentation and

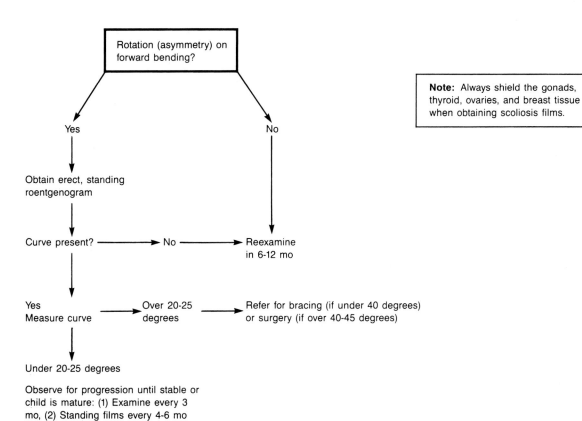

Note: Always shield the gonads, thyroid, ovaries, and breast tissue when obtaining scoliosis films.

**Fig. 8–20.**
Algorithm for decision making for genetic scoliosis in the growing child.

maintenance of the correction by spinal fusion along the entire length of the curve are usually performed. This may be preceded by corrective casts or traction.

In the adult patient, the spinal deformity may progress and eventually become painful. This is especially true of curves of more than 40 to 50 degrees. Occasionally, instrumentation and spinal fusion may also be indicated in these cases.

Female patients with curves over 25 degrees may experience a few degrees of increase in their curve with each pregnancy. In most patients, however, neither pregnancy nor delivery are complicated by the presence of scoliosis.

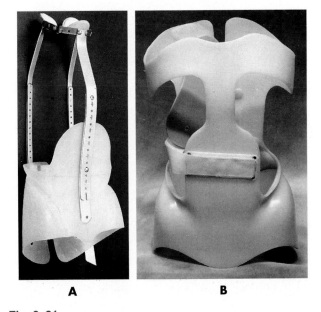

**Fig. 8–21.**
A, The Milwaukee brace. B, The thoracolumbosacral orthosis (TLSO). The newer underarm braces have largely replaced other orthoses when the outrigger is not required because they are as effective and cosmetically more acceptable.

# KYPHOSIS

Curvature of the spine in the anteroposterior direction in which the convexity is directed posteriorly is termed *kyphosis*. This curvature exists in the normal spine at the thoracic and sacral regions. Abnormal thoracic angulation can occur from several pathologic states. Diseases of the discs and vertebral bodies are the most common causes. Congenital kyphosis is rare and is usually secondary to a localized malformation of the spine.

## Senile Kyphosis

Senile kyphosis results from multiple areas of disc degeneration at the thoracic level. It is relatively common in the elderly patient and may be symptomatic. Roentgenograms will often reveal thinning of the discs and osteoporosis with mild wedging deformities (Fig. 8-22). Treat-

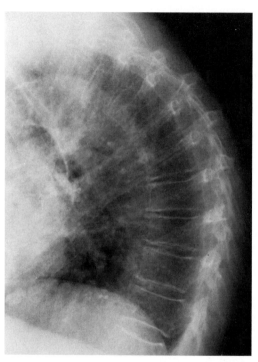

**Fig. 8–22.**
Roentgenogram of an elderly patient with senile kyphosis.

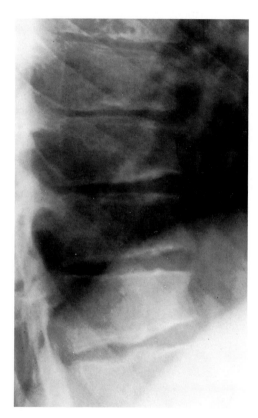

**Fig. 8–24.**
Roentgenogram of Scheuermann's disease. End-plate irregularities and mild wedging deformities are present. There is also increased AP diameter.

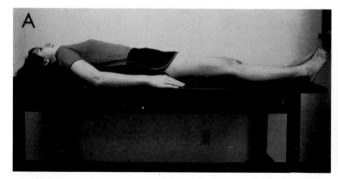

**Fig. 8–23.**
Exercises for postural round back. **A,** The resting position with a pillow under the dorsal spine. **B,** Scapular adduction and thoracic hyperextension exercise that stretches the pectoral muscles and contracted anterior soft tissues. In addition, the low back exercises previously described are performed to correct excessive lumbar lordosis.

ment is directed toward maintaining good posture. Exercises that strengthen the back and abdominal muscles are often helpful. The use of a light spinal brace will often relieve the symptoms.

## Postural Round Back

"Faulty posture" is common in adolescents and young children. It probably occurs as a result of minor muscular imbalances and weakness. The typical picture is one in which the patient, often a teenager, shows an increase in the normal dorsal kyphosis, lumbar lordosis, and an increased pelvic inclination. The parent often complains that the child does not sit straight but there is generally no pain. The patients are often asthenic. Commonly there are no specific findings, but sometimes the shoulders are rounded and drooped and the abdomen may be protuberant. The scapulae are commonly prominent. The kyphosis is typically supple and corrects with hyperextension, in contrast to the nonflexible, fixed kyphosis in Scheuermann's disease. Roentgenograms of the dorsal spine are usually unremarkable. No wedging or end-plate irregularities tend to be present.

After ruling out other causes of kyphosis, the patient is reassured and started on an exercise program to overcome any contractures and decrease the lumbar lordosis (Fig. 8-23). The disorder usually responds well to the exercises.

## Scheuermann's Disease

Scheuermann's kyphosis is a *fixed* kyphosis that develops near the time of puberty. The cause is unknown, but the deformity is caused by typical wedging abnormalities in the dorsal and dorsolumbar spine that result in a decrease in the anterior height of the vertebrae. Mild forms may clinically resemble postural round back.

### Clinical Features

Poor posture is a common complaint, and fatigue and pain often accompany the deformity. The family history may be positive. Examination reveals an increase in the normal kyphosis of the dorsal spine that is usually associated with local tenderness. There may be tightness of the hamstring, pectoral, and iliopsoas muscles. In contrast to postural round back, this kyphosis is usually fixed. That is, the kyphosis does not flatten with spine extension as it does with postural round back. The abdomen may be protuberant, and there is usually a compensatory increase in the lumbar lordosis. A mild scoliosis may also be present. The results of neurologic examination are usually normal.

A positive diagnosis is possible only with a roentgenographic examination. Wedging of the vertebrae, irregularity of the end plates and typical Schmorl's nodules are seen on the lateral view, usually between T2 and T12 (Fig. 8-24). Synostoses and osteophyte formation are not uncommon in the adult patient.

### Treatment

If the patient is immature with growth remaining, conservative treatment consisting of a brace and postural exercises will usually result in a cure. The brace is worn full time for approximately 1 year and is used at night for an additional year. Hamstring stretching and pelvic tilt exercises are initiated. Pain often resolves when growth ceases; however, severe deformity with pain or neurologic symptoms is an indication for surgery at any age. The surgery is similar to that performed for scoliosis.

Long-term results of conservative treatment are generally favorable when the disease is confined to the dorsal spine. There is an increased incidence of back pain with curves that are low in the dorsal spine or upper lumbar spine. The working capacity for the patient is usually not affected, however.

# DISCITIS (VERTEBRAL OSTEOMYELITIS)

Discitis is an infectious or inflammatory disease of unknown cause. An infectious basis is strongly suggested, but disc cultures are positive in less than 50% of cases. Viral infection has also been suggested as a cause. The process most commonly occurs in the midlumbar spine of children at the age of about 6 years. A history of trauma or infection elsewhere may be present. The process may affect the disc and both adjacent vertebrae.

### Clinical Features

The symptoms consist of low back pain that often radiates into the abdomen or lower extremities. The child has difficulty walking and standing and may even refuse to walk or sit at all. A slight limp may be present.

Examination reveals restriction of motion in the lumbar spine in association with hamstring spasm and a flattening of the normal lumbar lordosis. Local tenderness in the midlumbar region is usually present. The child is often irritable and may run a low-grade fever. Nausea and vomiting occasionally occur. Young children may even perceive their pain as abdominal in origin.

There is a positive blood culture in approximately 50% of patients, and the organism is usually *Staphylococcus*. Needle aspiration of the affected disc will sometimes reveal the same organism. There is usually an increase in the sedimentation rate and white blood cell (WBC) count. The bone scan is usually abnormal, and plain roentgenograms commonly reveal single disc space narrowing with irregularity of the adjacent end plates. MRI may be needed to rule out other conditions. Eventually, fusion may even occur between the involved vertebrae.

### *Treatment*

Treatment is controversial but usually consists of antibiotics, bed rest, and sometimes the application of a brace. Treatment is continued until the systemic signs of infection (such as the sedimentation rate, temperature, and WBC count) are normal. The prognosis is usually good. Surgery is rarely necessary.

## LUMBOSACRAL ANOMALIES

A variety of minor congenital abnormalities may exist in the lumbar spine and at the lumbosacral junction. The majority of these occur at the lumbosacral region, and most are asymptomatic. Facet joint asymmetry, variations in the number of lumbar vertebrae, spina bifida occulta, and transitional lumbosacral vertebrae are among the more common anomalies seen on routine roentgenograms. Only the transitional vertebra appears to be possibly related to low back pain.

The transitional vertebra (lumbarized S1 or sacralized L5) may produce pain at the false joint that forms at the articulation between its elongated transverse process and the sacrum (Fig. 8-25). The disc between this vertebra and the sacrum is usually markedly thinned but is rarely the cause of symptoms. The treatment is usually conservative. A lumbosacral corset may be beneficial by restricting motion at this area.

In general, congenital anomalies of the spine are seldom the cause of back pain in the pediatric age group. Inspection of the back is important to identify other congenital anomalies that may have significant neurologic deficits associated with them. (For example, Faun's beard is a doughy, fatty mass in the midline of the back, sometimes covered by excessive hair; this is evidence for a lipoma that may extend to the spinal cord and produce neurologic symptoms.)

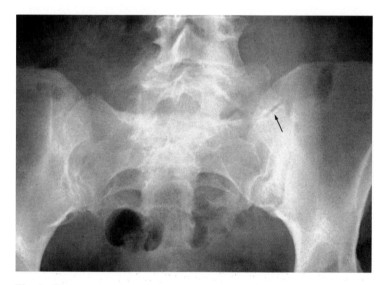

**Fig. 8–25.**
Transitional lumbosacral vertebra. A false joint is present *(arrow).*

## MEDICAL CAUSES OF BACK PAIN

Lower back pain may be caused by a variety of diseases not typically considered musculoskeletal in nature. A complete history and physical examination may not always be possible on the initial visit; but if a low back pain is not improving as expected, or if the symptoms are atypical, reevaluation is necessary with the possibility of other disorders always in mind. Because the "nonorthopedic" conditions tend to fall into a few distinct categories, the history, system review and examination should be performed with these other disorders in mind.

### History

The characteristics of the pain are often typical for certain disorders, and enough time must be taken to obtain a clear idea of its nature. Benign mechanical low back pain, for example, is usually worse with activity and relieved by rest, whereas the pain of spinal malignancy is often constant and even worse at night and during rest. The pain of ankylosing spondylitis is usually most noticeable in the morning upon arising but often improves during the day. Genitourinary pain often radiates into the groin and testicle or vulva while the cramps of ulcerative bowel disease may refer pain to the inner thigh. Osteoporosis may first manifest itself with a thoracic spine fracture after a seemingly minor event, such as opening a window. Any associated symptoms, such as numbness or tingling, should always be noted.

General systemic symptoms should be sought, especially weight loss, malaise, and fever. The smoking history is critical. Any previous injuries or surgery (especially for cancer) should be recorded. The status of the gastrointestinal and genitourinary systems should be evaluated, especially incontinence. Present medications and their doses are recorded. Skin disorders should be assessed, particularly if they suggest psoriasis or collagen vascular disease. The involvement of any peripheral joints should be determined. Previous hospitalizations and/or procedures such as myelography are noted.

Finally, any psychological or socioeconomic factors should be recorded and any positive responses developed.

## Physical Examination

The examination must be completed with the patient undressed. Age, height, and weight are recorded, and the patient is observed for general appearance, coordination, and gait. The skin should be examined for pallor, clubbing, cyanosis, and any diagnostic rashes.

### Chest, Heart, and Lungs

Examination of the heart should include auscultation for murmurs, especially that of aortic insufficiency, which may be seen in ankylosing spondylitis. Examination of the lungs should include auscultation for wheezes, especially localized ones, which could suggest tumor obstruction. Diaphragmatic excursion is evaluated for possible air trapping. Diminished excursion may also be a result of ankylosing spondylitis, which results in a decrease in chest expansion to less than 2.5 cm. (The average male's expansion is over 5.0 cm.) In addition to measuring chest expansion, the external evaluation should include a breast examination.

### Abdomen and Pelvis

Examination should include palpation for aneurysm, hepatomegaly, and/or splenomegaly. Any areas of tenderness are noted, and a rectal examination of the prostate is always included for males. Evaluation of women should include pelvic and rectal examinations with a Papanicolaou smear, Thayer-Martin culture (if indicated), and bimanual examination for full evaluation of both tubes and ovaries and rectal shelf area. The external genitalia are always examined, and the rectal examination should include guaiac testing of the stool.

### Back and Extremities

The patient is observed getting in and out of the chair and walking across the room. The back is inspected for atrophy, masses, scoliosis, and dorsal kyphosis. The hips and back are examined for range of motion and the gait pattern is observed. The back, pelvis, and hips are palpated for point tenderness. The peripheral pulses are also evaluated.

A neurologic examination including Babinski tests and tendon reflexes is then performed (Fig. 8-26). Clonus or reflex hyperactivity may indicate an intraspinous lesion such as a metastatic lesion in the cord area. Sensory deficits should be tested, but these are sometimes difficult to evaluate because of the patient's subjective assessment of this particular examination.

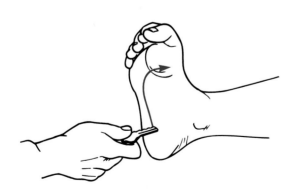 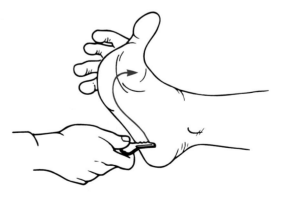

**Fig. 8–26.**
Babinski test. A sharp instrument is lightly scraped along the plantar aspect of the foot from the calcaneus along the outer border. The leg should be relaxed. If the ankle dorsiflexes or the foot withdraws, reduce the intensity of the stimulus. **A**, In a negative response the toes bunch together or do not move. **B**, An abnormal response includes extension of the great toe, while the other toes may splay and flex. The Babinski test is normally positive in the newborn but disappears soon after birth. An abnormal response indicates an upper motor neuron lesion. However, the response may be absent if there is damage to the reflex arc at the nerve or root level.

However, lower extremity numbness, loss of sensation in the perianal area, and a history of incontinence should suggest the possibility of spinal cord compression.

# SERONEGATIVE SPONDYLOARTHROPATHIES

These conditions comprise a group of interrelated disorders that are distinct entities but which share several clinical, roentgenographic, and genetic characteristics. Specific common features are inflammation (enthesitis) and pain (enthesopathy) at sites of tendon or ligament insertion. (An enthesis is the junction of ligament to bone.) Nonarticular inflammation of varying degrees may also involve the eyes, skin, mucous membranes, bowel, and heart.

These disorders are typically seronegative for the rheumatoid factor. It is sometimes difficult to differentiate among them because they may occur simultaneously. The disorders have been sometimes called rheumatoid variants. The spondyloarthropathies consist of four disorders: (1) ankylosing spondylitis, (2) psoriatic arthritis, (3) the arthritis associated with inflammatory bowel disease, and (4) Reiter's syndrome and other forms of reactive arthritis.

These diseases may even present under the age of 16. In this age group, they are often called "juvenile" spondyloarthropathies and must be distinguished from JRA. Peripheral joint involvement is more common in the young.

## Ankylosing Spondylitis

Ankylosing spondylitis is a chronic inflammatory condition of the joints of the axial skeleton that characteristically manifests itself by morning stiffness in the low back and progressive loss of spinal movement. It is the oldest and most easily recognized of the spondyloarthropathies. The disorder is 10 times more common in men and is commonly familial. Sacroiliitis is the classic lesion. The sacroiliac and spinal apophyseal joints are usually involved first, and the disorder commonly has its onset between the ages of 15 and 30 years. The disorder is also known as *Marie-Strümpell disease.*

An early diagnosis is often difficult because of the insidious onset of the disease. Years may pass between the onset of symptoms and the ultimate diagnosis as a result of the occurrence of nonspecific back pain from other disorders. The pain is usually located low in the buttocks and thigh region but rarely radiates into the hip, calf, or foot. Often the disease is mild, and there may be few systemic symptoms; however, in a severe form, fatigue, weight loss, anorexia, fever, and other systemic complaints may accompany the onset. Even though peripheral joint involvement may be present before the development of pain in the sacroiliac region, the diagnosis can only be presumptive until the sacroiliac joints are involved to such a degree as to be demonstrated roentgenographically. Although this disease is more common in men, women who have ulcerative colitis have an extremely high incidence of developing this disorder.

### Clinical Features

Clinical signs include bilateral sacroiliac tenderness and limited motion of the lumbar spine. An important physical finding is the loss of chest expansion to under 2.5 cm because of costosternal involvement, and this can be easily checked by measuring chest expansion at the nipple line before and after deep inspiration.

Virtually any of the other joints of the skeleton may be involved, but most commonly the hips, knees, and shoulders are the secondary joints affected. When there is involvement of the hips and shoulders, permanent damage may develop, but in the other joints the process often resolves without any residual disability or deformity, and this is similar to the arthritis that may be seen with inflammatory bowel disease.

Usually no skin lesions occur with ankylosing spondylitis, but an anterior uveitis occurs in approximately 25% of the patients. There is usually no urethritis that helps distinguish it from Reiter's syndrome. Aortitis develops in 5% of cases.

### Roentgenographic Findings

The early roentgenographic features are usually those of bilateral sacroiliitis. Initially there are erosions of these joints, and they lose their clear-cut demarcation because of cystic changes and subchondral sclerosis. The vertebral bodies may also become demineralized, and a typical "squaring off" of the anterior vertebral bodies develops. Apophyseal joint irregularities and paraspinal ligamentous calcifications develop later, and eventually there may be complete fusion of the sacroiliac and hip joints as healing takes place after the inflammation. As the disease progresses, calcifications of the anulus fibrosis and ossification of the anterior longitudinal ligament develop, which give rise to the so-called "bamboo-spine" appearance characteristic of ankylosing spondylitis (Fig. 8-27).

### Laboratory Findings

The current availability of the HLA-B27 system is important in the diagnosis of ankylosing spondylitis. This antigen occurs in over 90% of patients with ankylosing spondylitis, and the test may provide a useful method to screen those patients with either a familial history of the disease or low back pain suggestive of the disorder. Other laboratory findings suggestive of the disorder include an elevated sedimentation rate and a mild anemia.

### Extraskeletal Manifestations

The extraskeletal manifestations are those of uveitis, aortic insufficiency, and restrictive pulmonary disease.

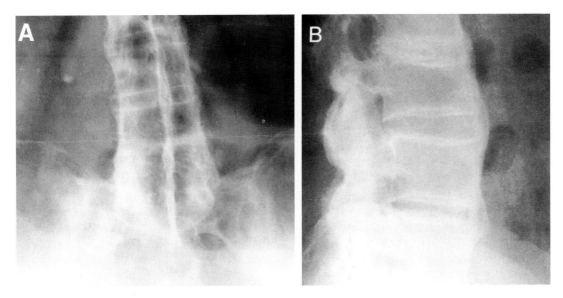

**Fig. 8–27.**
Ankylosing spondylitis. **A,** On the anteroposterior view the sacroiliac (SI) joints and the lumbar spine are fused. **B,** A lateral view shows the typical bamboo-spine appearance.

Because this is a chronic disease, the development of secondary amyloidosis is not uncommon and should be considered in those patients in whom chronic renal disease develops. On rare occasions, severe spinal deformity may lead to such kyphosis that the patient is unable to see forward.

### Differential Diagnosis

The differential diagnosis of ankylosing spondylitis includes the other spondyloarthropathies and rheumatoid arthritis. *Psoriatic arthropathy,* although similar, usually has late involvement of the sacroiliac joints, involves both the small and the large joints (particularly of the upper extremity), and has very specific skin lesions associated with it. Although aortitis may occur in psoriatic arthropathy, urethritis is absent, as is pulmonary fibrosis.

*Reiter's syndrome* is similar to psoriatic arthropathy in that sacroiliac joint involvement usually occurs late. The small and large joints (particularly of the lower extremity) are affected, and skin lesions are usually specific. Uveitis may occur, and urethritis is present at least at some point in the illness. Aortitis may occur, but pulmonary fibrosis has not been reported.

The arthritis associated with *inflammatory bowel disease* usually involves the large joints (particularly hips and shoulders), and sacroiliitis may be present early in the illness. Skin manifestations may be nonspecific or pathognomonic. In the patient with chronic ulcerative colitis, the skin lesion of pyodermic gangrenosum is at least suggestive of the chronic underlying illness. In chronic inflammatory bowel disease, uveitis may occur but is uncommon. Urethritis is usually not present, and aortitis is rare.

*Rheumatoid arthritis* usually affects the peripheral joints and is more common in females. The tenosyn-ovium and bursae are also commonly involved with the inflammatory process. It rarely affects the axial skeleton.

### Treatment

1. Medication. In general, the drugs utilized in the treatment are all NSAIDs such as indomethacin. Occasionally, disease-modifying antirheumatic drugs (DMARDs) are used when the response to other medication is inadequate.
2. Exercise. Next to drug therapy, exercise is the most important aspect of care. Swimming, general sports activities, and maintenance of ideal body weight are all important.
3. Postural training is especially important. Patients must be instructed to avoid stooping and to sit in an erect position. Otherwise, a flexion contracture of the spine may develop and cause the patient to be unable to look straight forward. The chair should have a hard, straight back and seat. Sleeping should be in the supine position on a firm mattress, and pillows should not be placed under the head or knees.
4. Surgery. Despite optimal management, the disease may progress to irreversible deformities of the spine and hips. Surgical techniques are available to correct the flexion deformity of the spine, and hip replacement is used for relief of the chronic hip pain. Re-ankylosis may occur after hip surgery, and the decision to undergo hip arthroplasty must be made with this possibility in mind.
5. Genetic counseling is often appropriate.

### Prognosis

Early diagnosis, good long-term management, regular follow-up examinations (including helping the patient understand the disease), exercise, and the appropriate medications will usually provide the patient with a normal life span. Death may occur as a result of the development of aortic insufficiency or secondary amyloidosis with chronic renal disease. If valvular disease develops, the patient should be educated regarding the use of prophylactic antibiotics to prevent subacute bacterial endocarditis. The usual course of the disease is not life-threatening, however, and a relatively normal lifestyle and work load are generally possible.

## Psoriatic Arthritis

Psoriasis may occasionally be accompanied by an inflammatory arthritis that affects both the axial skeleton and the peripheral joints. Spondyloarthropathy develops in 20% to 40% of cases. The prevalent age is between 30 and 55 years. The skin disorder usually precedes the arthritis by several years. Males and females are equally affected. Some 5% to 10% of patients with psoriasis will develop arthritis. The peripheral arthritis is usually polyarticular, involving the small joints of the hands and feet, and although it often runs a benign course in many patients, a destructive form can occur, especially in the hands (arthritis mutilans). Dystrophic changes in the nails with pitting and ridging develop in many patients with DIP involvement.

The HLA-B27 antigen is often positive in patients with axial involvement. Treatment is similar to other spondyloarthropathies.

## Reiter's Syndrome

This is a disorder of unknown etiology first described as a triad of nongonococcal urethritis, conjunctivitis, and arthritis. Many enteric and sexually acquired agents (for example, *Campylobacter* and *Chlamydia*) appear capable of inducing the disorder, which is now referred to as a form of reactive arthritis. This latter term denotes a sterile arthritis that develops in a joint as a result of an infection at a site distant from the inflamed joint itself. Reactive arthritis encompasses Reiter's syndrome. It does not usually include the arthritis associated with other infectious agents such as those caused by *Borrelia* (Lyme disease) and *Streptococcus* (rheumatic fever).

The syndrome is often incomplete. Inflammatory eye disease (uveitis, conjunctivitis) may occur. Low back pain is common. The patients are usually young and the joint symptoms generally appear within 3 to 4 weeks of the infection, but often there is no obvious evidence of previous infection. The lower extremities are mainly affected. Heel pain (enthesitis) from Achilles tendinitis or plantar fasciitis is common.

Sacroiliitis similar to that seen in ankylosing spondylitis is common. The HLA-B27 antigen is present in over 85% of cases, and the erythrocyte sedimentation rate is usually elevated. Laboratory evaluation is not otherwise helpful. The offending agents are difficult to culture.

Symptomatic treatment including the use of NSAIDs is advised. The use of antibiotics is controversial but many authorities recommend tetracycline for 10 to 14 days if urethritis is present. The arthritis is often self-limited and commonly resolves in a few months. The joint symptoms do not appear to be affected by the use of antibiotics.

## DIFFUSE IDIOPATHIC SKELETAL HYPEROSTOSIS

This is a common disorder of unknown cause characterized by excessive ossification at ligamentous and tendinous attachment sites to bone. DISH, sometimes called Forestier's disease or ankylosing hyperostosis of the spine, is a condition primarily affecting men over 60. Bony proliferation causes a characteristic pattern of excessive calcification and ossification that primarily involves the spine but may affect peripheral joints as well.

### Clinical Features

Many patients have had minor symptoms for years before the condition is diagnosed. The primary complaints are those of low grade spinal stiffness and pain, although the symptoms and signs are often relatively minor in spite of extensive hypertrophic spur formation. The thoracic spine is most commonly affected. The presence of large anterior osteophytes may lead to dysphagia (Fig. 8-28). Cervical myelopathy may result from

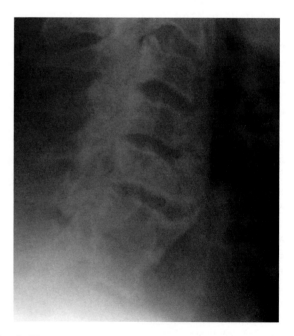

**Fig. 8–28.**
Diffuse idiopathic skeletal hyperostosis involving the cervical spine producing only minimal symptoms. Roentgenographic findings usually look worse than the disease.

ossification of the posterior longitudinal ligament. Peripheral joint symptoms are usually mild, although heel and elbow pain may occur.

The roentgenographic findings are those of bridging anterior osteophytes fusing at least four vertebral bodies while preserving disc space. The condition is differentiated from ankylosing spondylitis by lack of involvement of the SI and apophyseal joints and negative HLA testing.

### Treatment

Treatment consists of NSAIDs and an exercise program (walking and stretching). Symptoms are usually mild. The rare case of myelopathy or dysphagia may require surgical intervention.

## MULTIPLE MYELOMA

This disorder, sometimes called plasma cell myeloma, is a neoplastic proliferation of the plasma cell of the bone marrow. It may present as a systemic process or, less commonly, as a solitary lesion. Multiple myeloma is found in increasing incidence in patients over 40 years of age, and men are affected twice as often as women. It is usually associated with a rise in serum globulin content, often because of abnormal globulins. It is the most common primary tumor of bone.

### Clinical Features

The early manifestations of the disorder are weakness, anorexia, weight loss, and bone pain, especially involving the spine. The majority of patients initially present with back pain. This often leads to the detection of a destructive skeletal lesion. As the disease progresses, other organ systems become involved and result in more bone pain, anemia, renal insufficiency, and/or bacterial infections. The infections, which often take the form of recurrent bouts of pneumonia or urinary tract infection, are usually a result of the dysproteinemia. They are often pneumococcal in origin and are apparently related to the patient's inability to synthesize normal amounts of specific antibody in response to the bacterial challenge.

Secondary amyloidosis is also sometimes associated with the disorder. Amyloid deposition may be manifested in several patterns. Involvement of the heart or kidney may lead to cardiac failure or nephrotic syndrome.

### Roentgenographic Features

The classic finding is the "punched-out" lesion with sharply demarcated edges (Fig. 8-29). Usually, multiple lesions are found, but in 10%, only a single skeletal defect may be present. Diffuse osteoporosis because of generalized demineralization is the only finding in about 25% of cases. The typical lesions may occur in any part of the skeleton, but are most common in the spine, skull, ribs, and pelvis. Pathologic fractures are common. Intervertebral body collapse may result in nerve root or cord compression. Diffuse bony involvement may even result in hypercalcemia.

Using the bone scan to assess the disorder is helpful, but a negative scan can be misleading. This tumor is often "cold" on a bone scan because of its rapid destruction. Plain films are often better for evaluation. CT and MRI are also helpful.

### Laboratory Findings

In approximately half of the cases, the urine contains the Bence Jones protein, which has the unique property of precipitating in an acid pH when the temperature is between 4.4° C and 15.6° C and redissolving when the temperature is 32.2° C. Anemia is often present, and the sedimentation rate is usually elevated. Serum protein electrophoresis usually displays the characteristic dysproteinemia. The serum calcium concentration is occasionally elevated, but the alkaline phosphatase level is usually normal.

### Treatment and Prognosis

Because patients with multiple myeloma may have hypercalcemia, hypercalciuria, and hyperuricemia, the importance of ambulation and adequate hydration in their treatment cannot be overstressed. Every effort should be made not to immobilize the patient. Because plasma cell tumors are characteristically radiosensitive, x-ray therapy has been shown to be of extreme help in the control of localized symptomatic lesions. An oncologist should be consulted. Response to chemotherapy is measured by objective signs of improvement, including decrease in concentration of abnormal M-type serum

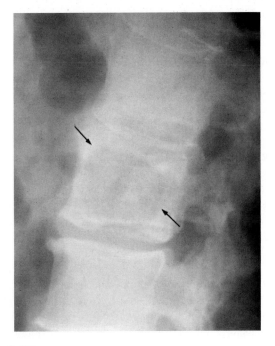

**Fig. 8–29.**
Multiple myeloma *(arrows)*. (This patient had a normal bone scan.)

globulins, decreased Bence Jones proteinuria, hematologic improvement of the anemia, and cessation of further skeletal destruction.

The prognosis remains poor, even with newer therapies. Complete remissions are uncommon. Most patients succumb after a median of 3 years, although a small percentage will survive 10 years. At present, no treatment is curative. Autologous bone marrow transplantation may offer some hope.

## OSTEOPOROSIS

Osteoporosis is a disorder of the skeleton in which the total skeletal bone mass is decreased, resulting in bony fragility. This may lead to fracture, often with little or no trauma. The primary form is usually considered a disease of older, thin, white females, although the condition may be seen in men, young amenorrheic athletes, or those with eating disorders. Some 15% to 18% of postmenopausal women have osteoporosis. It is the most common metabolic disease in the United States and has become even more prevalent as the average life span has increased. It is estimated that 1.5 million fractures occur yearly because of osteoporosis, at a cost exceeding $13 billion ($8 billion in hip fractures alone).

Elderly patients who experience a hip fracture have a 12% to 20% mortality rate within the first year of fracture from related complications. Approximately one third of the rest will not be able to return to their previous living arrangements. Half of the patients who fracture a hip will never regain functional weight-bearing status after their injury. Osteoporosis can largely be prevented, however, by attaining and maintaining the maximum bone mass. Even if the disorder is established, newer and more promising therapies are now available.

### Etiology and Classification

Bone growth occurs over the first decades of life with the peak in total body bone mass occurring at the end of the second or third decade. At skeletal maturity, the male peak bone mass is 10% to 15% greater than the female, and blacks have 10% more than whites. With the cessation of gonadal function, many females can experience a rapid loss of bone over a period of 3 to 5 years as a result of increased osteoclastic activity. This is more noticeable first in trabecular bone than cortical bone, and vertebral bodies are commonly involved. Other factors that influence further bone loss are lack of physical exercise and low calcium intake. With further aging, there can also be a progressive decline in osteoblastic activity as well as a net loss in bone mass.

Osteoporosis is of multifactorial etiology and is usually classified as either primary or secondary. The primary form is the type commonly seen in the older population. It is divided into Type I and Type II, although there is con-siderable overlap between the two forms. Type I osteoporosis develops as a result of estrogen loss after menopause, which allows increased osteoclastic bone resorption. It is typically seen in females but can occur in the hypogonadal male. This form is seen in the 50 to 70 years age group and females are affected six times as often as males. It is the most common form of symptomatic osteoporosis and is usually referred to as "postmenopausal." Accelerated loss of trabecular bone occurs and may result in crush fractures of vertebrae and fractures of the distal radius. Although all women become estrogen deficient at menopause, only a small number will develop Type I osteoporosis. Genetic factors may play a role.

Type II osteoporosis is associated with normal aging and is often called "senile" or involutional. The male to female ratio is 2:1 and this type occurs over age 60 to 70. This form is the result of a slow, progressive decline in osteoblastic activity without any increase in osteoclastic activity. Diminished calcium intake may play a role. Bone loss is both trabecular and cortical and may lead to wedge fractures of the vertebrae and hip fractures. Accelerated loss of trabecular bone occurs and may result in wedge fractures of the vertebrae and hip fractures. The proximal humerus, distal femur, and pelvis are other common sites for fractures. Unfortunately, the elderly female often suffers from the additive effects of both types of osteoporosis.

Secondary osteoporosis has multiple etiologies (Table 8-2). It may occur in the course of various diseases or as a result of complications from the use of certain medications. Lack of activity and immobilization may also result in osteoporosis (disuse). In elderly patients, intestinal lactase deficiency may also be associated with osteoporosis. It may be seen in developmental disturbances such as osteogenesis imperfecta or nutritional problems such as a lack of protein or vitamin C. Endocrine disorders such as hypopituitarism, acromegaly, thyrotoxicosis, Cushing's disease, and long-standing diabetes may also cause osteoporosis.

**Risk factors.**   A number of factors can influence peak bone mass or contribute to bone loss in the adult in addition to hormonal deficiency (Table 8-3). Some of these factors are modifiable and some are not.

**TABLE 8–2.**

Causes of Secondary Osteoporosis

Drugs (alcohol, steroids, heparin, anticonvulsants)
Disuse-prolonged immobilization
Malignancy (multiple myeloma)
Endocrine disease (diabetes, thyroid disease, eating disorders, exercise-induced amenorrhea)

### Clinical Features

The disease is insidious in onset, with the clinical disorder preceded by asymptomatic "silent" bone changes over many years. Spontaneous vertebral fractures may develop early after menopause but osteoporosis is often discovered as an incidental roentgenographic finding (Fig. 8-30). Vertebral fractures develop first because the vertebral body is primarily composed of cancellous bone, which undergoes loss earlier than cortical bone. The fractures often occur with little or no trauma. Local pain and tenderness are present and may last 6 to 8 weeks. In the early post-menopausal state, the incidence of fracture of the distal radius is also high. Even the young female athlete may be at risk for stress fracture if her bone mass is low as a result of athletic amenorrhea.

Because the femur is composed of both cortical and cancellous bone, hip fractures usually develop years later, after age 65. Metaphyseal fractures of the upper humerus and insufficiency fractures of the pelvis may also occur.

The physical findings reflect the residuals of the bony injury. Eventually, vertebral collapse may cause the characteristic loss of body height and dorsal kyphosis called "Dowager's hump." Chronic spine pain is not uncommon. Excessive kyphosis may even allow the rib cage to shift downward, preventing comfortable expansion of the stomach after eating and further limiting nutritional intake. Restrictive lung disease may also develop. Additional fractures are not uncommon, especially in older patients whose balance may be impaired.

The results of laboratory analysis are usually normal in primary osteoporosis. Laboratory testing may be useful in ruling out secondary causes. The rate of bone resorption or formation can be assessed by new methods of measuring certain biochemical markers (such as serum procollagen and osteocalcin) in blood or urine, but these tests are not in general use at this time and do not determine bone mass or fracture risk. They can be helpful in following response to treatment because the markers can determine the response to therapy within a few weeks. Changes in these markers are seen much quicker than the changes that occur in bone density studies, which may take 2 to 3 years.

### Special Studies

The first indication of osteoporosis is often noticed on plain films. Demineralization may be present in the spine and pelvis. Typically, there is loss of the horizontal trabeculae of the vertebral bodies and the density of the end plates appears accentuated in contrast. With extensive involvement, the discs may bulge into the adjacent vertebrae, causing a biconcave shape to the vertebral body called the "codfish vertebra." There are usually no osteophytes or cortical erosions. Crush or anterior wedge deformities of the vertebral bodies may be present. Increased dorsal kyphosis is a late finding.

**TABLE 8–3.**

Risk Factors in Osteoporosis

Small, thin frame
White or Asian race
Tobacco use (smoking is especially a problem because nicotine further decreases estrogen levels and may also induce earlier menopause)
Lack of exercise
Low calcium intake
Low weight relative to height
Excessive alcohol, caffeine intake
Strong family history of osteoporosis
Poor general nutrition
Estrogen deficiency
Prolonged immobilization
Chronic renal disease
Late menarche
Early menopause

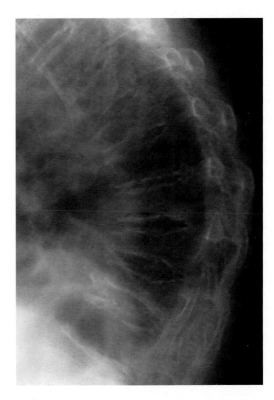

**Fig. 8–30.**
Osteoporosis. Multiple compression fractures are present.

### Bone Density Measurements

The determination of bone density is among the best measurements of any disease process. Several non-invasive techniques are available. Bone mass measurement is commonly used to detect bone loss and assess fracture risk. DEXA (dual-energy x-ray absorptiometry) has become the measurement of choice and is becoming more generally available. There is some controversy as to whether it is cost effective as a screening procedure, and women who elect hormone replacement therapy at menopause probably do not need the study.

A number of guidelines for the use of bone mineral density (BMD) studies are available, but in general, the test is most useful for the following: (1) to determine if a compression fracture is a result of osteoporosis, (2) to assess treatment, and (3) to decide if hormone replacement therapy (HRT) is indicated. The principle of the test is that a scanning device detects absorption from a roentgenographic source, providing a measurement of bone mineral density at a given site (often the spine and femoral neck). The results are then compared statistically to the bone mass of young normal adults. Osteoporosis is defined as a T-score greater than 2.5 SD (standard deviations) below the adult reference mean. A value within 1 SD is considered normal. Patients whose standard deviations are greater than 2.5 are at high risk for future fractures.

### Treatment

The prevention and treatment of osteoporosis begins at youth and should address the two most important bone processes: (1) the acquisition in the young of maximum peak bone mass that occurs at the end of the third decade, and (2) the loss of bone developing after menopause and continuing into later years. Certain factors (race, heredity) cannot be modified, but several

modifiable factors that affect peak bone mass can be addressed: (1) adequate calcium and vitamin D intake, (2) proper amount of exercise, and (3) nutrition. Young women should be discouraged from becoming overly concerned with the thin body image. A certain amount of extra weight may actually be healthy for the skeleton in both young and old. Smoking should be avoided, and caffeine and alcohol intake should be minimized. Young patients should avoid exercise-induced amenorrhea. Proper exercise, however, may help the young "bank" extra bone to help prevent adult osteoporosis. After menopause, all modifiable risk factors need to be identified and minimized. Safety issues may also need to be addressed (Table 8-4). Among the currently available therapeutic measures are the following:

1. *Exercise.* Although there is no clear evidence regarding the role of exercise in the prevention or treatment of osteoporosis, it is reasonable to include a regular *weight-bearing* program. General conditioning regimens, especially those designed to develop better body mechanics, may be useful in that they improve balance and thus decrease the chance of falling.

2. *General nutrition.* If the patient's dietary intake is inadequate, calcium (1 to 1.5 g/day) and vitamin D (400 to 800 IU/day) should be added. Calcium carbonate is preferred because of its low cost, but generic brands should be avoided because of poor absorption. If carbonate causes GI distress, calcium citrate may be used. Adequate intake is as important in the premenopausal female as it is in the older individual, and an accurate dietary history is therefore important. The diet should also contain adequate protein.

3. *Estrogen.* Hormone replacement therapy (HRT) has been proven to be the most effective means of preserving skeletal mass, preventing bone resorption, and decreasing fracture rates. It is usually started at menopause, but may still be effective if begun as late as 10 to 15 years after menopause. (The benefit may be minimal this late, however, because the rate of bone turnover is so low.) Adequate preservation of bone mass requires 10 to 15 years of therapy, and some researchers recommend continuing it forever. (Bone loss accelerates if HRT is discontinued, eventually reversing the protective influence of previous estrogen treatment.) Many gynecologists prefer to treat all women for general reasons, including the protection estrogen gives against cardiovascular disease. However, some investigators suggest that women with high bone density measurements at menopause may not be at risk for osteoporosis and thus might not require estrogen replacement.

**TABLE 8–4.**
Prevention and Treatment of Osteoporosis

| General | Specific |
| --- | --- |
| Avoid smoking, caffeine and alcohol | Estrogen |
| Exercise regularly | Salmon calcitonin |
| Maintain adequate calcium, vitamin D intake at all ages | Pain control (mild narcotics, NSAIDs, etc.) |
| Consider environmental aspects (good lighting, remove loose rugs, electrical cords, etc.) | Light braces |
| | Prompt treatment of fractures with early mobilization |
| | Calcium 1500 mg/d |
| Compensate for physical hazards (poor hearing, confusion, poor eyesight) | Vitamin D 400-800 IU/d |
| | Avoid prolonged bed rest |
| | Biphosphonates |
| Eliminate medications that might necessitate trips to the bathroom at night or that could cause falls | |
| Eat a balanced diet | |
| Always wear glasses if they are prescribed | |
| Use a cane and handrails if unsteady | |
| Wear shoes and slippers with skid-resistant soles | |
| Avoid social isolation | |

Estrogen therapy has a number of risks as well as benefits. Endometrial carcinoma is one of the potential adverse effects of long-term estrogen therapy. The addition of progesterone in the last days of the cycle appears to negate this risk. The question of whether or not to use progesterone in patients who have had hysterectomies remains unanswered. Another risk of estrogen therapy may be the possible increased incidence of breast cancer. All patients receiving hormone replacement should have regular examinations.

*Alternative Therapies.* The use of lower (one half) doses of estrogen combined with calcium supplementation has also been shown to protect against bone loss, although the findings are preliminary. Estrogen substitutes or analogues are also becoming popular. Referred to as SERMs (selective estrogen receptor modulators), these drugs may become alternatives to standard estrogen therapy. Raloxifene is the most popular. It fits estrogen receptors in bone and lowers lipids. It apparently carries no increased risk of breast cancer and does not stimulate the endometrium. Tamoxifen citrate, a chemical relative, is also being studied, but its use may be limited because of its stimulant effect of the uterus.

BMD studies may help the patient who is uncertain about hormonal replacement therapy. They may also improve the notoriously poor rate of compliance with estrogen replacement if the patient is made aware of the risk of osteoporosis. The patient whose bone density study is more than 2.5 standard deviations below the mean is considered at high risk for future fractures, and HRT should be recommended. A study between 1 and 2.5 is below normal and replacement therapy can be offered. If these patients decline, the study can be repeated every 1 to 2 years.

4. *Calcitonin.* This polypeptide hormone is secreted by the thyroid gland in mammals. It appears to act mainly on bone and can cause an inhibition of the normal ongoing resorptive process. It is most effective on bone disorders with an accelerated rate of resorption (such as Paget's disease), but also appears helpful in preventing osteoclast activity associated with osteoporosis. Salmon calcitonin can be given by subcutaneous injection or by nasal spray. Compliance with frequent injections can be a problem, partly because of injection site pain. It is used primarily in the nasal spray form. Systemic effects include nausea, vomiting, and flushing. It appears to have a beneficial analgesic effect and is often used to treat acute fracture pain. The high cost of the drug may prohibit its use in many older patients, especially those on a fixed income. Antifracture data is inconclusive. In early postmenopause, it appears to reduce trabecular bone loss in the spine but it may have no effect on the peripheral skeleton.

5. *Biphosphonates.* These drugs, also called diphosphonates, are synthetic analogs of pyrophosphate, a naturally occurring substance that is an inhibitor of bone mineralization. These drugs are also potent inhibitors of bone resorption and are becoming increasingly useful as an alternative to estrogen for women concerned about the side effects of HRT. Etidronate was the first to become widely used, but there has been concern that its mineralization-inhibiting effect could actually weaken bone further.

The later generation biphosphonates such as alendronate have a wider margin between their undesired effects (inhibition of mineralization) and their wanted effects (inhibition of bone resorption). Alendronate is FDA approved for use in osteoporosis. It improves bone mass and decreases the rate of spine and hip fractures. Lifetime use is usually recommended. GI side effects are common: the drug must be taken with water at least 30 minutes before food and the patient must remain upright for 30 minutes afterwards.

6. *Fluoride.* By an unknown mechanism, fluoride appears capable of increasing bone mass. Unfortunately, the bone produced is abnormal bone. Fluoride appears to have different effects on different types of bone. While increasing trabecular bone in vertebrae, it may actually decrease mineral content in cortical bone such as the upper part of the femur. As a result, the rate of vertebral compression fractures appears to decrease significantly, but the hip fracture rate increases. A slow-release product may be available soon that could be helpful, but further studies are needed to determine whether fluorides have any role in the management of osteoporosis.

7. *Miscellaneous.* Among the other products being investigated are vitamin $D_3$ (and its metabolite, calcitriol); thiazide diuretics; growth factors; parathyroid hormone in small doses; and androgens. Like fluorides, these are being used mainly in research centers, and their effectiveness is unknown.

Once a fracture has occurred, overimmobilization should be avoided. Analgesics should always be used in doses large enough for good pain relief to maintain a high level of activity. Light braces may be needed temporarily for compression fractures. Acute spinal fractures may benefit from intercostal or epidural nerve blocks.

## Other forms

An unusual type of regional osteoporosis is the so-called *Sudek's atrophy*, a result of reflex sympathetic dystrophy (RSD) that is commonly found in the hands and feet (see Chapter 18). This localized osteoporosis is characteristically associated with the other findings of RSD, such as swelling, excessive sweating, and pain. Bone scanning may reveal increased flow to the affected area, a finding that may confirm the diagnosis of reflex dystrophy.

*Idiopathic transient osteoporosis* of the hip is another local form of osteoporosis. It is a rare, self-limited condition of unknown cause characterized by diffuse mineralization, usually of the hip, although similar lesions have been reported elsewhere in the lower extremities. It was first described in women in late pregnancy, but is also seen in middle-aged men. The clinical features are those of hip pain and limitation of motion. Almost all patients recover, although there have been reported cases of pathologic fractures. The bone scan also shows increased uptake.

## Tumors of the Spine

### Primary

Excluding multiple myeloma, primary tumors (either benign or malignant) of the spinal column are relatively rare. Of the benign tumors, osteoid osteoma, eosinophilic granuloma, aneurysmal bone cyst, and osteoblastoma occur occasionally. Osteoid osteoma is an interesting benign vascular lesion characterized by night pain that is often relieved by aspirin. Malignant tumors are quite rare, with sarcomas of several origins being the most common.

In young patients, spinal neoplasms commonly cause local discomfort and scoliosis. Therefore, any young patient with a painful spinal curvature should be carefully assessed for tumor.

### Metastatic Bone Disease

Bone is the third most common site for distant spread of neoplastic disease, behind only the liver and the lung. The major sources are myeloma and breast, lung, kidney, prostate, and thyroid carcinomas. The tumor usually disseminates by the hematogenous route, commonly through Batson's plexus, a vertebral venous system.

Pain is the most common complaint and usually is a result of the expanding nature of the lesion and/or a pathologic fracture. There may be a referred or radicular element to the discomfort that gives the problem the appearance of a herniated disc. *Night pain*, either aggravated or not relieved by rest, often occurs. With progression of the disease, neurologic dysfunction may progress to complete paralysis.

Roentgenographs will often reveal the lesion, but 30% to 50% of the bone must be destroyed before the lesion is visualized on plain films. The bone scan is positive in 90% of cases. False negatives commonly occur in myelomas and many carcinomas. This is because these tumors produce such rapid and extensive bone destruction that new bone formation and the reparative process does not occur. CT and magnetic scans will usually reveal the lesion.

Laboratory studies commonly reveal an elevated alkaline phosphatase level. Acid phosphatase levels are usually increased in prostate metastases. Serum calcium levels may also be elevated. Bone marrow aspiration or biopsy is usually necessary to establish the diagnosis.

Treatment of the skeletal metastasis depends on biopsy confirmation of the type of tumor that is present and the appropriate use of radiation therapy, chemotherapy, or hormonal therapy as indicated.

## Back Pain of Abdominal or Pelvic Origin

Visceral pain is often referred to the more posterior parts of the spine that innervate the diseased organ. In general, disease of the upper portion of the abdomen may refer pain to the shoulder and dorsolumbar spine; lower abdominal disorders refer pain to the lower lumbar spine; and pelvic disease refers pain to the sacrum. Usually there are no findings related to the back, such as loss of motion.

### Abdominal Disorders

Peptic ulcer disease or tumor of the stomach or duodenum may induce pain in the lower thoracic and upper

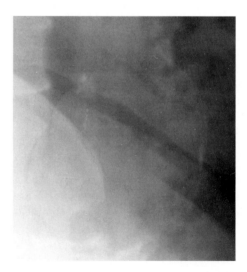

**Fig. 8–31.**
Lateral lumbar spine film revealing an abdominal aneurysm measuring 7 × 10 cm.

lumbar spine if the posterior wall is involved. If intense, it may radiate around to the front of the abdomen. The ulcer pain tends to retain its original character of response to antacids and food.

Thoracolumbar and left shoulder pain referral from pancreatitis is not uncommon. The pain may be quite intense. Previous episodes may have occurred, and a recent history of alcohol or dietary excess may be present. Tumor and peptic ulceration with extension to the pancreas commonly cause back and flank pain. The patient may seek relief by bending forward. The pain is more likely to be to the left of the spine if the tail of the pancreas is involved and to the right if the head is involved. Nausea, vomiting, prostration, and diaphoresis may be present, and the abdomen is usually distended and tender. There is commonly a leukocytosis and elevation of serum and urinary amylase levels.

An aneurysm of the aorta may cause not only acute abdominal pain and collapse with abdominal rigidity but also back pain (Fig. 8-31). Generally, the pain is thoracic, but may be higher or lower depending on location. There may be an absence or reduction of pulses in one of the lower extremities, and a pulsatile mass is often present.

In addition to aneurysms, disorders of other retroperitoneal structures may evoke back pain. The pain commonly radiates to the lower portion of the abdomen, groin, labia or testicles, and anterior aspect of the thighs. Iliopsoas tumors or abscess, lymphomas, or acute bleeding resulting from anticoagulation may all produce symptoms sometimes confused with hip, back, or abdominal disorders. Commonly, there is pain with hip motion in extension but not in flexion because the iliopsoas is relaxed in flexion.

Colon disorders (tumor, colitis, diverticulitis) may cause pain felt in the lower portion of the abdomen, lumbar spine, and groin. Transverse colon lesions may refer to L2 or L3, and sigmoid lesions may refer to the sacrum.

### Genitourinary Disorders

Renal diseases are among the most common nonorthopedic disturbances to simulate back disease. The pain of renal colic—caused by the passage of a small stone, clot, pus, or crystals—is usually ipsilateral and felt in the flank and lumbar area. It often radiates into the corresponding groin and testicle or vulva. Vomiting and restlessness are common, and there may be frequency and pain on urination. It is sometimes accompanied by hematuria. A positive Murphy's punch is diagnostic. Renal stones are rare in children, and when they occur, the patient should be evaluated for underlying metabolic disorders such as cystinuria.

Acute pyelonephritis commonly causes low back pain, but systemic and urinary symptoms usually clarify the diagnosis. Chills, fever, urinary frequency and urgency, and pain and tenderness in the costovertebral angle are usually present.

Renal vein thrombosis may also present as back and flank pain. Compression or invasion by local or metastatic tumor, proximal extension of a distal thrombus, and severe dehydration are among the common causes. The presence of unexplained edema (especially if unilateral) and the development of collateral abdominal veins may suggest the diagnosis. Recurrent pulmonary emboli may also occur. Palpable enlargement of the kidney, hematuria, and proteinuria are usually present. The proteinuria sometimes leads to nephrotic syndrome.

Back pain occasionally accompanies prostate disorders. Prostatitis may evoke sacral pain, sometimes radiating into one leg. It is usually accompanied by frequency, and there may be prostatic discharge. Prostate carcinoma with metastases to the lower portion of the back is another cause of lumbar or sacral pain. Most prostatic disorders are diagnosed by rectal examination, which should always be performed, especially for those patients whose back pain is unexplained.

Low back pain is also a common complaint in gynecologic practice. Simple menstrual pain may cause low lumbar and sacral pain. It is commonly crampy and radiates down the legs. Uterine colic or dysmenorrhea may cause similar symptoms. Vomiting sometimes occurs. Pain from endometriosis may also cause cyclical discomfort. The menstrual history is often suggestive of these disorders.

Retrodisplacement of the uterus, especially if associated with retroflexion, may cause a nagging sacral pain, particularly after the patient has been upright for several hours. Tension on the utero-sacral ligaments is the usual etiology of back pain as a result of enlargement, tumors, or malposition of the uterus. Large posterior pelvic tumors may be painful because of pressure or involvement of the sacral plexus. Backache of this type, in conjunction with pelvic malignancies (especially carcinoma of the cervix), usually indicates that the disease has advanced to involve the iliac nodes. This pain often becomes more severe and worse at night.

Pregnancy, ectopic or otherwise, should always be ruled out in women of childbearing years, especially if invasive or roentgenographic studies are being planned. A well-performed pelvic examination will help separate the majority of these disorders (Fig. 8-32).

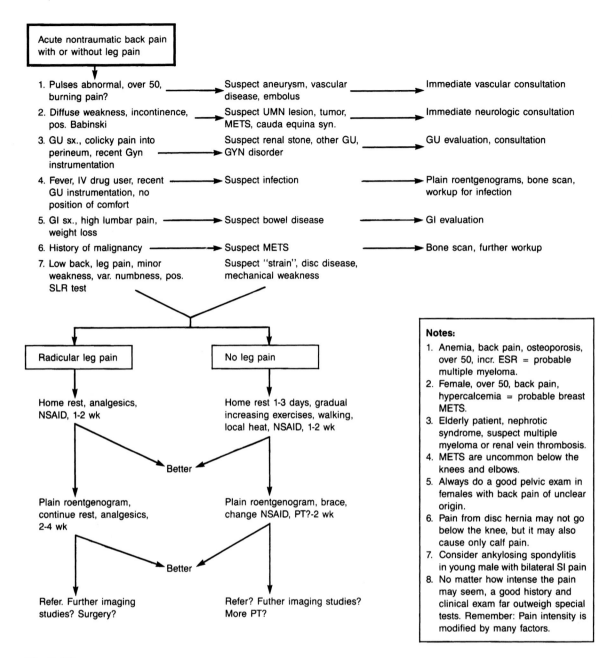

**Fig. 8–32.**
Algorithm for low back and/or leg pain.

# BIBLIOGRAPHY

Aho K et al: HLA antigen 27 and reactive arthritis, *Lancet* 2:157, 1973.

Ansell BM: Rheumatic disorders in childhood, *Clin Rheum Dis* 2:303, 1976.

Appelrouth D, Gottlieb NL: Pulmonary manifestations of ankylosing spondylitis, *J Rheumatol* 2:446, 1975.

Arnett FC: The implications of HL-A W27, *Ann Intern Med* 84:94, 1976.

Avioli LV: Osteoporosis, pathogenesis and therapy. In Avioli LV, Vrane SM, editors: *Metabolic bone disease*, New York, 1977, Academic Press.

Avioli LV: Senile and post-menopausal osteoporosis, *Adv Intern Med* 21:391, 1976.

Avioli LV: Significance of osteoporosis: a growing national health care problem, *Orthop Rev* 21:1126-1129, 1992.

Bauer DC, Browner WS, Cauley JA, et al: Factors associated with appendicular bone mass in older women, *Ann Int Med* 118:657-665, 1993.

Bargolie B et al: Plasma cell myeloma—new biological insights and advances in therapy, *Blood* 73:865, 1989.

Benson MKD, Byrnes DP: The clinical syndromes and surgical treatment of thoracic intervertebral disc prolapse, *J Bone Joint Surg Br* 57:471, 1975.

Bernat JL: A dangerous backache, *Hosp Pract* 12:36, 1977.

Berstein DS et al: Prevalence of osteoporosis in high and low fluoride areas of North Dakota, *JAMA* 198:499, 1966.

Bingham WF: The role of HLA B27 in the diagnosis and management of low back pain and sciatica, *Neurosurg* 47:561, 1977.

Birdi N, Allen U, D'Astous J: Poststreptococcal reactive arthritis mimicking acute septic arthritis: a hospital-based study, *J Pediatr Orthop* 15:661-665, 1995.

Blount WP, Moe JH: *The Milwaukee brace,* Baltimore, 1973, Williams & Wilkins.

Blumberg B, Ragan C: The natural history of rheumatoid spondylitis, *Medicine (Baltimore)* 35:1, 1956.

Boden SD et al: Abnormal magnetic resonance scans of the lumbar spine in asymptomatic subjects, *J Bone Joint Surg Am* 72:403, 1990.

Boden SD, Weisel SW: Lumbar spine imaging: role in clinical decision making, *J Am Acad Orthop Surg* 4:238-248, 1996.

Bolender NF, Schonstrom NSR, Spengler DM: Role of computed tomography and myelography in the diagnosis of central spinal stenosis, *J Bone Joint Surg Am* 67:240, 1985.

Bondilla KK: Back pain: osteoarthritis, *J Am Geriatr Soc* 25:62, 1977.

Bough B et al: Degeneration of lumbar facet joints, *J Bone Joint Surg Br* 72:275, 1990.

Bradford DS et al: Scheuermann's kyphosis: results of surgical treatment by posterior spine arthrodesis in 22 patients, *J Bone Joint Surg Am* 57:439, 1975.

Brewerton DA et al: Reiter's disease and HLA-27, *Lancet* 2:996, 1973.

Brown MD: Diagnosis of pain syndromes of the spine, *Orthop Clin North Am* 6:233, 1975.

Brown MD: *Intradiscal therapy with chymopapain or collagenase,* Chicago, 1982, Year Book Medical Publishers Inc.

Buchanan JR et al: Assessment of the risk of vertebral fracture in menopausal women, *J Bone Joint Surg Am* 69:212, 1987.

Bulkey BH, Roberts WC: Ankylosing spondylitis and aortic regurgitation, *Circulation* 48:1014, 1973.

Calabro JJ, Amante CM: Indomethacin in ankylosing spondylitis, *Arthritis Rheum* 11:56, 1968.

Caldwell AB, Chase C: Diagnosis and treatment of personality factors in chronic low back pain, *Clin Orthop* 129:141, 1977.

Calin A: Raised serum creatine phosphokinase activity in ankylosing spondylitis, *Ann Rheum Dis* 34:244, 1975.

Carman DL et al: Measurement of scoliosis and kyphosis radiographs. Intraobserver and interobserver variation, *J Bone Joint Surg Am* 72:328, 1990.

Carrette S et al: A controlled study of corticosteroid injections into facet joints for chronic low back pain, *N Engl J Med* 325:1002-1007, 1991.

Chapuy MC et al: Vitamin $D_3$ and calcium to prevent hip fractures in elderly women, *N Engl J Med* 327:1637-1642, 1992.

Cuellar ML, Espinoza LR: Management of spondyloarthropathies, *Curr Opin Rheumatol* 8:288-295, 1996.

Curtis P: Low back pain in the primary care setting, *J Fam Pract* 4:381, 1977.

Deen HG: Diagnosis and management of lumbar disk disease, *Mayo Clin Proc* 71:283-287, 1996.

Dickson RA: Conservative treatment for idiopathic scoliosis, *J Bone Joint Surg Br* 67:176, 1985.

Duncan H, Frame B, Frost HM, Arnstein AR: Migratory osteolysis of the lower extremities, *Ann Int Med* 66:1165-1167, 1967.

Dyck P et al: Intermittent cauda equina compression syndrome, *Spine* 2:75, 1977.

Eisenstein SM, Perry CR: The lumbar facet arthrosis syndrome: clinical presentation and articular surface changes, *J Bone Joint Surg Br* 69:3, 1987.

Eismont FJ, Currier B: Current concepts review: surgical management of lumbar intervertebral disc lesions, *J Bone Joint Surg Am* 71:1266, 1989.

Engleman EG, Engleman EP: Ankylosing spondylitis: recent advances in diagnosis and treatment, *Med Clin North Am* 61:347, 1977.

Fast A: Low back disorders: conservative management, *Arch Phys Med Rehabil* 69:880-891, 1988.

Ferris B, Edgar M, Leyshon A: Screening for scoliosis, *Acta Orthop Scand* 59:417, 1988.

Ginsberg GM, Bassett GS: Back pain in children and adolescents: evaluation and differential diagnosis, *J Am Acad Orthop Surg* 5:67-78, 1997.

Godfrey RB et al: A double-blind crossover trial of aspirin, indomethacin and phenylbutazone in ankylosing spondylitis, *Arthritis Rheum* 15:110, 1972.

Greipp PR: Prognosis in myeloma, *Mayo Clin Proc* 69:895-902, 1994.

Guck TP et al: Prediction of long term outcome of multidisciplinary pain treatment, *Arch Phys Med Rehabil* 87:293, 1986.

Haddad JG et al: Effects of prolonged thyrocalcitonin administration in Paget's disease of bone, *N Engl J Med* 283:549, 1970.

Hart FD: The ankylosing spondylopathies, *Clin Orthop* 74:7, 1971.

Harvey MA, James B: *Differential diagnosis,* Philadelphia, 1972, WB Saunders.

Heaney RP: A unified concept of osteoporosis, *Am J Med* 39:877, 1965.

Heaney RP: Nutrition and catch-up bone augmentation in young women, *Am J Clin Nutr* 68:523-524, 1998.

Henley EN, Shapiro DE: The development of low back pain after excision of a lumbar disc, *J Bone Joint Surg Am* 71:719, 1989.

Hensinger RN: Current concepts review. Spondylolysis and spondylolisthesis in children and adolescents, *J Bone Joint Surg Am* 71:1098, 1989.

Hurley DL, Khosla S: Update on primary osteoporosis, *Mayo Clin Proc* 72:943-949, 1997.

Hurme M, Alaranta H: Factors predicting the result of surgery for lumbar intervertebral disc herniation, *Spine* 12:933-938, 1987.

Jackson RP et al: Facet joint injection in back pain: a prospective statistical study, *Spine* 13:966, 1988.

Jausey J et al: Some results of the effects of fluoride on bone tissue in osteoporosis, *J Clin Endocrin* 28:869, 1969.

Jayson MIV, Bouchier LAD: Ulcerative colitis with ankylosing spondylitis, *Ann Rheum Dis* 27:219, 1968.

Jonsson B, Stromquist B: Symptoms and signs in degeneration of the lumbar spine, *J Bone Joint Surg Br* 75:381-386, 1993.

Kertesz A, Kormos R: Low back pain in the workman in Canada, *Can Med Assoc J* 115:901-903, 1976.

Kiel DP et al: Hip fractures and the use of estrogen in postmenopausal women: the Framingham study, *N Engl J Med* 317:1169, 1987.

Kostiuk JP et al: Cauda equina syndrome and lumbar disc herniation, *J Bone Joint Surg Am* 68:386, 1986.

Krupp MA, Chatton MJ: *Current diagnosis and treatment*, Los Altos, Calif, 1972, Lange Medical Publications.

Lane JM, Nydick M: Osteoporosis: current modes of prevention and treatment, *J Am Acad Orthop Surg* 7:19-31, 1999.

Lane JM, Vigorita VJ: Osteoporosis: current concepts review, *J Bone Joint Surg Am* 65:274, 1983.

Lauerman WC, Cain JE: Isthmic spondylolisthesis in the adult, *J Am Acad Orthop Surg* 4:201-208, 1996.

Leutwek L, Whedon GD: Osteoporosis, *DM*, April 1963.

Macnab I: *Backache*, Baltimore, 1977, Williams & Wilkins.

Malpas JS: Problems in the management of myeloma, *Postgrad Med J* 65:468, 1989.

Manniche C et al: Clinical trial of intensive muscle training for chronic low back pain, *Lancet* 24:1473, 1988.

McBryde AM, McCollum DE: Ankylosing spondylitis in women, *N C Med J* 34:34, 1973.

McCullock JA: Chemonucleolysis, *J Bone Joint Surg Br* 59:45, 1977.

McEwen C et al: Ankylosing spondylitis and spondylitis accompanying ulcerative colitis, regional enteritis, psoriasis, and Reiter's disease, *Arthritis Rheum* 14:391, 1971.

McGoey BV et al: Effect of weight loss on musculoskeletal pain in the morbidly obese, *J Bone Joint Surg Br* 72:322, 1990.

Meyerding HW: Spondylolisthesis, *Surg Gynecol Obstet* 54:371, 1932.

Millard PS, Rosen CJ, Johnson KH: Osteoporotic vertebral fractures in postmenopausal women, *Am Fam Physician* 55:1315-1322, 1997.

Miller GM, Forbes GS, Onofrio BM: Magnetic resonance imaging of the spine, *Mayo Clin Proc* 64:986, 1989.

Moe JH, Kettleson DN: Idiopathic scoliosis, *J Bone Joint Surg Am* 52:1509, 1970.

Montgomery SP, Erwin WE: Scheuermann's kyphosis: long-term results of Milwaukee brace treatment, *Spine* 6:5, 1981.

Mooney V: Percutaneous discectomy, *Spine* 3:103, 1989.

Mooney V et al: Chronic low back pain: evaluation and therapy, *Orthop Clin North Am* 9:543, 1978.

Morrissy RT et al: Measurement of Cobb angle on radiographs of patients who have scoliosis. Evaluation of intrinsic error, *J Bone Joint Surg Am* 72:320-327, 1990.

Murray PM, Weinstein SL, Spratt KF: The natural history and long-term follow-up of Scheuermann's kyphosis, *J Bone Joint Surg Am* 75:236-248, 1993.

Nachenson AL: The lumbar spine, an orthopedic challenge, *Spine* 1:59, 1976.

Nash CL: Scoliosis bracing, *J Bone Joint Surg Am* 62:848, 1980.

Nelson MA: Lumbar spinal stenosis, *J Bone Joint Surg Br* 55:506, 1973.

Novak RE, Jones SG, Jones MW: *Novak's textbook of gynecology*, ed 8, Baltimore, 1970, Williams & Wilkins.

O'Connor MI, Carrier BI: Metastatic disease of the spine, *Orthopedics* 15:611-620, 1992.

Ogryzlo MA: Ankylosing spondylitis. In Hollander JL, McCarty DJ Jr, editors: *Arthritis and allied conditions*, ed 8, Philadelphia, 1972, Lea & Febiger.

Ogryzlo MA, Rosen PS: Ankylosing (Marie-Strümpell) spondylitis, *Postgrad Med* 45:182, 1969.

Peterson LE, Nachemson AL: Prediction of progression of the curv in girls who have adolescent idiopathic scoliosis of moderate severity, *J Bone Joint Surg* 77:823-827, 1995.

Petrie RS, Sinaki M, Squires RW, Bergstralh EJ: Physical activity but not aerobic capacity correlates with back strength in healthy premenopausal women from 29 to 40 years of age, *Mayo Clin Proc* 68:738-742, 1993.

Radin EL: Reasons for failure of L5-S1 intervertebral disc excisions, *Int Orthop* 11:255, 1987.

Ramirez LF, Thisted R: Complications and demographic characteristics of patients undergoing lumbar discectomy in community hospitals, *Neurosurgery* 25:226-230, 1989.

Recker RR et al: Effect of estrogen and calcium carbonate on bone loss in post-menopausal women, *Ann Intern Med* 87:649, 1977.

Resnick NM, Greenspan SL: "Senile" osteoporosis reconsidered, *JAMA* 261:1025, 1989.

Riggs BL et al: Short- and long-term effects of estrogen and synthetic anabolic hormone in post-menopausal osteoporosis, *J Clin Invest* 51:1659-1663, 1972.

Riggs BL, Melton LJ III: The prevention and treatment of osteoporosis, *N Engl J Med* 327:620-627, 1992.

Riggs BL, Melton LJ III: Involutional osteoporosis, *N Engl J Med* 314:1676, 1986.

Riggs BL, Melton LJ III: *Osteoporosis. Etiology, diagnosis and management*, New York, 1988, Raven Press.

Rosenberg E et al: Effect of long-term calcitonin therapy on the clinical course of osteogenesis imperfecta, *J Clin Endocrinol Metab* 44:346, 1977.

Ruge D, Wiltse LL: *Spinal disorders: diagnosis and treatment*, Philadelphia, 1977, Lea & Febiger.

Scheuman DJ, Nagel DA: Low back and leg pain, *Primary Care* 1:549, 1974.

Schlosstein L et al: High association of an HL-A antigen, W27, with ankylosing spondylitis, *N Engl J Med* 288:704, 1973.

Sewell KL: Modern therapeutic approaches to osteoporosis, *Rheum Dis Clin North Am* 15:583, 1989.

Sim FH: Metastatic bone disease. Philosophy of treatment, *Orthopedics* 15:541-543, 1992.

Simons GW, Sty JR, Storshak RJ: Retroperitoneal and retrofascial abscesses, *J Bone Joint Surg Am* 65:1041-1058, 1983.

Singer FR: *Paget's disease of bone*, New York, 1977, Plenum Publishing Corp.

Smith L: Enzyme dissolution of the nucleus pulposus in humans, *JAMA* 187:137, 1964.

Spiegel PS et al: Intervertebral disc-space inflammation in children, *J Bone Joint Surg Am* 54:284, 1972.

Steinbach HL, Dodds WJ: Clinical radiology of Paget's disease, *Clin Orthop* 57:277-297, 1968.

Steinbach ML: The roentgen appearance of osteoporosis, *Radiol Clin North Am* 2:191, 1964.

Thompson GH: Back pain in children, *J Bone Joint Surg Am* 75:928-938, 1993.

Tribus CB: Scheuermann's kyphosis in adolescents and adults: diagnosis and management, *J Am Acad Orthop Surg* 6:36-43, 1998.

Turner PG, Green JH, Galasko CS: Back pain in childhood, *Spine* 14:812, 1989.

Turner RH, Bianco AJ: Spondylolysis and spondylolisthesis in children and teen-agers, *J Bone Joint Surg Am* 53:1298, 1971.

Voss LA, Fadale PD, Hulstyn MJ: Exercise-induced loss of bone density in athletes, *J Am Acad Orthop Surg* 6:349-357, 1998.

Waldenstrom J: *Diagnosis and treatment of multiple myeloma,* New York, 1970, Grune & Stratton Inc.

Walson AH, Rohwedder JJ: Upper lobe fibrosis in ankylosing spondylitis, *AJR* 124:466, 1975.

Wedgewood RJ, Schaller JG: The pediatric arthritides, *Hosp Pract* 12:83, 1977.

Weinerman SA, Bockman RS: Medical therapy of osteoporosis, *Orthop Clin North Am* 21:109, 1990.

Weinstein SL: Adolescent idiopathic scoliosis: prevalence and natural history, *Am Acad Orthop Surg Lect* 38:115, 1989.

Wenger DR, Bobechko WP, Gilday DL: The spectrum of intervertebral disc-space infection in children, *J Bone Joint Surg Am* 60:100, 1978.

Wheeler M: Osteoporosis, *Med Clin North Am* 60:1213, 1976.

Williams PC: The conservative management of lesions of the lumbosacral spine, *Am Acad Orthop Surg Lect* 10:90, 1953.

Wiltse LL, Widell EH, Jackson DW: Fatigue fracture: the basic lesion in isthmic spondylolisthesis, *J Bone Joint Surg Am* 57:1722, 1975.

# CHAPTER 9

# The Pelvis and Sacrum

Except for ankylosing spondylitis, painful disorders of the pelvis are uncommon. Most are secondary to trauma and usually respond to conservative treatment.

## ANATOMY

The bony pelvis is formed by the innominate bones, the sacrum, and the coccyx. Each hip (innominate) bone is composed of three elements: the ischium, the ilium, and the pubis. These three components meet at the acetabulum and are united by the triradiate cartilage until the age of 16 years, when fusion takes place. The sacrum is composed of five vertebrae, and the coccyx usually consists of four. The coccyx and sacrum are situated more posteriorly in women than in men and thus are more exposed to trauma.

Little motion occurs at the sacroiliac and interpubic joints because of strong ligamentous structures at these areas. Some motion occurs at the sacrococcygeal joint, but little is present between coccygeal segments.

## ROENTGENOGRAPHIC ANATOMY

The pelvis can be well visualized by a routine anteroposterior roentgenogram (Fig. 9-1). In addition, the sacrum and coccyx may be studied by lateral views and anteroposterior views angled 15 degrees cephalad and caudad.

## OSTEITIS PUBIS

Osteitis pubis is a painful inflammation of the pubic symphysis that is usually self-limited. The cause is unknown, but the condition often develops after urologic procedures or infections, after childbirth, or after repetitive stresses associated with certain athletic activities.

### Clinical Features

The onset is gradual, with symptoms developing a few days after the traumatic event. Pain and tenderness over the symphysis pubis are usually present. Coughing may aggravate the pain, which radiates along the adductor and rectus abdominis muscles. Stretching these muscles is painful.

Examination reveals local tenderness over the symphysis pubis and adjacent soft tissue. Passive abduction of the hips and active adduction of the hips against resistance are painful.

Roentgenograms of the pelvis taken early in the disease may be normal. Later, variable amounts of spotty demineralization, widening of the symphysis pubis, and sclerosis are noted (Fig. 9-2). Bone scanning is often positive. Reossification eventually occurs over several months.

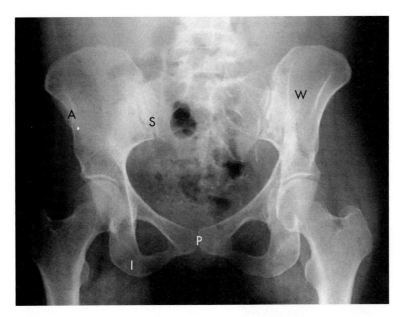

**Fig. 9–1.**
Pelvic roentgenogram: *S* = sacroiliac joint; *A* = anterior superior iliac spine; *P* = pubic symphysis; *I* = ischium; *W* = wing of the ilium.

### Treatment

Treatment consists of NSAIDs, rest, and stretching exercises. This may be supplemented by deep heat or ice. A local steroid/lidocaine injection may also be helpful. The disease has a tendency toward spontaneous recovery, but this may take several weeks. The activity level of the patient is allowed to increase as tolerated.

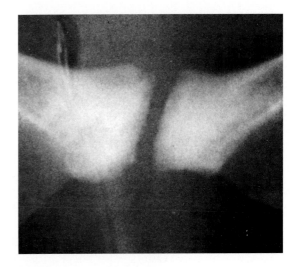

**Fig. 9–2.**
Osteitis pubis.

## DISORDERS OF THE SACROILIAC JOINT

The sacroiliac (SI) joints consist of large, broad, irregular articular surfaces made of depressions and ridges. This interlocking nature, along with extensive capsular and ligamentous support, contributes to its considerable inherent stability. Little movement occurs in these joints.

There is considerable controversy surrounding conditions that may affect the SI joints. Although these joints may occasionally be involved with inflammatory diseases, they are rarely the source of other pathology. Al-

though some textbooks continue to discuss various disorders, "dysfunctions," and injuries ("going out"), most have never been proven. Pain from the lumbar spine is often referred to this area, which can be a further source of confusion. Lastly, except for the presence of local tenderness, there are no good, reliable clinical tests or maneuvers that can be used as a part of the physical examination to localize pain to this joint. Provocative testing using joint injection has been used with inconclusive results, and except in late cases, roentgenographic evaluation is usually of limited value as well.

## Osteitis Condensans Ilii

This is a lesion of unknown etiology in which bilateral sclerosis occurs in a fairly large area of ilium adjacent to the sacroiliac joints (Fig. 9-3). It is most common in multiparous women. Its importance lies in distinguishing it from ankylosing spondylitis (Marie-Strümpell disease). Ankylosing spondylitis is usually associated with an increase in the sedimentation rate and roentgeno-

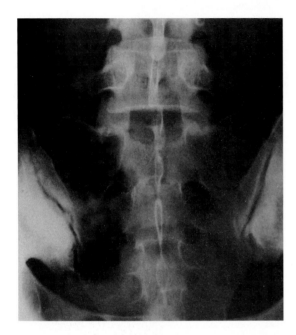

**Fig. 9–3.**
Osteitis condensans ilii. The iliac portions of the sacroiliac joints are sclerotic and white. The joints themselves are not involved.

graphic involvement on both sides of the sacroiliac joint. It occurs primarily in men and is associated with pain. However, there is disagreement as to whether osteitis condensans ilii is ever a painful condition. It may be associated with lesions similar to those seen in the pubic bones near the symphysis pubis in osteitis pubis.

## Sacroiliitis

Bilateral sacroiliitis occurs in conjunction with a group of diseases called seronegative spondyloarthropathies (see Chapter 8). The SI joints are involved early in the course of these diseases. The HLA-B27 antigen is usually present in these disorders, which often involve the spinal joints as well.

## Infection

Unilateral bacterial involvement of the SI joint is uncommon and often overlooked because of poorly localizing symptoms. The SI joint is a common site for pyarthrosis associated with parenteral drug abuse, and organisms involved are often unusual (commonly *Pseudomonas*). The signs and symptoms may suggest sepsis of the hip, kidney, or even the retroperitoneal area. Bone scanning and joint aspiration are often required to confirm the diagnosis.

## Degenerative Joint Disease

Symptomatic involvement of these joints by osteoarthritis is unusual. Even when findings are present roentgenographically, symptoms may be minimal or absent completely (Fig. 9-4). Treatment is symptomatic in these rare cases and, partly because of the difficulty in the diagnosis, surgery is almost never recommended.

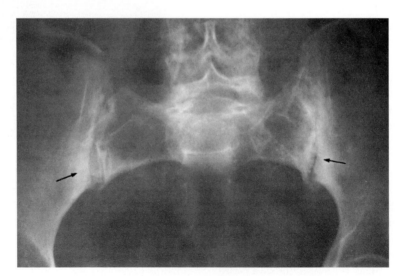

**Fig. 9–4.**
Pelvic roentgenogram showing bilateral osteoarthritic joint changes.

# DISORDERS OF THE SACROCOCCYGEAL REGION

The coccyx consists of three to five segments and usually angulates forward to a variable degree. The sacrococcygeal (SC) junction is a symphysis. In the normal, erect sitting position with weight on the thighs, the coccyx does not have pressure against it. With flattening of the lumbar lordosis and sitting in the slumping position, however, the coccyx can reach the seat, and pain may develop over its tip (coccygodynia). Coccygodynia is not really a disease but simply a symptom. Disorders of the coccyx are uncommon.

Fracture of the coccyx can occur, usually from a fall on the more exposed coccyx of the female. It has been described during obstetric procedures. During childbirth, the coccyx is forced backward up to 2 cm or more. This is allowed by a healthy SC joint. Sometimes forceful movement of the coccyx is recommended during difficult deliveries when a stiff SC segment impedes delivery. Injury to the coccyx may occur and lead to fibrosis and stiffness. Manipulation or fracture of this stiffened segment may be required in future deliveries.

Chronic strains and osteoarthritis may also result from repetitive trauma. Joint motion is usually restricted, and activities that move the coccyx are painful. Complete bony ankylosis may even result, with the coccyx fusing in a deformed position. Fractures of the tip of the sacrum or coccyx also occur, but usually do not produce long-term symptoms unless a painful pseudarthrosis or traumatic arthritis ensues. "Tailbone" (sacrum or coccyx) fractures are actually quite uncommon. The roentgenogram is often misinterpreted because of the normal sacrococcygeal and intercoccygeal spaces.

The sacrum and coccyx are commonly the site of pain referral from visceral structures or lumbar disc degeneration. However, the exact etiology of coccygodynia is unknown in most cases.

## Clinical Features

Pain on sitting is the most common complaint. This pain is aggravated by slumping, by sitting on a hard seat, or by activity. Many symptoms begin with an injury and may be aggravated by constipation or rectal disease. The symptoms are more common in women. Local pain and tenderness at the sacrococcygeal joint and adjacent soft tissues are common physical findings. A rectal examination should always be performed and often reveals pain on sacrococcygeal motion. This pain often radiates into the buttocks.

Depending on the history, the roentgenogram may reveal recent injury or degenerative arthritis. Fractures, when they occur, usually involve the lower part of the sacrum or first sacrococcygeal segment (Fig. 9-5). Osteoarthritis may be noted at the sacrococcygeal joint.

The alignment or configuration of the sacrum or coccygeal segments visualized roentgenographically seems to have little importance in coccygodynia.

### Treatment

All forms of painful coccyx are treated with warm sitz baths and a soft doughnut-shaped pillow. Constipation should be avoided. Analgesics and antiinflammatory drugs are prescribed as necessary. A local injection of steroid is often beneficial for chronic inflammation or osteoarthritis.

Because the coccyx is often the site of exaggerated symptoms in patients who somatize, and because it is difficult to pinpoint the exact source of coccygeal pain in many patients, surgery is rarely indicated. The occasional patient with painful osteoarthritis or a rigid, deviated coccyx who does not respond to conservative measures may benefit from coccygectomy, but even this procedure is rarely performed any longer. Acute injuries are all treated conservatively for at least 6 months, even when significant anterior angulation of the coccyx is present.

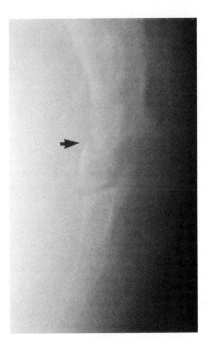

**Fig. 9–5.**
Fracture of the lower portion of the sacrum (arrow) just above the sacrococcygeal joint.

# BACK AND PELVIC PAIN IN PREGNANCY

More than half of all women develop low back pain during pregnancy. It usually begins around the fifth month and the exact cause is unknown. It is more common in multiparous patients and in those with a previous history of back pain. Postpartum pain may also develop in some patients.

Several theories have been advanced to explain this pain, but much of the information regarding the problem is only anecdotal. Most of these theories relate to changes (hormonal, vascular and mechanical) that may occur during pregnancy.

One theory suggests that lumbar spine pain develops because of the forward shift of the center of gravity with development of an increase in the lumbar lordosis. Combined with the increased pelvic tilt, this could explain the midline lumbar discomfort that occurs in many women. The development of pain does not seem to follow the distribution of weight gain during pregnancy, however. Although lumbar disc herniation is rare, disc "protrusion" may also play some role. The intervertebral joints could also be more relaxed than normal, leading to lumbar strain.

Another explanation involves the production of relaxin and the relaxation of the sacroiliac joints and the symphysis pubis. The symphysis pubis widens from a normal of 0.5 mm to a maximum of 12.0 mm. after delivery. The SI joint is normally stable as a result of its broad, interlocking surfaces, and most studies show that little motion occurs at the joint. Excess pelvic relaxation and symphysiolysis may rarely lead to "instability" at the SI joint or symphysis pubis and result in inflammation, although physical tests to assess SI motion are generally unreliable.

Direct pressure by the gravid uterus may also play some role in the onset of pain, especially in late pregnancy.

A vascular cause for back pain has also been theorized. It is known that the relaxed, gravid uterus can compress the aorta and vena cava. It is also known that venous return is increased at night when the dependent edema of the lower extremities returns to the vascular space at rest with the legs elevated. This could lead to some compromise of the circulation to the lumbar neural elements and produce the back and leg pain with cramping that is seen at night during some pregnancies.

The presence of scoliosis does not seem to have any adverse effects on the outcome of pregnancy, although some studies suggest that there may be a slight progression of the curve during pregnancy. Unless the curve is severe, it does not appear to contribute to back pain.

## Prevention and Treatment

Although no specific treatment has much scientific validity, the following suggestions may be offered to the pregnant patient with low back pain:

1. Practice good lifting habits. Flat shoes could help lumbar lordosis. Keep the knees higher than the hips when sitting.
2. Do general conditioning exercises, especially low-impact aerobics or walking.
3. Try lumbar stretching exercises for lordosis; they may help. Pelvic tilt and hip flexion (knee to chest) are advised.
4. Stretch and strengthen the hamstrings to compensate for weakened abdominals.
5. Maintain abdominal muscle tone. However, some suggest avoiding standard sit-ups, which require the supine position and can increase intraabdominal pressure from the Valsalva maneuver. Instead, do lateral bending and trunk rotation exercises in the standing position.
6. If the SI joint or symphysis pubis is clearly involved, try wearing an SI corset or trochanteric belt while walking or standing. Acute pain may need bed rest and a pelvic binder.
7. To avoid the night pain from vascular pressure, wear good support hose during the day; this may decrease the development of edema. Special pillows are available to elevate the abdomen, and positional changes at night may help.
8. Remember that most symptoms resolve a few months after delivery. Lumbosacral corsets may be helpful for residual symptoms postpartum.

# EPISACRAL LIPOMAS

Two types of pain in the fatty tissue of the low back have been described. The most common is the tender, fatty nodule in the SI area, sometimes called the *episacroiliac lipoma* or "back mouse." It has been speculated that some fatty tissue may herniate through the normal deep fascia and become edematous and the source of pain. The significance of these nodules is disputed. Clinically, the patient complains of pain in the tender nodules, which are palpable and often bilateral. The mass is usually palpable as a mobile, soft tumor that slips beneath the examining finger. The treatment ranges from ignoring the lesion as insignificant to multiple puncturing and injection of the nodule with local anesthetic, followed by massage. Surgical removal does not seem justified because of the uncertainty regarding their significance.

A less common area of pain is the normal presacral fat pad. The patient is most often female and the pain may be related to the menstrual cycle. There may even be complaints of a sense of "swelling" in the area, although none is usually present on examination. Most likely, pain in this normal fat pad is referred from elsewhere, but the cause remains obscure.

## FRACTURES OF THE PELVIS

The pelvic ring is essentially a rigid circle with little motion at the interpubic or sacroiliac areas. Fractures involving the ring are generally classified as stable or unstable (see Chapter 16). Stable fractures are those in which the ring is completely broken only at one point (for example, superior and inferior pubic ramus fractures on the same side). With unstable fractures, the ring is broken in two or more areas (for example, both pubic rami on the same side plus an SI dislocation).

Stable fractures commonly result from minor falls, especially in elderly, osteoporotic females. These fractures may be treated symptomatically with a short period (1 to 2 days) of rest followed by ambulation and weightbearing as tolerated, usually with a walker.

Unstable fractures (Fig. 9-6) are often serious and potentially life threatening. They may be accompanied by genitourinary or other visceral injuries. Posterior fractures, in particular, may damage the adjacent venous and arterial system and produce massive retroperitoneal bleeding. The initial care is therefore directed at general stabilization of the patient. The fracture usually requires prolonged immobilization and, occasionally, surgical repair.

Fractures of the acetabulum occasionally involve the main weight-bearing surface of the hip joint (Fig. 9-7). Reduction, either surgically or by traction on the femur, may be needed to restore a smooth surface and prevent the development of traumatic arthritis.

### Pelvic Insufficiency Fractures

This injury is a type of stress fracture that almost exclusively occurs in elderly females. Stress fractures can be of two types: (1) fatigue and (2) insufficiency. Fatigue fractures develop when unusually high stress is applied to a normal bone. Insufficiency fractures occur in weak bone undergoing normal stress.

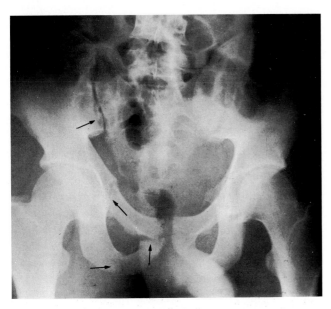

**Fig. 9–6.**
An unstable fracture of the pelvis. In addition to the fractures of the pubic bones, a sacroiliac separation is present on the ipsilateral side. Whenever displacement is present in a fracture at the pubic ramus, injury to another point in the pelvic ring is likely.

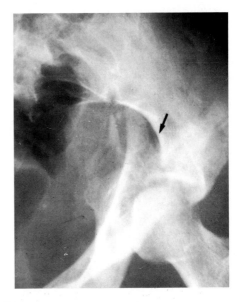

**Fig. 9–7.**
Fracture of the acetabulum (arrow). Reduction of the weight-bearing portion was obtained by skeletal traction.

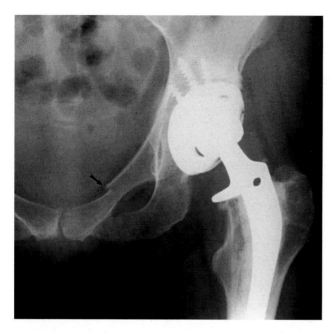

**Fig. 9–8.**
Insufficiency fracture of the pubic bone *(arrow)*. The patient had recently been able to increase her walking activity after successful joint replacement.

Osteoporosis is the usual predisposing cause, but inactivity, long-term steroid use, and other types of metabolic bone disease may also play a role. The usual sites of fracture are the pubic bones, ilium, and sacrum (Fig. 9-8). Because there is usually no history of trauma, the injury is often overlooked or misinterpreted as metastatic disease. Multiple areas may even be involved. (Compression fractures of the vertebrae and femoral neck fractures may act in a similar fashion, but are generally easier to recognize.)

### Roentgenographic Findings

When the fracture involves the sacrum, it is usually vertical and may be bilateral. The findings of early resorption or late sclerosis may be easily missed because of superimposed bowel gas as well as the subtle appearance of the fracture. Iliac involvement is usually above the acetabulum.

Bone scanning is extremely sensitive for this injury as well as other similar conditions. Fractures may be detected as early as 3 days after the onset. (Scans may also remain slightly positive for 1 to 2 years.) Computed tomographic evaluation will usually allow differentiation from metastatic disease.

## BIBLIOGRAPHY

Berg G et al: Low back pain during pregnancy, *Obstet Gynecol* 71:71-75, 1988.

Curtis P: In search of the "back mouse," *J Fam Pract* 36:657-659, 1993.

Dittrich RJ: Coccygodynia as referred pain, *J Bone Joint Surg Am* 33:715, 1951.

Failinger MS, McGanety PL: Current concepts review: unstable fractures of the pelvic ring, *J Bone Joint Surg Am* 74:781-791, 1992.

Gotis-Graham I, Mcguigen L, Diamond T et al: Sacral insufficiency fractures in the elderly, *J Bone Joint Surg* 16B:882-886, 1994.

Grasland A, Pouchot J, Mathieu A et al: Sacral insufficiency fractures: an easily overlooked cause of back pain in elderly women, *Arch Intern Med* 156:668-674, 1996.

Hauge MD, Cooper KL, Litin SC: Insufficiency fractures of the pelvis that simulate metastatic disease, *Mayo Clin Proc* 63:807, 1988.

Heckman JD, Sassard R: Current concepts review: musculoskeletal considerations in pregnancy, *J Bone Joint Surg Am* 76:1720-1730, 1994.

Howorth B: The painful coccyx, *Clin Orthop* 14:145, 1959.

Kristiansson P, Svardsudd K, von Schoultz B: Back pain during pregnancy: a prospective study, *Spine* 21:702-709, 1996.

Macnab I: *Backache*, Baltimore, 1977, Williams & Wilkins.

Mooney V: Can we measure function in the sacroiliac joint? In Vleeming A et al, editors: *The first interdisciplinary world congress on low back pain and its relation to the sacroiliac joint*, Rotterdam, the Netherlands, 1992, ECO.

Postacchini F, Massobrio M: Idiopathic coccygodynia: analysis of 51 operative cases and a radiographic study of the normal coccyx, *J Bone Joint Surg Am* 65:1116-1124, 1983.

Resnik CS, Resnik D: Radiology of disorders of the sacroiliac joints, *JAMA* 253:2863, 1985.

Rungee JL: Low back pain during pregnancy, *Orthopedics* 16:1339-1344, 1993.

Schnute WJ: Osteitis pubis, *Clin Orthop* 20:187, 1961.

Shipp FL, Haggart GE: Further experience in the management of osteitis condensans ilii, *J Bone Joint Surg Am* 32:841, 1950.

Sturesson B: Mobility of pelvis in living persons. In Vleeming A et al, editors: *The first interdisciplinary world congress on low back pain and its relation to the sacroiliac joint*, Rotterdam, the Netherlands, 1992, ECO.

Swezey RI: Non-fibrositic lumbar subcutaneous nodules: prevalence and clinical significance, *Br J Rheumatol* 30:376-378, 1991.

Traycoff RB, Crayton H, Dodson R: Sacrococcygeal pain syndromes: diagnosis and treatment, *Orthopedics* 12:1373, 1989.

Wray CC, Eason S, Hoskinson J: Coccydynia. Aetiology and treatment, *J Bone Joint Surg Br* 73:335-338, 1991.

# CHAPTER 10

# The Hip

The hip is a ball-and socket joint in which the femoral head articulates deeply into the acetabulum. This deep fit, combined with thick ligamentous and muscular supporting structures, makes the hip extremely stable but relatively inaccessible. Therefore the diagnosis of disorders of the hip is sometimes difficult.

## ANATOMY

The proximal portion of the femur consists of a head, neck, and greater and lesser trochanters. The axes of the neck and femoral shaft form an angle in the anteroposterior plane known as the neck-shaft angle or "angle of inclination." This normally measures 125 to 130 degrees. An increase in this angle is termed coxa valga; a decrease is termed coxa vara. The neck and shaft also form an angle in the transcondylar plane that is referred to as the angle of femoral torsion (Fig. 10-1). Normal femoral torsion is 40 degrees in the child, and this decreases to 15 to 20 degrees in the adult. Excessive femoral torsion is termed anteversion or antetorsion and is sometimes responsible for in-toeing. A decrease in the normal femoral torsion is termed retroversion or retrotorsion and may cause an out-toeing gait.

The vascular anatomy of the femoral head is of critical importance in many disorders of the hip. The main sources of blood supply are the retinacular and intramedullary vessels, both of which course from the intertrochanteric region proximally to nourish the femoral head (Fig. 10-2). Diseases or injuries that compromise the circulation may damage the viability of the femoral head and lead to avascular necrosis.

Among the nerves that supply the hip joint is the obturator nerve. This nerve also supplies a sensory branch to the medial side of the thigh and motor supply to some of the hip adductors. Irritation of this nerve from hip joint disease may result in referred pain along the inner aspect of the knee and thigh that may cause confusion with disorders of the knee joint. Therefore complaints of pain in this area (in the absence of physical findings in the knee) should always draw attention to the hip joint.

## EXAMINATION

Several bony landmarks are available for orientation on physical examination. The anterior and posterior superior iliac spines and iliac crest are easily palpable because they are not crossed by any muscles (Fig. 10-3). The proximal portion of the iliac crest lies at the level of the fourth lumbar vertebra. The greater trochanter is palpable laterally, and the pubic symphysis is palpable anteriorly.

The femoral head lies approximately 2.5 cm distal and lateral to the point where the femoral artery passes beneath the inguinal ligament. This relationship should be recalled when performing venipuncture from the femoral vein. A needle passed through the vein may enter the hip joint and introduce infection into the hip. All femoral venipuncture sites should therefore be meticulously scrubbed and prepared prior to needle insertion.

## ROENTGENOGRAPHIC ANATOMY

The roentgenographic study of the hip joint should include views in the anteroposterior and lateral planes (Fig. 10-4). The lateral view may be either a "true" lateral or a "frog-leg" exposure that is taken with the hips in maximum external rotation.

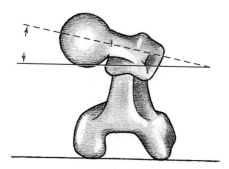

**Fig. 10–1.**
The angle of femoral torsion.

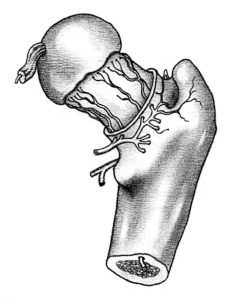

**Fig. 10–2.**
Blood supply to the head of the femur. Fracture through the neck can seriously disrupt the circulation to the head.

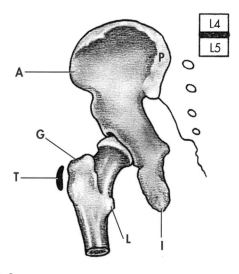

**Fig. 10–3.**
Bony landmarks of the hip: *A* = anterior superior iliac spine; *G* = greater trochanter; *T* = trochanteric bursa; *P* = posterior superior iliac spine; *L* = lesser trochanter; *I* = ischial tuberosity. The upper level of the iliac crest lies at the level of the fourth lumbar vertebra. Adjacent to the posterior superior iliac spine is the sacroiliac joint.

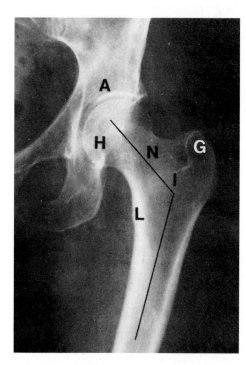

**Fig. 10–4.**
Anteroposterior roentgenogram of the normal hip: *A* = rim of the acetabulum; *H* = head of the femur; *N* = neck of the femur; *L* = lesser trochanter; *G* = greater trochanter; *I* = intertrochanteric region. The angle of inclination is marked.

## CONGENITAL DYSPLASIA OF THE HIP

Congenital dysplasia of the hip (CDH) is a common disorder in which the femoral head may be displaced out of the acetabulum to varying degrees. The condition is often bilateral, and although the cause is unknown, heredity appears to play a role. Females are affected nine times more often than males, and although the condition may affect both hips, the left is more commonly involved. Firstborn children, or children born by breech deliveries, also have a higher incidence of the disorder. It is occasionally present in association with clubfoot and congenital muscular torticollis deformities. The hip may be frankly dislocated at birth or "dislocatable." The child may even be born with simple hip dysplasia without dislocation. In this case dislocation may occur months later, a situation sometimes called developmental hip dislocation rather than congenital dislocation. The minimally subluxed hip with inadequate coverage by the acetabulum may even cause the late onset of osteoarthritis in adulthood.

Pathologically, abnormalities are seen in both the acetabulum and femoral head. The acetabulum may be shallower in contour and more vertically inclined than normal. This results in insufficient coverage and inadequate containment of the femoral head. The femur is often excessively anteverted, and the hip joint capsule may also be lax.

### Clinical Features

The clinical picture will range from minimal findings to obvious frank dislocation depending on the age of the child. In the newborn, provocative maneuvers such as Barlow's and Ortolani's tests are commonly used to detect instability. The tests are similar. The Ortolani test refers to the gentle reduction of the dislocated hip by abduction of the flexed hip (Fig. 10-5). This is often accompanied by a soft "clunk." In Barlow's test, the hip is purposely dislocated by gentle downward pressure of the flexed, adducted hip. With posterior pressure, the femoral head will be displaced out of the acetabulum if the hip is unstable. The head is then reduced by gentle abduction of the flexed hip. Barlow's test should not be performed excessively as it could make the problem worse. Asymmetric skin folds are often unreliable as indicators of CDH as are the presence of "clicks," which simply may be transmitted noise from the knee or trochanter.

Within a few weeks, the hip is less flexible and the ability to reduce the dislocated hip by the provocative maneuvers is lessened. At this time, the only finding may be limited abduction (Fig. 10-6). If the hip is dislocated, it may not be reducible and other signs, such as shortening of the extremity, are present (Fig. 10-7).

If weight bearing has begun, a painless limp is often the initial symptom. Hip motion, especially abduction, is limited and abnormal piston mobility or "telescoping" may be present. The Trendelenburg test is usually positive. This test takes advantage of the fact that normally, when standing on one leg, contraction of the abductor muscles on the side bearing weight will cause the opposite side of the pelvis to be elevated. If the hip is dislocated, these muscles no longer work effectively, and when the child stands on the affected leg, the opposite side of the pelvis moves downward instead.

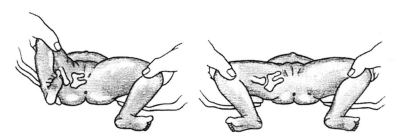

**Fig. 10–5.**
Ortolani's sign for congenital dislocation of the hip. A "click" is palpable or audible as the hip is reduced by abduction. If the test is negative, the examination should always be repeated in 2 to 4 months.

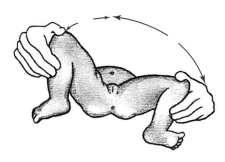

**Fig. 10–6.**
Restricted abduction of the right hip.

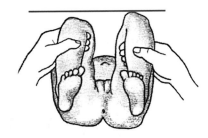

**Fig. 10–7.**
Galeazzi's or Allis' sign. The child is placed on a firm surface with the hips and knees flexed. The knee will appear lower on the dislocated side.

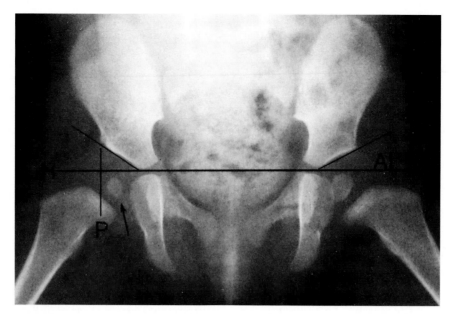

**Fig. 10–8.**
Roentgenogram of the pelvis: *P* = Perkin's vertical line; *H* = Hilgenreiner's horizontal line; *AI* = acetabular index. The ossification center of the capital femoral epiphysis should lie in the inferior medial quadrant formed by Perkin's and Hilgenreiner's lines. The AI normally measures less than 30 degrees. Here, ossification of the capital epiphysis on the dysplastic hip *(arrow)* has been delayed as compared with the left.

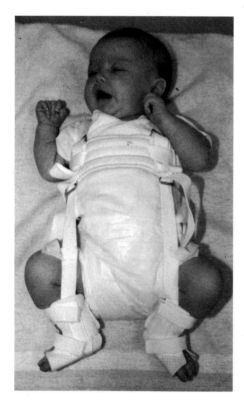

**Fig. 10–9.**
The Pavlik harness.

The roentgenographic examination is usually not helpful when the patient is under 3 months of age unless a complete dislocation is present. After this age, a delay in the ossification of the femoral head is often noted (Fig. 10-8). The acetabulum may be more inclined vertically, and the acetabular index is often increased. If subluxation or dislocation has occurred, upward and outward displacement of the femoral head will be seen.

Ultrasonography is useful in congenital hip dysplasia, especially in high-risk infants (such as those who are breech-delivered or who have a positive family history) or those with uncertain clinical findings. Among its benefits is the elimination of exposure to radiation. Magnetic resonance imaging (MRI) may eventually be helpful, but the diagnosis can usually be established by other means.

### Treatment

Any suggestion of instability in the hip of the newborn warrants treatment. The treatment is initiated as soon as possible and varies with the age of the patient and the degree of dysplasia. *Early detection* is of utmost importance because conservative treatment is more likely to succeed in the infant. The more the child's age exceeds the weight-bearing age, the more likely surgery will be necessary and the less likely a normal functional result will ensue. Whenever any doubt exists, treatment and follow-up are indicated.

The objective of treatment is to reduce the femoral head into the acetabulum and maintain that reduction. By maintaining the hip in the reduced position, normal development of the hip joint structures and acetabulum is encouraged. A variety of external devices are available for the treatment of the hip with moderate instability and stiffness. The most functional is the Pavlik harness, which maintains the hip in a more natural "human" position, allows active motion, and prevents full extension in the adducted position (Fig. 10-9). The har-

ness is usually worn for several weeks until the hip is stable. This device does not force the hip into the excessive abduction that can occur when using triple diapers or many of the other abduction splints. This position of extreme abduction may actually harm the hip by exerting too much pressure on the femoral head, which may lead to avascular necrosis.

Failure to obtain or maintain a stable reduction necessitates surgical intervention. The objective is to reduce the hip by either closed or open methods and maintain the reduction by casting or osteotomy. Children are usually kept under observation until the capital epiphysis is properly located in a well-formed acetabulum.

## LEGG-CALVÉ-PERTHES DISEASE

Perthes' disease, or coxa plana, is a self-limited disorder of the hip in which a portion of the ossific nucleus of the femoral head undergoes avascular necrosis. Eventually, the infarcted, necrotic bone is absorbed and replaced by normal bone. The cause of this condition is unknown, but some cases follow transient synovitis of the hip. The disorder usually occurs between the ages of 4 and 10 years, and males are four times more commonly affected than females. Fifteen percent of cases are bilateral, and the condition is rare in blacks.

The disease is often divided into three stages. The early stage of the disease is characterized by inflammation and synovitis of the hip joint and early ischemic changes in the ossific nucleus of the femoral head. Roentgenograms taken at this stage reveal joint swelling that may result in lateral displacement of the femoral

head. An increase in the opacity of the ossific nucleus is usually present (Fig. 10-10).

In the second stage, called the regenerative or fragmentation stage, the necrotic area begins to be replaced by viable bone. This phase lasts from 1 to 2 years. The roentgenographic appearance during this stage is one of fragmentation and compression of the femoral head with secondary widening of the femoral neck.

Reossification and healing occur in the third stage, which varies in duration beyond 1 year. The roentgenogram in this stage shows a disappearance of the rarefaction while normal bone continues to re-form. The final roentgenographic appearance depends on several factors, including the age of the patient and the degree of involvement. The femoral head may end up normal in shape or irregular and flat (coxa plana) as a result of

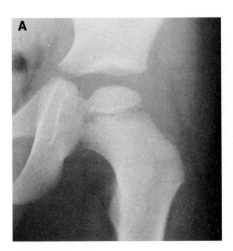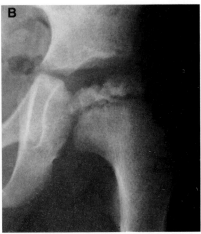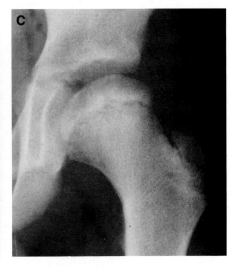

**Fig. 10–10.**
Roentgenographic changes in Legg-Calvé-Perthes disease. **A,** In the early stages the joint space is widened, and the head is dense. **B,** The head is fragmented, and the metaphysis is widened. **C,** End result after treatment. Normal function was restored.

collapse of the osteonecrotic bone and overlying cartilage. The end result may be osteoarthritis if coxa plana develops.

### Clinical Features

The onset is gradual, and the initial complaint is usually a mildly painful limp. The pain is often referred down the inner aspect of the thigh to the knee (via the obturator nerve). The discomfort is often relieved by rest and aggravated by weight bearing. Examination reveals moderate restriction of motion secondary to the synovitis. Abduction and internal rotation are especially limited. Pain is present at the extremes of motion, and tenderness is usually noted over the anterior hip joint.

Plain roentgenograms are usually abnormal, but MRI or bone scanning may be helpful in equivocal cases.

### Treatment and Prognosis

The ultimate goal of treatment is to prevent deformity of the femoral head while healing is progressing. If deformity can be prevented, the chances of degenerative joint disease developing at a later date are lessened. The initial goals of treatment are the relief of pain and maintenance of joint motion (accomplished by rest) to control synovitis. Then the femoral head must be centered and kept in the acetabulum. If the head is contained in the acetabulum while it is re-forming, the acetabulum will "mold" the head and prevent significant deformity from occurring. These goals of treatment are usually accomplished by the use of an abduction brace that allows motion but contains the head in the acetabulum (Fig. 10-11). The brace must be worn continuously for up to 2 years, although the results of specific forms of treatment remain inconclusive and some investigators advocate only nighttime bracing. Surgery may be necessary in certain selected cases.

The prognosis depends on the age of the patient, the degree of involvement, and the adequacy of treatment. Young patients with minimal involvement who are treated early do well with few sequelae. Patients over the age of 8 years often have some permanent restriction of motion, a slight limp, and a more irregular or flattened femoral head. A few patients will later develop degenerative arthritis.

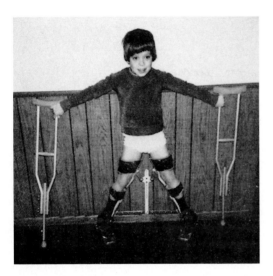

**Fig. 10–11.**
Abduction brace.

## SLIPPED CAPITAL FEMORAL EPIPHYSIS

Slipped capital femoral epiphysis is a disorder of unknown cause in which weakening of the epiphyseal plate of the upper portion of the femur occurs and results in upward and anterior displacement of the femoral neck. The actual amount of displacement will vary. In most cases, the slippage is gradual, and some elements of healing are usually present.

The condition is seen most commonly in boys between the ages of 11 and 16 years during their rapid growth spurt. The disorder is bilateral in 25% of cases and often occurs in two distinct body types. The first is the slender, tall, rapidly growing boy; the second is the large, obese boy with underdeveloped sexual characteristics. The presence of the disorder in these two body types suggests a hormonal cause, but none has ever been proved.

### Clinical Features

The onset is generally gradual, and symptoms usually occur even when little displacement is present. Discomfort in the hip, groin, and knee and a painful limp with activity are the most common initial complaints.

Examination reveals tenderness over the hip joint capsule. An external rotation (toeing-out) deformity of the lower extremity may be present, and internal rotation, abduction, and flexion are usually restricted. Pain is present at the extremes of motion, and the hip tends to rotate externally and abduct as it is flexed (Whitman's sign).

In the early "preslipping" stage, the roentgenogram characteristically reveals irregular widening of the epiphyseal plate and joint swelling (Fig. 10-12). As displacement occurs, a line drawn along the superior or anterior neck of the femur will transect less of the femoral head than normal. This may be more readily seen on the lateral view. More severe degrees of slippage are usually easily diagnosed.

A condition similar to slipped capital femoral epiphysis is termed *acute traumatic separation* of the upper femoral epiphysis (Fig. 10-13). This is actually an epi-

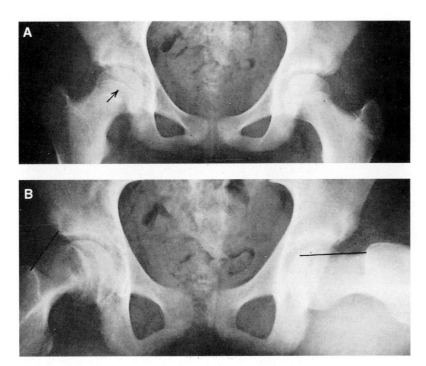

**Fig. 10–12.**
Slipped capital femoral epiphysis. **A**, Widening of the epiphyseal plate on the right side *(arrow)* and **B**, displacement of the femoral head are present. Displacement is best seen on the lateral view.

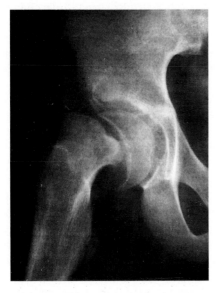

**Fig. 10–13.**
Acute traumatic separation of the upper femoral epiphysis.

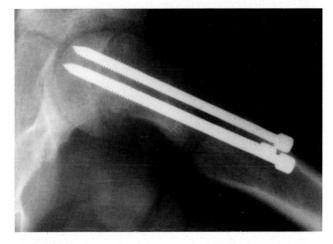

**Fig. 10–14.**
Postoperative roentgenogram after pinning for slipped capital femoral epiphysis.

physeal fracture and has a much poorer prognosis than the gradual slippage that occurs in slipped capital femoral epiphysis.

### Treatment

As soon as the diagnosis is made, surgery is indicated. The patient is immediately placed on crutches, and weight bearing is prohibited. Traction in the hospital may be necessary to reduce the acute component of the slippage. To prevent further slippage from occurring, the femoral head is fixed to the neck, generally by using small pins (Fig. 10-14). Weight bearing is prohibited for several months until the epiphyseal plate closes. Severe deformities may also require osteotomy of the femur.

The prognosis is usually good, except in those cases with acute traumatic separation. Slight shortening of

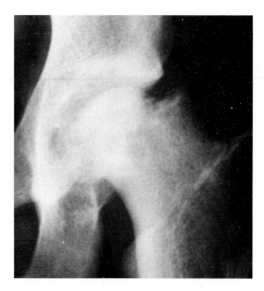

**Fig. 10–15.**
Avascular necrosis and osteoarthritis after acute traumatic slipped capital femoral epiphysis. Reconstructive surgery was eventually required.

less than 1.25 cm may result, along with a mild external rotation deformity. In cases with acute traumatic separation, avascular necrosis of the femoral head is a common complication, and this usually results in severe traumatic arthritis of the hip (Fig. 10-15).

## Acute Cartilage Necrosis (Chondrolysis)

An occasional complication of slipped capital femoral epiphysis is acute necrosis or lysis of the articular cartilage of the hip joint. The articular surfaces of both the acetabulum and femoral head may be involved up to 1 year after the slippage. This condition appears to be directly related to the severity of the slippage. The cause of this process is unknown, but destruction and degeneration of the hyaline cartilage occur. A painful fibrous ankylosis of the hip joint is often the end result.

# TRANSIENT SYNOVITIS (IRRITABLE HIP)

Transient or "toxic" synovitis is a self-limited, nonspecific inflammation of the synovium of the hip joint that occurs in children. It is the most common cause of pain in the hip in children under 10 years of age. The cause is unknown, but a viral infection is suspected. Its importance lies in its similarity to other hip joint disorders, especially septic arthritis. The diagnosis is one of exclusion.

### Clinical Features
The onset is often acute and may follow a traumatic event or a recent upper respiratory infection. A painful limp is characteristic, and the pain is often referred to the inner aspect of the thigh and knee joint. A few patients will have night pain.

The hip is typically held in a position of slight flexion, abduction, and external rotation so that the hip joint capsule is under the least amount of tension. Pressure and discomfort are thereby reduced. Passive motions, especially internal rotation and abduction, are restricted. Temperatures of 37.3° C to 38.3° C may be present.

Roentgenograms are usually normal but may reveal swelling of the capsule and adjacent soft tissue. Slight widening of the joint space may also be present, but there are no changes in bone texture. Ultrasonography may help determine the presence of joint fluid.

Laboratory findings are usually minimal, although there may be a slight increase in the white blood cell count. Aspiration and culture of the hip joint fluid are negative, although fluid examination is required only if septic arthritis is suspected.

### Treatment
Bed rest, gentle skin traction, and the elimination of weight bearing are indicated. The relief of pain and discomfort is usually rapid, and motion is restored in 2 to 4 days. Crutches are used for 2 to 4 weeks, and the patient is observed closely for up to 2 years. This is because Perthes' disease may develop in some cases, although the exact relationship is unclear. Antibiotics are used only when the disorder is associated with an infection elsewhere. Recurrences are possible.

# SEPTIC ARTHRITIS IN CHILDHOOD

Pyogenic infection of the hip may result from an osteomyelitis of the femoral neck or from a bacteremia. It may even develop from contamination by a faulty femoral venipuncture. If improperly treated, complete destruction of the hip joint may occur.

### Clinical Features
The onset is usually rapid and develops over 24 hours. The child appears acutely ill and refuses to bear weight. The hip is held flexed and externally rotated, and movement is painful. Fever, leukocytosis, and an ele-

**TABLE 10–1.**

The Limping Child—Differential Diagnosis of Common Causes*

| Disorder | Symptoms/History | Findings |
| --- | --- | --- |
| Congenital dislocated hip | Painless. Usually noticed when child first begins to walk (12-18 mo). May be bilateral | Trendelenburg sign positive. Leg shortened if unilateral. "Telescoping" of leg at hip. Abnormal roentgenogram |
| Perthes' disease (or other AVN) | Minimal pain (groin, anteromedial thigh). Age 4-8 yr. Family history positive if due to rare sickle cell or other hereditary anemia. No fever | Decreased hip ROM, especially abduction, and IR. Roentgenogram may show early joint widening. Later (2-4 wk) bony changes. Lab normal (except if a result of blood disorder) |
| Toxic synovitis | Irritable. Slight fever, groin and anteromedial thigh pain. Age 4-8 yr | Diminished hip movement. Slightly painful with motion. Roentgenogram may show slight joint space widening, fluid. Slight increase in ESR, WBC. Hip aspirate shows increased WBC, no bacteria |
| Septic hip | Painful! Septic, febrile, unable to ambulate. Groin pain (may be difficult to localize findings in young child) | Pain on slightest hip movement. Roentgenogram shows hip joint swelling. Hip aspirate positive for bacteria. Lab reflects infection |
| Slipped upper femoral epiphysis | Age 10-14 yr. Mild ache in groin, thigh. Leg often externally rotated | Limited IR. Roentgenogram shows slippage |
| "Low-grade" osteomyelitis, lower limb | Fever, irritable. Moderate pain with weight bearing (may be difficult to localize findings in young child) | Local bony tenderness and soft tissue swelling. Protected motion. Early plain roentgenogram normal. Bone scan abnormal |
| Inflammatory joint disease | Single or multiple joints. May be mildly febrile | Joint swelling, heat. Some limitation of motion. Serum studies sometimes abnormal. Often diagnosis of exclusion |
| Neurologic disorders (CP, etc.) | Often bilateral. No pain. Gait is wide based. Delay in motor development. History of perinatal problems | Abnormal neurologic findings |

* **Notes:** Always consider (1) battered child (especially if history of prior injuries, such as burns), (2) tumor, and (3) occult fractures. *IR* = internal rotation; *ROM* = range of motion.

vated sedimentation rate are common. Plain roentgenograms may show only widening of the joint space as a result of swelling, and bone scanning is usually not helpful in the initial stages.

### Treatment

Hip sepsis in the child is an emergency. Aspiration of the hip before the administration of antibiotics is the most diagnostic procedure. This is usually performed under fluoroscopic guidance and general anesthesia. *Staphylococcus aureus* and *Streptococcus* are the most common offending organisms. If infection is confirmed, intravenous antibiotics are started, and the hip is usually drained surgically.

### Differential Diagnosis

Differentiation of mild cases from toxic or rheumatoid synovitis may be difficult. A child with toxic or rheumatoid synovitis generally appears well except for the hip, the fever is usually mild, and the hip is more "irritable" than painful. The white blood count and sedimentation are only slightly elevated. The hip aspirate may show an increase in white blood cells, especially polymorphonucleocytes, but the Gram stain and culture will be negative. Complete bed rest and symptomatic care usually cause considerable improvement in 24 hours, in contrast to a septic hip, which usually gets worse (Table 10-1).

## COXA VARA

Coxa vara is an abnormality of the upper portion of the femur that consists of a decrease in the normal angle of inclination below 110 to 125 degrees (Fig. 10-16). This may be caused by a variety of acquired and congenital conditions and usually results in a shortened extremity.

### Acquired Forms

Acquired forms are the most common types of coxa vara. Included in this category are Perthes' disease, slipped

capital femoral epiphysis, rickets, osteomalacia, and various injuries to the upper part of the femur. Each disease has its own clinical and roentgenographic features.

### Congenital Forms

Congenital local disturbances in the growth of the proximal aspect of the femur may also lead to shortening and a significant coxa vara deformity. These disorders usually fall into three distinct classifications: (1) congenital

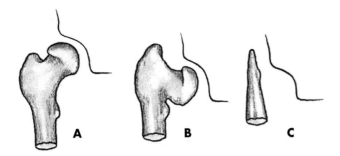

**Fig. 10–16.**
**A,** The normal neck-shaft angle. **B,** Coxa vara. **C,** Proximal focal femoral deficiency.

coxa vara, (2) congenital bowed femur with coxa vara, and (3) congenital short femur with coxa vara.

### Congenital Coxa Vara (Infantile, Cervical, Developmental)

In this disorder, a faulty development of the femoral neck leads to the varus deformity. The cause is unknown. The disorder is often bilateral and becomes manifested after weight bearing has begun.

The child usually presents with a painless limp. If the disorder is bilateral, a "duck-waddle" gait may be present. In this gait pattern, the body sways from side to side. Abduction and internal rotation of the affected extremity are usually restricted, and the leg may be from 2.5 to 5 cm shorter than normal. The lumbar lordosis is usually exaggerated, and with continued weight bearing the varus deformity may progress.

Roentgenographic examination usually reveals a decrease in the neck-shaft angle. In addition, a triangular defect in the inferior aspect of the femoral neck may be present.

The treatment of mild deformities in which the neck-shaft angle is greater than 100 degrees consists of a shoe lift, exercises to release contractures, and periodic reexamination. A brace that prohibits weight bearing may be necessary. More severe deformities require an osteotomy of the upper portion of the femur to correct the angulation.

### Congenital Bowed Femur With Coxa Vara

This type of coxa vara is characterized by lateral bowing of the femur. The coxa vara is usually not as severe as that found with congenital coxa vara, but the shortening of the extremity may reach 10 to 15 cm. Treatment consists of equalizing the extremities by shoe lifts.

### Congenital Short Femur With Coxa Vara

This uncommon disorder is also known as proximal focal femoral deficiency. Portions of the proximal aspect of the femur are either completely absent or severely underdeveloped, and shortening of the limb may reach 25 to 37.5 cm by adulthood. Bracing is necessary in the young child, and amputation of the lower part of the leg, followed by prosthetic fitting to equalize the leg lengths, is usually the definitive treatment.

# DEGENERATIVE ARTHRITIS (OSTEOARTHRITIS)

Degenerative arthritis confined to the hip joint is a common affliction in the middle and later years of adult life. The cause is not completely understood, but trauma, congenital hip dysplasia, avascular necrosis of the femoral head, and slipped capital femoral epiphysis can be factors in its onset.

Pathologically, the articular cartilage becomes progressively thinned and worn away. New bone proliferation around the femoral head and acetabulum occurs, and the synovium becomes chronically thickened and congested.

### Clinical Features

The clinical course is gradual and both hips may be affected. The onset of symptoms may be precipitated by a relatively minor injury. Pain after activity and stiffness after rest are characteristic. The stiffness often subsides with activity and the pain often subsides with rest. The pain is often referred to the knee joint region. The pain increases with the passage of time, sometimes occurring even at rest. Crepitus and grating in the hip may develop, and a painful limp is common. Patients often complain that they cannot flex and externally rotate the hip to put on their stockings.

Examination reveals tenderness over the anterior and posterior hip joint and restriction of motion, especially

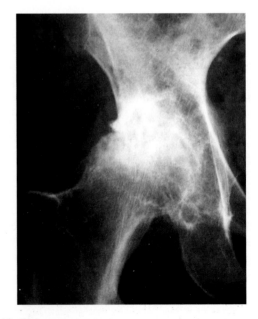

**Fig. 10–17.**
Degenerative arthritis of the hip.

rotation and abduction. Pain is usually present at the extremes of motion. A flexion contracture often develops. This can be measured by the Thomas test. In this test, the patient is placed in a supine position and the opposite thigh is flexed up to the chest to eliminate motion at the pelvis and lumbar spine. The angle formed between the affected thigh and the examining table is the amount of flexion contracture of the hip.

The roentgenographic findings are characteristic (Fig. 10-17). Irregular sclerosis, joint space narrowing, and osteophyte formation are prominent features.

### Treatment

Conservative treatment will often relieve symptoms and improve motion. The regimen requires a cooperative patient. NSAIDs are often helpful and the joint is unloaded. Weight reduction is recommended when indicated and the use of a cane is encouraged. The cane is usually held in the hand opposite the affected extremity (although it may be used in the ipsilateral hand) and pressure is applied to the cane while weight is borne on the painful hip (see Chapter 18). Moist heat is sometimes helpful. Gentle range-of-motion exercise such as swimming will often overcome contractures and restore motion. The treatment plan may have to be repeated at intervals. Intraarticular hip joint injection with steroid is rarely performed as a result of the relative inaccessibility of the joint

A variety of surgical options are available for those patients who fail to respond to conservative treatment. Osteotomy or arthrodesis may be considered, but the most popular is total hip arthroplasty. The goal is the elimination of pain. In addition, joint replacement will often improve hip joint motion. The indications for each procedure will vary according to the age and occupation of the patient.

## AVASCULAR NECROSIS (OSTEONECROSIS)

Avascular or aseptic necrosis of the femoral head is an uncommon condition that occurs in the third to fifth decade. It is characterized by the development of an area of bone necrosis in the anterosuperior weight-bearing portion of the femoral head. The cause is unknown ("idiopathic") in most cases, but the condition is often bilateral and is more common in men. It may be seen in association with gouty arthritis, chronic alcoholism, and chronic renal disease; in divers and workers who use compressed air; and in those patients who have undergone long-term steroid therapy. It can develop after dislocation of the hip. It probably occurs secondary to a circulatory disturbance to the femoral head. After the initial infarction, collapse and fragmentation may occur, which lead to deformity of the femoral head and degenerative arthritis.

### Clinical Features

The onset is gradual, with pain and a slight limp being common. A history of trauma is usually absent in the usual idiopathic type. Joint motion becomes progressively restricted, mainly as a result of chronic synovitis.

The roentgenogram reveals an increase in the density of the superior portion of the femur (Fig. 10-18). A radiolucent zone is often present between the avascular segment and the surrounding bone. The joint space is usually well preserved until late in the disease when collapse of the head occurs. This can cause irregularity and later degenerative arthritis. Avascular necrosis is one of the main indications for MRI, which usually reveals the lesion quite clearly (Fig. 10-19).

### Treatment

The goal of treatment is to prevent collapse of the femoral head and to encourage repair of the necrotic

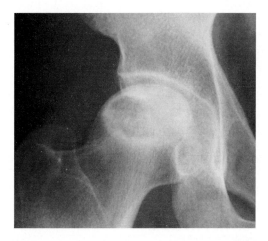

**Fig. 10–18.**
Avascular necrosis of the femoral head.

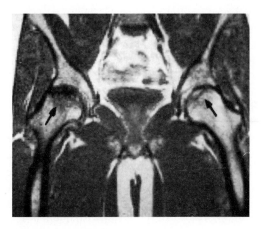

**Fig. 10–19.**
MRI showing bilateral avascular necrosis.

area. With minimal involvement, prolonged abstinence from weight bearing through the use of crutches may allow regeneration of the avascular segment, although considerable time is required. Later in the disease, when collapse has occurred, prosthetic replacement is indicated.

## BURSITIS

Several bursae are present about the hip joint. The one most subjected to irritation and pain is the trochanteric bursa. This sac lies between the greater trochanter and the overlying tendinous portion of the gluteus maximus muscle. Inflammation of the sac is common in the elderly patient and is characterized by local pain over the trochanter that often radiates down the lateral aspect of the thigh to the knee. This pain pattern may cause confusion with lumbar disc disease. Local tenderness usually is present, and hip motion, especially internal rotation and abduction, may be painful. It is difficult for the patient to lie on the affected side. Roentgenograms are usually normal, although irregularity and calcification over the trochanter have been observed.

Treatment consists of moist heat, rest, and antiinflammatory agents. Ultrasound to the affected area may be beneficial, and a local injection of a steroid/lidocaine mixture into the area of maximum tenderness is often curative (Fig. 10-20).

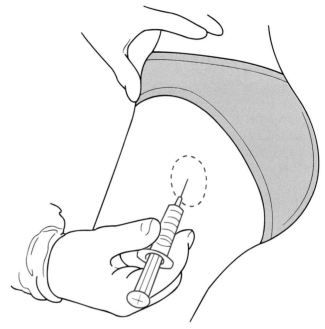

**Fig. 10–20.**
Injection for trochanteric bursitis. The point of maximal tenderness is injected with 1 ml of steroid and 5 ml of lidocaine. A spinal needle may be required in the obese patient. The needle tip should encounter bone and the area should be widely infiltrated.

## THE SNAPPING HIP

This is a condition in which a palpable snapping sensation occurs with hip motion, usually during rotation in adduction. The snap may even be audible and visible. The most common cause is a tightness of a portion of the iliotibial band, which catches on the prominent greater trochanter during movement. The condition may be associated with trochanteric bursitis. Rare causes include snapping of the iliopsoas tendon over the head of the femur; and intraarticular pathology. The sensation often can be reproduced by the patient. Usually there is little discomfort.

Treatment is generally symptomatic for the common trochanteric bursitis. Heat, local cortisone injections, reassurance, and modification of activities are usually curative.

## MERALGIA PARESTHETICA

Meralgia paresthetica is a common disorder characterized by pain and paresthesias occurring along the course of the lateral femoral cutaneous nerve of the thigh. This nerve enters the leg beneath the inguinal ligament and supplies sensation to the anterolateral aspect of the thigh (Fig. 10-21). Painful involvement of the nerve may be confused with hip and low back disorders. The cause of this condition is unknown, but direct pressure or constriction of the nerve at its point of exit into the thigh is thought to play a role. The condition is more common in joggers and in gymnasts (possibly as a result of repeated excessive hip extension exercises). Rarely the disorder can be traced to an intraabdominal or pelvic mass (because of the retroperitoneal course of the nerve). The condition may be confused with an L3-L4 disc problem.

### Clinical Features

The disorder is sometimes seen in obese patients or those who wear tight corsets or undergarments. Hypersensitivity, burning, tingling, and pain that occurs with activity or direct pressure over the nerve are characteristic. The symptoms are often relieved by rest and hip flexion.

The pain may be aggravated by passive extension of the hip. A slight decrease in sensation over the anterolateral aspect of the thigh is sometimes noted, and pain may be reproduced with pressure on the nerve medial to the anterior superior iliac spine. A good pelvic and abdominal examination should be performed. Electrodiagnostic studies are not helpful except to rule out other causes.

### Treatment

Painful symptoms often subside spontaneously over a variable length of time although numbness may be permanent. Weight loss and the avoidance of constricting garments are advised. Injection of the nerve distal to the inguinal ligament 1.25 cm medial and 2.5 cm below the anterosuperior iliac spine with a local anesthetic may relieve symptoms. Surgical release or even removal of

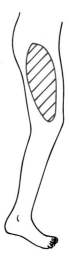

**Fig. 10–21.**
Sensory area of the anterolateral thigh affected in meralgia paresthetica.

the nerve may occasionally be necessary for intractable cases, but the surgical results are only fair.

## PROTRUSIO ACETABULI (OTTO PELVIS)

Abnormal intrapelvic protrusion of the acetabulum is a relatively uncommon disorder of unknown cause. It may be present on a congenital basis or develop secondary to trauma or arthritis. It is often bilateral and is characterized by abnormal deepening of the acetabulum, which allows the femoral head to be displaced further into the pelvis.

### Clinical Features

The onset is usually gradual, with progressive restriction of hip motion occurring over several years. Eventually, with the onset of degenerative arthritis, pain becomes a prominent symptom. Complete ankylosis of the joint often occurs. The roentgenogram reveals abnormal protrusion of the medial wall of the acetabulum with thinning and degenerative changes (Fig. 10-22).

### Treatment

Treatment is the same as for osteoarthritis. Surgery is usually required for disabling pain.

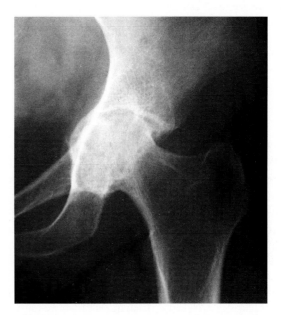

**Fig. 10–22.**
Protrusio acetabuli. The medial acetabular wall protrudes and the femoral head has migrated medially.

## DISLOCATIONS OF THE HIP

Dislocations of the hip are the result of severe trauma and are usually posterior in direction (Fig. 10-23). They commonly result from the knee being struck while the hip and the knee are in a flexed position. This force drives the femoral head out of the joint posteriorly. These injuries are often associated with fractures of the posterior acetabular wall. Anterior dislocations are less common and usually result from a force on the knee with the thigh abducted. The

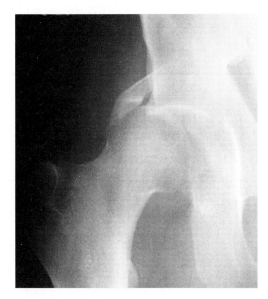

**Fig. 10–23.**
Posterior dislocation of the hip (with fracture of acetabulum).

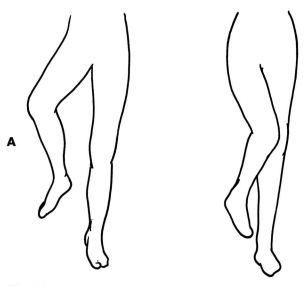

**Fig. 10–24.**
Appearance of hip dislocations: **A,** Anterior (hip is externally rotated). **B,** Posterior (hip is internally rotated).

neck of the femur impinges on the posterior rim of the acetabulum, and the head is levered out the front.

### Clinical Features

With posterior dislocation the hip is characteristically held in a position of flexion and internal rotation (Fig. 10-24). All motions are painful. There may be an associated injury of the ipsilateral knee. In anterior dislocations the leg usually rests in external rotation.

### Treatment

Hip dislocation is an emergency. In the dislocated position, great tension is placed on the blood supply to the femoral head and avascular necrosis may result if the dislocation is not promptly reduced. To prevent this complication, early reduction is indicated. Weight bearing is often prohibited after reduction.

## FRACTURES OF THE HIP

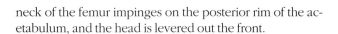

The femoral head receives its blood supply from vessels that course proximally up the femoral neck. Fractures that occur distal to these vessels (intertrochanteric) do not disturb the blood supply to the femoral head, but fractures that occur proximally (intracapsular) may destroy the blood supply. With disruption of the blood supply, nonunion of the fracture and avascular necrosis of the femoral head are much more common.

Intracapsular and intertrochanteric fractures are both common in the elderly patient and usually result from a fall on the hip. Both fractures are characterized by shortening and external rotation of the affected leg with pain in the region of the hip joint (Fig. 10-25). Osteoporosis clearly plays a significant role (see Chapter 8). Occasionally, the patient may actually fracture the hip before falling, the fracture representing the completion of an insufficiency injury. Femoral neck fractures may also be occult and show up only with repeated examinations, bone scan, or MRI.

### Treatment

The objective of management is the return to the pre-injury level of function as soon as possible. If external immobilization or prolonged bed rest were required in the treatment of these fractures in this age group, the mortality would be high as a result of pneumonia, DVT, and urinary tract infections. For this reason, early surgery within 24 to 48 hours is indicated to allow the patient to be out of bed at the earliest possible time. Displaced *intracapsular* fractures in the elderly are best treated by early prosthetic replacement (Fig. 10-26). This allows early weight bearing and eliminates the possibility of nonunion and avascular necrosis that could necessitate secondary surgical procedures. (If osteoarthritis is present, total hip replacement is often performed.) Undisplaced or impacted fractures are often treated nonoperatively or by simple internal fixation to add stability. These fractures have a much better prognosis regarding healing and avascular necrosis.

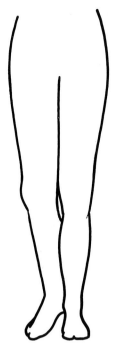

**Fig. 10–25.**
External rotation deformity typical of hip fractures.

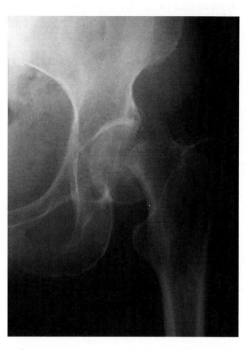

**Fig. 10–26.**
Roentgenogram of the hip showing a displaced femoral neck fracture.

Young, healthy patients are treated by reduction of the fracture (if needed) and internal fixation. It is best to try to preserve the femoral head in this age group if it is possible because the long-term results are better than with prosthetic replacement.

*Intertrochanteric* fractures are treated by open reduction and internal fixation (Fig. 10-27). This allows early activity by eliminating the pain at the fracture site. Nonunion in this fracture is much less common than with the intracapsular fracture. Weight bearing is usually restricted for 3 months until union of the fracture has occurred, however.

**Nonsurgical treatment.** Intertrochanteric and intracapsular fractures occasionally occur in nonambulatory patients, sometimes as a result of a fall during a transfer. These fractures are usually treated nonsurgically, especially in the demented patient with limited pain perception. Early bed-to-chair mobilization and vigilant nursing care are important to prevent complications. The fracture usually becomes pain-free in a short time and even if solid bony healing does not occur, a painless fibrous union develops with a satisfactory end result.

Occasionally, an isolated fracture of either trochanter may occur after a minor injury (Fig. 10-28). Treatment is symptomatic, with crutches and weight-bearing activity as tolerated.

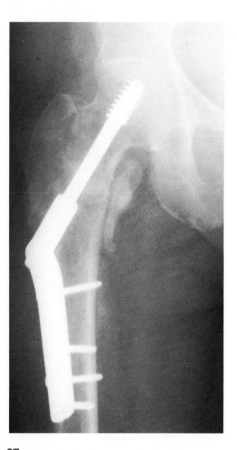

**Fig. 10–27.**
Roentgenogram after reduction and nailing of an intertrochanteric fracture.

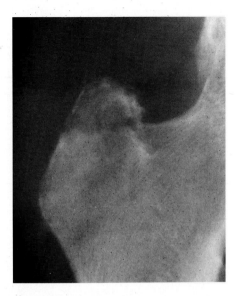

**Fig. 10–28.**
Avulsion fracture of the greater trochanter.

## The Occult Hip Fracture

Some fractures about the hip are difficult to diagnose. This is especially true of the fatigue fracture of the femoral neck or pelvis. There may be no history of injury, particularly when the femoral neck is involved. El-derly females with osteoporosis are susceptible. Vague groin pain may be present and, as with other disorders involving the hip region, the pain may be referred down the medial thigh to the knee. In the absence of displacement there is no deformity, and there is often full range of motion, although there may be pain with movement, especially "rolling" the leg in the supine patient. Weight bearing is usually painful as well. There may be some local tenderness.

The initial roentgenograms may be negative, although a true lateral view will occasionally reveal a femoral neck fracture not obvious on other views.

If the diagnosis is suspected, the patient should be admitted to the hospital and placed on non–weight-bearing status to prevent displacement of the fracture in case one is present. Bone scanning is helpful. It may show evidence of the fracture as early as 24 hours but is often not diagnostic until 48 to 72 hours. Magnetic imaging is also helpful, and although more costly, it can allow more early diagnosis and treatment. A "limited" study is available in many radiology departments at less cost. However, in most patients, the hip pain has been present for 2 or 3 days, and bone scanning is usually sufficient to establish the diagnosis. Treatment is usually surgical for femoral neck fractures to prevent displacement, which could require a more complicated operation.

## DIFFERENTIAL DIAGNOSIS OF BACK AND LEG PAIN (TABLE 10-2)

**TABLE 10–2.**
Differential Diagnosis of Common Causes of Back, Hip, and Leg Pain (see Fig. 10-29)

| Disorder | Common Pain Location or Radiation | Findings Present | Findings Absent |
|---|---|---|---|
| Disc disease | Low back, high buttock. May radiate to posterior thigh (posterior or lateral calf if nerve root impingement). May have paresthesias in foot (Fig. 10-29) | Limited low back movement. Often no history of injury. May have positive SLR. Neurologic deficit if nerve root under pressure | Normal hip movement. No local tenderness other than low back |
| Hip disease (osteoarthritis, AVN, etc.) | Groin, low buttock. Anteromedial thigh to knee | Groin pain with hip movement. Decreased hip movement | No back pain, no pain below knee. No neurologic symptoms or findings |
| Hamstring strain | Posterior thigh | Painful SLR but local tenderness, swelling, and hemorrhage in hamstring. History of acute strain to muscle | Back motion normal. No low back pain. No paresthesias or pain below knee |
| Trochanteric bursitis | Lateral hip, lateral thigh to knee | Tender greater trochanter. May have pain on adduction with IR | Full range of hip and back motion. No paresthesias. No low back pain |
| Spinal stenosis | Variable. Both buttocks, legs. Older patient "pseudoclaudication" pain—worse with walking, better with rest. Long history of back pain. Pain often relieved by flexion of spine | Back extension may reproduce pain. May have minimal variable neurologic abnormalities. Usually advanced degenerative disc disease on roentgenogram | Straight leg raising usually negative. Hips move normally |

*AVN* = avascular necrosis; *SLR* = straight leg raising; *IR* = internal rotation.

**A**          **B**          **C**

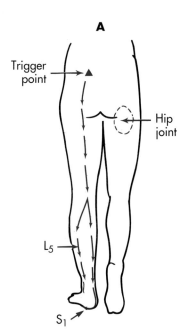
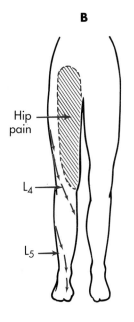
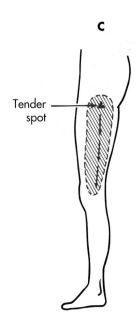

**Fig. 10–29.**
**A,** Typical lumbar disc pain when herniation is far enough to cause radicular (L5 or S1) pain. If herniation is minor, only unilateral low back pain may occur. **B,** Anterior distribution of hip joint pain. (Hip disease may also cause low buttock pain.) Also shown are nerve roots L4 and L5. **C,** Pain distribution of trochanteric bursitis. **Note:** Calf or general leg symptoms may be the first and only sign of lumbar disc herniation with radiation. Chronic "hamstring" pain lasting longer than 3 to 4 weeks, especially in the absence of an obvious injury, should suggest a radiculopathy.

## BIBLIOGRAPHY

Aadalen RJ et al: Acute slipped capital femoral epiphysis, *J Bone Joint Surg Am* 56:1473-1487, 1974.

Aegerter E, Kirkpatrick JA: *Orthopedic diseases*, ed 3, Philadelphia, 1968, WB Saunders.

Allen WC, Cope R: Coxa saltans: the snapping hip revisited, *J Am Acad Orthop Surg* 3:303-308, 1995.

Allwright SJ, Cooper RA, Nash P: Trochanteric bursitis: bone scan appearance, *Clin Nucl Med* 13:561, 1988.

Amstutz HC, Wilson PD Jr: Dysgenesis of the proximal femur (coxa vara) and its surgical management, *J Bone Joint Surg Am* 44:1, 1962.

Anderson GH et al: Preoperative skin traction for fractures of the proximal femur. A randomized prospective trial, *J Bone Joint Surg Br* 75:794-796, 1993.

Aronson DD, Karal LA: Stable slipped capital femoral epiphysis: evaluation and management, *J Am Acad Orthop Surg* 4:173-181, 1996.

Boeree NR, Clarke NM: Ultrasound imaging and secondary screening for congenital dislocation of the hip, *J Bone Joint Surg* 76(4):525-533, 1994.

Bos CF, Bloem JL: Treatment of dislocation of the hip, detected in early childhood based on magnetic resonance imaging, *J Bone Joint Surg Am* 71:1523, 1989.

Bowen JR, Foster BK, Hartzell CR: Legg-Calvé-Perthes disease, *Clin Orthop* 185:97, 1984.

Cattaral A: The natural history of Perthes' disease, *J Bone Joint Surg Br* 53:37, 1971.

Clarke NM et al: Real-time ultrasound in the diagnosis of congenital dislocation and dysplasia of the hip, *J Bone Joint Surg Br* 67:406, 1985.

Coleman BG et al: Radiographically negative avascular necrosis: detection with MR imaging, *Radiology* 168:528, 1988.

Coleman SS: Treatment of congenital dislocation of the hip, *J Bone Joint Surg Am* 47:590, 1965.

Curtis BH et al: Treatment for Legg-Perthes disease with the Newington ambulation-abduction brace, *J Bone Joint Surg Am* 56:1135, 1974.

Davies SJ, Walker G: Problems in the early recognition of hip dysplasia, *J Bone Joint Surg Br* 66:479-484, 1984.

Engesaeter LB et al: Ultrasound and congenital dislocation of the hip, *J Bone Joint Surg Br* 72:197-201, 1990.

Epstein HC: Posterior fracture-dislocations of the hip, *J Bone Joint Surg Am* 56:1103, 1974.

Ficat RP: Idiopathic bone necrosis of the femoral head, *J Bone Joint Surg Br* 67:3, 1985.

Friedenberg ZB: Protrusio acetabuli, *Am J Surg* 85:764, 1953.

Gage JR, Winter RB: Avascular necrosis of the capital femoral epiphysis as a complication of closed reduction of congenital dislocation of the hip, *J Bone Joint Surg Am* 54:373, 1972.

Genez BM et al: Early osteonecrosis of the femoral head. Detection in high risk patients with MR imaging, *Radiology* 168:521, 1988.

Gore DR: Iatrogenic avascular necrosis of the hip in young children, *J Bone Joint Surg Am* 56:493, 1974.

Grant JCB: *A method of anatomy*, ed 6, Baltimore, 1958, Williams & Wilkins.

Hauzeur JP et al: The diagnostic value of magnetic resonance imaging in non-traumatic osteonecrosis of the femoral head, *J Bone Joint Surg Am* 71:641, 1989.

Hermel MB, Albert SM: Transient synovitis of the hip, *Clin Orthop* 22:21, 1962.

Hernandez RS, Cornell RG, Hensinger RN: Ultrasound diagnosis of neonatal congenital dislocation of the hip, *J Bone Joint Surg Am* 76:539-543, 1994.

Ilfeld FW, Makin M: Damage to the capital femoral epiphysis due to Frejka pillow treatment, *J Bone Joint Surg Am* 59:654, 1977.

Iwasaki K: Treatment of congenital dislocation of hip by the Pavlik harness, *J Bone Joint Surg Am* 65:760, 1983.

Kennie DC et al: Effectiveness of geriatric rehabilitative care following fractures of the proximal femur in elderly women: a randomized clinical trial, *Br Med J* 297:1083, 1988.

Koval KJ, Zuckerman JD: Functional recovery after fracture of the hip. Current concepts review, *J Bone Joint Surg Am* 76:751-758, 1994.

Landin LA, Danielson LG, Wattsgard C: Transient synovitis of the hip: its incidence, epidemiology and relation to Perthes disease, *J Bone Joint Surg Br* 69:238, 1987.

Lennox IA, McLauchlan J, Murali R: Failures of screening and management of congenital dislocation of the hip, *J Bone Joint Surg Br* 75:72-76, 1993.

Marcus ND, Enneking WF, Massan RA: The silent hip in idiopathic aseptic necrosis (treatment by bone-grafting), *J Bone Joint Surg Am* 55:1351, 1973.

Marks DS, Clegg J, al-Chalabi AN: Routine ultrasound screening for neonatal hip instability, *J Bone Joint Surg Br* 76(4):534-538, 1994.

Meyers MH: *Fractures of the hip*, Chicago, 1985, Year Book Medical Publishers.

Mitchell GP: Problems in the early diagnosis and management of congenital dislocation of the hip, *J Bone Joint Surg Br* 54:4, 1972.

Petrie JG, Bitenc I: The abduction weight-bearing treatment in Legg-Perthes' disease, *J Bone Joint Surg Br* 53:56, 1971.

Poul J et al: Early diagnosis of congenital dislocation of the hip, *J Bone Joint Surg Br* 74:695-700, 1992.

Ramsey PL, Lasser S, MacEwen GD: Congenital dislocation of the hip: use of the Pavlik harness in the child during the first six months of life, *J Bone Joint Surg Am* 58:1000, 1976.

Rizzo PF et al: Diagnosis of occult fractures about the hip. Magnetic resonance imaging compared with bone-scanning, *J Bone Joint Surg Am* 75:395-401, 1993.

Schulte KR et al: The outcome of Charnley total hip arthroplasty with cement following a minimum of twenty-year follow-up, *J Bone Joint Surg Am* 75:961-975, 1993.

Shbeeb MI, Matteson EL: Trochanteric bursitis (greater trochanter pain syndrome), *Mayo Clin Proc* 71:565-569, 1996.

Shin AY, Gillingham BL: Fatigue fractures of the femoral neck in athletes, *J Am Acad Orthop Surg* 5:293-302, 1997.

Skaggs DL, Tolo VT: Legg-Calve-Perthes Disease, *J Am Acad Orthop Surg* 4:9-16, 1996.

Smith K, Bonfiglio M, Dolan K: Roentgenographic search for avascular necrosis of the head of the femur in alcoholics and normal adults, *J Bone Joint Surg Am* 59:391, 1977.

Solomon L: Drug-induced arthropathy and necrosis of the femoral head, *J Bone Joint Surg Br* 55:246, 1973.

Somerville EW: Perthes' disease of the hip, *J Bone Joint Surg Br* 53:639, 1971.

Stewart MJ, Milford LW: Fracture-dislocation of the hip, *J Bone Joint Surg Am* 36:315, 1954.

Sucato DJ, Schwend RM, Gillespie R: Septic arthritis of the hip in children, *J Am Acad Orthop Surg* 5:249-260, 1997.

Sunberg SB, Savage JP, Foster BK: Technetium phosphate bone scan in the diagnosis of septic arthritis in childhood, *J Pediatr Orthop* 9:379, 1989.

Swointkowski MF: Intracapsular fractures of the hip, *J Bone Joint Surg Am* 76:129-138, 1994.

Tachdjian MO: *Pediatric orthopedics*, Philadelphia, 1972, WB Saunders.

Terjesen T, Bredland T, Berg V: Ultrasound for hip assessment in the newborn, *J Bone Joint Surg Br* 71:767, 1989.

Tinetti ME, Speechley M, Ginter SF: Risk factors for falls among elderly persons living in the community, *N Engl J Med* 319:1701-1707, 1988.

Toalt V et al: Evidence for viral aetiology of transient synovitis of the hip, *J Bone Joint Surg Br* 75:973-974, 1993.

Tornetta P, Mostafavi HR: Hip dislocation: current treatment regimens, *J Am Acad Orthop Surg* 5:27-36, 1997.

Urbaniak JR, Harvey EJ: Revascularization of the femoral head in osteonecrosis, *J Am Acad Orthop Surg* 6:44-54, 1998.

Viere RG et al: Use of the Pavlik harness in congenital dislocation of the hip. An analysis of failures of treatment, *J Bone Joint Surg Am* 72:238, 1990.

Williamson DM, Glover SD, Benson MK: Congenital dislocation of the hip presenting after the age of three years, *J Bone Joint Surg Br* 71:745, 1989.

Wilson NI, DiPaola M: Acute septic arthritis in infancy and childhood, *J Bone Joint Surg Br* 68:584, 1986.

Wopper JM et al: Long-term follow-up of infantile hip sepsis, *J Pediatr Orthop* 8:322, 1988.

# CHAPTER 11

# The Knee

The knee is the largest joint in the body. The lower portion of the femur and upper aspect of the tibia articulate at only two points where the rounded femoral condyles bear weight on the flat tibial plateaus. The knee joint is subject to a variety of traumatic, mechanical, and inflammatory disorders.

## ANATOMY

The knee joint consists of medial and lateral, femoral and tibial condyles; and the patella. It is essentially a round bone sitting on a flat bone with no intrinsic bony stability and depends completely on its ligaments, muscles, menisci, and capsule for support. The most important ligaments of the knee are the medial and lateral collateral ligaments along with their associated posterior capsular structures and the anterior and posterior cruciate ligaments (Fig. 11-1). The medial collateral ligament originates below the adductor tubercle and attaches to the upper medial tibia. It limits abduction and assists in controlling rotation. The lateral collateral ligament (LCL) attaches to the lateral epicondyle of the femur and head of the fibula and controls adduction. The cruciate ligaments attach to the intraarticular portions of the femur and tibia. The anterior cruciate ligament (ACL) prevents anterior displacement of the tibia and helps control rotation of the tibia on the femur. The posterior cruciate ligament (PCL) prevents backward displacement of the tibia on the femur.

The muscles about the knee also play important roles in its function. The quadriceps group is the most important. These muscles control extension and prevent dislocation of the patella. The medial and lateral hamstrings provide posterior support to the knee and control flexion. Additional support is provided by the popliteus muscle and the iliotibial band.

Normal knee motion consists of a combination of rotation and either extension or flexion. Normally, as the knee flexes, the tibia internally rotates. Extension of the knee is accompanied by lateral or external rotation of the tibia. These rotational motions are controlled by the ligaments and menisci of the knee. This rotation is reflected in the course that the patella takes with flexion and extension movements (Fig. 11-2). Thus damage to the knee (such as a torn meniscus, which prevents normal tibial rotation) can cause patellar symptoms resulting from abnormal patellar excursion. These patellar symptoms are typically aggravated by walking up and down stairs, an activity that puts the greatest strain on the patella and knee extensors.

## ROENTGENOGRAPHIC ANATOMY

Anteroposterior and lateral views are essential in the diagnosis of knee disorders (Fig. 11-3). A tunnel view will visualize the intercondylar notch, and tangential views are helpful in diagnosing patellar disorders. Over the age of 40, the AP view should always be performed with the patient standing. This may reveal subtle joint space narrowing if osteoarthritis is present.

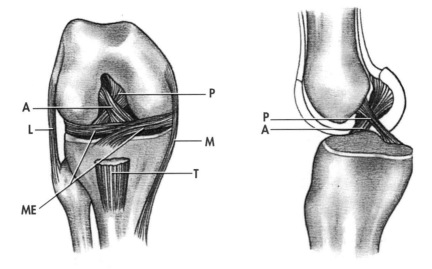

**Fig. 11–1.**
Ligaments of the knee: *A* = anterior cruciate ligament; *P* = posterior cruciate ligament; *L* = lateral collateral ligament; *M* = medial collateral ligament; *T* = patellar tendon; *ME* = medial and lateral menisci.

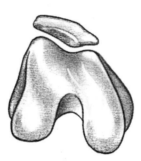

**Fig. 11–2.**
Excursion of a patella with knee flexion.

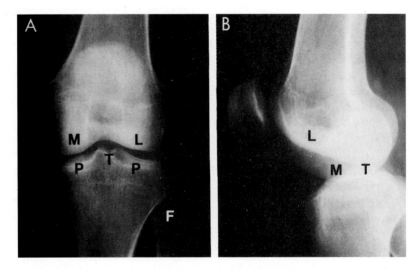

**Fig. 11–3.**
Roentgenograms of a normal knee: *M* = medial femoral condyle; *L* = lateral femoral condyle; *T* = tubercles of the intercondylar eminence; *P* = medial and lateral tibial plateaus; *F* = head of the fibula. Note that the medial femoral condyle projects more distally on both views.

# LESIONS OF THE MENISCUS

## Injuries of the Meniscus

The menisci, or semilunar cartilages, are two C-shaped structures composed of fibrocartilage that help act as cushions between the femur and tibia. They also assist in the control of normal knee motion. If the normal rotation of the tibia is forcibly prevented as the knee is flexed or extended (that is, if flexion occurs with external rotation or extension occurs with internal rotation), a tear in the meniscus can occur. The injury may be isolated or in conjunction with ligamentous ruptures.

Meniscus tears are the most common of all knee injuries, and the pathologic characteristics of the tear are variable (Fig. 11-4). When an injury occurs that produces free fragments or tears, these do not heal to the main body of the meniscus. The fragment often remains permanently detached but viable because nourishment for the meniscus is provided by the joint fluid. This joint fluid circulates around the tear and prevents healing from taking place. Persistent symptoms are the result. The medial meniscus is injured ten times more often because it is more firmly attached and less mobile than the lateral meniscus. In long-standing disease, articular cartilage erosion and degenerative changes at the tibiofemoral and patellofemoral joints may even result.

### Clinical Features

The history is usually one of a twisting injury to the knee with the foot in the weight-bearing position. Occasionally, the injury is slight. Often a "popping" or "tearing" sensation is felt, followed by severe pain. The pain is often well localized medially or laterally, depending on which meniscus is injured. Locking, from mechanical blockage of motion by the meniscus, may occasionally occur, but restricted motion after meniscus injury is usually a result of other causes (such as hamstring guarding or swelling) that produce a pseudolocking effect. Swelling from joint effusion occurs gradually over several hours. This is in contrast to ligamentous injury, where the swelling is immediate because of hemorrhage. The swelling from meniscus injury is commonly at the maximum on the day after the injury.

The acute symptoms may subside within a few days only to be replaced by intermittent episodes of locking, buckling, giving out, swelling, and mild pain. Walking up and down stairs is often difficult, and squatting may be painful.

The examination usually reveals a joint effusion (Fig. 11-5). Its presence indicates acute or chronic synovial irritation. Its absence by history or examination should cause another diagnosis to be considered. This fluid may cause the patella to be ballottable. A click may also be present when the patella is pressed against the femur.

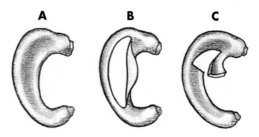

**Fig. 11–4.**
A, Normal meniscus. B, Longitudinal, or "bucket-handle," tear. C, Tear of the posterior horn.

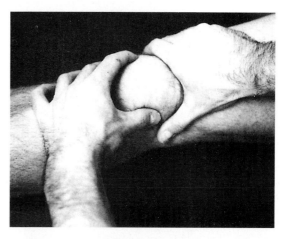

**Fig. 11–5.**
Checking for joint effusion. Milking the suprapatellar pouch with downward pressure will often reveal fluid that might not otherwise be apparent. Pressure against the patella may produce a "click" as the patella strikes the femur.

Pain and tenderness at the joint line, either medially or laterally, may be present. The range of motion is often limited. This may be as a result of swelling, pseudolocking, or occasionally the interposition of the torn meniscus. In long-standing disease, atrophy of the quadriceps muscle, especially the vastus medialis, occurs rapidly (Fig. 11-6).

The McMurray test is sometimes helpful in detecting a meniscus tear, although it is difficult to perform on a painful, swollen knee and the results are often inconsistent (Fig. 11-7). Full knee flexion, which increases pressure on the posterior horns, may cause pain with many meniscus tears.

### Special Studies

1. Plain roentgenograms are usually normal, but should always be performed to rule out other disorders.

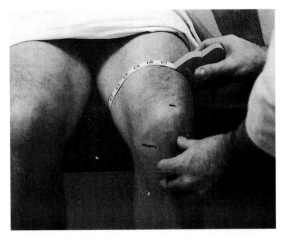

**Fig. 11–6.**
The circumference of the thigh is measured 10 cm above the proximal pole of the patella (the medial joint line is marked).

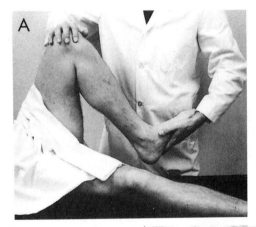

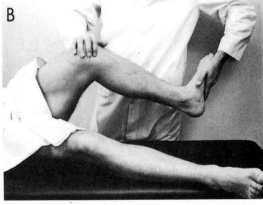

**Fig. 11–7.**
McMurray test. **A,** To test for medial meniscus injury, the hip and knee are flexed maximally, and a valgus (abduction) force is applied to the knee. **B,** The foot is externally rotated, and the knee is passively extended. An audible or palpable snap during extension suggests a tear of the medial meniscus. To test for lateral meniscus injury, the procedure is performed with a varus, internal rotation stress applied.

2. Magnetic resonance imaging (MRI) is replacing most of the special studies used to evaluate knee pathology. Ligament and meniscal injuries as well as osteonecrosis are accurately visualized. It should not be used as a "screening test" however, and meniscus injuries should first have an adequate clinical trial of conservative management for several weeks. In addition, meniscal abnormalities on MRI do not always correlate with symptoms, especially in older patients. (Joint line tenderness plus a positive history are as reliable as magnetic imaging.)

### Treatment

The initial treatment is conservative, except for those rare cases in which the knee is truly locked. Many meniscus tears, especially peripheral ones, can heal spontaneously in a few weeks. A bulky compression dressing and ice are applied if the injury is acute, and the knee is elevated. The patient is placed on crutches and started on quadriceps-strengthening exercises (Fig. 11-8). These exercises will help compress out the joint effusion and maintain strength, and they should always be performed with the knee near complete extension to prevent patellofemoral pain from developing. Gentle range-of-motion exercises are started in 2 to 3 days. Swimming is an excellent exercise for increasing motion and decreasing discomfort. As pain subsides and motion returns, weight-bearing activities are gradually resumed, but quadriceps exercises are continued for 2 to 4 weeks.

There are few indications for aspiration of the knee and even fewer indications for the injection of steroids in the treatment of an acute injury. The protective responses of the patient should be maintained, and it is better to reduce swelling by quadriceps contractions and to rehabilitate the knee through exercises.

Surgery is reserved for those cases of true irreducible locking, or cases with recurrent or persistent signs and symptoms of meniscus injury. The meniscus is removed or repaired, often arthroscopically. The results are usually excellent, and most patients are able to resume normal activities 3 to 6 weeks after surgery.

## Discoid Meniscus

Because of a failure in normal development, a meniscus (usually the lateral) may be elliptical rather than semilunar. The most common clinical finding in this disorder is an audible click that occurs with motion of the knee joint. The click may be present in infancy, but the disorder is usually not otherwise symptomatic at this age. The meniscus often wears away, so the clicking disappears.

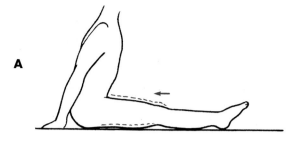
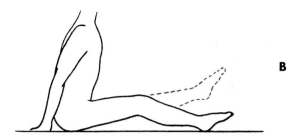
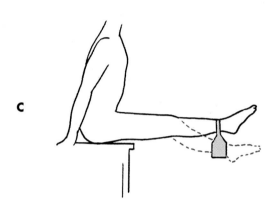
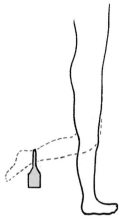

**Fig. 11–8.**
Knee exercises. **A**, Isometric quadsetting. The muscle is tightened and the knee stiffened and relaxed several times. **B** and **C**, Isotonic short-arc knee extension. The knee is straightened through the last 30 degrees (to prevent peripatellar pain). Weights are gradually added beginning with 2 kg and progressing to 10 kg. **D**, Isotonic knee curls for hamstring strengthening. Weight is increased as with quad strengthening. All exercises are performed as five sets of ten lifts each, three times a day. Exercises should not cause pain or swelling.

Occasionally, however, symptoms persist into adulthood, with clicking and aching pain at the lateral joint margin being common complaints. A palpable degenerative *cyst* may even form in the meniscus. Local tenderness at the lateral joint space is usually present.

Meniscectomy may be necessary in an adult with persistent symptoms. Infants usually require no treatment.

## Calcification of the Menisci

The meniscus can become calcified from a variety of causes (Fig. 11-9), the most common being degeneration and trauma. However, calcification can also occur in several other conditions, including degenerative arthritis, ochronosis, and pseudogout. The calcification itself is usually not painful. The symptoms are those that result from the primary disorder, and treatment is directed at that disorder.

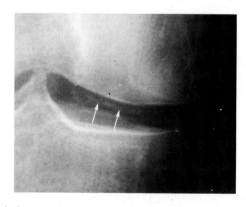

**Fig. 11–9.**
Calcification of the meniscus.

# CYSTS

Only two types of cystic lesions, the popliteal cyst and the cyst of the semilunar cartilage, occur with any frequency around the knee joint. The *popliteal* or *Baker's cyst* is an enlargement of the semimembranous bursa that is normally present in the medial aspect of the popliteal space. This bursa usually connects with the knee joint.

Cysts develop in any age group. In children, the cyst appears to be a primary lesion, in contrast to adults in whom most of these cysts are secondary to an intraarticular abnormality of the knee. This abnormality, often a posterior tear of the medial meniscus or rheumatoid arthritis, causes an increase in joint fluid. This chronic effusion opens the normal anatomic communication between the joint and cyst and allows fluid to escape into the semimembranous bursa. The cyst may reach an enormous size in rheumatoid patients and even dissect distally into the calf.

Occasionally the Baker's cyst may rupture in the adult, allowing the escape of the fluid into the soft tissues. The fluid can be irritating and can cause the development of a clinical picture (pain, swelling, tenderness) resembling thrombophlebitis and referred to as the "pseudothrombophlebitis syndrome." Homan's sign may even be positive. Differentiation is critical in that thrombophlebitis may require anticoagulation, which is contraindicated in the ruptured cyst (or rupture of the medial head of the gastrocnemius muscle, which can present with similar findings). Venous ultrasound or venography is usually diagnostic.

### Clinical Features

In children, the symptoms are usually related to the effects of direct pressure of the cyst on the adjacent soft tissues. Local discomfort may be present. In adults, the symptoms are related not only to the effects of the pressure of the cyst but also to the primary intraarticular abnormality. (Many cysts are *asymptomatic*, however.) The cyst commonly changes in size, depending on the activity of the patient and the amount of swelling in the knee.

Examination will reveal a cystic mass of variable size lateral to the medial hamstrings in the popliteal fossa (Fig. 11-10). The lesion may be locally tender. Other findings of primary joint disease may be present, especially in adults.

Except for occasional osteoarthritis, the roentgenogram is usually normal. Arthrographic and ultrasound studies as well as MRI will usually reveal the cyst (Fig. 11-11). Magnetic imaging may also be useful in deter-

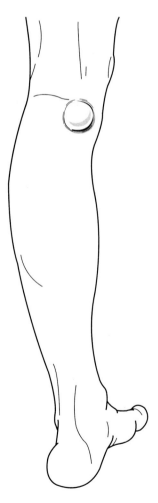

**Fig. 11–10.**
The popliteal cyst in its usual medial location inferior to the knee crease and lateral to the medial hamstrings.

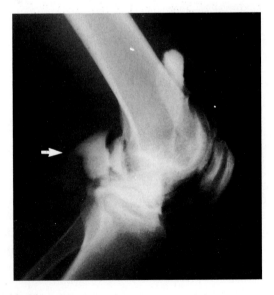

**Fig. 11–11.**
Arthrogram revealing a large popliteal cyst.

mining the presence of coexisting intraarticular lesions. Occasionally, the cyst may even form multiple calcific loose bodies (Fig. 11-12).

### Treatment

In children with primary cysts, treatment should be conservative. There is a high rate of spontaneous disappearance of the cyst in this age group and an equally high rate of recurrence after surgical excision. Aspiration and injection of the cyst may be attempted, but it is usually not necessary because the cyst often disappears in 1 to 2 years.

Adult patients are primarily treated nonsurgically. The cyst may be aspirated to reassure the patient of its benign nature. Aspiration, sometimes with injection of 1 cc of steroid, is sometimes performed to relieve symptoms. (Although recurrence is common, the symptoms are often more tolerable.) If surgery is being considered, every attempt should be made to detect any underlying joint abnormality. Cyst excision without correction of the intraarticular abnormality is followed by a high rate of recurrence of the cyst. Correction of the intraarticular condition will also often make cyst excision unnecessary because the cyst becomes asymptomatic after elimination of the cause of the chronic effusion. Many patients are treated successfully by aspiration alone, or with simple observation if the cyst is not symptomatic.

## Cysts of the meniscus

Cysts may also develop in a *meniscus* (usually the lateral) as a result of degeneration or trauma. The patient is generally a young adult who has a history of pain and a gradually enlarging mass over the lateral joint line (Fig. 11-13). A knee effusion may be present. Treatment consists of aspiration or meniscectomy and cyst excision if the patient is symptomatic.

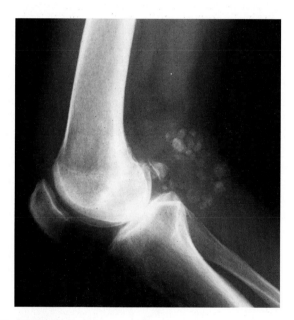

**Fig. 11–12.**
Multiple calcific loose bodies in a Baker's cyst.

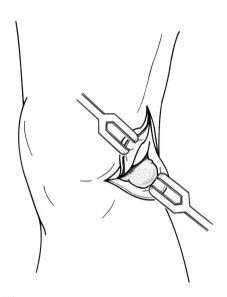

**Fig. 11–13.**
Cyst of the lateral meniscus.

## LESIONS OF THE LIGAMENTS

Ligamentous injuries to the knee are among the most serious of all knee disorders. The management of these injuries has changed over the years and continues to evolve. These injuries may occur alone or in combination and are sometimes associated with meniscal tears. The ACL is injured eight times more often in females than in males.

### Clinical Features

The mechanism is usually one of forceful stress against the knee when the extremity bears weight. Direct contact may be involved, although the ACL in particular is often injured without contact. A valgus stress against the knee may sprain or tear the medial collateral ligament, and a varus stress will injure the lateral collateral ligament. Cruciate injuries often occur as a result of a twisting injury and a "pop" or tearing sensation is often described, especially with ACL ruptures.

After the injury, the ability to bear weight on the extremity is often lost. Swelling from an acute ligament or capsular tear is usually immediate as a result of hemorrhage. If a cruciate injury has occurred, the joint fills rapidly with blood. If a collateral or capsular tear has occurred, localized ecchymosis may become visible in a few days. Incomplete tears or sprains are often more painful than complete ligamentous ruptures.

The examination is of utmost importance in the acute injury. Any swelling or discoloration is noted. The lesion can often be localized by palpation alone. Palpation should begin away from the suspected area to promote cooperation. A point of maximum tenderness is often present along the course of the collateral ligament or capsule.

The knee should always be tested for stability with the patient relaxed in the supine position. The injured knee is always compared with the opposite, uninvolved knee. The tests are performed in the following sequence:

1. Valgus-varus stress testing at 30 degrees of knee flexion. With the knee flexed 30 degrees, the cruciate ligaments are relaxed. This prevents them from producing a false negative test result. The medial and lateral ligaments can then be tested by applying valgus and varus stresses to the knee (Fig. 11-14). If laxity exists in either direction, the test reflects an injury to the involved collateral ligament. Sometimes, the test is graded according to the amount of laxity. A grade I injury is present when the joint opens 5 mm more than the normal

and a grade III or "complete" rupture is present when the joint opens greater than 1 cm.

2. Valgus-varus stress testing at 0 degrees. Valgus and varus stresses are applied in the same manner as when the knee was tested at 30 degrees of flexion. If the knee was stable at 30 degrees, it will also be stable at 0 degrees because the collateral ligaments are intact. However, with the knee in extension, the cruciate ligaments tighten and by themselves can prevent the joint from opening in spite of a collateral ligament tear. Therefore if the knee is unstable in extension, a more serious knee injury has occurred. Posterior capsular and cruciate damage may also be present in this case. (When the knee is extended, the cruciate and posterior capsular structures play a greater role in preventing varus and valgus opening.)

3. Drawer signs. Anteroposterior instability and rotatory instability are tested by determining how much abnormal excursion of the tibia is present when anterior and posterior stresses are applied to the tibia with the knee in a flexed position (Fig. 11-15). Anterior drawer testing is performed with the foot in external rotation, neutral rotation, and internal rotation. Abnormal forward excursion of the tibia with the foot in either position is highly suggestive of a significant injury to the anterior cruciate ligament and joint capsule. The posterior drawer test is then performed by applying backward pressure against the tibia. Abnormal laxity with this test is present with posterior cruciate and posterior capsular injuries. The tibia will also "sag" posteriorly with the hip and knee flexed 90 degrees if the PCL is ruptured.

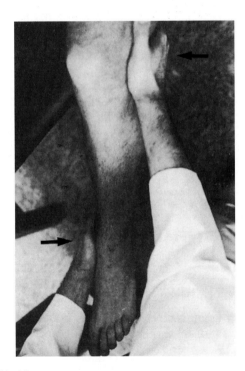

**Fig. 11–14.**
Abduction (valgus) stress test at 30 degrees of knee flexion. To test the lateral collateral ligament, a varus stress is applied. The test is repeated in full extension. Collateral ligament injuries are graded by the amount of joint space opening.

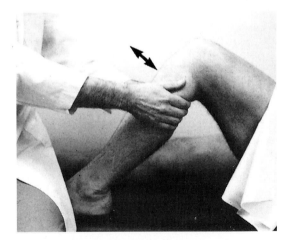

**Fig. 11–15.**
The drawer tests are performed with the hip flexed 45 degrees and the knee flexed 90 degrees. The hamstrings should always be relaxed.

4. The anterior cruciate ligament can also be assessed by the Lachman test (Fig. 11-16). This is essentially an anterior drawer test performed with the knee close to full extension. The femur is stabilized with one hand while firm pressure is applied to the proximal portion of the tibia in an attempt to translate it forward. A positive test result is one in which there is palpable and visual anterior movement of the tibia with a characteristic soft end point. This test is probably more accurate than the traditional anterior drawer sign and has another advantage in that it can be performed with the acutely injured knee in the position of comfort.

Roentgenographic examination may reveal avulsion fractures pulled off by the injured ligament (Fig. 11-17). Roentgenograms should always be obtained, especially in the growing child (below the age of 15 years) with open epiphyses. This will rule out a fracture of the distal femoral epiphysis, which may simulate collateral ligament injury (Fig. 11-18). MRI is helpful in assessing cruciate ligament status.

### Treatment

Most isolated collateral ligament injuries are now treated nonsurgically, even those that are complete (except severe LCL ruptures). Rest, ice, compression, protection, and early rehabilitation are recommended. Functional hinged braces are used, and healing is usually good.

Treatment of cruciate injuries varies depending on the age and activity of the patient and the presence of any additional injuries. Isolated ACL and PCL ruptures are generally treated nonsurgically, at least initially, in most cases. Reconstruction may be required in patients with high demands. A well-constructed brace may pro-

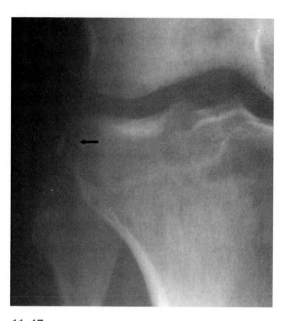

**Fig. 11–17.**
The lateral capsular fracture. A small avulsion fracture of the lateral ligament usually signals a severe joint injury, commonly in combination with an ACL rupture.

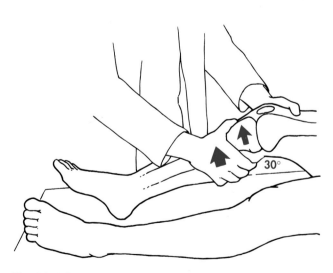

**Fig. 11–16.**
Lachman's test. This is essentially an anterior drawer test performed with the knee in approximately 30 degrees of flexion. The femur is stabilized with one hand, and the tibia is drawn forward with the other. An increase in the forward motion and lack of a definite end point suggests a rupture of the anterior cruciate ligament.

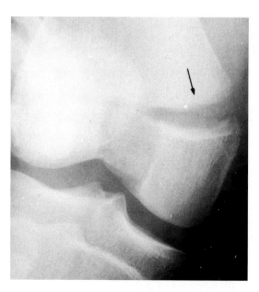

**Fig. 11–18.**
Stress roentgenography of the knee reveals an epiphyseal fracture of the lower portion of the femur that may be misdiagnosed clinically as a ligamentous injury.

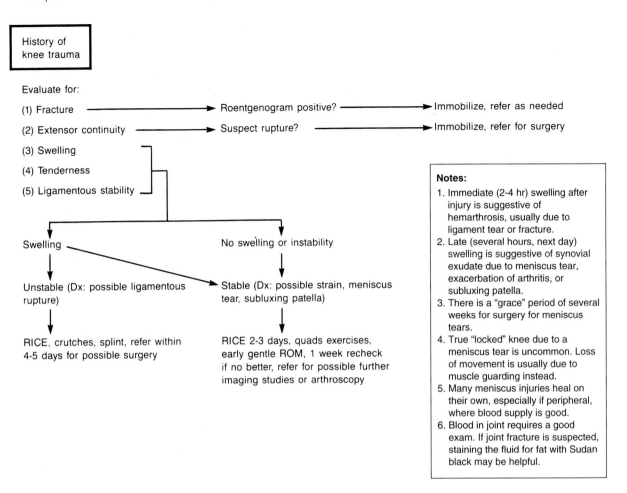

**Fig. 11–19.**
Algorithm for investigation of the acute knee injury.

vide an option in some patients. The treatment of combined injuries is unsettled. Surgery may be required to improve joint stability.

Minor ligament sprains are treated in the same manner as meniscus injuries (Fig. 11-19). Immobilization in a compression dressing, with ice and elevation for 2 to 3 days, is followed by exercises to promote absorption of swelling and restoration of motion and strength.

## Chronic Instability

Patients often present with episodes of the knee "giving way" or "going out," especially with activities that require cutting or changing directions. A chronic effusion may be present in the knee. Although a torn meniscus can cause similar symptoms, the most common cause of this problem is chronic instability as a result of ACL deficiency. Although the initial disability from an isolated ACL injury may seem minimal, the injury often results

in progressive deterioration with increasing knee laxity, tears in either meniscus, and articular cartilage degeneration. The ACL rupture has been referred to as "the beginning of the end" of the athlete's knee.

Older injuries often cause the knee to "give out," a term usually called the "pivot shift." This usually occurs when the patient comes to a sudden stop or changes directions quickly. The pivot shift is a sign that the tibia is subluxing on the femur. A synovitis is often present. The findings are often suggestive of meniscal injury (which may also be present), but the pivot shift test is usually diagnostic (Fig. 11-20).

### Treatment

The treatment is individualized. The athlete usually needs referral for evaluation (MRI, arthroscopy) followed by surgical reconstruction and augmentation or ligament replacement. This is followed by several months of rehabilitation and exercise.

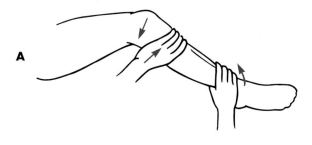

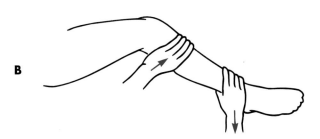

**Fig. 11–20.**
The pivot shift test. **A**, With the knee slightly flexed, the proximal portion of the tibia is lifted forward and internally rotated, and the knee is then extended. (This subluxes the tibia forward, and the femur falls backward.) **B**, Valgus force is then applied, and the knee is flexed. At about 30 degrees, the subluxation will suddenly be reduced with a palpable sensation and reproduce the patient's symptoms of instability.

Treatment of the recreational athlete is often nonsurgical. Exercises, bracing, and occasionally, modification of activities will usually allow a relatively normal lifestyle. If sufficient symptoms of instability develop

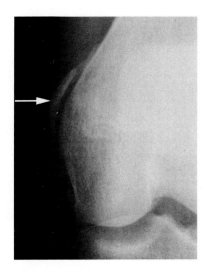

**Fig. 11–21.**
Pellegrini-Stieda disease.

later, surgical reconstruction to prevent subluxation is indicated. Surgery in these cases does not relieve pain but may eliminate symptoms of "giving out" and prevent arthritis from developing.

## Pellegrini-Stieda Disease

Occasionally, a sprain of the medial collateral ligament is followed by the formation of a calcified mass at the site of the ligament injury (Fig. 11-21). This area of dystrophic calcification may remain tender and swollen for an extended period. Ossification of the mass may even occur. The symptoms gradually subside, and symptomatic treatment is usually all that is necessary. The mass rarely needs to be removed.

# DISORDERS OF THE EXTENSOR MECHANISM

The extensor mechanism of the knee consists of the quadriceps muscles and tendon, the patella, and the patellar tendon. Several painful disorders may alter its function, and some of them are difficult to cure.

## Patellofemoral Pain (Chondromalacia)

Chondromalacia of the patella is a term that has commonly been used to describe anterior knee pain. Strictly speaking, the term chondromalacia should probably be used to describe only the pathologic lesion of cartilaginous softening and fibrillation that had previously been thought to cause this clinical syndrome. Actually, the anatomic lesion of chondromalacia is a common find-

ing in the normal knee and it is unclear whether or not it is associated with symptoms. The same syndrome of anterior knee pain is often present when the articular cartilage is normal. Thus the term "chondromalacia of the patella" is gradually being replaced by terms such as *patellofemoral pain syndrome* or *anterior knee pain syndrome* when describing the condition of anterior knee pain.

The syndrome is one of the most common causes of pain in adolescents and young adults, but it can occur at any age. Its cause is unknown, but several factors may play a role in its onset.

Any injury or anatomic abnormality that predisposes to an irregular pattern of movement of the patella can

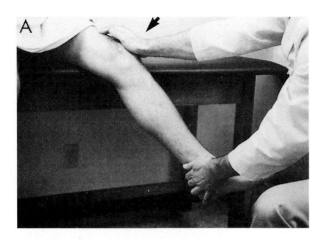

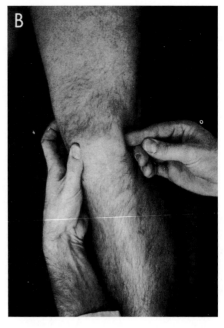

**Fig. 11–22.**
Examination for retropatellar pain. **A**, With the knee slightly flexed, pressure against the patella as the knee is actively extended may produce typical pain. **B**, With the knee extended, the patella is displaced medially or laterally. Pain is reproduced by digital pressure under either the medial or lateral patellar facet.

lead to this syndrome. Recurrent subluxation of the patella, quadriceps imbalance (weak vastus medialis), a high riding patella (patella alta), and angular deformities about the knee may be associated with this syndrome. Direct trauma, such as that which occurs with a fall or a dashboard injury to the patella, may also predispose to patellofemoral pain. It may develop as a result of repeated trauma such as vigorous squatting during weightlifting.

In some patients, it does appear that the chondromalacia may cause pain. Grossly, the cartilage loses its normal, smooth, glistening appearance and becomes fibrillated and frayed. It may even be completely denuded, thereby exposing the underlying subchondral bone. Fewer than 20% of patients with patellofemoral pain will have gross chondromalacia, however.

### Clinical Features

The majority of patients are teenagers or young adults. Crepitus is often the symptom of most concern. Pain beneath or near the patella is usually present. It is characteristically aggravated by walking up and down stairs, an activity that puts the patella under the greatest flexion load. Squatting and prolonged sitting with the knee flexed are also uncomfortable. This discomfort is often relieved by extension of the knee. Symptoms of giving way or locking may be present, and a history of previous trauma is common. The disease is often bilateral and may be confused with a meniscus injury.

Examination will reveal generalized tenderness around the patella, but the site is often not consistent or specific compared with the tenderness seen when quadriceps or patellar tendinitis is present. Direct pressure against the patella may be painful, and contraction of the quadriceps against patellar pressure is often uncomfortable (Fig. 11-22). Effusions are uncommon unless the condition is associated with another problem such as a meniscal injury. Crepitus may be present, although there is no direct correlation between the presence of crepitus and the pain. There may also be findings of malalignment or an unstable patella, but commonly the examination is normal except for tenderness around and beneath the patella. Roentgenographic examination is usually normal unless patellar subluxation is present.

### Treatment

Most management programs emphasize conservative treatment. The patient is reassured of the benign nature of the problem. Treatment is directed toward the underlying cause, if any is present. "Flexion loads" should be avoided, especially improperly performed quadriceps exercises. Otherwise, treatment consists of aspirin, moist heat, and intensive short arc quadriceps exercises (Table 11-1). Most cases eventually recover spontaneously. If symptoms persist, surgery may rarely be indicated. If needed, it usually consists of some procedure to realign the patella to prevent abnormal motion

**TABLE 11–1.**

Treatment for Anterior Knee Pain

| | |
|---|---|
| Stretch | Quads, hamstrings, triceps, heel cord |
| Strengthen | Quads (short arc) |
| Modalities | Ice, heat, massage? |
| Medication | NSAIDs |

**Note:** Eliminate overuse, flexion loads.

or to release abnormal lateral pressure. Shaving or removal of "abnormal" articular cartilage is often only of limited value. Arthroscopy may even trigger a sympathetic dystrophy in some cases. Anterior knee pain itself does not appear to lead to patellofemoral arthritis, but symptoms may persist for years.

## Recurrent Subluxation of the Patella

Recurrent subluxation of the patella (patellofemoral instability) is a common disorder that is often undiagnosed because the symptoms are similar to other derangements of the knee. The patella usually subluxes or dislocates laterally. The onset is usually without any specific trauma although the condition may follow an acute patellar dislocation that fails to heal properly. The disorder is often bilateral. The cause is often complex. Conditions that predispose the patella to not remain centralized in the femoral groove and track too far laterally are: (1) a shallow lateral femoral condyle, (2) a high Q angle (see Chapter 15), (3) inadequate development of the oblique portion of the vastus medialis muscle, (4) genu valgum, and (5) internal femoral torsion.

### Clinical Features

The symptoms are pain, swelling, and a sensation of the knee giving out. Acute dislocation may even occur, but more commonly, the symptoms are a result of recurrent subluxation.

Physical examination usually reveals local tenderness over the medial facet of the patella and in the soft tissue medial to the patella. The patella may appear laterally displaced and higher than normal when the knee is slightly flexed (patella alta). Passive hypermobility with lateral displacement is often noted when pressure is applied against the patella with the knee relaxed (Fig. 11-23). A joint effusion and mild quadriceps atrophy may be present. Malalignment and thigh atrophy may be present.

Roentgenographic studies are often helpful. A "sunrise" view taken with the knee relaxed in slight flexion will often reveal lateral displacement (Fig. 11-24).

### Treatment

Treatment is directed at improving extensor muscle tone. Short arc quadriceps exercises will often strengthen the

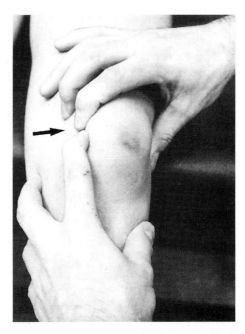

**Fig. 11–23.**
The "apprehension" test. Abnormal lateral hypermobility, sometimes with reflex quadriceps activation, may be noted when attempting to displace the patella laterally with the knee relaxed and slightly flexed. The patient may even become apprehensive and grab the examiner's arm to prevent further displacement.

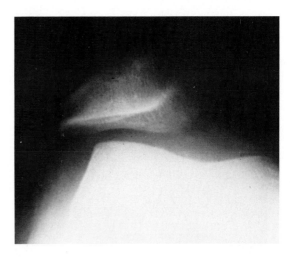

**Fig. 11–24.**
A "sunrise" view of the knee reveals abnormal lateral displacement of the patella.

vastus medialis portion of the quadriceps enough to prevent recurrent lateral subluxation. The hamstrings are stretched if needed.

Surgery may be indicated to reconstruct the extensor mechanism to prevent recurrence. A variety of procedures are available. All of them attempt to realign the patella to prevent abnormal lateral excursion from occurring. Exercise seems as successful as surgery, with either treatment having a 10% to 15% failure rate.

## Acute Dislocation of the Patella

A sudden valgus strain to the knee or a direct blow against the medial aspect of the patella may cause the patella to dislocate laterally. The deformity is usually obvious, with the patella displaced in the lateral position and the knee held in slight flexion. There are usually no predisposing anatomic factors such as those seen with recurrent subluxation. Roentgenographic examination should always be performed to rule out any associated osteochondral fracture.

Reduction is easily accomplished by lifting the heel of the extremity off the table. This extends the knee and flexes the hip, thereby relaxing the entire quadriceps mechanism. Gentle pressure against the patella may be necessary to complete the reduction. The knee is immobilized for 2 to 3 weeks by a knee immobilizer. Quadriceps exercises are begun as soon as possible. Traumatic dislocation is always accompanied by a partial rupture of the medial retinaculum and supporting structures of the patella. This may rarely lead to recurrent episodes of subluxation or dislocation. If it does, surgical reconstruction of the extensor mechanism may be necessary.

## Ruptures of the Extensor Mechanism

The extensor mechanism occasionally ruptures as a result of attrition. Often, the rupture occurs with normal activities, such as stair climbing. The rupture may take place in the quadriceps or patellar tendon. Active extension is immediately lost, but pain may be minimal, especially in an older patient with chronic degeneration of the muscle-tendon unit.

### Clinical Features

Clinically, hemorrhage and a palpable sulcus are present in the area of the rupture. Extension of the knee is markedly weakened or even completely absent.

A lateral roentgenogram taken with the knee in 90 degrees of flexion will usually reveal proximal displacement of the patella when the rupture has occurred in the patellar tendon (Fig. 11-25). Roentgenograms are usually not helpful when the rupture has occurred proximal to the patella in the quadriceps mechanism.

### Treatment

Treatment is usually surgical repair, followed by immobilization and rehabilitation.

## Osgood-Schlatter Disease

Osgood-Schlatter disease is a disorder that involves the growing tibial tuberosity of adolescents. The cause is unknown, but the disorder is generally considered to be a traumatically produced lesion that occurs at the attachment of the patellar tendon to the tibial tuberosity. It is a self-limited condition that ends with closure of the upper tibial epiphyseal plate. The disorder usually becomes evident between the ages of 8 and 15 years and is often bilateral. Males are affected three times as often as females.

### Clinical Features

Local pain, swelling, and tenderness over the tibial tubercle are characteristic clinical features. The pain is accentuated by activity. Stair climbing and squatting on the knees may be especially uncomfortable. The pain is also increased by extension of the knee against resistance.

Although usually normal, a lateral roentgenogram of the upper portion of the tibia with the leg slightly internally rotated may reveal variable degrees of separation and fragmentation of the upper tibial epiphysis. Occasionally, the fragmented area fails to unite to the tibia and persists into adulthood (Fig. 11-26).

### Treatment

Removing the stress on the tendon is usually sufficient treatment. Stretching, NSAIDs, and ice after exercise are advised. Simple abstinence from physical activity will relieve the symptoms in most cases although several months may be needed. On the other hand, adverse outcomes are rare even if the patient remains active in

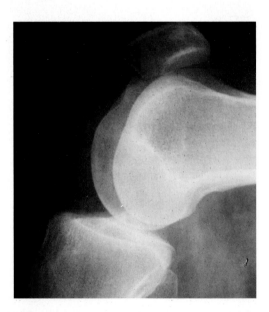

**Fig. 11–25.**
Rupture of the patellar tendon with marked proximal displacement of the patella.

spite of the discomfort. Temporary immobilization in a knee splint may be necessary in resistant cases. Surgery is rarely indicated. The prognosis for complete restoration of function and relief from pain is excellent. The condition usually heals when the epiphysis closes, which may take 1 to 2 years. The prominence of the tibial tubercle often persists into adulthood but symptoms are rare other than minor pain when kneeling.

### Larsen-Johansson Disease

This is another disorder that can present as anterior knee pain in the adolescent. It appears to be the result of chronic traction (overuse) at the cartilaginous junction of the patella and either the quadriceps tendon or patellar tendon. Most commonly it occurs at the junction with the patella and thus resembles "jumper's knee" in the adult. Clinically, tenderness is present at the affected site. Roentgenograms may occasionally reveal ossification of the tendon at its attachment to the patella.

The treatment is similar to that for Osgood-Schlatter disease, and the symptoms usually cease at the time of skeletal maturation.

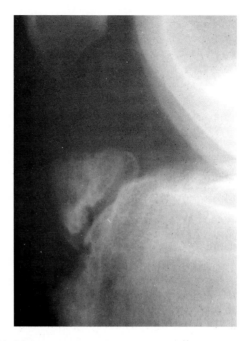

**Fig. 11–26.**
Osgood-Schlatter disease. A portion of the epiphysis has failed to unite.

## OSTEOCHONDRITIS DISSECANS

Osteochondritis dissecans is a condition of unknown cause in which a segment of subchondral bone undergoes avascular necrosis. This segment of bone, with its overlying articular cartilage, may even separate or become detached from the joint surface and produce a loose body. The knee is the most common joint affected (the talar dome and elbow are other sites) and the lateral surface of the medial femoral condyle is the area most often involved, although usually not the weight-bearing surface. The condition is primarily a disorder of young adults, but it may also be seen in children. Males are more commonly affected, and the disorder may be bilateral. Juvenile and adult forms are described. The term is probably a misnomer in that no inflammation is present.

### *Clinical Features*

The symptoms consist of pain, stiffness, and swelling that are worsened with activity. A painful limp is often present, and locking may even occur if the fragment has become detached. Diminished motion, swelling, and medial joint tenderness are usually present. This tenderness may be well localized and is best elicited by deep local pressure over the affected area with the knee flexed 90 degrees. Thigh atrophy may be seen and Wilson's sign may be abnormal (pain with knee extension and internal rotation of the foot).

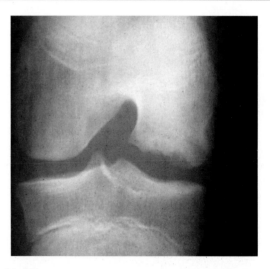

**Fig. 11–27.**
Osteochondritis dissecans of the knee. The "tunnel" view is often helpful in visualizing the defect. This fragment may become detached and form a loose body. This area should not be confused with the normal irregularity of the distal femoral epiphysis in young children.

The roentgenogram is usually diagnostic (Fig. 11-27). A fragment of avascular bone is seen that is demarcated from the adjacent femur by a radiolucent line. Occasionally, a loose body may be present. Bone scanning and MRI may be helpful in management decisions.

### Treatment

Undisplaced lesions in children are treated conservatively and the prognosis is usually good. The joint is protected from weight bearing by the use of crutches. Several months are required for complete healing.

In the older child or adult, the lesion is less likely to heal, and surgery is often indicated.

## LOOSE BODIES

Loose bodies, commonly referred to as "joint mice," are often found in the knee joint. They may be present as the result of osteoarthritis, osteochondral fractures, or osteochondritis dissecans; or secondary to primary disease of the synovium.

### Clinical Features

Loose bodies may cause swelling and intermittent locking of the joint. There is often a feeling of weakness and instability. The loose body is occasionally palpable and freely movable.

The roentgenogram is usually diagnostic (Fig. 11-28). A primary lesion such as osteochondritis dissecans may be detected, but often no joint abnormality other than the loose body is visualized.

### Treatment

Treatment is surgical if symptomatic. Sometimes the loose body will become attached to the synovium.

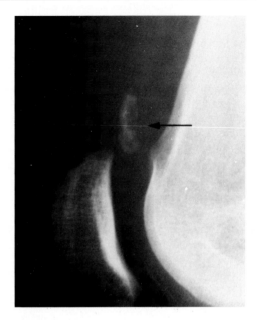

**Fig. 11–28.**
Osteocartilaginous loose body *(arrow)* in the suprapatellar pouch.

## DEGENERATIVE ARTHRITIS

The knee is the joint most commonly affected by osteoarthritis. Although the cause is unknown, obesity, trauma, ligamentous instability, and malalignment of the lower extremity all play significant roles. The pathologic features were described in Chapter 10.

### Clinical Features

The symptoms are similar to those that occur with osteoarthritis in any other joint. The medial compartment is most commonly involved; this typically leads to increased bowing over time. Pain with activity that is relieved by rest is characteristic. Morning stiffness that is relieved by activity is also usually present. A chronic effusion is not uncommon. Crepitus and grating are also common complaints. Restriction of motion, joint swelling, local tenderness, and deformity are common clinical findings. Late stages are associated with pain at rest.

The roentgenographic features consist of joint space narrowing, osteophyte formation, and sclerosis in the subchondral region (Fig. 11-29).

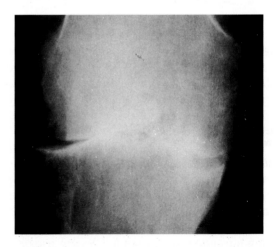

**Fig. 11–29.**
Degenerative arthritis of the knee. The joint space is severely narrowed.

### Treatment

Symptoms are often relieved by conservative treatment consisting of weight loss, rest, NSAIDs, and quadriceps exercises. A cane is often helpful to relieve the weight-bearing stress. An occasional intraarticular injection of steroid may be indicated to relieve pain. When pain is diminished, gentle range-of-motion exercises are begun to overcome contractures. Viscosupplementation and unloading braces have been tried with variable benefits.

Surgical treatment involves elimination of the painful weight-bearing articulation. Arthrodesis in the active young adult will eliminate the pain, but the patient may find the permanent stiffness disturbing. Realignment osteotomy and joint replacement are often indicated.

## OSTEONECROSIS

Avascular necrosis of bone occurs in many joints and under many conditions. The femoral head, humeral head, and talus are common sites. It may be spontaneous (idiopathic) or secondary to known causes such as chronic steroid therapy, gout, and chronic alcoholism. It may be seen in divers and workers who use compressed air (caisson disease). Most of the time, the cause is unknown. As in osteochondritis dissecans, the medial femoral condyle is the most common site of involvement in the knee. Secondary osteoarthritis often develops.

### Clinical Features
This disorder is more common over the age of 50 years. The onset is usually gradual with progressive pain and swelling. The medial femoral condyle may be locally tender.

### Roentgenographic Findings
Initially, films are usually normal or show minimal degenerative arthritis consistent with the patient's age. An early bone scan may show well-localized increased uptake over the involved area. MRI will also reveal the lesion.

Eventually, radiolucency from a subchondral zone of sclerosis appears. The necrotic area often fragments and collapses, and this results in secondary osteoarthritis (Fig. 11-30).

### Treatment
Strengthening exercises, NSAIDs, and reduction of weight bearing will allow healing within a few months

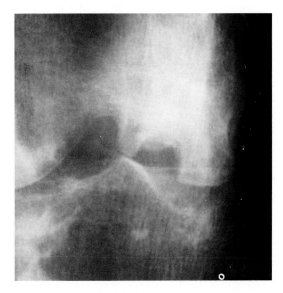

**Fig. 11–30.**
Osteonecrosis of the distal femur. Note the large defect in the femoral articular surface. Also present are diffuse sclerotic bone changes in other regions of the knee. The patient was on long-term steroid use for scleroderma. Joint replacement was necessary.

in more than half the cases. In the rest surgery is eventually required, usually in the form of an osteotomy or joint replacement.

## BURSITIS

Protective bursal sacs are present wherever soft tissue, such as muscle or tendon, moves over a bony prominence. They can become painful as a result of irritation or direct trauma. One such bursa that is often symptomatic in the knee is the *anserine bursa*. This bursa is located deep to the insertions of the semitendinosus, gracilis, and sartorius tendons medially (Fig. 11-31). Anserine bursitis is often difficult to separate from medial joint osteoarthritis. (They sometimes occur together.) The tenderness from anserine bursitis is *below* the joint line.

Treatment measures include moist heat, rest, and the injection of a steroid/lidocaine mixture into the tender

bursa (Fig. 11-32). NSAIDs are given to control pain and inflammation. Recurrent anserine bursitis is often related to osteoarthritis of the knee.

The *prepatellar bursa* lies between the skin and the patella. Direct trauma may cause it to fill with blood acutely. It often becomes irritated from recurrent trauma, especially kneeling (housemaid's knee), and it is occasionally involved in infection. Chronic traumatic changes may occur with permanent thickening of the bursa, which makes it more prone to recurrent injury.

Acute traumatic prepatellar bursitis usually responds to rest and aspiration. The fluid should be cultured if

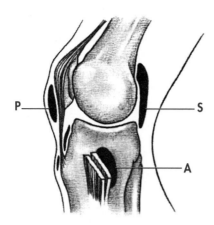

**Fig. 11–31.**
Bursae of the knee: *A* = anserine bursa; *P* = prepatellar bursa; *S* = semimembranous bursa. The last may become enlarged and form a Baker's cyst.

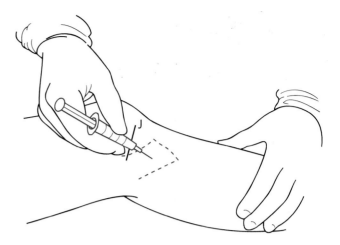

**Fig. 11–32.**
Pes bursitis injection. Approximately 2 FB below the joint line *(J)* is the usual site of maximum tenderness. One ml of steroid plus 3 to 4 ml of lidocaine are used. The needle should encounter bone, and half of the injection is given there. The remainder is injected throughout the general area of pain.

suspicious for infection. If infection develops, aspiration or open drainage followed by the appropriate antibiotic coverage is indicated. Incision and drainage should never be performed for sterile recurrent swelling because a chronic draining sinus tract may result. Recurrent bursal effusions may be aspirated repeatedly. Even-

tually, most will "dry up" on their own. A chronic, swollen bursa that is vulnerable to repeated injuries may need to be excised.

## TENDINITIS

Several tendons adjacent to the knee joint may become chronically inflamed. The patellar and quadriceps tendons are most commonly involved. The disorder is often seen in weightlifters and athletes who jump, and is a result of overuse. The quads tendon may be affected at its insertion. The patellar tendon may be involved anywhere along its length (jumper's knee). Flexor tendons are less often affected. Pain with activity and local point tenderness are characteristic clinical features. Pa-

tients often complain of stiffness after sitting with the knees flexed for a long period. As in most cases of tendinitis, the pain is aggravated by passive stretching of the tendon as well as by forceful contraction of the muscle-tendon unit against resistance.

The treatment is symptomatic, with rest, heat, stretching, and antiinflammatory medication. Steroid injections may be helpful, but the patellar tendon should never be injected.

## ARTHROSCOPY

Arthroscopy is a valuable tool in the diagnosis and treatment of many disorders of the knee. The procedure has also been used in the shoulder, elbow, hip, and ankle joint but is most useful in problems of the knee. The procedure is safe and relatively minor with little morbidity. It may be performed on an outpatient basis, with ambulation being possible shortly afterward. Its diagnostic accuracy approaches 100%, and by using separate puncture holes of entrance, small instruments may be passed into the knee to perform a variety of functions. The most common are removal or repair of meniscus tears and removal of loose bodies. It is used

to evaluate the knee of patients with Baker's cyst to determine whether any intraarticular abnormality is present that may have caused the cyst to develop. In this case the intraarticular problem, rather than the Baker's cyst, might require treatment. Arthroscopic surgery is also commonly used to remove damaged articular cartilage from the patella in patients with chondromalacia, but the results in these patients are often inconsistent and unpredictable.

Diagnostic arthroscopy is helpful in evaluating acute injuries of the knee to determine whether ligamentous repair may be necessary. It is also useful in difficult diagnostic problems in those symptomatic knees with vague symptoms and few physical findings. There is some risk of overuse of the procedure, especially in these patients, and it should be kept in mind that the procedure is still a surgical one that requires an anesthetic and should be undertaken only with proper indications.

## Plica Syndrome

The synovial plicae are four (suprapatellar, infrapatellar, medial, and lateral) membranous folds or bands that may be an occasional source of chronic knee pain. They have become items of interest mainly because of the increasing use of arthroscopy. The plica may become symptomatic when irritated by direct trauma, overuse, or inflammatory disorders, although the relationship between plicae and disease and symptoms remains unclear. The most common clinical features are chronic aching (usually medial to the patella) and local tenderness. When the medial plica is visualized arthroscopically, it is released by partial excision. The other folds are not commonly symptomatic.

# FRACTURES OF THE KNEE

Many fractures about the knee are intraarticular. They may occur through the femoral condyles or tibial plateaus. Open reduction with internal fixation is usually indicated if any displacement is present that would cause the articular surface to be irregular or that would lead to instability. Otherwise, traumatic arthritis may develop.

## Fractures of the Tibial Plateau

A common fracture in the knee is an injury to the lateral tibial plateau (Fig. 11-33). This injury results from a force applied to the lateral aspect of the knee with the leg in the extended weight-bearing position. Undisplaced, impacted fractures are easily treated by a compression dressing and early motion with avoidance of weight bearing for 6 to 8 weeks. Unimpacted fractures in good position are treated by a long leg cast for 6 weeks. Displaced fractures require open reduction and internal fixation with elevation of the depressed plateau fragment.

## Fractures of the Patella

Fractures of the patella are usually transverse and result from a direct blow to the knee. They are classified as undisplaced or displaced (Fig. 11-34).

Undisplaced (under 8 mm) fractures are easily treated nonoperatively. A compression dressing followed by a removable splint may be all that is necessary in the conscientious patient. Otherwise, a cylinder cast or brace is applied and maintained for 5 to 6 weeks. This is followed by an active exercise program to restore strength and mobility.

Displaced fractures usually require surgery. Comminuted fragments are removed, and the patellar fracture and extensor mechanism of the knee are repaired.

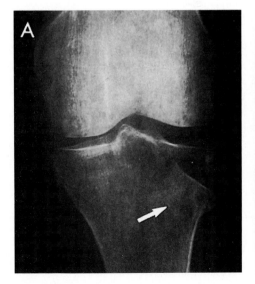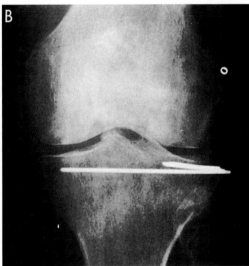

**Fig. 11–33.**
**A,** Depressed fracture *(arrow)* of the lateral tibial plateau. **B,** The fragments have been elevated and internally fixed.

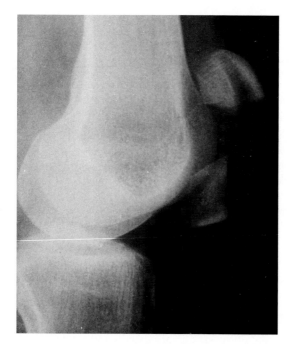

**Fig. 11–34.**
Displaced fracture of the patella.

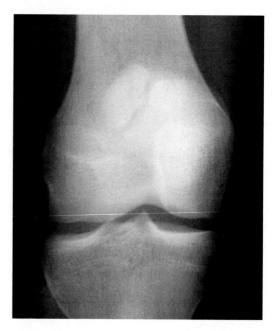

**Fig. 11–35.**
Bipartite patella.

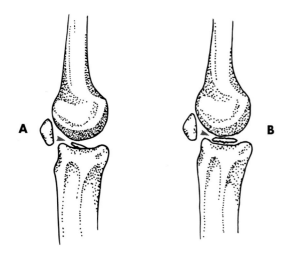

**Fig. 11–36.**
Fractures of the intercondylar eminence of the tibia. **A**, The displaced fracture that is still attached. Conservative treatment is usually adequate. **B**, The avulsed fragment is completely separated from its bed. Surgery is usually necessary for this injury.

Patellar fractures are not to be confused with a *bipartite patella* (Fig. 11-35). This is a developmental variant that is often bilateral and usually asymptomatic. It is most often located in the superolateral pole of the patella and represents failure of this ossification center to unite with the main patella.

## Fractures of the Tibial Eminence

Fractures of the intercondylar region of the tibia are more common in children than adults. They usually occur in the area of attachment of the anterior cruciate ligament. If the fragment is only partially displaced, conservative treatment with a long leg cast for 8 weeks is usually sufficient treatment (Fig. 11-36). Only the fracture that is completely avulsed and displaced from its bed requires surgical repair (Fig. 11-37) to restore strength to the cruciate ligament and prevent any mechanical blocking from occurring.

## TRAUMATIC DISLOCATION OF THE KNEE

This is an uncommon injury but one that can be extremely disabling. It usually results from severe trauma. Associated neurovascular injuries are common, especially peroneal nerve damage. The dislocation is more commonly anterior (Fig. 11-38). Some injuries reduce spontaneously, which makes recognition of the exact nature of the injury difficult.

### Evaluation and Treatment

Occasionally, if the dislocation has spontaneously reduced, there may be an absence of obvious gross deformity, except for swelling. Usually, however, there is gross deformity, and there are always signs of severe

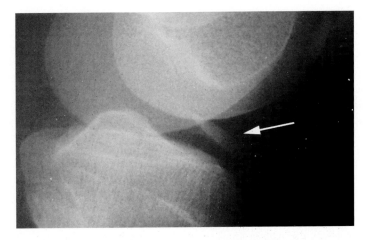

**Fig. 11–37.**
Roentgenogram of completely avulsed intercondylar fracture *(arrow)*.

ligamentous disruption. The neurovascular status of the extremity is always recorded.

The knee should be reduced as soon as possible. The neurovascular status is then reevaluated. Angiography is indicated if there are any concerns about the vascular status of the limb. Definitive ligament repair is probably helpful in young patients, but older patients may be treated nonsurgically. Nerve repair may be attempted, but the results are poor. Rehabilitation with bracing is helpful in restoring function.

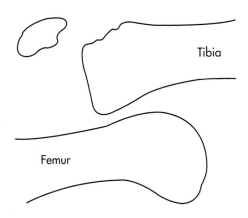

**Fig. 11–38.**
Traumatic dislocation of the knee.

# BIBLIOGRAPHY

Abernathy PJ et al: Is chondromalacia patellae a separate clinical entity? *J Bone Joint Surg Br* 60:205-210, 1978.

Aegerter E, Kirkpatrick JA: *Orthopedic diseases*, ed 3, Philadelphia, 1968, WB Saunders.

Aglietti P et al: Idiopathic osteonecrosis of the knee: aetiology, prognosis and treatment, *J Bone Joint Surg Br* 65:588, 1983.

Ahuja SC, Bullough PG: Osteonecrosis of the knee: a clinicopathological study in twenty-eight patients, *J Bone Joint Surg Am* 60:191, 1978.

Allman FL: Clinical diagnosis of anterior cruciate ligament instability in the athlete, *Am J Sports Med* 4:84, 1976.

Andrish JT: Meniscal injuries in children and adolescents: diagnosis and management, *J Am Acad Orthop Surg* 4:231-237, 1996.

Arnbjornson A et al: The natural history of recurrent dislocation of the patella. Long-term results of conservative and operative treatment, *J Bone Joint Surg Br* 74:140-142, 1992.

Boden BP et al: Patellofemoral instability: evaluation and management, *J Am Acad Orthop Surg* 5:47-57, 1997.

Bourne MH et al: Anterior knee pain, *Mayo Clin Proc* 63:482, 1988.

Brantigan OC, Voshell AF: The mechanics of the ligaments and menisci of the knee joint, *J Bone Joint Surg* 23:44, 1941.

Cahill BR: Osteochondritis dissecans of the knee: treatment of juvenile and adult forms, *J Am Acad Orthop Surg* 3:237-247, 1995.

Carpenter JE, Kasman R, Mathews LS: Fractures of the patella, *J Bone Joint Surg Am* 73:1550-1561, 1992.

Childress HM: Popliteal cysts associated with undiagnosed posterior lenses of the medial meniscus, *J Bone Joint Surg Am* 52:1487, 1970.

Covey CD, Sapega AA: Injuries of the posterior cruciate ligament, *J Bone Joint Surg Am* 75:1376-1386, 1993.

Cramer KE, Moed BR: Patellar fractures: contemporary approach to treatment, *J Am Acad Orthop Surg* 5:323-331, 1997.

Crawford EJ, Emery RJ, Archroth PM: Stable osteochondritis dissecans—does the lesion unite?, *J Bone Joint Surg Br* 72:320, 1990.

Crosby EB, Insall J: Recurrent dislocation of the patella, *J Bone Joint Surg Am* 58:9, 1976.

Curl WW: Popliteal cysts: historical background and current knowledge, *J Am Acad Orthop Surg* 4:129-133, 1996.

Cutbill JW et al: Anterior knee pain: a review, *Clin J Sports Med* 7:40-45, 1997.

Dandy DJ, Jackson RW: The impact of arthroscopy on the management of disorders of the knee, *J Bone Joint Surg* 57:346, 1975.

Dinham JM: Popliteal cysts in children, *J Bone Joint Surg Br* 57:69, 1975.

Dye SF et al: Factors contributing to function of the knee joint after injury or reconstruction of the anterior cruciate ligament, *J Bone Joint Surg* 80(A):1380-1393, 1998.

Ecker ML, Lotke PA: Spontaneous osteonecrosis of the knee, *J Am Acad Orthop Surg* 2:173-178, 1994.

Edeen J et al: Results of conservative treatment for recalcitrant anterior knee pain in active young adults, *Orthop Rev* 21:593-599, 1992.

Eifert-Mangine M et al: Patellar tendinitis in the recreational athlete, *Orthopedics* 15:1359-1367, 1992.

Ewing JW: Plica: pathologic or not? *J Am Acad Orthop Surg* 1:117-121, 1993.

Feagin JA Jr, Curl WW: Isolated tear of the anterior cruciate ligament: 5 year follow-up study, *Am J Sports Med* 4(3):95-100, 1976.

Ficat RP, Hungerford DS: *Disorders of the patello-femoral joint*, Baltimore, 1977, Williams & Wilkins.

Fischer RL: Conservative treatment of patellofemoral pain, *Orthop Clin North Am* 17:269, 1986.

Galway HR, MacIntosh DL: The lateral pivot shift: a symptom and sign of anterior cruciate insufficiency, *Clin Orthop* 147:45-50, 1980.

Garth WB: Current concepts regarding the anterior cruciate ligament, *Orthop Rev* 21:565-575, 1992.

Good L, Johnson RJ: The dislocated knee, *J Am Acad Orthop Surg* 3:284-292, 1995.

Goodfellow J, Hungerford DS, Woods C: Patello-femoral joint mechanics and pathology: chondromalacia patellae, *J Bone Joint Surg Br* 58:291, 1976.

Goodfellow J, Hungerford DS, Zindel M: Patello-femoral joint mechanics and pathology: functional anatomy of the patello-femoral joint, *J Bone Joint Surg Br* 58:287, 1976.

Guhl JF: Update in the treatment of osteochondritis dissecans, *Orthopedics* 7:1744, 1984.

Harvell JC et al: Diagnostic arthroscopy of the knee in children and adolescents, *Orthopedics* 12:1561, 1989.

Hede A, Hempel-Poulson S, Jensen JS: Symptoms and level of sports activity in patients awaiting arthroscopy for meniscal lesions of the knee, *J Bone Joint Surg Am* 72:550, 1990.

Helfet AJ: *Disorders of the knee*, Philadelphia, 1974, JB Lippincott.

Hillard-Sembell D et al: Combined injuries of the anterior cruciate and medial collateral ligaments of the knee, *J Bone Joint Surg* 78(2):169-176, 1996.

Hughston JC et al: The classification of knee ligament instabilities: I. The medial compartment and cruciate ligaments, *J Bone Joint Surg Am* 58:159, 1976.

Hughston JC et al: The classification of knee ligament instabilities: II. The lateral compartment, *J Bone Joint Surg Am* 58:173, 1976.

Huston U, Wojtys EM: Neuromuscular performance characteristics in elite female athletes, *Am J Sports Med* 24:427-436, 1996.

Indelicato PA et al: Isolated medial collateral ligament rupture in the knee, *J Am Acad Orthop Surg* 3:9-14, 1995.

Insall J: Patellar pain, *J Bone Joint Surg Am* 64:147, 1982.

Insall J, Falvo KA, Wise DW: Chondromalacia patellae, *J Bone Joint Surg Am* 58:1, 1976.

Jackson RW: The painful knee: arthroscopy or MRI imaging? *J Am Acad Orthop Surg* 4:93-99, 1996.

Jensen DB et al: Tibial plateau fractures, *J Bone Joint Surg Br* 72:49, 1990.

Johnson DP, Eastwood DM, Witherow PJ: Symptomatic synovial plicae of the knee, *J Bone Joint Surg Am* 75:1485-1496, 1993.

Jordan MJ: Lateral meniscal variants. Evaluation and treatment, *J Am Acad Orthop Surg* 4:191-200, 1996.

Katz MM, Hungerford DS: Reflex sympathetic dystrophy affecting the knee, *J Bone Joint Surg Br* 69:797, 1987.

Koval KJ, Helfet DL: Tibial plateau fractures: evaluation and treatment, *J Am Acad Orthop Surg* 3:86-94, 1995.

Kujula UM et al: Patellofemoral relationships in recurrent patellar dislocation, *J Bone Joint Surg Br* 71:788, 1989.

Larson RL, Taillon M: Anterior cruciate insufficiency: principles of treatment, *J Am Acad Orthop Surg* 2:26-35, 1994.

Laurin CA et al: The abnormal lateral patellofemoral angle: a diagnostic roentgenographic sign of recurrent patellar subluxation, *J Bone Joint Surg Am* 60:55, 1978.

Lee JK et al: Anterior cruciate ligament tears: MR imaging compared with arthroscopy and clinical tests, *Radiology* 166:861, 1988.

Lipscomb PR Jr, Lipscomb PR Sr, Bryan RS: Osteochondritis dissecans of the knee with loose fragments, *J Bone Joint Surg Am* 60:235, 1978.

Losee RE, Johnson TR, Southwick WO: Anterior subluxation of the lateral tibial plateau. A diagnostic test and operative repair, *J Bone Joint Surg Am* 60:1015-1030, 1978.

Lotke PA, Ecker ML: Osteonecrosis of the knee, *J Bone Joint Surg Am* 70:470-473, 1988.

Lundburg M, Messner K: Long-term prognosis of isolated partial medial collateral ligament ruptures: A ten-year clinical and radiographic evaluation of a prospectively observed group of patients, *Am J Sports Med* 24:160-163, 1996.

Maenpaa H, Lehto MU: Patellar dislocation: the long-term results of nonoperative management in 100 patients, *Am J Sports Med* 25:213-217, 1997.

Matava MJ: Patellar tendon ruptures, *J Am Acad Orthop Surg* 4:287-296, 1996.

Meyers MH, McKeever FM: Fractures of the intercondylar eminence of the tibia, *J Bone Joint Surg Am* 52:1677, 1970.

Mink JH, Levy T, Crues JV III: Tears of the anterior cruciate ligament and menisci of the knee: MR imaging evaluation, *Radiology* 167:769, 1988.

Natri A, Kannus P, Jarvinen M: Which factors predict the long-term outcome in chronic patellofemoral pain syndrome? A 7-year prospective follow-up study, *Med Sci Sports Exer* 30:1572-1577, 1998.

Nicholas JA: The five-one reconstruction for anteromedial instability of the knee, *J Bone Joint Surg Am* 55:899, 1973.

Noble J, Erat K: In defense of the meniscus. A prospective study of 200 meniscectomy patients, *J Bone Joint Surg Br* 62:7, 1980.

Noyes FR, Barber-Westin SD: The treatment of acute combined ruptures of the anterior cruciate and medial ligaments of the knee, *Am J Sports Med* 23:380-391, 1995.

O'Donoghue DH: *Treatment of injuries to athletes*, ed 4, Philadelphia, 1984, WB Saunders.

Papagelopoulos PJ, Sim FH: Patellofemoral pain syndrome: diagnosis and management, *Orthopedics* 20:148-157, 1997.

Rezing PM, Insall J, Bohne WH: Spontaneous osteonecrosis of the knee, *J Bone Joint Surg Am* 62:2, 1980.

Rougraff BT, Reek CC, Essenmacher J: Complete quadriceps tendon ruptures, *Orthopedics* 19:509-518, 1996.

Sandberg R, Balkfors B: Partial rupture of the anterior cruciate ligament. Natural course, *Clin Orthop* 220:176-178, 1987.

Sandow MJ, Goodfellow JW: The natural history of anterior knee pain in adolescents, *J Bone Joint Surg Br* 67:36, 1985.

Shelbourne KD, Patel DV: Management of combined injuries of the anterior cruciate and medial collateral ligaments, *J Bone Joint Surg* 77(A):800-806, 1995.

Shelton WR, Barrett GR, Dukes A: Early season anterior cruciate ligament tears. A treatment dilemma, *Am J Sports Med* 25:656-658, 1997.

Sherman OH et al: Arthroscopy—"no-problem surgery": an analysis of complications in two thousand six hundred and forty cases, *J Bone Joint Surg Am* 68:256-265, 1986.

Simonet WT, Sim FH: Current concepts in the treatment of ligamentous instability of the knee, *Mayo Clin Proc* 59:67, 1984.

Sisto DJ, Warren RF: Complete knee dislocation, *Clin Orthop* 198:94, 1985.

Slocum DB, Larson RL: Rotatory instability of the knee: its pathogenesis and a clinical test to demonstrate its presence, *J Bone Joint Surg Am* 50:211, 1968.

Small NC: Complications in arthroscopic surgery of the knee and shoulder, *Orthopedics* 16:985-988, 1993.

Spiers AS et al: Can MRI of the knee affect arthroscopic practice? *J Bone Joint Surg Br* 75:49-52, 1993.

Stanitski CL: Anterior knee pain syndromes in the adolescent, *J Bone Joint Surg Am* 75:1407-1416, 1993.

Traina SM, Bronberg DF: ACL injury patterns in women, *Orthopedics* 20:545-552, 1997.

Watanabe AT et al: Common pitfalls in magnetic resonance imaging of the knee, *J Bone Joint Surg Am* 71:857, 1988.

Wolfe RD, Colloff B: Popliteal cysts, *J Bone Joint Surg Am* 54:1057, 1972.

Yang SS, Nisonson B: Arthroscopic surgery of the knee in the geriatric patient, *Clin Orthop Related Res* 316:50-58, 1995.

# CHAPTER 12

# The Ankle and Foot

The ankle and foot perform the major functions of supporting the body and propelling it forward. In the process of filling these roles, several painful conditions may develop. Most of these develop in the forefoot, and many of them are caused by poorly fitted shoes.

## ANATOMY

The ankle is a hinge joint composed of the articular surfaces of the lower portion of the tibia, talus, and medial and lateral malleoli (Fig. 12-1). The stability of this joint or "mortise" is maintained by the malleoli and their ligaments, which grasp the talus and prevent medial and lateral displacement. The talus and socket are both broader in front, an arrangement that provides maximum stability when the ankle is in dorsiflexion or neutral and that prevents posterior displacement. Only movements of dorsiflexion and plantar flexion occur at the ankle.

The foot is composed of 26 bones, 12 of which are components of the medial and lateral longitudinal arches (Fig. 12-2). Strong fascial supports maintain these arches and prevent collapse (Fig. 12-3). Eversion and inversion movements of the foot take place in the hindfoot at the subtalar joint. Injury or disease that affects this joint will cause pain in the region of the heel when walking on uneven or irregular surfaces. Abduction and adduction movements occur in the midfoot or midtarsal joints.

## FLATFOOT

Flatfoot is a common disorder that is defined as a depression or loss of the medial longitudinal arch of the foot. It is usually combined with valgus or eversion of the heel and abduction of the forefoot. An apparent flatfoot is present in many children up to the age of 2 years. This is as a result of the presence of a fat pad in the area of the longitudinal arch. As the fat pad atrophies with weight bearing, the normal arch usually becomes visible. Flatfoot is usually one of two types, flexible or rigid, but it can also be caused by a ruptured posterior tibial tendon.

### Flexible Flatfoot

Flexible or hypermobile flatfoot is a disorder often seen in both adults and children. The condition is often hereditary and varies in severity. It is occasionally associated with a tight Achilles tendon (heel cord). The tight heel cord tends to hold the heel in eversion. With growth, stretching of the medial ligaments of the foot and ankle may then occur.

### Clinical Features

Symptoms are rare but may consist of pain, burning, and easy fatigability. With weight bearing, the heels are everted, and the forefoot appears pronated and abducted (Fig. 12-4). The child often "breaks down" the medial counter of the shoe. When it is not bearing weight, the foot often looks normal. Absence of the medial arch is apparent, and the foot is mobile without any fixed deformity. A mild genu valgum (knock-knee) or internal tibial torsion may be present. With the heel in-

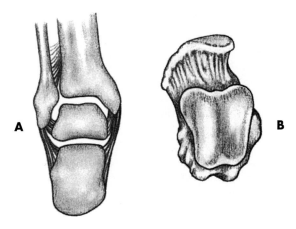

**Fig. 12–1.**
Bones of the ankle and heel. **A,** The talus is held in position in the mortise by the malleoli and ankle ligaments. **B,** The talus's articular surface is wider anteriorly than posteriorly. The ankle is therefore more stable in neutral or slight dorsiflexion when the wider anterior portion of the talus fits in the mortise. It is unstable in plantar flexion. Wearing high-heeled shoes may therefore lead to chronic ankle and calf pain. Eversion and inversion movements take place in the subtalar (talocalcaneal) joint.

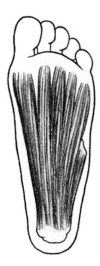

**Fig. 12–3.**
The plantar fascia. It may be affected by Dupuytren's contracture in a similar manner to the hand. It may also become inflamed, especially at the medial attachment to the calcaneus (plantar fasciitis).

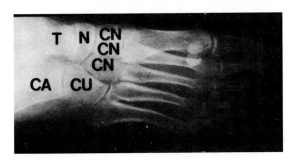

**Fig. 12–2.**
Roentgenogram of the foot: *N* = navicular; *T* = talus; *CA* = calcaneus; *CU* = cuboid; *CN* = cuneiforms, medial, intermediate, and lateral. The foot is divided into the forefoot (phalanges and metatarsals), midfoot (tarsals), and hindfoot (talus and calcaneus).

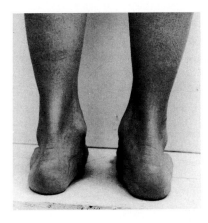

**Fig. 12–4.**
Flatfoot deformity with eversion of the heels and loss of the normal longitudinal arch.

verted, passive dorsiflexion of the ankle will be limited if the heel cord is tight.

A lateral roentgenogram taken with the foot bearing weight may reveal a loss of the normal arch and plantar flexion of the talus (Fig. 12-5). Some secondary bony changes may be present in the adult.

### Treatment

The treatment of flexible flatfoot is controversial. The natural history in most cases is spontaneous correction with maturity. Symptoms are rare during childhood and uncommon even in the adult with moderately severe deformity. Actually, most foot pain in young adults is as a result of an abnormally high rather than an abnormally

low arch. Shoe corrections and orthotics used for this condition have never been scientifically proved to be of benefit. An arch cannot be "created" by supporting it. Exercises are of doubtful value, except for those that stretch the tight heel cords (Fig. 12-6). These exercises will cure many cases associated with heel cord contractures. A soft arch support may be tried if symptoms are present. Surgery is reserved for symptomatic cases but is rarely necessary. No treatment is needed in most cases.

## Rigid Flatfoot

Rigid or peroneal spastic flatfoot differs from flexible flatfoot in that the deformity is not passively correctable

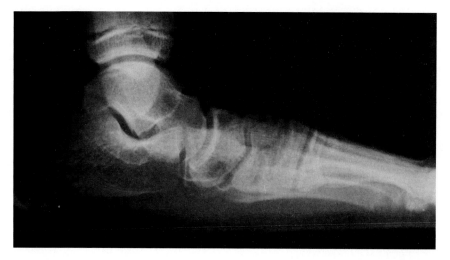

**Fig. 12–5.**
Lateral weight-bearing roentgenogram revealing plantar flexion of the talus.

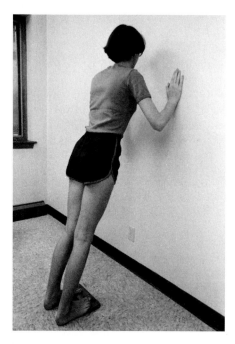

**Fig. 12–6.**
Heel cord stretching exercises. The legs are internally rotated; the forefeet are placed on a 2.5-cm board, and the patient leans forward.

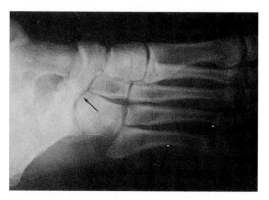

**Fig. 12–7.**
Tarsal coalition. An incomplete calcaneonavicular bar is present *(arrow)*. The anterior process of the calcaneus is abnormally prolonged.

and is present whether weight bearing or not. This condition is usually secondary to a tarsal coalition or arthritis in the hindfoot. Tarsal coalitions are congenital cartilaginous or bony bridges that may be found between the two bones of the hindfoot or between either of these bones (usually the calcaneous) and the navicular. The resultant loss of motion in the hindfoot leads to local irritation and protective spasm in the peroneal muscles, producing the flatfoot appearance. The condition is bilateral in half of the cases.

### Clinical Features

The onset of the disorder is usually gradual and begins in early adolescence if it is the result of a coalition. Stiffness and a painful limp are the most common initial symptoms. Tenderness and pain may be present over the peroneal tendons or in the hindfoot. The heel is often everted, and subtalar motion is limited and painful. The forefoot may be abducted. Passive stretching of the peroneal tendons by forefoot adduction and inversion often reproduces the pain. Swelling will be present if the disorder is secondary to a rheumatoid process.

Roentgenograms may reveal arthritic changes in the hindfoot or the presence of a coalition (Fig. 12-7).

### Treatment

Symptomatic treatment is indicated in early cases. Rest, heat, and NSAIDs are usually helpful. A short leg walking cast may be worn intermittently to relieve symptoms. Surgery is often necessary, however. If the disorder is secondary to arthritis, arthrodesis of the hindfoot and navicular is indicated. When a tarsal coalition is present, the bony or cartilaginous bar may be resected. If this does not alleviate the symptoms, arthrodesis is usually performed.

## Posterior Tibial Tendon Rupture

Acquired flatfoot deformity can develop as a result of posterior tendon rupture, usually from attrition and failure. The diagnosis is difficult and often missed until the patient discovers the loss of the arch. Often there is a history of previous pain in the area, and the patient may have even had treatment for tendinitis. Clinically, the tendon sheath may be empty and the heel everts with weight bearing. The medial arch is lower. Inversion of the heel and forefoot against resistance is weak. The patient is unable to perform the single heel rise test in which the patient tries to rise on the tiptoe on the affected side.

Treatment may require NSAIDs, orthotics or longitudinal arch supports, and even surgical reconstruction.

# CLUBFOOT

Congenital clubfoot, or talipes equinovarus, is a fixed deformity that is present at birth. It is often bilateral, and a hereditary factor is often present. The cause is unknown.

### Clinical Features

The deformity consists of three major components, none of which is passively correctable. This lack of correctability distinguishes clubfoot from other common foot deformities (which may be a result of intrauterine molding and usually resolve without treatment). The three components are equinus of the ankle and forefoot, varus of the heel, and adduction of the forefoot (Fig. 12-8). The medial border of the foot is concave, and the lateral border is convex.

### Treatment

Treatment begins within the first few days of life and consists of manipulation of the foot to stretch the contracted soft tissues, followed by the application of a corrective cast. The cast is changed at weekly inter-

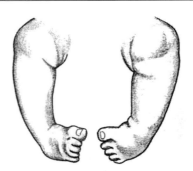

**Fig. 12–8.**
Bilateral clubfeet (talipes equinovarus).

vals, and the foot is further manipulated until complete correction is obtained. This method of treatment will often succeed if it is begun immediately. Surgery is required when casting fails. The procedures range from simple heel cord lengthening to wide soft-tissue releases.

# CALCANEOVALGUS

Talipes calcaneovalgus is the most common neonatal foot disorder. It is characterized by excessive eversion and dorsiflexion of the foot. The cause is unknown, but positional compression in utero is likely. In contrast to clubfoot, the deformity is not fixed and may be easily overcorrected.

### Clinical Features

The deformity is easily diagnosed shortly after birth. Marked laxity of the ligaments of the foot and ankle is obvious, and the foot can often be dorsiflexed so that the toes touch the anterior aspect of the tibia (Fig. 12-9). The heel cord may appear to be severely stretched.

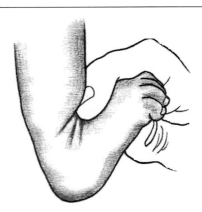

**Fig. 12–9.**
Talipes calcaneovalgus.

### Treatment

Mild cases require no treatment. More severe cases respond well to passive stretching exercises. Corrective casts may be necessary for a short period. A mild flatfoot deformity may persist but there is no evidence that a calcaneovalgus deformity will become a flexible flatfoot.

## KOHLER'S BONE DISEASE (OSTEONECROSIS OF THE TARSAL NAVICULAR)

The tarsal navicular may undergo avascular necrosis similar to what occurs in other bones. The cause of all of these disorders is not completely understood, but interference with the circulation to the bone is thought to be the usual cause of the ischemia.

The onset of this disorder is about the age of 5 years. A painful limp is the usual initial complaint. Local pain, tenderness, and swelling over the navicular bone are often present.

The roentgenographic appearance is usually characteristic. Flattening, sclerosis, and irregularity of the navicular are usually present (Fig. 12-10).

Protection from excessive trauma, sometimes by the use of a short walking cast for 7 to 8 weeks, is sufficient treatment in most cases. Spontaneous recovery is the rule, and complete reossification of the navicular usually occurs within 2 to 3 years.

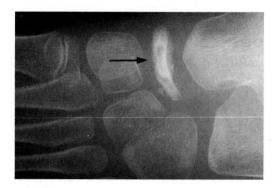

**Fig. 12–10.**
Kohler's disease *(arrow).*

## ANKLE SPRAINS

The sprain is the most common of all ankle injuries and may be the most common injury in sports. Most of these (85%) involve the lateral ligament complex as a result of excessive inversion. The anterior talofibular (ATF) ligament is usually injured first (Fig. 12-11). More severe injuries involve the calcaneofibular (CF) ligament. Only rarely is the posterior talofibular (PTF) ligament involved. The injuries are often graded I, II, and III, with I being mild and II being moderate. Grade III injuries are more severe, with instability resulting from rupture of the ATF and CF ligaments. Inversion (varus) sprains may also cause marked hemorrhage of the peroneal muscles and even peroneal nerve damage. The subtalar joint may also be injured.

Other ligamentous ankle injuries are much less common, but the anterior inferior tibiofibular (AITF) ligament, deltoid ligament, and interosseous membrane may be involved in eversion and rotational injuries. Damage to the tibiofibular syndesmosis is sometimes called a "high sprain" because of pain *above* the ankle from injury to the interosseous membrane. On rare occasions, the fibula may even be separated from the tibia.

### Clinical Features

The symptoms will depend on the severity of the injury. There is often a history of a "pop" at the time of injury. Mild sprains may cause only slight loss of function, but

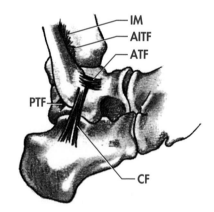

**Fig. 12–11.**
The lateral ankle ligaments, anterior and posterior talofibular and calcaneofibular. Also shown are the anterior inferior tibiofibular ligament and the beginning of the interosseous membrane *(IM).*

with more severe injuries, swelling and pain are significant and prohibit further use of the limb. Syndesmotic sprains often appear more benign because of minimal swelling. However, the pain and disability are greater than the clinical appearance would suggest, and the patient may be unable to bear weight.

Physical examination is important. Hemorrhage and local tenderness are present at the site of injury. The clinical assessment of stability is sometimes helpful as it may determine the course of treatment. Stability of lateral injuries should be assessed by the anterior drawer and talar tilt tests (Fig. 12-12). The anterior drawer is the most reliable and least painful in the acute stage. Positive tests indicate complete rupture of the ATF and CF ligaments and a grade III injury. Motor function should always be evaluated.

In syndesmotic injuries, the area of tenderness is more anterior and proximal. Dorsiflexion of the foot and compressing the ankle mortise (the "squeeze" test) may provoke pain, and the ankle may feel spongy.

Roentgenographic evaluation is always performed and should include the fifth metatarsal base to rule out fracture of the small toe. If the injury is in a child or adolescent with open growth plates, tenderness over the fibular malleolus (even with normal roentgenographic findings) implies the more likely *growth plate fracture* rather than a lateral sprain and a cast is usually necessary.

Opinions vary on the usefulness of arthrograms, tenograms, and stress films (Fig. 12-13). A good clinical examination is usually sufficient to determine stability.

### Treatment

Regardless of the severity, almost all sprains are treated nonoperatively. At first, all injuries are elevated and a soft compression dressing is applied for comfort and to help control swelling. Ice (1 hour on, 1 hour off) is applied, and crutches are used for ambulation. Rest, ice, compression, and elevation (RICE) are continued for 1 to 2 days. Antiinflammatory medication may be helpful, and crutches are often needed for 2 to 3 days. Heat is never used.

The next phase of treatment is rehabilitation, which includes early active range-of-motion exercises (circumduction) and weight bearing as tolerated (Fig. 12-14).

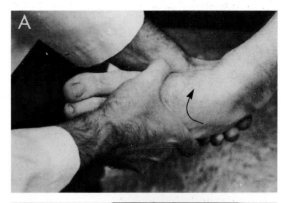
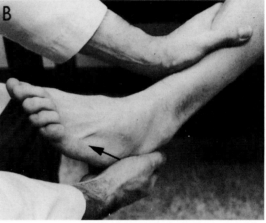

**Fig. 12–12.**
Tests for ankle instability. **A,** Inversion stress test. **B,** Anterior drawer test with the foot slightly plantar flexed.

"Alphabet" exercises (writing the alphabet in capital letters with the great toe) are begun, and exercise against resistance is added in 4 to 5 days. Wrapping or bracing with a stabilizing orthosis may also be helpful. Static bicycling may be added after 1 week, along with fast walking.

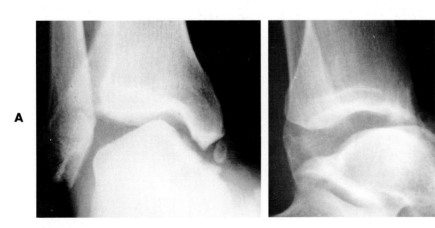

**Fig. 12–13.**
**A,** Stress roentgenography of the ankle revealing severe lateral instability, with tilting of the talus. **B,** The anterior drawer test.

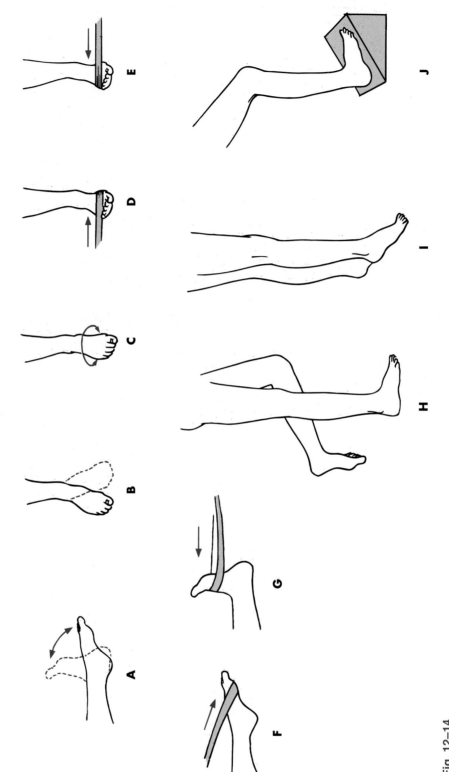

**Fig. 12–14.**
Ankle exercises. **A-C,** Range of motion (dorsiflexion, plantar flexion, circumduction, and writing the alphabet with the great toe). **D-G,** Strengthening exercises using a rubber strap (invertors, evertors, plantar flexors, dorsiflexors). **H,** Static one-leg standing with eyes closed. **I,** Toe raises. **J,** Heel cord stretches. Each exercise is performed 10 to 15 times. Ice is applied for a few minutes before and after each exercise period, and the exercises are performed three times a day.

If the pain is particularly severe, or if the patient requires independence, a short leg walking cast may be applied for 2 to 4 weeks. A cast brace is also a good option to control excessive pain.

Casting is used less often now because of concern over the temporary loss of motion and the atrophy that occurs. This requires some time for restoration of function after cast removal. However, cast treatment has many advocates and should still be considered, especially in those patients who might require independent walking. Other options for painful sprains include various short leg orthoses that immobilize the ankle and foot, such as the AFO (ankle-foot orthosis). These are usually weight-bearing appliances that can be removed for exercise. They are worn for about 4 weeks. A compression stocking can help control swelling.

The treatment of severe sprains with instability remains somewhat controversial, but they are usually treated in the same manner as other sprains: with a functional rehabilitation program. Although the results of surgical repair of unstable acute sprains are excellent, surgery is usually reserved for chronic instability in the high-level professional athlete or for those with significant syndesmotic separations.

**Note:** Lateral sprains of any severity may also cause symptoms that linger for weeks and months. Some syndesmotic sprains take even longer to heal (55 days vs. 35 days for lateral sprains), and heterotopic ossification may even develop in the interosseous membrane. (Unless symptoms occur, long-term results are not usually affected by such ossification.) If healing seems delayed, the following conditions should be considered: (1) talar dome fracture, (2) reflex sympathetic dystrophy, (3) chronic tendinitis, (4) peroneal tendon subluxation, (5) another occult fracture, such as that involving the anterior superior process of the calcaneous or the lateral process of the talus, and (6) poor rehabilitation. Repeat plain roentgenograms, bone scan, or MRI may be indicated (Fig. 12-15).

Ankles that are chronically unstable because of lateral ligamentous laxity may benefit from the application of a 0.3-cm lateral heel and sole wedge to prevent inversion. Taping or bracing during vigorous activities is also helpful, as are strengthening exercises. Continuing symptoms may require surgical reconstruction of the lateral ligaments to relieve symptoms of instability, although late traumatic arthritis and chronic instability are rare regardless of treatment.

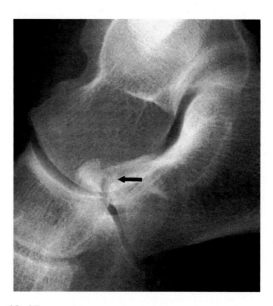

**Fig. 12–15.**
Fracture of the anterior superior process of the calcaneus. This injury may not unite and cause chronic pain.

## TARSAL TUNNEL SYNDROME

Rarely, nerve entrapment may occur in the foot by compression of the posterior tibial nerve beneath the flexor retinaculum at the ankle. This retinaculum arises from the medial malleolus and inserts into the medial aspect of the calcaneous (Fig. 12-16). Space-occupying lesions, traction injuries, fibrosis secondary to fractures, or deformities of the heel and foot can all compromise the tunnel and cause pressure on the posterior tibial nerve.

### Clinical Features
The symptoms are often vague in contrast to other compression neuropathies such as carpal tunnel syndrome. Burning pain, numbness, and tingling may be present in the sole of the foot. The Valleix phenomenon (proximal radiation of the pain) may occur. The exact location of these symptoms is variable. They are often

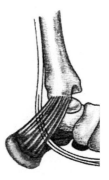

**Fig. 12–16.**
The tarsal tunnel. The posterior tibial nerve runs beneath the flexor retinaculum.

worse with activity. The pain may even radiate into the calf. Sensory loss and intrinsic muscle weakness are occasionally present. Tinel's sign may be positive over the tarsal tunnel. Sustained eversion or compression of the tunnel may reproduce symptoms. Nerve conduction studies may be abnormal in some cases but often are inconclusive.

## SUBLUXING PERONEAL TENDONS

Sudden, forceful dorsiflexion of the foot accompanied by contraction of the peroneal muscles may cause a tear in the retinaculum that holds these tendons in their groove behind the lateral malleolus. This may allow the tendons to acutely or chronically sublux over the lateral malleolus (Fig. 12-17).

### Clinical Features
Usually the diagnosis is easily made. The tendons are seen or felt to lie over the lateral malleolus. In chronic cases the subluxation can often be reproduced by the patient.

### Treatment
Acute cases are treated either by reduction and immobilization in a short leg walking cast for 4 weeks or by open repair of the retinaculum. Chronic cases are usually treated surgically by reconstruction of the retinaculum.

### Treatment
Hindfoot deformity may be treated with an orthosis. A medial heel wedge or heel seat may be used in an attempt to remove traction from the nerve. In selected patients with a clear diagnosis, surgical release of the entrapment may be indicated if symptoms persist; but often the results are mixed.

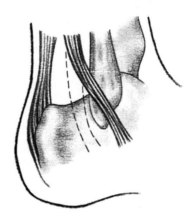

**Fig. 12–17.**
Subluxing peroneal tendons.

## OSTEOCHONDRITIS DISSECANS OF THE TALUS (TALAR DOME FRACTURE)

This condition is characterized by the formation of a small area of necrotic bone on the articular surface of the talus. The cause is usually traumatic, and the medial aspect of the talus is the area most commonly involved. It is often the lesion causing persistent symptoms after a "sprain" that does not heal.

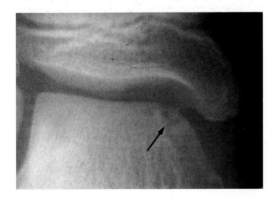

**Fig. 12–18.**
Osteochondritis dissecans of the talus (talar dome fracture *[arrow]*).

### Clinical Features
The onset is gradual, and a history of the injury is often absent. The disorder usually occurs during adolescence or early adulthood. A painful limp and chronic swelling in the ankle with activity are common complaints. Examination of the ankle with the foot in plantar flexion may reveal an area of point tenderness over the articular surface of the talus. Ankle motion is often restricted.

Roentgenographic examination usually reveals the characteristic lesion (Fig. 12-18). The necrotic fragment may even become detached into the joint cavity. MRI and CT are also helpful.

### Treatment
The undisplaced fragment is treated by prolonged abstinence from weight bearing until the lesion heals. Cast immobilization is often indicated. Persistent symptoms or detachment of the fragment may require surgical intervention.

# DISORDERS OF THE HINDFOOT

## Plantar Fasciitis ("Painful Heel Syndrome")

The plantar fascia extends from the calcaneus to the proximal phalanges of each toe and plays an important role in gait. Inflammation of this fascia is a common occurrence and leads to pain on the plantar aspect of the heel. The pain may be present anywhere along the plantar fascia, but it is often found near the medial tubercle of the calcaneus and along the medial longitudinal arch. It is a nonspecific inflammation that is probably secondary to repetitive strain. Both heels are often affected. This bilateral involvement may be an early symptom of other inflammatory disorders, such as ankylosing spondylitis, rheumatoid arthritis, or gouty arthritis. It may be seen in association with tight heel cords.

### Clinical Features

The pain is usually felt directly beneath the calcaneus but may be present in the area of the medial arch. The discomfort is characteristically worse with the first steps in the morning and after weight-bearing activities. Examination reveals local point tenderness in the area of involvement, usually the medial tubercle of the calcaneous. The pain may be aggravated by direct pressure or by maneuvers that place the fascia under a strain, such as dorsiflexing the toes and ankle. Some patients have a tight heel cord.

Roentgenographic findings are usually normal but may reveal a traction spur on the os calcis that is directed distally (Fig. 12-19). The significance of this osteophyte in the etiology of symptoms is unknown. It may be a response to muscle tension and is often found in the asymptomatic foot. A stress fracture or other bony disorder may need to be ruled out in chronic cases (Fig. 12-20).

### Treatment

Taping, relief pads, heel cups, cushions, and various orthoses have all been used with only modest success. OTC pads and cups are as effective as more expensive orthoses. No treatment designed to cushion the heel seems to help, probably because heel strike may not be the cause of the problem. Exercises that stretch the heel cord and plantar fascia may help, but they should not be performed in the acutely painful foot. Only a gentle pulling sensation should be felt. Cold or ice as counterirritants may promote temporary relief. A heel lift or high-heeled shoe may relieve pain in some cases. Oral antiinflammatory medication is used as necessary. Many patients will benefit from local infiltration of the tender area with a steroid/lidocaine mixture (Fig. 12-21). The injection may be repeated three or four times. Application of a short leg walking cast for 6 weeks is often beneficial. Custom-fitted tension night splints that hold the foot in slight dorsiflexion are used in some resistant cases. Physical therapy is not usually recommended.

The prognosis is usually good, although healing may be slow (requiring as much as 1 to 2 years in some cases). Medical treatment is effective in 90% of cases. When conservative treatment fails, release of the plantar fascia at its attachment to the os calcis and excision

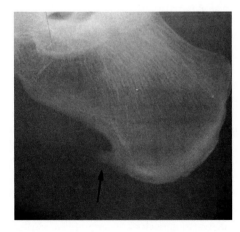

**Fig. 12–19.**
Roentgenography of the os calcis shows the distally directed spur on its inferior aspect *(arrow)*. The patient should be reassured that even though a "spur" may be present, it is not sharp as the name might suggest but rather it is round and smooth and that the relationship between heel pain and heel spurs has never been established.

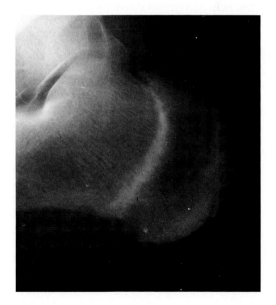

**Fig. 12–20.**
Stress fracture of the calcaneus.

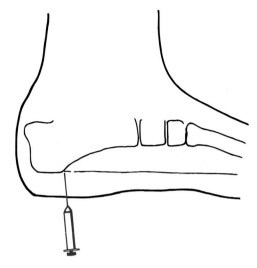

**Fig. 12–21.**
Injection site for plantar fasciitis. Injection should be through the sole into the area of maximum tenderness. A 25- or 27-gauge needle should be used and the medication injected slowly as some pain may occur. The total volume should be no greater than 1.5 ml.

of the bony prominence are indicated, but not before 6 to 12 months of medical management.

## Plantar Fibromatosis

This disorder is a fibrous tissue proliferation of the plantar fascia similar to Dupuytren's contracture in the palm. Clinically, the plantar lesion usually involves the medial half of the middle of the plantar fascia, but rarely causes a contracture (in contrast to Dupuytren's disease). The lesion generally begins as a painless subcutaneous nodule that slowly enlarges and eventually becomes tender. Treatment with a molded orthotic may allow transfer of the weight away from the nodule. Surgery is often indicated when weight bearing becomes painful. Recurrence after excision is common.

## Achilles Tendinitis

Overuse of the calf muscles may result in inflammation of the Achilles tendon, either acute or chronic. This disorder is often seen in the athlete. Pain, local tenderness, swelling, and a dry crepitus may be present. The tendon is often thickened in chronic cases. Passive stretching of the tendon by dorsiflexion of the ankle typically aggravates the pain. Calcification of the tendon may even occur.

Treatment consists of rest, heat, gentle stretching exercises, and antiinflammatory medications. A 1 cm heel lift may help diminish stress on the heel cord. A short leg walking cast or removable rigid brace may be nec-

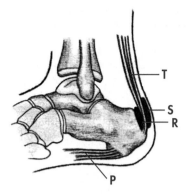

**Fig. 12–22.**
Bursae of the heel: *S* = superficial calcaneal bursa; *R* = retrocalcaneal bursa; *T* = Achilles tendon; *P* = plantar fascia.

essary. Local steroid injections probably should be avoided.

## Bursitis

Two bursae are consistently present near the insertion of the Achilles tendon (Fig. 12-22). The superficial bursa is often irritated by the constant rubbing of the counter of the shoe. The retrocalcaneal bursa may be irritated by a prominent posterosuperior angle of the calcaneus (Haglund's disease).

The treatment of both conditions is similar: relief pads, heat, and elevation of the heel of the shoe with a soft cushion are usually sufficient. Deep bursitis may respond to steroid injection, avoiding the tendon. Occasionally, the bursa and any underlying bony prominence may have to be resected.

## Calcaneal Apophysitis

A low-grade inflammatory reaction at the insertion of the Achilles tendon is often seen in association with irregular ossification and sclerosis of the calcaneal apophysis (Fig. 12-23). This disorder, sometimes referred to as *Sever's disease*, usually occurs in boys between the ages of 8 and 14 years. Local pain, tenderness, and swelling that are aggravated by activity are common. Passive stretching of the heel cord may reproduce the pain.

The roentgenographic changes seen in this disorder are probably not related to the presence of pain in the heel because these same findings are often found in the normal, asymptomatic foot.

Treatment includes NSAIDs, local heat, and the avoidance of activity. A 1.25-cm heel lift may diminish the stress on the heel cord. Stretching exercises may also help. A short leg walking cast applied with the foot

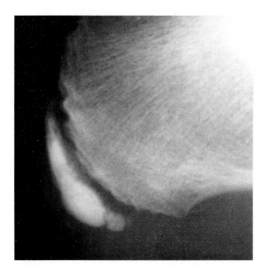

**Fig. 12–23.**
Roentgenogram of the heel in Sever's disease. Sclerosis of the apophysis is a normal finding.

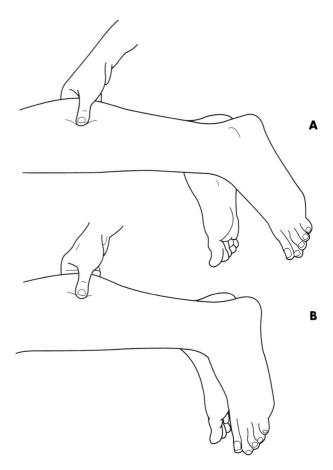

**Fig. 12–24.**
Thompson's test. The normal foot will automatically plantar flex when the calf is squeezed (**A**). This movement is absent when the heel cord is ruptured (**B**).

in slight equinus may be necessary in resistant cases. The disease is always self-limited.

## Achilles Tendon Rupture

Spontaneous rupture of the heel cord is an injury that usually results from gradual degeneration of the tendon. (A normal tendon is difficult to pull apart.) The rupture usually occurs 2.5 to 5 cm from the insertion of the tendon into the os calcis. The injury is missed by the initial treating physician up to 25% of the time.

### Clinical Features

The injury often occurs during an activity that puts stress on the tendon, such as jumping or pushing off with the weight on the forefoot. The acute injury is often associated with a "pop" and the patient often describes the feeling that the heel was shot. After the injury, the patient walks flatfooted and is unable to stand on the ball of the foot. Tenderness and hemorrhage are present, and a sulcus is usually palpable at the site of the rupture. However, this sulcus may be obscured by an organizing clot if the examination is delayed (a fact that may explain the difficulty in early diagnosis). Although active plantar flexion is usually lost, some flexion occasionally remains because of the activity of the other posterior compartment muscles. Thompson's squeeze test is usually positive (Fig. 12-24). Excessive passive dorsiflexion of the ankle will also be present.

### Treatment

The best results of treatment are obtained by immediate surgical repair. Nonoperative treatment by applying a short leg cast with the foot in equinus will also allow healing in many cases. Recurrence of the rupture is not uncommon regardless of treatment, and protection from excessive activity must be maintained for up to 1 year. Competitive athletes are rarely able to perform as well as before the injury. Neglected ruptures usually require reconstruction.

## Plantaris Tendon Rupture

The plantaris tendon lies medial to the heel cord in the calf. Traditionally, the cause of a sudden sharp pain in the calf with no loss of calf strength was always attributed to rupture of this tendon. Opinions differ as to whether or not the plantaris tendon actually ruptures. This entity may actually be the result of a partial rupture of the *gastrocnemius* muscle. The injury always occurs with activity. Treatment is symptomatic, but differentiation from complete Achilles tendon rupture is important. It may also present with symptoms similar to a ruptured Baker's cyst.

# DISORDERS OF THE FOREFOOT

## Morton's Neuroma

A common cause of pain in the forefoot is the interdigital neuroma. This lesion results from perineural fibrosis of the plantar nerve where the medial and lateral plantar branches communicate (Fig. 12-25). It may represent an entrapment neuropathy similar to carpal tunnel syndrome. The condition is probably secondary to repetitive trauma, and the fibrosis results in a painful fusiform swelling of the nerve. Females are more commonly affected. Tight footwear may be a cause.

### Clinical Features

The clinical picture is one of severe burning pain that is accentuated by activity. The pain is reported most often in the region of the third web space (rarely, the second) and may radiate into the third and fourth toes. Tight shoes aggravate the discomfort, and the pain is often relieved by removing the shoe and massaging the foot. Numbness may be present in the affected toes.

The examination is usually unremarkable except for exquisite tenderness on digital pressure between the third and fourth metatarsal heads. Compression of the forefoot transversely may also reproduce the pain. Sometimes while applying compression, a "click" may be felt in the web when bursa or neuroma is caught between the metatarsal heads. Some decrease in sensation may be present on the opposing surfaces of the two affected toes. Roentgenographic and electrical studies are not helpful. The diagnosis is usually clinical.

### Treatment

A pad that separates the heads of the third and fourth metatarsals may be helpful. NSAIDs may be tried, and the local injection of a steroid/lidocaine mixture into the tender web area from a dorsal approach may give some relief. The patient should avoid tight-fitting shoes. Surgical removal of the neuroma is often necessary.

## Metatarsalgia

Pain beneath the metatarsal head is referred to loosely as metatarsalgia. The term is used to describe a nonspecific symptom usually involving the lesser toes. Often no obvious cause is found but a variety of abnormalities may be responsible for the pain. These include an abnormally high arch, synovitis of the second MP joint, improper shoe selection (especially a high-heeled shoe), and a tight Achilles tendon. The disorder is often associated with hammertoes, clawed toes, and a hallux valgus deformity.

### Clinical Features

The symptoms consist of a typical burning or cramping pain in the region of the metatarsal heads, usually the middle ones. These symptoms are worse with activity and relieved by rest. Tender calluses often develop under the metatarsal heads. Variable degrees of dorsal contractures of the metatarsophalangeal joints may be present.

### Treatment

The object of treatment is to transfer the weight-bearing pressure away from the affected metatarsal heads onto the metatarsal neck and shaft. The calluses that form secondary to the abnormal pressure will usually disappear with time. Trimming or paring them with a pumice stone will only provide temporary relief if the pressures are not removed from the affected metatarsal heads. A low-heeled shoe with sufficient room in the forefoot is recommended. A metatarsal bar may be added to transfer the weight behind the metatarsal heads (Fig. 12-26). Warm soaks are prescribed as necessary. Surgery is reserved for those patients who have a clearly defined cause and who fail to respond to conservative treatment.

## MTP Synovitis

Painful synovitis of unknown etiology can affect the MP joints of the toes, usually the second. Subluxation and even dislocation can eventually occur. Most cases are idiopathic, although disproportionate length of the second ray and malalignment may be causative. Chronic stretching of the plantar soft tissue from wearing high-heeled shoes may also play a role.

Examination will reveal swelling and tenderness. Instability or even frank dislocation may be present.

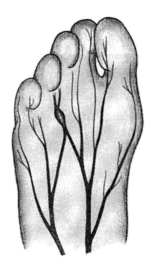

**Fig. 12–25.**
Morton's neuroma.

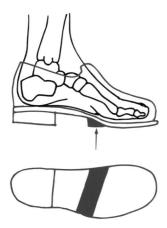

**Fig. 12–26.**
The anterior metatarsal bar *(arrow)*. It is placed behind the metatarsal heads so that weight is transferred to the metatarsal necks.

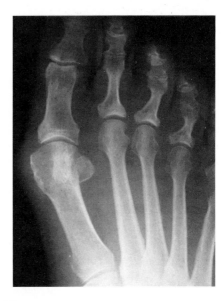

**Fig. 12–28.**
Hallux valgus with bunion exostosis.

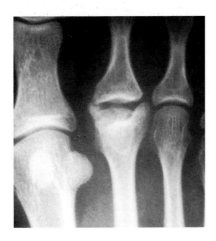

**Fig. 12–27.**
Freiberg's disease, second toe.

Treatment includes NSAIDs, shoe modifications, and occasional steroid injections. Surgery may be required for permanent relief.

## Freiberg's Disease

Freiberg's disease is a disorder of unknown cause in which aseptic necrosis occurs in one of the metatarsal heads, usually the second. The condition is most common in adolescents and girls are more often affected.

### Clinical Features
The disease appears as pain, swelling, and restriction of motion of the metatarsophalangeal joint. The metatarsal head is usually palpably enlarged. Roentgenographic examination reveals widening and irregularity of the metatarsal head (Fig. 12-27). Loose bodies may be present.

### Treatment
The inflammation is treated with NSAIDs, warm soaks, and local steroid injections. An anterior metatarsal bar will often relieve pressure on the metatarsal head. Persistent pain necessitates arthroplasty of the involved joint.

## Hallux Valgus

Hallux valgus is a lateral deviation of the great toe at the metatarsophalangeal joint. This is usually associated with a bony and soft tissue enlargement over the medial aspect of the first metatarsal head that is referred to as the bunion. Females are most commonly affected. The cause is unknown, but heredity and the wearing of tight shoes play major roles.

### Clinical Features
Pain and deformity are the main initial symptoms. The soft tissue over the prominence may become inflamed and tender. Sometimes the bunion bump will even ulcerate and drain. Painful calluses often develop on the second toe, which is forced into hyperextension by the deviated great toe.

Roentgenographic findings include lateral displacement of the proximal phalanx and the presence of a medial exostosis (Fig. 12-28). Degenerative changes may also be present in the metatarsophalangeal joint.

### Treatment
Conservative treatment is directed at relieving the pressure over the painful bunion prominence. Properly fitted, low-heeled shoes with the toe portion stretched to

accommodate the bunion are effective. An "extra depth" shoe may be needed to accommodate a dorsiflexed second toe. A splint that separates the first and second toes may also be beneficial. Tight hose should be avoided. Local measures such as rest and moist heat are indicated when acute pain is present. Disabling pain and deformity are indications for surgery. Excision of the exostosis and realignment of the great toe are usually performed.

## Hallux Rigidus

Hallux rigidus is a painful condition affecting the metatarsophalangeal joint of the great toe and characterized by restriction of motion. It is usually secondary to traumatic osteoarthritis. The condition may develop at any age but is most common in the third and fourth decades.

### Clinical Features

Gradually increasing pain and stiffness are typical and are often precipitated by a minor injury. The pain occurs with ambulation, especially when the patient's toe is dorsiflexed late in the stance phase of walking. Examination reveals swelling, tenderness, and restricted motion of the metatarsophalangeal joint. Attempts at passive motion, especially dorsiflexion, are painful. Osteophytic buildup is easily palpable on the dorsum of the joint. The toe is held in a protective position of slight flexion, and as the patient walks, more weight is borne on the outer metatarsal heads and lateral border because of the lack of ability to extend the great toe.

The roentgenogram usually reveals typical findings of degenerative arthritis with joint narrowing and spur formation (Fig. 12-29).

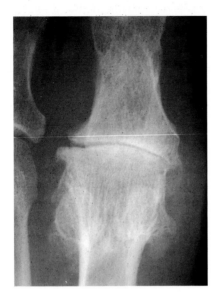

**Fig. 12–29.**
Hallux rigidus. Narrowing and sclerosis are present at the metatarsophalangeal joint of the great toe.

### Treatment

Symptomatic relief can be obtained by rest, moist heat, and antiinflammatory medication. An intraarticular injection of steroid may provide additional relief (Fig. 12-30). A shoe with sufficient room in the forefoot is worn, and an anterior metatarsal bar is applied to the shoe. A rockerbottom shoe may also be tried. This shoe will allow the foot to roll over without dorsiflexion of the toes, but is awkward looking. Arthroplasty or arthrodesis of the metatarsophalangeal joint is indicated in resistant cases.

## Hallux Varus

Hallux varus is a deformity usually seen in children in which medial angulation of the great toe occurs at the metatarsophalangeal joint. It is usually congenital and associated with other foot deformities, but it may be seen in adults after surgical overcorrection of a hallux valgus deformity.

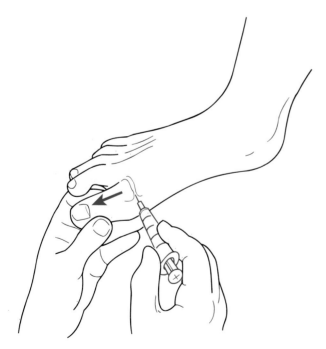

**Fig. 12–30.**
Injecting the MP joint of the great toe. Palpate the joint line and apply distal traction to distract the space. A 25-gauge needle is used from a dorsal approach; 1 to 2 ml of fluid is injected.

Mild cases in children may respond to passive stretching exercises and proper shoe wear. More severe cases in both adults and children usually require surgical correction.

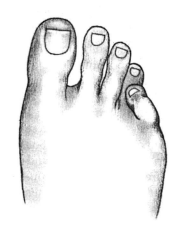

**Fig. 12–31.**
Congenital overlapping fifth toe.

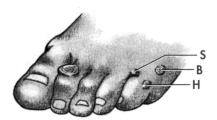

**Fig. 12–32.**
Hammered second toe with a dorsal callus. Also shown are the soft corn *(S)*, bunionette *(B)*, and hard corn *(H)*.

## Congenital Overlapping Fifth Toe

This is a common familial deformity, often bilateral, in which the small toe is dorsiflexed and may come to lie on the top of the fourth toe (Fig. 12-31). The capsule and extensor tendon on the dorsum of the metatarsophalangeal joint are shortened and do not allow passive correction of the deformity. Calluses may develop on the dorsum of the toe secondary to chronic irritation by the shoe.

Passive stretching of mild deformities is indicated, but usually does not completely correct the problem. Surgical realignment or even amputation may be necessary in symptomatic cases.

## Hammertoe

A hammertoe is one in which a flexion deformity develops at the proximal interphalangeal joint and causes the tip of the toe to be depressed downward (Fig. 12-32). A mild hyperextension deformity at the metatarsophalangeal joint may be present. Painful calluses develop over the tip of the toe, over the dorsum of the proximal interphalangeal joint, and under the metatarsal heads. The second toe is most commonly affected, and the disorder is often seen in association with a hallux valgus deformity of the great toe. The cause is often improperly fitted, tight shoes.

Mild flexible deformities may be corrected by stretching exercises and "over-and-under" taping to adjacent toes (Fig. 12-33). Toe caps or pads may also be helpful. Properly fitted shoes are important. Extra depth shoes may be needed. Resistant cases usually require surgical correction.

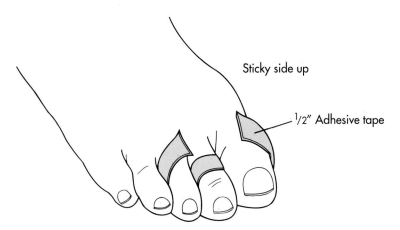

Sticky side up

½" Adhesive tape

**Fig. 12–33.**
Over-and-under taping for a hammered or clawed second toe. The second toe is most often clawed, often because it is too long. Before taping, stretching exercises are performed to improve the MP extension and IP flexion contractures. The tape is applied to the proximal phalanx in most cases.

## Corns and Calluses

Corns and calluses develop in response to abnormal pressures against the skin of the foot. External pressure resulting from improper shoe wear combined with internal pressure from abnormal bony protuberances will often lead to the production of thickened, painful, hard skin over the bony prominence. In areas where moisture and perspiration collect, the skin becomes macerated, and a *soft corn* (clavus mollis) develops and may even ulcerate.

*Hard corns* (clavus durus) are most commonly found on the dorsolateral aspect of the proximal interphalangeal joint of the fifth toe, whereas soft corns are most common in the fourth web space. The tailor's bunion or bunionette occurs on the dorsolateral aspect of the metatarsophalangeal joint of the fifth toe. Calluses are often seen under the weight-bearing portion of the metatarsal heads or sesamoid bones of the great toe.

Removal of the external pressure is essential in the conservative management of all of these soft tissue lesions in the forefoot. A low-heeled shoe with adequate width in the forefoot is worn. Relief pads and metatarsal bars are usually helpful. Warm soaks in soapy water, followed by the application of a keratolytic medication such as salicylic acid salve, will help eliminate the callus or corn. (Normal skin should be avoided when applying the salve. The salve should remain in place, covered by adhesive tape, for 3 to 5 days. The patient should watch for skin maceration. After the tape is removed, the hard callus or corn may be shaved in layers.) A pumice stone may also be used to pare down the callus. This procedure is often helpful, but deep excision of any corn or callus should be avoided because an infected ulcer may result. Soft corns may be eliminated in 1 to 2 weeks, but hard calluses may take

longer. A cotton pad or lamb's wool may be placed between the toes if a soft corn is present, and a doughnut-shaped pad is always worn around a hard corn or callus to shift weight from the lesion to the adjacent normal skin. The toes should be kept as dry as possible at all times.

Surgical correction may be advised in resistant cases to eliminate the bony prominence.

*Plantar warts* also occur near the metatarsal heads, but usually not directly on the weight-bearing surface. The wart is generally surrounded by a callus and may look exactly like a simple callus. Characteristic papillary tips are usually present. Paring or curettage of the wart and the use of a keratolytic agent such as salicylic acid salve will often effect a cure. Relief pads are worn as necessary. The lesion has a high incidence of spontaneous disappearance in several months.

## Disorders of the Toenail

The ingrown nail is a common condition that mainly affects the great toe. In this disorder, the nail does not actually grow into the soft tissue; instead, the soft tissue overgrows and obliterates the nail sulcus (Fig. 12-34). The nail itself is usually normal, although some older patients have incurved nails. The causes are probably multiple, but incorrect nail trimming, the use of sharp tools to clean the nail gutters, improperly fitted tight shoes and stockings, and bony deformities have all been implicated. Roentgenograms should be obtained to rule out unusual causes such as subungual exostosis. Because of improper trimming, a small nail spike may be formed that continues to grow and irritate the soft tissue (Fig. 12-35). A chronic infection is usually the end result.

In most mild early cases, soaks, antibiotics, and proper shoes and stockings may be curative. The nail edge should be kept elevated with a soft cotton wad or metal shield until it grows out beyond the soft-tissue re-

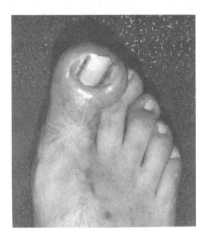

**Fig. 12–34.**
A typical ingrown great toenail.

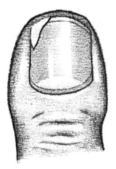

**Fig. 12–35.**
The ingrown toenail often results from improper trimming that produces a nail spike. The nail should always be trimmed transversely.

action. Unfortunately, this can be a slow process because the nail takes approximately 3 months to grow 1 cm. Proper transverse trimming of the nail should prevent recurrences.

Surgery may be necessary in resistant cases. Among the procedures used, removal of the central portion of the nail does not seem to allow the lateral margin of the nail to elevate away from the sulcus as theorized. Avulsing the whole nail is usually not effective either. When the nail regrows, it usually runs into the soft tissues again and causes recurrence in up to 70% of cases. The surgical procedures most commonly used involve removing (1) one or both nail margins, (2) the entire nail, or (3) the entire nail plus a tuft of the distal phalanx. Removing one or both nail margins is the most popular. Removing the whole nail sometimes leaves an unsightly nail plate area, and amputating the distal tuft causes some shortening. Soft-tissue procedures are rarely used because of a high recurrence rate.

Surgery for nail margin removal is as follows (Fig. 12-36):

1. Local anesthesia and a Penrose drain as a tourniquet are used.
2. A short, angled incision is made in the eponychium down to the nail.
3. With heavy scissors, the section of nail to be removed is cut proximally to separate it from the remaining nail.
4. A knife blade is then used to separate the nail and matrix to be removed from the remaining nail and matrix. Along with the nail, the dorsal and inferior matrix is excised from its origin to distal to the edge of the lunula, and the nail margin plus matrix is removed.

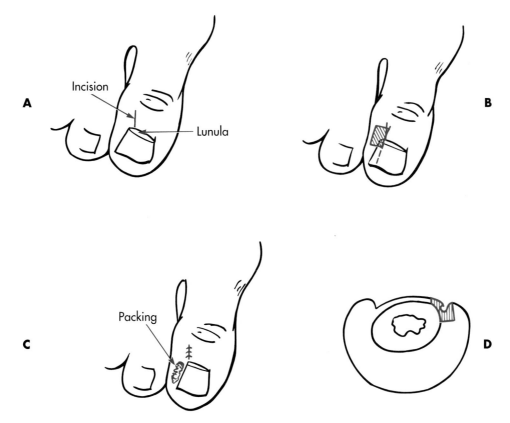

**Fig. 12–36.**
Ingrown toenail removal. **A**, A short, angled skin incision is made in the eponychium down to the nail. **B**, With heavy scissors, the portion of the nail to be excised *(dotted line)* is separated from the remaining nail. (The important area of soft tissue and nail growth matrix to be removed is crosshatched.) **C**, A curet is used to remove any granulation tissue and remaining soft tissue in the periosteal area of the phalanx, and the incision is closed. A small pack is left in the gutter. **D**, Approximate cross section of a toe showing the area to be removed under the skin. It is not necessary to remove tissue very far beyond the lunula, but be certain to remove all necessary growth matrix to prevent any spikes of nail from regrowing at the margin. (**Note:** The nail grows from a dorsal and deep matrix that envelops the base of the nail and extends just beyond the lunula. This area also extends proximally beneath the eponychium.) Both sides may be done if necessary.

5. Curettage is performed on the area to remove any granulation tissue and remaining matrix, and the incision is closed with a single suture.

6. A small pack is left in the sulcus and removed in 2 to 3 days when dressings are changed.

Phenol cauterization and sodium hydroxide have also been used to eliminate the germinal matrix itself. The results are about the same as those obtained with surgical removal.

Surgery for an older, thickened, incurved nail usually involves removing the entire nail because, as a rule, the whole nail is involved.

Two other common conditions, the hypertrophied nail and the ram's-horn nail, may result from poor local hygiene. Both are most common in the elderly. A hypertrophied nail is usually caused by a low-grade fungus infection. The affected nail is thickened, and a yellow, powdery substance is present beneath it. A ram's horn nail is characterized by massive overgrowth. The nail may even curl over to the plantar aspect of the toe. Both disorders will usually respond to soaks and proper local care. Removal of the entire nail is occasionally required.

## ACCESSORY BONES

Many accessory and sesamoid bones are present in the normal foot (Fig. 12-37). Most are asymptomatic. However, an unusually large accessory navicular bone may cause pain from local pressure (Fig. 12-38). It is often associated with weakness in the longitudinal arch and a mild flatfoot deformity. Relief pads may eliminate symptoms, but surgical excision of the accessory bone is sometimes necessary to completely relieve the pain.

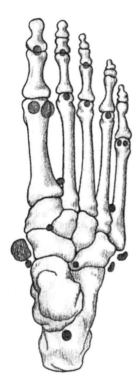

**Fig. 12–37.**
Accessory and sesamoid bones of the foot.

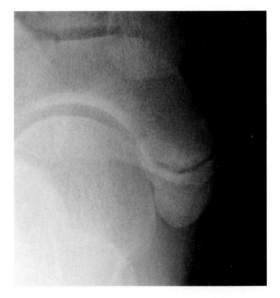

**Fig. 12–38.**
Accessory navicular. The medial navicular is also enlarged.

## FRACTURES OF THE ANKLE

The ankle joint or "mortise" is shaped like an inverted U with the dome of the talus fitting between the medial and lateral malleoli. The posterior margin of the tibia is often called the third or posterior malleolus.

The talus is held in its position by bony and ligamentous structures and occupies a special position in the ankle joint. Any deviation from that position through injury could result in traumatic arthritis.

Most common ankle fractures are the result of eversion or lateral rotation forces on the talus (in contrast to common sprains, which are usually a result of inversion).

### Physical Findings

The amount of deformity usually depends upon the extent of displacement. Pain, tenderness, and hemorrhage are usually present at the site of the injury. The ligamentous structures (especially the deltoid ligament) should be gently palpated to determine the extent of the soft tissue injury.

### Imaging Studies

Accurate roentgenographic assessment of ankle injuries requires standard AP and lateral views accompanied by an AP taken 15 degrees internally rotated. The last view is taken to properly visualize the mortise.

### Treatment

The two most important clinical and roentgenographic assessments that will determine the treatment of ankle fractures are: (1) the position of the talus in the mortise and (2) the stability of the fracture. If the talus is already displaced, referral is indicated because reduction will be required, sometimes by surgical means, to restore the ankle mortise (Fig. 12-39). Any deviation of the position of the talus in the joint could lead to traumatic arthritis.

If there is no widening of the ankle mortise (talar displacement), many injuries can be safely treated with simple casting without reduction or surgical intervention. There is, however, the potential for displacement if both sides of the joint are significantly injured (for example, the common oblique fracture of the lateral malleolus

with rupture of the deltoid ligament). It is important to determine by clinical examination (presence of tenderness) if ligamentous injury might be present. If that is the case, the injury can still be treated with casting, but it is considered unstable and weight bearing is prohibited to prevent displacement in the cast. All ankle fractures should be routinely evaluated roentgenographically at 1 to 2 weeks to determine if there is any sign of displacement of the talus. Some of the more common ankle fractures and their treatments are as follows:

1.  Undisplaced or avulsion fractures of either malleolus below the ankle joint line. Stability of the joint is not compromised and a short leg walking cast or walking cast boot would be sufficient. Weight bearing is allowed as tolerated. Protection may be discontinued in 4 to 6 weeks.
2.  Isolated undisplaced fractures of the medial, lateral, or posterior malleolus are usually stable and require only a short leg walking cast for 8 weeks. The fracture line of the lateral malleolus may persist roentgenographically for several months, but immobilization beyond 8 weeks is unnecessary. Undisplaced bimalleolar fractures are treated with a long leg cast flexed 30 degrees at the knee to prevent displacement of the fracture fragments. In 4 weeks, a short leg walking cast may be applied for an additional 4 weeks.
3.  Isolated fractures of the lateral malleolus that are slightly displaced may be treated with casting if no medial (deltoid) ligament injury is present (Fig. 12-40). A below-knee walking cast is applied

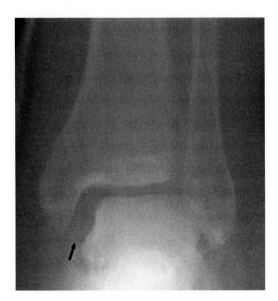

**Fig. 12–39.**
Fracture of the lateral malleolus with widening of the ankle mortise *(arrow)*, sometimes called the medial clear space (MCS).

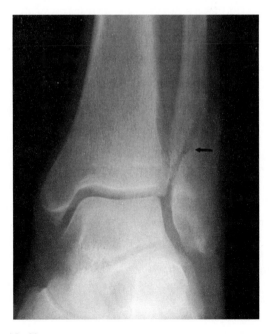

**Fig. 12–40.**
Minimally displaced fracture of the lateral malleolus *(arrow)* with no widening of the ankle mortise.

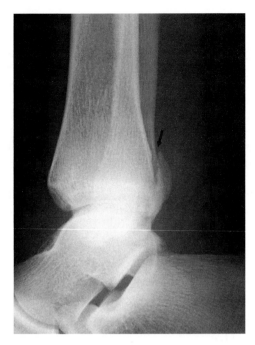

**Fig. 12–41.**
Minimally displaced fracture of the posterior malleolus (*arrow*).

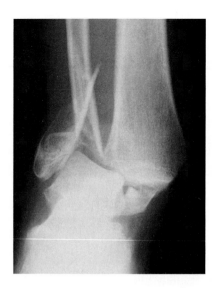

**Fig. 12–42.**
Fracture-dislocation of the ankle.

with the ankle in neutral and weight bearing is allowed as tolerated. Immobilization for 6 to 8 weeks is sufficient. If medial tenderness is present (suggesting deltoid ligament rupture), a carefully molded cast should suffice if weight bearing is not allowed and the patient is followed closely for signs of instability, especially after swelling recedes. If there develops any significant widening of the medial ankle mortise (increase in the "medial clear space") as a result of lateral displacement of the talus, referral for possible reduction is appropriate.

4. The undisplaced fracture of the distal fibular growth plate is diagnosed clinically. There is tenderness over the epiphyseal plate. Roentgeno-graphic examination is usually negative. A short leg walking cast for 4 weeks is sufficient. Growth disturbance is rare.

5. Isolated displaced fractures of the posterior malleolus involving less than 25% of the articular surface can be safely treated with a short leg cast (Fig. 12-41). Fractures involving more than 25% of the articular surface should be referred.

Fractures with dislocation of the talus should be reduced as soon as possible (Fig. 12-42). If the dislocation is not promptly reduced, severe soft-tissue injury with blistering and skin breakdown may result. Definitive surgical treatment of the fractures may also have to be delayed. The dislocation is reduced by traction and manipulation with the patient under local anesthesia. After the reduction, the ankle is placed in a soft, bulky compression dressing reinforced with plaster splints. Any necessary surgery can then be performed on an elective basis.

## FRACTURES OF THE FOOT

### Fractures of the Calcaneus

Fractures of the calcaneus usually result from a fall on the heel. Ten percent are associated with a compression fracture of the lumbar spine. (The heel is usually so painful that the back pain may not be noticed until much later.) The os calcis is usually crushed, and the fragments are displaced in varying amounts (Fig. 12-43).

Fractures of the os calcis are painful injuries characterized by severe swelling so intense that blistering and even skin necrosis may occur. To control the swelling and hemorrhage, all calcaneus fractures are treated ini-tially with a soft compression dressing, ice, and elevation. A cast is never applied immediately after the injury. The pain from the fracture and swelling is only intensified if a constricting circular cast is present over the heel.

Minimally displaced fractures are treated by cast immobilization for 2 to 3 weeks or with crutches and the avoidance of bearing weight. The cast is removed as soon as possible to begin mobilization of the ankle and heel. Eversion and inversion movements are begun, but weight bearing is not allowed for 6 to 8 weeks until the fracture has healed. Displaced fractures may be

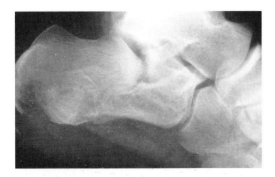

**Fig. 12–43.**
Fracture of the calcaneus with moderate displacement.

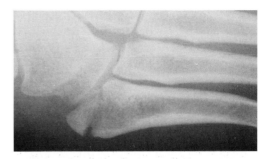

**Fig. 12–45.**
Fracture of the base of the fifth metatarsal.

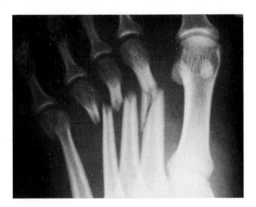

**Fig. 12–44.**
Displaced fractures of the metatarsals.

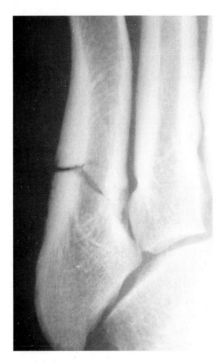

**Fig. 12–46.**
Fracture of the shaft of the fifth metatarsal.

treated in the same manner or by either closed or open reduction.

Regardless of treatment, prolonged immobilization is inadvisable. Temporary disability after this injury may persist for 1 to 2 years, and some permanent impairment is common. Early motion without weight bearing appears to be most beneficial. Some restriction of eversion and inversion is usually permanent, which makes walking on rough, irregular surfaces difficult. The heel is often widened permanently. Late surgery is often helpful.

## Fractures of the Metatarsals

Fractures of the necks or shafts of the metatarsals usually result from compression injuries of the foot. Undisplaced fractures require little treatment other than a soft compression dressing and crutches for 4 to 6 weeks. A short leg walking cast or hard-soled sandal may be preferable in a few days to allow the patient to discard the crutches.

Displaced fractures of the necks of the metatarsals may need reduction to prevent pain from developing under the metatarsal heads (Fig. 12-44). Manipulation is sometimes effective, but maintenance of the reduction is often difficult. Open reduction with internal fixation is sometimes necessary.

Fractures of the *base* or styloid of the fifth metatarsal are common and result from an inversion injury to the foot (Fig. 12-45). They are usually undisplaced and require little treatment. A light compression dressing and hard-soled sandal are usually sufficient. Crutches may be necessary for 7 to 10 days, and healing is usually complete in 5 to 6 weeks. Nonunion is rare.

Fractures of the *shaft* of the fifth metatarsal, especially proximal ones, heal slowly and may require a short leg walking cast for 6 to 8 weeks (Fig. 12-46). The cortex of the proximal diaphysis is normally thick and often relatively avascular (especially in long distance runners, a result of high stresses). The relatively poor circulation in this area may lead to delayed union and even nonunion. Surgical intervention may even be required.

## Fractures of the Phalanges

Fractures of the toes are common and usually require little treatment. Undisplaced fractures may be treated by taping the injured toe to the adjacent toe for 3 to 4 weeks. Displaced fractures can usually be reduced without anesthesia. Open reduction is rarely necessary. However, fractures of the proximal phalanx of the great toe should be reduced accurately.

## FOOT CARE

Most foot problems develop in the forefoot, and many have been previously discussed. For the treatment of painful conditions of the forefoot, the patient should avoid high heels and keep the foot in a soft shoe with a wide toe box (the portion covering the forefoot). The simple addition of an anterior heel (anterior metatarsal bar) will improve many of the problems that develop under the metatarsal heads.

The diabetic patient with or without vascular disease has the potential for far more serious problems, and special care must be taken to avoid them. The following general principles are helpful:

1. The feet should be inspected and cleaned daily. The feet should be washed with a mild soap in lukewarm water and patted dry. Overzealous rubbing should always be avoided. The feet are inspected for any cracks or fissures, and a mirror is used if necessary. The shoes should also be inspected for any areas that could cause skin irritation.

2. Stockings should always be worn and should fit comfortably. They should be kept dry at all times to prevent skin maceration. Tight, constricting stockings should not be worn, but loose stockings that may wrinkle should also be avoided.

3. Smoking and temperature extremes should be avoided.

4. "Home surgery" should be avoided, especially by the diabetic patient or the patient with vascular disease. Nails should be left long and cut straight across. A pumice stone may be used on thick calluses in the healthy patient, but these same calluses place the diabetic patient's foot at risk for infection because they often crack and develop open sores. Diabetic patients should not use the pumice stone but should attempt to soften the calluses by changing the weight-bearing stresses on the foot.

5. Diabetic patients should also avoid applying strong chemical agents to calluses or corns.

6. A mild moisturizing cream should be applied daily, but the web spaces should be kept dry. Powder may be used there, and small pieces of cotton may be placed between the toes if necessary.

7. Shoes should fit comfortably. Soft leather or canvas is preferred because these materials "breathe" better and cause fewer pressure areas. Foam rubber soles cause fewer plantar calluses. The toe box should be wide and high enough to accommodate any contractures or exostosis. The patient with more severe forefoot deformities may require a specially constructed shoe or an in-depth (extra depth) shoe. This has a wider, deeper toe box that is helpful for hammered or clawed toes.

8. Full-length, soft, molded inlays can be used when pressure sores or painful calluses are present. An in-depth shoe is usually required to provide enough room for the insole, which is usually the full length of the shoe. Insoles reduce and spread the repetitive stress on the foot. Many good over-the-counter materials are available. Excellent materials such as polyethylene foam can be heat-molded to conform to the individual's foot. Relief areas can then be cut out of the material wherever pressure sores are present on the corresponding part of the foot. These often require an in-depth shoe to allow for the size of the insert. These materials have to be replaced occasionally because they will lose their volume and flatten to some degree.

When ulcers do develop, they are most common on the weight-bearing surface of the foot or on the medial aspect of the great toe. These are often referred to as mal-perforans (Fig. 12-47). At this stage vigorous local care, minor debridement, and control of infection are indicated. Excessive heat, which places a great demand on the soft tissue, should be avoided. The previously mentioned metatarsal bars and insoles are used to re-

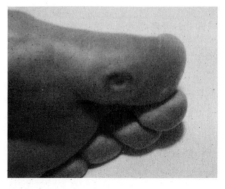

**Fig. 12–47.**
Healing mal-perforans ulcer of the great toe.

lieve the pressure on the ulcer. If the foot is warm and has pulses, amputation is usually not necessary, and healing of these ulcers will commonly occur with proper care.

## Shoes

Because the majority of foot problems are caused by tight-fitting shoes (especially the toe box), the first treatment is addressing the source of the problem. Women's shoes, especially high-heeled ones, are the source of many difficulties. For the typical high-heeled shoe or even pump to stay in place, excessive pressures must be applied to the forefoot, requiring a shoe that is often smaller than the foot. Lowering the heel and widening the forefoot of the shoe could help, but this often results in a shoe that won't stay on because the heel is too wide. The only option is a lace-up shoe. Although less attractive, this shoe is more comfortable because more room can be allowed in the toe box for the forefoot and the shoes won't feel loose in the heel. "Orthopedic" prescription shoes are expensive and usually unnecessary. A soft, low-heeled, lace-up shoe of any type will often provide symptomatic relief of many forefoot problems. In general, shoes should be fitted while standing and at the end of the day, when the feet are the largest. The foot spreads with age, and shoe sizes should increase as well.

The same pragmatic approach may be taken regarding children's shoes. Only rarely are special shoes ever needed, and there are absolutely no advantages for children to wear the traditional, expensive, high-topped leather shoe. (Societies in which shoes are not worn at all actually experience fewer foot deformities.) Children may outgrow two to four pairs each year, and the total cost of such shoes would be considerable even if they were of some benefit. Children wear shoes to keep the feet warm and to prevent harm from sharp objects. Otherwise, they may go barefooted as much as they like or wear any inexpensive brand as long as the shoes are comfortable.

## BIBLIOGRAPHY

Anderson IF et al: Osteochondral fractures of the dome of the talus, *J Bone Joint Surg Am* 71:1143, 1989.

Beskin JL: Nerve entrapment syndromes of the foot and ankle, *J Am Acad Orthop Surg* 5:261-269, 1997.

Bleck EE: The shoeing of children: sham or science?, *Dev Med Child Neurol* 13:188, 1971.

Bleck EE, Berzins UJ: Conservative management of pes valgus with plantar flexed talus, flexible, *Clin Orthop* 122:85, 1977.

Cass JR, Morrey BF: Ankle instability: current concepts, diagnosis and treatment, *Mayo Clin Proc* 59:165, 1984.

Churchill JA, Mazur JH: Ankle pain in children: diagnostic evaluation and clinical decision making, *J Am Acad Orthop Surg* 3:183-193, 1995.

Cowell HR: Talocalcaneal coalition and new causes of peroneal spastic flat foot, *Clin Orthop* 85:16, 1972.

DeMaio M et al: Plantar fasciitis, *Orthopedics* 16:1153-1163, 1993.

Downs DM, Jacobs RL: Treatment of resistant ulcers on the plantar surface of the great toe in diabetics, *J Bone Joint Surg Am* 64:930, 1982.

DuVries HL: *Surgery of the foot*, ed 2, St Louis, 1965, CV Mosby Co.

Eastwood DM, Gregg PJ, Atkins RM: Intra-articular fractures of the calcaneum, *J Bone Joint Surg Br* 75:183-189, 1993.

Eckert WR, Davis EA Jr: Acute rupture of the peroneal retinaculum, *J Bone Joint Surg Am* 58:670, 1976.

Furey JG: Plantar fasciitis: the painful heel syndrome, *J Bone Joint Surg Am* 57:672, 1975.

Gill LH: Plantar fasciitis: diagnosis and conservative management, *J Am Acad Orthop Surg* 5:109-117, 1997.

Greenfield GB: *Radiology of bone diseases*, Philadelphia, 1969, JB Lippincott.

Greig JD: Results of surgery for ingrowing toenails, *J Bone Joint Surg Br* 71:859, 1989.

Heifitz CJ: Ingrown toenail: a clinical study, *Am J Surg* 37:298, 1937.

Helfet AJ: A new way of treating flat feet in children, *Lancet* 1:262, 1956.

Ho K et al: Using tomography to diagnose occult ankle fractures, *Ann Emerg Med* 27:600-605, 1996.

Hopkinson WJ et al: Syndesmotic sprains of the ankle, *Foot Ankle* 10:325-330, 1990.

Inglis AE et al: Ruptures of the tendo Achilles: an objective assessment of surgical and non-surgical treatment, *J Bone Joint Surg Am* 58:990, 1976.

Johnson KA: *Surgery of the foot and ankle*, New York, 1989, Raven Press.

Keats TE: *An atlas of normal roentgen variants that may simulate disease*, Chicago, 1977, Year Book Medical Publishers.

Konradsen L, Halmer P, Sondergard L: Early mobilizing treatment for grade III ankle ligament injuries, *Foot Ankle* 12:69-72, 1991.

Korkala O et al: A prospective study of the treatment of severe tears of the lateral ligament of the ankle, *Int Orthop* 11:13, 1987.

Lea RB, Smith L: Non-surgical treatment of tendon Achilles rupture, *J Bone Joint Surg Am* 54:1398, 1972.

Lee TH, Wapner KL, Hecht PJ: Plantar fibromatosis. Current concepts review, *J Bone Joint Surg Am* 75:1080-1085, 1993.

Mann RA: Disorders of the first metatarsophalangeal joint, *J Am Acad Orthop Surg* 3:34-43, 1995.

Marcus RE, Goodfellow DB, Pfister ME: The difficult diagnosis of posterior tibial tendon rupture in sports injuries, *Orthopedics* 18:715-721, 1995.

McComis GP, Nawoczenski DA, DeHaven KE: Functional bracing for rupture of the Achilles tendon: clinical results and analysis of ground-reaction forces and temporal data, *J Bone Joint Surg* 79(12):1799-1808, 1997.

Michelson JD: Fractures about the ankle. Current concepts review, *J Bone Joint Surg* 77(1):142-152, 1995.

Michelson JD et al: Examination of the pathologic anatomy of ankle fractures, *J Trauma* 32:65-70, 1992.

Milgram JE: Office measures for relief of the painful foot, *J Bone Joint Surg Am* 46:1095, 1964.

Mizel MS, Michelson JD: Nonsurgical treatment of monarticular nontraumatic synovitis of the second metatarsophalangeal joint, *Foot Ankle Int* 18:424-426, 1997.

Mosier KM, Asher M: Tarsal coalitions and peroneal spastic flat foot, *J Bone Joint Surg Am* 66:976, 1984.

Myerson M, Quill GE: Late complications of fractures of the calcaneus, *J Bone Joint Surg Am* 75:331-342, 1993.

Paley D, Hall H: Intra-articular fractures of the calcaneus, *J Bone Joint Surg Am* 75:342-355, 1993.

Parmar HV, Triffitt PD, Gregg PJ: Intra-articular fractures of the calcaneum treated operatively or conservatively, *J Bone Joint Surg Br* 75:932-937, 1993.

Pedowitz WJ, Kovatis P: Flatfoot in the adult, *J Am Acad Orthop Surg* 3:293-302, 1995.

Pfeiffer WH, Cracchiolo A: Clinical results after tarsal tunnel decompression, *J Bone Joint Surg Am* 76:1222-1230, 1994.

Prichasuk S: The heel pad in plantar heel pain, *J Bone Joint Surg Br* 76:140-142, 1994.

Rao UB, Joseph B: The influence of footwear on the prevalence of flatfoot, *J Bone Joint Surg Br* 74:525-528, 1992.

Robb JE, Murray WR: Phenol cauterization in the management of ingrowing toenails, *Scott Med J* 27:236, 1982.

Rockwood CA, Green DP: *Fractures in adults*, ed 2, Philadelphia, 1984, JB Lippincott.

Sachithanandam V, Joseph B: The influence of footwear on the prevalence of flatfoot, *J Bone Joint Surg Br* 77(2):254-257, 1995.

Saltzman CL, Tearse DS: Achilles tendon injuries, *J Am Acad Orthop Surg* 6:316-325, 1998.

Sarmiento A, Wolf M: Subluxation of peroneal tendons, *J Bone Joint Surg Am* 57:115, 1975.

Schon LC, Glennon TP, Baxter DE: Heel pain syndrome. Electrodiagnostic support for nerve entrapment, *Foot Ankle* 14:129-135, 1993.

Severance HW Jr, Bassett FH III: Rupture of the plantaris: does it exist? *J Bone Joint Surg Am* 64:9, 1982.

Staheli LT, Chew DE, Corbett M: The longitudinal arch: a survey of eight hundred and eighty-two feet in normal children and adults, *J Bone Joint Surg Am* 69:426, 1987.

Staples OS: Ruptures of the fibular collateral ligaments of the ankle: result study of immediate surgical treatment, *J Bone Joint Surg Am* 57:101, 1975.

Stone JW: Osteochondral lesions of the talar dome, *J Am Acad Orthop Surg* 4:63-73, 1996.

Sullivan JA: Pediatric flatfoot: evaluation and management, *J Am Acad Orthop Surg* 7:44-53, 1999.

Sykes PA: Ingrowing toenails: time for critical appraisal? *J R Coll Surg Edinb* 31:300, 1986.

Tachdjian MO: *Pediatric orthopedics*, Philadelphia, 1972, WB Saunders.

Taylor GS: Prominence of the calcaneus: is operation justified, *J Bone Joint Surg Br* 68:467, 1986.

Thompson FM, Coughlin MJ: The high price of high-fashion footwear, *J Bone Joint Surg Am* 76:1586-1593, 1994.

Thompson TC, Terwilliger C: The terminal Syme operation for ingrown toenail, *Surg Clin North Am* 31:575, 1951.

Turco CJ: Surgical correction of the resistant clubfoot, *J Bone Joint Surg Am* 53:477, 1971.

Vincent KA: Tarsal coalition and painful flatfoot, *J Am Acad Orthop Surg* 6:274-281, 1998.

Wapner KL, Sharkey PF: The use of night splints for the treatment of recalcitrant plantar fasciitis, *Foot Ankle* 12:135-137, 1992.

Weinfield SB, Myerson MS: Interdigital neuritis: diagnosis and treatment, *J Am Acad Orthop Surg* 4:328-335, 1996.

Wenger DR et al: Corrective shoes and inserts as treatment for flexible flatfoot in infants and children, *J Bone Joint Surg Am* 71:800, 1989.

Wuest TK Injuries to the lower extremity syndesmosis, *J Am Acad Orthop Surg* 5:172-181, 1997.

Zadik FR: Obliteration of the nailbed without shortening of the terminal phalanx, *J Bone Joint Surg Br* 32:66, 1950.

Zinman C, Wolfson N, Reis ND: Osteochondritis dissecans of the dome of the talus. Computed tomography scanning in diagnosis and follow-up, *J Bone Joint Surg Am* 70:1017, 1988.

# CHAPTER 13

# Infections of Bone and Joint

Although bone and joint infection remains a serious problem, acute, fulminating bone involvement is seen much less often than in the past. The cause of most bone infection is bacterial. Treatment of the established chronic infection remains a challenging problem in spite of the development of more effective antibiotics.

## OSTEOMYELITIS

Osteomyelitis is an infection of the bone or bone marrow. It is often classified as either acute, subacute, or chronic. Acute and subacute osteomyelitis are usually disorders of childhood and are less common in the adult. The subacute form represents an altered host-organism response and is often the result of antibiotics given for other infections. Chronic osteomyelitis, in contrast, is primarily a disease of adults and usually develops as a result of an open wound, either traumatic or surgical.

### Acute Osteomyelitis

The most common site of involvement in childhood is the metaphyseal end of a single long bone, often near the knee joint. The route of infection is usually hematogenous, although local direct extension from a neighboring soft-tissue infection occasionally occurs. A history of trauma may be elicited. A primary site of infection is rarely found.

The metaphyseal area of growing bone is most often involved. This is because as enchondral ossification proceeds, the blood vessels that normally invade the growth zone are looped, resulting in sluggish circulation. This can allow a nidus of infection to become established. The metaphyses also have fewer phagocytes, which may make this area more susceptible.

In patients over the age of 50, the spine becomes the most common site of infection. These patients often have a history of genitourinary disease and/or manipulation, and the onset of the infection can be insidious.

#### Cause

Most cases of acute hematogenous osteomyelitis are caused by *Staphylococcus aureus*. In infants and chil-dren, other important causes are group B streptococci, gram negative coliforms, and *Haemophilus influenza*. Although *H. influenza* is becoming less common as a result of vaccination, it can still be a problem in the period from infancy to 4 years, when the child has lost passive immunity from the mother. Gram-negative bacilli are an important cause of osteomyelitis involving the vertebral bodies in adults. In socioeconomically deprived individuals there is a higher incidence of osteomyelitis caused primarily by *Staphylococcus* and tuberculosis. Tuberculous and fungal causes of osteomyelitis can usually be traced to the pulmonary system. Blacks afflicted with sickle cell disease have a particularly high susceptibility to *Salmonella* osteomyelitis. Osteomyelitis may follow infections of the genitourinary or biliary tracts, or any type of surgical manipulation (particularly colorectal surgery).

With the current incidence of intravenous (IV) drug abuse, there is a much higher rate of osteomyelitis that is predominantly spondylitis or intervertebral disc infection. Involvement of the lumbar vertebrae or sacroiliac joints is peculiar to this type of development of osteomyelitis. The cause of the infection is often *Pseudomonas aeruginosa*, although the causative organism may vary from one locale to another.

In general, acute hematogenous staphylococcal osteomyelitis occurs primarily in late infancy and also at puberty. In some cases, the source of the infection can be discovered by inspection of the skin. Occasionally, a furuncle is found to be the cause.

#### Clinical Features

Acute osteomyelitis in the child is often preceded for several days by signs of systemic disease and/or general sepsis. Anorexia, nausea, malaise, irritability, and fever are present, usually during the acute phase. This stage of the disease may last for several days before bone pain and local overlying inflammation appear. Fever, chills, and diaphoresis are the usual systemic complaints. Pain, bone tenderness, swelling of the soft tissue, and limitation of joint motion are usually apparent on physical examination.

In infants the disease may be alarming and life-threatening in its onset. The involved area will usually show limitation of motion (pseudoparalysis) and there may be *tenderness* in the involved bone well before swelling and redness occur.

In the adult the onset is usually less acute. Constitutional symptoms may be considerably less marked or even absent. In the older child and the adult it is not uncommon for the first symptoms of osteomyelitis to be those of bone involvement. Usually there will be limitation of joint motion, especially if the osteomyelitis involves the spine or if the primary lesions are particularly close to joint spaces where sympathetic effusions may occur.

Tuberculous, fungal, and rickettsial causes of osteomyelitis generally have a chronic, insidious onset. These diseases are more common in patients who are immunologically depressed, who have other underlying diseases such as alcoholism, or whose immune systems have been altered by immunosuppressive therapy or human immunodeficiency virus. As previously mentioned, the primary source of these infections is often pulmonary, and a low-grade fever, weight loss, anorexia, and chronic cough or sputum production may be present. Tuberculous osteomyelitis may involve the vertebral column and cause pathologic fractures of the involved vertebrae. This usually results in angular kyphosis of the spine or so-called Pott's disease (Fig. 13-1).

In the drug-abusing patient who is afebrile and presents with an onset of back pain that is aggravated by moving, coughing, sneezing, or straining at stool, pyogenic spondylitis and gram-negative osteomyelitis should be suspected.

### *Roentgenographic Features*

The classic roentgenographic finding of acute osteomyelitis in childhood is deep, circumferential soft-tissue swelling with obliteration of muscular planes. Spotty rarefactions representing early destruction may appear in the affected bone within 7 to 12 days. Shortly after this, periosteal new bone formation becomes evident and indicates that the infection has spread through the cortex (Fig. 13-2).

Plain roentgenograms are of less value in adult osteomyelitis because significant bony changes may not be apparent until at least 50% of bone destruction has occurred, which may be 2 to 4 weeks into the illness. In the spine, infection can involve the vertebral body or the disc space. Disc space infections are uncommon but occasionally do occur in children and in patients who have undergone surgery on the intervertebral disc. In these cases, the roentgenographic changes are vertebral end-plate irregularities and disc space narrowing. Eventually new bone proliferation occurs, and complete fusion of the disc is often the result. In osteomyelitis of the vertebral body, the roentgenographic changes are those of bone destruction with loss of vertebral height. Occasionally paravertebral swelling and/or paraspinal masses may also be demonstrated.

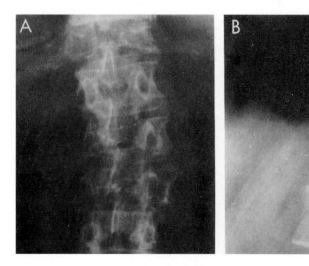

**Fig. 13–1.**
Pott's disease. Angulation is present on both the anteroposterior (**A**) and the lateral (**B**) views.

Radioisotope bone scans are the mainstay in the early diagnosis of bone infection. The technetium scan is nonspecific, however. An advantage of the technetium scan is that it can be performed within a few hours. An isotope-labeled *WBC scan* is more specific for infection.

Magnetic resonance imaging (MRI) and computed tomographic (CT) scanning may also be helpful when there are minor destructive changes present. MRI is more likely to be of assistance in detecting *subtle* changes.

## Subacute Osteomyelitis

This form may now be more common than the acute form and often results when the patient has been treated with antibiotics for other reasons. These children typically present at least 2 weeks after the onset of the infectious process. Staphylococcus organisms are the most common cause. Clinical signs are generally less severe than with the acute form, and although pain is usually present, systemic signs are often absent. The erythrocyte sedimentation rate (ESR) may be elevated and bone tenderness is present. The condition is often confused with neoplasm. The bone scan is positive and biopsy is usually required, with curettage of the lesion being helpful in resolving the condition.

## Chronic Osteomyelitis

This disorder can occasionally be the end result of an acute hematogenous osteomyelitis, but it is more commonly caused by an open fracture or wound (and,

rarely, by a surgical procedure). It is often seen in the lower extremities of the diabetic patient. All forms of chronic osteomyelitis are difficult to eradicate. The cause is often polymicrobial.

### *Clinical Features*

This disorder is characterized by the onset of inflammation and cellulitis after an open fracture; or by persistent drainage after an episode of acute osteomyelitis. Occasionally it develops in the postoperative period after orthopedic procedures. Often systemic signs from previous infection have subsided.

Fever, pain, and mild systemic symptoms are typical. External physical findings may be minimal, but soft-tissue inflammation and tenderness will usually develop.

Often the infection becomes latent after treatment. The nidus of infection may become surrounded by dense bone and fibrous tissue. This often prevents antibiotic penetration. A minor trauma occurring later (*sometimes years*) may reactivate the inflammation, cellulitis, and drainage. *Exacerbations* may occur for years and some chronic wounds even drain persistently.

### *Roentgenographic Features*

Chronic osteomyelitis usually appears as irregular, sclerotic bone that may contain several areas of radiolucency. Irregular areas of destruction are commonly present, and there is often periosteal thickening (Fig. 13-3). Small, dense areas of dead bone (called *sequestra*) may be present. If the acute hematogenous osteomyelitis has been extensive, the entire shaft may become a *sequestrum*. This dead bone is then surrounded by a new shell of bone called the *involucrum*.

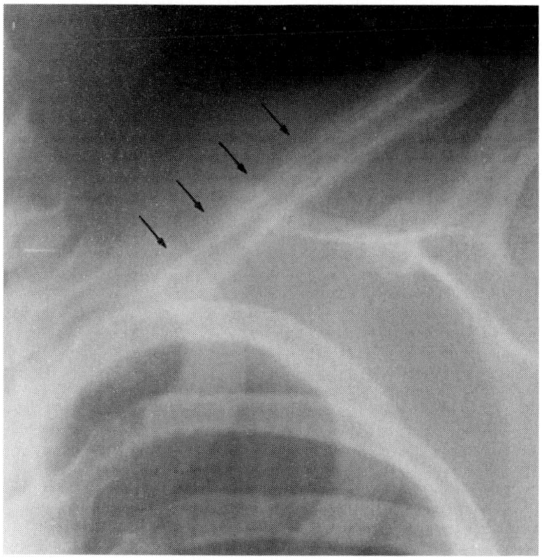

**Fig. 13–2.**
Acute osteomyelitis of the clavicle. Note the periosteal reaction.

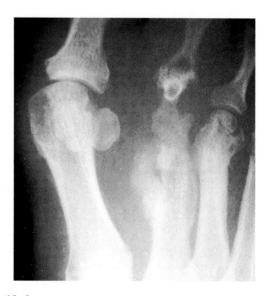

**Fig. 13–3.**
Chronic osteomyelitis of the second toe.

Fortunately, this extensive involvement is rarely seen in Western society.

## Complications

The most common complications of acute osteomyelitis are soft-tissue abscess formation, septic arthritis from extension to the adjacent joints, and metastatic infections from the initial focus. Occasionally, chronic osteomyelitis can be a complication of acute osteomyelitis. However, this is relatively uncommon in children because growing bone is a more active substance and has the ability to "turn over" and clear itself of infection. Overgrowth of bone because of stimulation, and shortening as a result of growth plate destruction, can also occur in the young.

The most common complication of chronic osteomyelitis is recurrent episodes of inflammation and drainage (or even chronic drainage). If this occurs after the insertion of an orthopedic implant, it is often necessary to remove the implant before the infection will subside. In weight-bearing joints this often results in less-than-optimal function, but removal of the foreign body does increase the chances of curing the infection.

Development of a chronically draining sinus can also be mildly debilitating because of the extensive protein loss. On rare occasions, squamous cell carcinoma can even develop at the drainage site. Occasionally amputation is even necessary in diabetic patients or other individuals with poor local tissue health. Extensive spinal involvement may lead to paraplegia, and pathologic fractures may even occur in weight-bearing bones.

## Diagnosis

Cultures of the blood or of the lesion are essential to determine the exact causative agent and to institute the proper antimicrobial therapy. Blood cultures are positive in the majority of children with acute osteomyelitis but are often negative in adults. Every attempt should be made to isolate the organism. Needle aspiration of the site may be attempted, but this is sometimes inadequate. If a primary focus can be identified, a smear, Gram stain, and culture and sensitivity should be taken from this site. Cultures of chronic sinus tract drainage often are not representative of the cause of the chronic osteomyelitis, and deep cultures of the involved bone should be obtained.

The laboratory work-up should include a determination of the sedimentation rate and a complete blood cell count (CBC) in addition to the above cultures. There is usually a leukocytosis and an elevation of the erythrocyte sedimentation rate (ESR). The ESR and C-reactive protein are sometimes useful in following the patient's progress while undergoing treatment.

## Differential Diagnosis

The differential diagnosis must include: (1) acute suppurative arthritis, (2) rheumatic fever, (3) cellulitis, and (4) tumor.

The most common cause of acute septic arthritis in young adults is *Neisseria gonorrhoeae*, whereas *S. aureus* is the major nongonococcal pathogen in older adults. Also, septic arthritis in the older population is often superimposed on some other bone disease, most commonly rheumatoid arthritis. In general, the clinical manifestations of septic arthritis are variable and related to the type of organism causing the underlying infection. Most patients with gonococcal septic arthritis have prominent prodromal symptoms such as fever, chills, headaches, anorexia, and malaise, followed by the development of monoarticular septic arthritis. In gonococcal arthritis, an important portion of the diagnosis lies in the history of a migratory polyarthralgia. A tenosynovitis may be present, but cultures from this involved synovium are usually sterile; the skin lesions and small joint effusions, however, are generally positive for the offending organism. The arthritis seen in gonococcal disease is that of involvement of the large joints, primarily the knee, followed by the wrists, ankles, and elbows.

The clinical picture of patients with acute rheumatic fever, gout, and rheumatoid arthritis may mimic that seen in acute septic arthritis. Synovial fluid examination is helpful. The diagnosis of acute rheumatic fever is still best obtained by adhering to the Jones criteria of major and minor manifestations (Table 13-1).

Cellulitis may sometimes be difficult to differentiate from septic tissue swelling on roentgenographic ex-

**TABLE 13–1.**
Modified Jones Criteria (Revised)

**Major Manifestations**

Carditis
Polyarthritis
Chorea
Erythema marginatum
Subcutaneous nodules

**Minor Manifestations**

Arthralgia
Fever
Prolonged PR interval
Elevated ESR, C-reactive protein

**Supporting evidence of previous group A streptococcal infection**

- Positive throat culture or rapid streptococcal antigen test
- Elevated or rising streptococcal antibody titer

**Note:** The presence of two major or one major and two minor manifestations indicates a high probability of acute rheumatic fever if supported by evidence of preceding group A streptococcal infection.

amination. The soft-tissue swelling is primarily superficial, usually involving skin and subcutaneous tissue. The offending organism is usually hemolytic streptococcus. Occasionally, the cellulitis can evoke a *sympathetic effusion* in an adjacent joint, but passive and active movements of that joint are generally not as painful as they are in acute septic arthritis. In addition, the clinical response to treatment is usually dramatic. If there is a sympathetic effusion in an adjacent joint and there is a problem in differentiation among cellulitis, septic arthritis, and acute osteomyelitis, the joint may be aspirated through an area of healthy skin, but great care must be taken to avoid contaminating a normal joint. MRI is useful in separating cellulitis from osteomyelitis. The condition is commonly confused with vascular disorders in the lower leg. The rubor goes away with elevation if as a result of PVD but not if cellulitis is present.

To establish the diagnosis of tumor, special roentgenographic studies and biopsy are necessary.

## Treatment and Prognosis

### Acute Osteomyelitis

After proper cultures are obtained, the treatment of acute osteomyelitis should begin immediately and not be delayed while waiting for the identification of the offending organism. Because the majority of cases in the young are caused by *S. aureus*, it is appropriate to use an IV antibiotic to cover this pathogen as well as group B streptococcus, enteric rods, and probably *H. influenza* as well. In addition to the proper antibiotic coverage, the patient should have general supportive measures. Dehydration and anemia should be corrected, and the diet should be high in vitamins and protein. Early surgical drainage and debridement is indicated in acute osteomyelitis unless there has been a rapid clinical response within 24 hours. The extremity should be properly immobilized for a period of 3 to 4 weeks.

If necessary, changes are made in the antibiotic coverage when the offending organism is identified. The sedimentation rate and C-reactive protein levels are followed during treatment. IV antibiotic coverage is usually continued for 4 weeks, but each case should be treated individually and there is no consensus regarding the route and length of antibiotic coverage. Treatment for the subacute form is essentially the same.

Sometimes fever may recur after an initially good response to the appropriate antibiotic treatment. When this happens, a careful clinical reevaluation is necessary, and the following conditions should be considered: (1) laboratory error in identification of the organism, (2) drug fever (usually as a result of a cephalosporin or a penicillin), (3) superinfection, (4) abscess formation, or (5) inadequate drainage.

In general, the prognosis for acute osteomyelitis is good, although complications have been reported in as many as 25% of cases. A delay in diagnosis and treatment may lead to chronic osteomyelitis or multiple recurrences. These recurrences can be as late as 30 years later and are usually as a result of the same organism. They are often reactivated by local trauma.

### Chronic Osteomyelitis

The treatment of chronic osteomyelitis is similar to that of the acute form, but prevention remains the most important aspect of this disease. All open fractures are frequently and meticulously debrided and great care is taken to eliminate contamination. Chronic osteomyelitis may be treated by incision and drainage, radical debridement, and appropriate antibiotic coverage for 4 to 6 weeks. However, once it is established it is difficult to cure. Recurrent drainage and residual deformity both add to the morbidity.

A local infection that develops when a prosthetic device is being used by the patient will usually require removal of the device before the infection can be controlled.

Infection of the bones of the feet is common in diabetic patients, who often have coincidental peripheral vascular disease. Painless ulcers may develop secondary to diabetic polyneuropathy and diabetic vascular disease. Hyperemia and swelling are often noted clinically. If a fracture occurs in the foot of a diabetic patient, it may be accompanied by a similar redness and swelling and be a source of some confusion. A roentgenogram will usually clarify the diagnosis.

## PYOGENIC ARTHRITIS

Septic or pyogenic arthritis may occur in any age group but is more common in the young. It is usually monoarticular, and large peripheral joints (usually the knee or hip) are most often involved. Polyarticular disease is rare but may occur in patients with preexisting inflammatory disease or chronic illness. Unusual sites (sacroiliac, sternoclavicular joints, and symphysis pubis) may be involved in IV drug abusers.

Gonococcal infection often leads to a separate clinical syndrome and is discussed separately.

### Pathogenesis

The offending organism is usually *N. gonorrhoeae* or *S. aureus*, but a variety of other bacteria may be causative. *H. influenzae* may still be seen in children, but the prevalence is decreasing because of vaccination.

Gram-negative rods are often involved in IV drug users. Entrance to the joint is usually gained by hematogenous seeding, rarely by direct extension from an adjacent infection. In the hip, it may be introduced by an improperly performed venipuncture from the groin. The disorder is more common in patients with underlying chronic disease states and those undergoing immunosuppressive therapy.

Upon invasion of the joint by the pathogenic bacteria, the organisms seed the synovial membrane, which becomes swollen and hyperemic. It begins to produce large amounts of fluid that distend the joint capsule. Frank pus eventually accumulates, and destruction of articular cartilage may even occur.

### Clinical Features

The onset is usually acute, with pain being the most common early symptom. A history of infection elsewhere is occasionally obtainable. If a weight-bearing joint is involved, ambulation is usually difficult and may become impossible because of the pain. Fever and other signs of systemic infection are usually present.

Examination generally reveals a warm, swollen, diffusely tender joint. The joint is usually held in slight flexion because, in this position, the intracapsular pressure is decreased and discomfort is thereby minimized. Attempts at passive motion tend to be extremely painful.

### Special Studies

Roentgenographic findings early in the disease process are usually minimal and consist primarily of distention of the joint capsule. The peripheral WBC count is markedly elevated as a rule, and blood cultures may be positive. The sedimentation rate is generally high, but the neonate and geriatric patient may show only minimal laboratory abnormalities. Bone scanning and other studies are of limited value but may be helpful in the evaluation of the patient whose symptoms are of uncertain cause.

Confirmation of the diagnosis is best made by joint aspiration under sterile conditions. Most joints are best aspirated on the extensor side (except the hip, which may be aspirated from the anterior or lateral aspect). Because the joint is usually distended, aspiration is ordinarily not difficult. The fluid is initially cloudy and thin but may be purulent. The joint glucose level is decreased, and the WBC count is markedly increased. A Gram stain is performed, and cultures are taken. The specimen should always be inspected for crystals.

### Treatment

Treatment should begin immediately after cultures to prevent joint destruction and, in the case of the hip joint, dislocation. Rest and immobilization will diminish the pain. The definitive antibiotic therapy will depend on Gram stain and culture results. The IV route should always be used. Intraarticular injection is unnecessary because most antibiotics readily pass through the synovial membrane. Direct instillation may even provoke an inflammatory synovitis.

Some *superficial* joints may respond to repeated aspiration, but surgical drainage may be indicated. This is especially true of the hip in children. Surgery may be delayed if a dramatic clinical response occurs with conservative treatment, but if such a response is not forthcoming, drainage should be performed. Surgery will diminish the intraarticular pressure, allow evacuation of the thick fibrous exudate, and prevent the articular destruction that may occur in pyarthrosis. It can often be done arthroscopically.

When irreversible joint destruction has occurred, arthrodesis may be necessary. Joint replacement might be attempted, but there is some risk of reactivating the dormant infection.

## Gonococcal infection

The disease states caused by the bacteria *N. gonorrhoeae* may range from asymptomatic carrier to the condition known as disseminated gonococcal infection (DGI). Gonococcal infection is the most common form of pyogenic arthritis in many areas. It often presents in the young, sexually active individual with a distinct clinical syndrome of polyarthritis, tenosynovitis, and dermatitis. In these patients, the gonococcal organism is often difficult to demonstrate. Blood cultures are usually negative and the organism can be recovered from joint fluid less than 50% of the time. Although most patients with gonococcal arthritis do not have genitourinary symptoms, gonococcus can be recovered from these sites about 80% of the time. These sites should always be cultured if gonococcal infection is suspected clinically. A rapid response to the appropriate antibiotic is almost diagnostic. NSAIDs will also help speed the resolution of symptoms. Joint destruction as a result of *N. gonorrhoeae* is uncommon.

## Viral "Arthritis"

Inflammatory changes with pain in the joints is sometimes seen after vaccination for rubella. Signs of bacterial infection are absent. The condition is diagnosed by exclusion and the treatment is symptomatic.

Arthralgias also accompany a number of viral illnesses, but the pathogenesis of these arthritis-like symptoms is not known. Rarely, viral illnesses may present as a monoarticular synovitis.

## SPECIAL PROBLEMS

### Brodie's Abscess

This is a subacute pyogenic osteomyelitis localized in the metaphysis (usually of long bones of the lower extremity) and appearing on the roentgenogram as a lucent lesion with some surrounding sclerosis. The primary symptom is pain, with fever and leukocytosis being rare. The offending organism is usually *S. aureus,* but occasionally gram-negative organisms have been identified. This disease is insidious in onset and lacks the systemic symptoms of hematogenous osteomyelitis. Treatment is curettage and antibiotics.

### Disc Space Infection

With the increase in drug abuse, disc space and adjacent vertebral body infection is not an uncommon cause of *back pain.* The chief complaint is usually localized to the area of the underlying infection, and there may be tenderness on palpation of the spine over the infected disc space. Early roentgenograms are usually not beneficial, although there may be occasional disc space narrowing. The bone scan is usually positive. There is usually mild leukocytosis and an elevated sedimentation rate. Management is through identification of the inciting bacterial agent and institution of appropriate antibiotic therapy. The offending organism may occasionally be isolated from the blood, but aspiration and culture of disc space material is often necessary to identify the etiologic organism.

### Anaerobic Infections

Anaerobes are becoming increasingly recognized as causes of significant clinical infection. The more common organisms involved are *Bacteroides fragilis, Peptococcus, Propionibacterium, Clostridium,* and *Fusobacterium.* They are often mixed with aerobes, and it is often difficult to tell which is the pathogen. These mixed infections are also more difficult to cure.

Anaerobic bone infections are also often associated with the presence of a metallic foreign body such as a prosthesis. When anaerobes are present in infections in the foot, they are almost always associated with diabetes or vascular insufficiency.

### Gas Gangrene

Clostridia organisms are widely distributed in nature, but only a few are severe pathogens. Several species can cause gas gangrene in humans. The most common is *C. perfringens (C. welchii).* Other causes are *C. novyi,*

*C. histolyticum, C. septicum, C. bifermentans,* and *C. fallax.*

Gas gangrene is an uncommon clinical infection in which a severe soft-tissue wound or surgical trauma allows the tissue to become contaminated with the *Clostridium* spore. Local anaerobic conditions (a closed wound) favor conversion from the spore form to the vegetative form, which produces the potent toxins typical of this disorder. These toxins destroy soft tissue and muscle and can cause severe septic shock and death. Other organisms, including group A β-hemolytic *Streptococcus,* may cause necrotizing soft-tissue infections.

#### Clinical Features

This disease can result from a small, seemingly innocuous wound, but usually results from a severe wound that is improperly cared for. It may also follow abdominal surgery because clostridia normally inhabit the gastrointestinal tract.

The presentation may vary from a mild local cellulitis to the lethal myonecrosis. Signs of infection are usually present within 24 hours after the trauma. Pain often precedes local or systemic signs and is often out of proportion to the severity of the injury. The wound is usually swollen and red and produces a dark, odorous exudate.

The more severe forms are accompanied by chills, fever, tachycardia, delirium, and all of the other signs of a rapidly progressing infection. Renal shutdown and death may even occur. The involved skin and muscle undergo further necrosis, and vesicles appear in the infected area.

Gas may be present in the soft tissue but is not diagnostic of clostridia. (It also may be a result of mechanical reasons such as open trauma or pulmonary injuries, or infection by other bacteria such as the coliforms or anaerobic streptococci.) The roentgenogram may reveal edema and gas within muscle groups. (In bacterial infections not caused by clostridia, the gas is often in the deeper tissue.)

#### Treatment

Prevention is accomplished by a thorough debridement of all potentially contaminated cases and by leaving the wound open if necessary. Mild local infection may need only modest debridement and drainage. The more severe forms require early and radical excision of all involved tissue. Amputation may even be necessary. The appropriate antibiotics are administered intravenously in large doses, and general supportive care is given.

Because moderate levels of oxygen have been shown to suppress bacterial activity, hyperbaric oxygen has been used as an adjunct to surgical debridement.

The oxygen is supplied by placing the patient in a special chamber several times a day until the symptoms improve. At this time, these chambers are only available at a modest number of medical facilities.

## Septic Bursitis

Infection of superficial bursae is a common occurrence. The bunion, olecranon, and prepatellar bursae are the most commonly affected. In contrast to septic arthritis, this disorder usually occurs in healthy individuals and commonly results from local spread. Occupations that predispose to chronic trauma and fluid collection in the bursa (carpet layers, plumbers, etc.) are more prone to sepsis in this area. There may be evidence of a recent local abrasion or break in the skin. *S. aureus* is the most common offending organism.

### Clinical Features

A painful localized bursal swelling is usually present and is often accompanied by an intense cellulitis. A partially healed skin abrasion may be seen nearby. Systemic signs of sepsis are commonly present, including regional lymphadenopathy.

A sympathetic joint effusion is fairly common, especially in the knee. The joint itself is not usually tender, and motion is only mildly restricted. The effusion may suggest joint involvement.

### Treatment

The bursa is aspirated and the fluid evaluated in the standard manner by Gram stain, culture, and sensitivity. Blood cultures, blood counts, and sedimentation rates are also performed as indicated. (**Note**: It is important not to aspirate the joint itself. Passing the needle through the area of cellulitis and then into the joint could spread the infection into the joint.)

Community-acquired septic bursitis is usually caused by *S. aureus* or β-hemolytic streptococcus sensitive to a penicillinase-resistant semisynthetic penicillin, such as oxacillin or nafcillin. Surgical drainage of the bursa may be necessary, but many patients respond well to repeated aspirations.

## Prosthetic Joint Infection

Fewer than 1% of joint replacements become infected, but the complication can be disastrous to the joint and difficult to cure. It may occur at any time after surgery. Early involvement is usually the result of skin contamination, often by coagulase-negative staphylococci. Later, the source is hematogenous, with a variety of pathogens being causative. Joints that have had previous surgery are also more predisposed to infection.

The diagnosis may be difficult. Pain is a common occurrence, but fever and systemic signs may be lacking. Various bone scans may be helpful but local aspiration with culture is usually necessary. Often, to cure the infection, all of the hardware must be permanently removed. Arthrodesis is often necessary; but in some cases the joint is simply left out, and this results in a "resection" arthroplasty. Because of the risk of reactivating the dormant infection, only occasionally is the joint replaced again, and then only after a long period of antibiotic therapy and local wound care.

## Penetrating Wounds

### Gunshot Wounds

The amount of damage done to tissues by gunshot wounds is dependent upon the velocity of the weapon. Low-velocity weapons usually cause minimal wound tract injury. Important structures are usually pushed away by the missile. These injuries are best treated on an outpatient basis by minimal local debridement of the entrance and exit wounds, irrigation, a sterile dressing, and a broad-spectrum antibiotic. Tetanus prophylaxis is administered, and if necessary, delayed closure is performed later. Associated fractures are usually undisplaced and are treated by external immobilization.

Bullet removal or operative exploration is undertaken only if the bullet is superficial or symptomatic or if minor fragment migration could cause damage to major adjacent structures. Missile wounds of the knee joint probably should be explored surgically and debrided if fragments are present or if the joint was traversed. The missile and osteochondral fragments are removed. It is possible for lead to be dissolved by synovial tissue and lead to arthritis and, rarely, chronic lead intoxication. Elsewhere the fragments are usually encapsulated by scar tissue, thereby eliminating their exposure to bodily fluids. Fragments near the spine are usually left alone unless a significant or progressive neural loss occurs.

Wounds caused by high-velocity weapons are managed the same way as those caused by low-velocity weapons, except that more extensive debridement is usually necessary. Their complication rate is much higher, and delayed closure is the rule.

Shotgun wounds also require more extensive debridement. They are often the most serious of missile wounds. The projectile consists of multiple pellets and a wadding (usually fiber or burlap) that transmits the force. Wounds inflicted from a weapon closer than 20 yards are assumed to contain some of this wadding, and exploration and removal are necessary. If the "scatter pattern" of the shotgun is wide, more damage is assumed, especially if the shotgun was fired at close range. A small wound can disguise extensive deeper destruction.

### Power Gun Nail Wounds

These injuries result from the use (mainly by carpenters) of air-powered gun systems to drive nails. Occasionally, the nails are accidentally driven into extremities, often directly into bone. They usually can be simply pulled out of the bone under local anesthesia. The wound is then treated similarly to any other low-velocity weapon injury. Small pieces that remain embedded in bone are probably best left alone.

### Bite Wounds

More than 1% of all emergency room visits are the result of bites, and the majority of these wounds are superficial. Dog bites account for most of these wounds. They usually present as small puncture wounds. The infection rate is low, and loose closure of any extensive wound is usually acceptable after thorough cleansing, irrigation, and debridement. Extremity wounds may be left open; however, small puncture wounds should not be opened. Prophylactic antibiotic therapy, usually with amoxicillin-clavulanate, is indicated. This agent will be active against *S. aureus* (except for methicillin-resistant *S. aureus*), β-hemolytic streptococci, anaerobic streptococci, and *Pasteurella multocida,* which is a common cause of infection after dog and cat bites. Antirabies therapy and tetanus prophylaxis are provided when indicated.

Human bites require especially careful evaluation and examination. The most common site of injury is a closed fist that has struck the mouth (see Chapter 7). The injury that often occurs is a laceration over the metacarpophalangeal joint that may disrupt the extensor tendon and even penetrate into bone (Fig. 13-4). The wound may be small, and if the hand is examined with the fingers extended, the true extent of the injury may be overlooked because the injury was sustained with the fingers flexed. If joint involvement is noted, extra care is taken to ensure good cleansing and debridement. The wound should be treated open. Antibiotics are administered, and the wound is followed closely. The most common infecting organisms are *S. aureus,* streptococci, and anaerobes found in the normal flora of the human mouth.

### Puncture Wounds

The most common site of this wound is the foot. The common clinical picture is that of early improvement followed in 1 to 2 weeks by worsening local signs. A foreign body is sometimes found in the wound, and the most common organism is *Pseudomonas*. Staphylococci and streptococci are also often involved. Osteomyelitis and even joint damage can result. Treatment involves drainage, removal of the foreign body (if present), and the appropriate antibiotic.

Local debridement in the emergency room at the time of the original injury may help prevent late infection. Roentgenograms are indicated to rule out foreign bodies. The decision to use antibiotics at the time of initial wound care remains controversial.

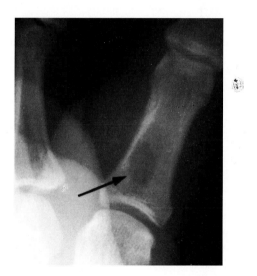

**Fig. 13–4.**
Osteomyelitis of the proximal phalanx secondary to a human bite *(arrow)*.

## ANTIBIOTICS IN ORTHOPEDICS

The initial therapy in severe infections should always be broad enough to cover the most common organisms. More specific therapy will depend upon the proper identification of the offending agent and its sensitivity to the various antimicrobial drugs. An ever-increasing number of antibiotics are available; the physician should become sufficiently familiar with several well-established ones. It is better to be familiar with several good ones than to try every new one that comes on the market. Cost and safety are also important factors to consider. The duration of antibiotic therapy (especially for bone, joint, and bursa infections) varies depending upon response and the bacteria involved. In general, antibiotic therapy is usually continued for 3 to 6 weeks. With the availability of home IV therapy, prolonged hospitalization is usually not required.

# BIBLIOGRAPHY

Altemeier WA, Fullen WD: Prevention and treatment of gas gangrene, *JAMA* 217:806, 1971.

Ashby M: Low velocity gunshot wounds involving the knee joint: surgical management, *J Bone Joint Surg Am* 56:1047, 1974.

Boll KL, Jurik AG: Sternal osteomyelitis in drug addicts, *J Bone Joint Surg Br* 72:328, 1990.

Brettler D et al: Conservative management of low velocity gunshot wounds, *Clin Orthop* 140:26, 1979.

Brown P: Gas gangrene in a metropolitan community, *J Bone Joint Surg Am* 56:1445, 1982.

Chuinard RG, D'Ambrosia RD: Human bite infections of the hand, *J Bone Joint Surg Am* 59:416, 1977.

Dormans JP, Drummond DS: Pediatric hematogenous osteomyelitis: new trends in prevention, diagnosis, and treatment, *J Am Acad Orthop Surg* 2:333-341, 1994.

Edson RS, Terrell CL: The aminoglycosides, *Mayo Clin Proc* 66:1158-1164, 1991.

Eismont FJ et al: Pyogenic and fungal vertebral osteomyelitis with paralysis, *J Bone Joint Surg Am* 65:19, 1983.

Eismont FJ et al: Vertebral osteomyelitis in infants, *J Bone Joint Surg Br* 64:32, 1982.

Emmons CW, Binford CH, Utz JP: *Medical mycology*, ed 2, Philadelphia, 1970, Lea & Febiger.

Freig BS et al: Imipenem and cilastatin in acute osteomyelitis and suppurative arthritis. Therapy in infants and children, *Am J Dis Child* 141:335, 1987.

Gaasch WH, editor: Guidelines for the diagnosis of rheumatic fever. Jones criteria, 1992 update, *JAMA* 268:2069-2073, 1992.

Gentry LO: Overview of osteomyelitis, *Orthop Rev* 16:255, 1987.

Green M, Myhan WL Jr, Fausek MD: Acute hematogenous osteomyelitis, *Pediatrics* 16:368, 1956.

Gustaferro CA, Steckelberg JM: Cephalosporin antimicrobial agents and related compounds, *Mayo Clin Proc* 66:1064-1073, 1991.

Hart GB et al: The treatment of clostridial myonecroses with hyperbaric oxygen, *J Trauma* 14:712, 1974.

Hoeprich PD: *Infectious diseases*, Hagerstown, Md, 1972, Harper & Row.

Holzman RS, Birkko F: Osteomyelitis in heroin addicts, *Ann Intern Med* 75:693, 1971.

Hughes SPF, Fitzgerald RH Jr: *Musculoskeletal infections*, Chicago, 1986, Year Book Medical Publishers Inc.

LaMont RL et al: Acute hematogenous osteomyelitis in children, *J Pediatr Orthop* 7:579, 1987.

Lifeso RM et al: Post-traumatic squamous cell carcinoma, *J Bone Joint Surg Am* 72:12, 1990.

May JW et al: Current concepts review. Clinical classification of post-traumatic osteomyelitis, *J Bone Joint Surg Am* 71:1422, 1989.

Rutstein DD et al: Jones criteria (modified) for guidance in diagnosis of rheumatic fever, *Mod Concepts Cardiovasc Dis* 24:291, 1955.

Sacato DJ, Schwend RM, Gillespie R: Septic arthritis of the hip in children, *J Am Acad Orthop Surg* 5:249-260, 1997.

Schmid FR: Principles of diagnosis and treatment of infectious arthritis. In Hollander JL, McCarty DJ Jr, editors: *Arthritis and allied conditions*, ed 8, Philadelphia, 1972, Lea & Febiger.

Smith DL et al: Septic and nonseptic olecranon bursitis, *Arch Intern Med* 149:1581, 1989.

Thompson GR, Ferreya A, Bracket RG: Acute arthritis complicating rubella vaccinations, *Arthritis Rheum* 14:19-26, 1971.

Thompson RL, Wright AJ: Cephalosporin antibiotics, *May Clin Proc* 58:79, 1983.

Uuzonian TJ et al: Evaluation of musculoskeletal sepsis with indium-111 white blood cell imaging, *Clin Orthop* 221:304, 1987.

Vu Quoc D, Nelson JD, Holtalin KC: Osteomyelitis in infants and children, *Am J Dis Child* 129:1273, 1975.

Warsman AD, Bryon D, Siemsen JK: Bone scanning in the drug abuse patient: early detection of hematogenous osteomyelitis, *J Nucl Med* 14:647, 1973.

Wilkowske CJ, Hermans PE: General principles of antimicrobial therapy, *Mayo Clin Proc* 62:789, 1987.

Wright AJ, Wilkowske CJ: The penicillins, *Mayo Clin Proc* 62:806, 1987.

Wright AJ, Wilkowski CJ: The penicillins, *Mayo Clin Proc* 66:1047-1063, 1991.

Yuh WTC et al: Osteomyelitis of the foot in diabetic patients: evaluation with plain films, 99 Tc-MDP bone scintigraphy and MR imaging, *AJR* 152:795, 1989.

# CHAPTER 14

# The Arthritides

Disorders of the joints are common and may cause considerable pain and disability. They are commonly classified as noninflammatory, inflammatory, or infectious. This chapter reviews the more common joint disorders.

## THE SYNOVIUM

A synovial lining encloses the joint space of all diarthrodial joints. This membrane is also present in bursae and tendon sheaths. It is normally one to three cells thick and is constructed of multiple villi. It will reflect not only local disturbances but also systemic disease and is responsible for the production of joint fluid.

Synovial fluid is a clear, slightly yellow liquid that is present only in small amounts in the normal joint. Its main functions are those of lubrication and nutrition. Its characteristic viscosity is as a result of the presence of high concentrations of hyaluronic acid, which is produced by the synovial lining cells. This mucopolysaccharide also contributes a portion of the matrix of the synovial lining and is partially responsible for the filtering properties of the synovium.

Joint fluid is a dialysate of blood plasma: that is, crystalloids are present, but colloids are not. Normal joint fluid does not clot because many of the coagulation factors are absent. Glucose is present in concentrations 10 mg/dL lower than serum. This difference increases to 30 mg/dL in rheumatoid and other inflammatory types of arthritis and may approach 70 mg/dL in infectious arthritis. Normal fluid also contains complement, lipids, and proteins in amounts much lower than the serum level. The white blood cell (WBC) count is usually under $200/mm^3$, with the majority being mononuclear. Inflammation increases the cell count and the percentage of polymorphonuclear leukocytes.

A great deal of information can be obtained from the examination of a joint aspirate (Table 14-1). How-ever, this examination is not indicated in every joint effusion and should be limited to those diagnostic problems that are not secondary to trauma. The joint is usually aspirated from the extensor side under sterile conditions. Three test tubes are sufficient for most determinations: (1) a plain tube for gross examination, clotting, and a mucin clot test; (2) one ethylenediaminetetraacetic acid (EDTA)-treated tube for cell and crystal analysis; and (3) one heparinized tube for bacteriologic study. Five milliliters of fluid are placed in each tube.

A quick bedside assessment of the fluid can be made prior to the more extensive laboratory analysis. The color and clarity of the sample are estimated by merely observing the fluid in the syringe. The viscosity can be roughly determined by the thread test. A drop of the fluid is placed between the apposed thumb and index finger. The fingers are gradually spread apart, and the length of the thread the fluid forms before it breaks is measured. Normal and osteoarthritic fluid may "string" out 2.5 to 5 cm before breaking, but the dilute fluid of inflammation will string little.

### The Mucin Clot Test

This test determines the amount of hyaluronate in the fluid. Acetic acid is added to the tube and the sample is observed for clot formation. A "poor" mucin clot indicates a decrease in hyaluronate. This results from dilution, depolymerization, and loss of filter function from either inflammation or infection. A "good" clot is present in normal fluid and osteoarthritis.

## Crystal Analysis

Reliable crystal examination requires the use of polarized light. The sodium urate crystals present in gout are needle-shaped and negatively birefringent (shine brightly) under polarized light. The calcium pyrophosphate crystal in pseudogout (chondrocalcinosis) is rhomboid in shape and positively birefringent.

(**Note**: From a practical standpoint, most of the useful information that can be obtained from the study of joint fluid is available from a simple Gram stain, cell count, crystal analysis, and culture and sensitivity.)

**TABLE 14–1.**
Synovial Fluid Analysis

| Disease | Appearance | Viscosity | Mucin Clot | WBC (%), Polymorphonuclear Leukocytes | Other Findings |
|---------|-----------|-----------|------------|---------------------------------------|----------------|
| **Noninflammatory** | | | | | |
| Normal | Clear, yellow | High | Good | Under 200, under 10% | |
| Traumatic arthritis | Cloudy, straw to red | High | Good | Under 2,000, under 25% | Cartilage debris |
| Osteoarthritis | Straw, yellow, clear | High | Good | Under 5,000, under 25% | Cartilage debris |
| **Inflammatory** | | | | | |
| Rheumatoid | Cloudy, green/gray | Low | Fair/poor | 15,000 50%-80% | Glucose difference 10-25 mg/dL, rheumatoid arthritis cells |
| Gout | Cloudy, white, flaky | Decreased | Fair/poor | 10,000, 25%-75% | Sodium urate crystals |
| Pseudogout | Cloudy | Decreased | Fair/poor | 5-15,000, 25%-75% | Calcium pyrophosphate crystals |
| Systemic lupus erythematosus | Cloudy, yellow | High | Good/fair | 5-10,000, under 25% | Lupus erythematosus cells |
| **Infectious** | | | | | |
| Bacterial | Cloudy, purulent | Low | Poor | 50-200,000, over 90% | Glucose difference over 50 mg/dL, culture + |

# OSTEOARTHRITIS

The most common type of noninflammatory arthritis is degenerative arthritis, or osteoarthritis. This condition is characterized by articular cartilage deterioration and bony overgrowth of the joint surface. The cause is unknown but it is strongly correlated with age. Two forms are usually recognized: primary (idiopathic) and secondary. The primary form may be localized or generalized. Secondary osteoarthritis may result from a number of disorders including trauma, metabolic conditions, and other forms of arthritis such as rheumatoid and gouty arthritis. Pathologically, the cartilage loses its normal glistening appearance and becomes roughened and irregular. Eventually the cartilage becomes completely worn away, thus exposing the subchondral bone. Secondary synovitis and osteophytic spur formation are common. The clinical course is slowly progressive.

## Clinical Features

Pain is the most common initial symptom. This often occurs with motion or activity and is relieved by rest. The source of discomfort is unknown. It may result from chemical mediators and possibly from mechanical factors. Joint stiffness typically occurs with rest and improves with activity. The physical findings include crepitus, swelling, restriction of motion, and joint enlargement from spur formation. In the hands, these osteophytic overgrowths are termed *Heberden's nodes* when they are present at the distal interphalangeal joint and *Bouchard's nodes* when they occur at the proximal interphalangeal joint. Pain is usually present on joint motion. Disuse atrophy of the adjacent musculature may develop rapidly, thus increasing the disability and pain. Although osteoarthritis is not considered an "inflammatory" disease, mild inflammation with heat is often present. This can be appreciated clinically in a superficial joint (such as the knee) by placing one hand on the front of each knee of the sitting patient and then switching the hands back and forth. Subtle differences in temperature suggestive of synovitis (which indicates an intraarticular problem) may become more apparent. This clinical test is often helpful in the obese patient in whom an effusion may be difficult to visualize.

The roentgenographic findings consist of joint space narrowing, spur formation, sclerosis, and subchondral cyst formation (Fig. 14-1). The laboratory findings and synovial analysis are normal except for occasional flakes of cartilage in the joint fluid.

### Treatment

The main objectives of treatment are the relief of pain and the prevention of progression. As with any joint disorder, the patient should not be told that arthritis is present unless the physical and laboratory findings are consistent with the diagnosis. The stigma of "arthritis" should not be attached to any condition merely to explain vague or nonspecific symptoms. However, once the diagnosis is established, the patient should be made to realize that whereas miracles cannot be expected, there is almost always something that can be done to relieve the pain and deformity, regardless of the cause.

Treatment for osteoarthritis begins with rest of the involved joint. This will help reduce inflammation and pain. Weight loss and temporary abstinence from weight bearing by the use of a cane or crutch will lessen the pressure on the involved lower extremity. Removable splints or braces are also helpful.

Stretching exercises are helpful and the joint should be passed through a full range of motion several times daily to reduce joint stiffness. The local application of moist heat is beneficial during the acute painful stage and may be especially helpful prior to exercise. Exercises designed to combat stiffness and restore muscle strength are important because the weakness will contribute to joint instability and disability. All exercise should be low impact. Biking, swimming, and cross-country ski machines are useful, but the treadmill and other repetitive weight-bearing exercise activities should be avoided. Antiinflammatory agents are often used but may be no more effective than acetaminophen for pain relief since the condition lacks a strong inflammatory component. Mild analgesics may even be indicated on an occasional basis. Intraarticular cortisone injections will often relieve a great deal of the pain. Their effect is usually only temporary, but pain relief may last several months. Various liniments may be useful for their counterirritant effect. Viscosupplementation (a series of joint injections using a hyaluronate-like material) has been tried but the results are inconclusive.

The surgical procedures most commonly employed are arthrodesis and arthroplasty (Fig. 14-2). Each is effective in eliminating the painful articulation. The realignment of faulty weight-bearing joints by osteotomy may also be beneficial.

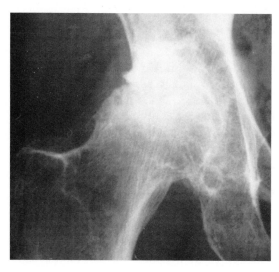

**Fig. 14–1.**
Degenerative arthritis of the hip. Joint space narrowing, sclerosis, and subchondral cyst formation are present.

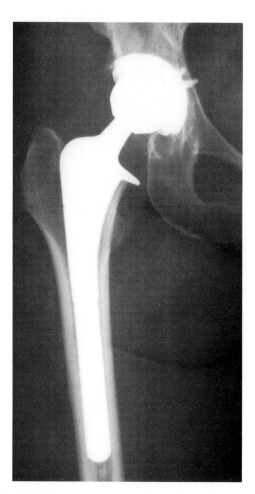

**Fig. 14–2.**
Total hip arthroplasty (uncemented).

# GOUT

Primary gouty arthritis is an inherited metabolic disease characterized by a disturbance of purine metabolism in which crystals of sodium urate are deposited in various soft tissues, primarily joints, synovium of tendons, and the kidneys. The crystals and the resultant symptoms are the result of an increase in the serum uric acid, a normal end product of purine metabolism. Hyperuricemia and gout can develop from excessive uric acid production, decreased renal excretion of uric acid, or both.

The majority of patients are men in the third and fourth decades and the incidence increases with age. The disorder is less common in women, and rare before menopause. Obesity, chronic exposure to lead, excessive alcohol intake, hypertension, and the management of hypertension with diuretics appear to be some of the risk factors involved in its development. Secondary gout may also follow hyperuricemia from many causes, including leukemia, hemolytic anemia, and other blood dyscrasias.

## Clinical Features

The initial attack is usually of sudden onset and occurs in a single joint or area of tenosynovium of the lower extremity (Table 14-2). The MP joint of the great toe is classically the first site of involvement (podagra), although any joint or area of tenosynovium can be involved. The extensor synovium on the dorsum of the midfoot is another common site of acute attack. The pain and inflammation are usually severe and may be precipitated by exercise, dietary indiscretion, and physical or emotional stress. Attacks are common after illness or shortly after surgery, and they typically begin at night. Swelling, heat, redness, and other signs of inflammation are usually present. The physical findings may even simulate cellulitis. The area is often tender to even the slightest touch. Fever, tachycardia, and other constitutional symptoms may accompany the attack. The initial episode may be followed by polyarticular involvement. Eventually deposits of urate crystals (termed tophi) may form in the subcutaneous tissue.

Early in the disease, roentgenogram findings are normal. Later, erosive changes appear that have a characteristic punched-out appearance (Fig. 14-3). Destruction and degeneration of the articular cartilage often follow.

Laboratory findings include a mild leukocytosis, elevated sedimentation rate, and hyperuricemia, although acute attacks are occasionally associated with a normal level of uric acid. The synovial aspirate is usually cloudy and mildly inflammatory in nature. Urate crystals are usually demonstrable. They are needle-shaped and negatively birefringent. A 24-hour urinary collection for uric acid may be helpful in determining the appropriate treatment.

## Treatment

The treatment will depend on the stage of the disease. The objectives in management are to terminate or prevent the acute attack, encourage mobilization of tophaceous deposits, and reduce the level of serum uric acid.

**TABLE 14–2.**

Joint Swelling—Differential Diagnosis*

| Disorder | Symptoms/History | Findings |
|---|---|---|
| Pyogenic arthritis | Usually painful but sometimes low grade. Fever, acute onset. Usually monoarticular | Febrile, increase heat, painful movement. Systemic signs of illness. Joint fluid positive for bacteria |
| Gouty arthritis | Knee, great toe, or generalized foot pain. Symptoms may be initiated by physical stress such as surgery. May be extremely painful but usually low grade. Usually monoarticular. Previous episodes? | Redness, increased heat. Crystals in joint fluid. Elevated serum uric acid. Fluid often cloudy |
| Osteoarthritis | Chronic, gradual. Monoarticular. May have history of mechanical injury. Stiffness after rest, pain after prolonged activity | Restricted movement but pain usually only at the extremes of movement. Fluid is clear, only excessive amounts |
| Pseudogout | Middle age to elderly. Usually monoarticular. Previous episodes? | Crystals in cloudy fluid (calcium pyrophosphate) |
| Rheumatoid arthritis | Multiple joints may be involved. Females most commonly affected. Usually subacute or insidious in onset but occasionally acute. Often symmetric. Metacarpophalangeal, proximal interphalangeal joints usually involved | Subcutaneous nodules in late cases. Laboratory studies may show positive rheumatoid test and increased ESR |
| Others | History may reflect skin rash or other skin changes. Note other system involvement (complete history, especially GI and pulmonary systems) | FANA, ESR may be abnormal. Many collagen disorders have polyarticular symptoms and act like rheumatoid arthritis |

*Notes: The workup should include aspiration of joint fluid. Fluid is observed for color, and the string test is performed. The fluid is analyzed for cell count. Gram stain, crystal analysis, and culture and sensitivity. The blood work should include complete blood cell count, uric acid, blood cultures if indicated, sedimentation rate, fluorescent antinuclear antibody (FANA), and rheumatoid factor. Blood cultures should include aerobic and anaerobic cultures. Roentgenographic evaluation is always performed to evaluate for osteoarthritis and calcific changes in soft tissues.

Prevention of the acute attack depends on modification of diet and lifestyle. Obesity should be avoided or treated and alcohol intake should be kept moderate, no more than two drinks per day. Hypertension and its management requires careful assessment, and nondiuretic drugs may be needed.

There is no indication to treat asymptomatic hyperuricemia. Less than half of those with hyperuricemia will ever develop gout, and the pharmacologic treatment of hyperuricemia can probably be delayed until the patient actually develops symptoms.

Nonsteroidal antiinflammatory drugs (NSAIDs) have generally replaced colchicine in the management of the acute attack, although it is still used on occasion. (Two 0.5-mg tablets are given initially, followed by one tablet every hour, up to 12 tablets, until the symptoms subside or diarrhea ensues.) Disappearance of symptoms with colchicine helps confirm the diagnosis, but its dosing is inconvenient and the gastrointestinal (GI) side effects can be severe. Intravenous colchicine has fewer side effects. Quick-acting drugs such as ibuprofen and indomethacin are often recommended, although most of the NSAIDs are effective. Aspirin may not be as useful. For those who are intolerant of NSAIDs, corticosteroids or ACTH can be used. The side effects of steroid use can be minimized by tapering the dose as soon as possible. When oral medication cannot be given (e.g., in the post-op patient), intraarticular cortisone injections are valuable. The medical management of the acute attack is accompanied by rest, elevation, moist heat, and narcotics as needed.

The first attack probably does not warrant prophylaxis, but one of two agents (probenecid or allopurinol) is commonly used for protection from further attacks. Probenecid is a uricosuric agent: that is, it increases the renal excretion of uric acid. It should not be used in the

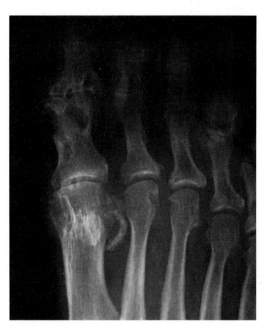

**Fig. 14–3.**
Gouty arthritis. Multiple punched-out lesions are present.

presence of renal disease. Probenecid is also effective in reducing the size of the tophaceous deposits. Allopurinol is a xanthine oxidase inhibitor that prevents the formation of uric acid from xanthine and hypoxanthine. It is especially valuable in the patient who forms urate stones because it directly decreases the production of uric acid. Although not always required, the 24-hour urine collection may give direction in deciding which agent to use. (Hypoexcretors are given probenecid to block absorption and overproducers are given allopurinol.)

Surgery is usually limited to excision of large tophi and, occasionally, arthroplasty.

## PSEUDOGOUT (CHONDROCALCINOSIS)

Pseudogout is one of the clinical patterns associated with a crystal-induced synovitis of unknown etiology resulting from the deposition of calcium pyrophosphate dehydrate crystals in joint hyaline and fibrocartilage. The crystal deposition is termed chondrocalcinosis. It is also called calcium pyrophosphate dehydrate (CPDD) deposition disease. The prevalence is uncertain but is probably similar to gout (3/1000 individuals). Chondrocalcinosis is present in over 20% of all people age 80 but most are asymptomatic. The condition resembles gout in its clinical manifestations except that large rather than small joints are more commonly involved.

### Clinical Features

The clinical presentation is variable but the symptoms are similar to those of chronic gouty arthritis. The age of onset is 60 to 70 years. Intermittent acute episodes occur, but the joint most commonly involved is the knee rather than the great toe. The condition is often familial and is occasionally associated with diabetes, renal disease, and other systemic conditions. Like gout, acute attacks may be triggered by a variety of surgical or medical events.

In addition to the goutlike symptoms, calcification of the cartilage of the knee, especially the meniscus, is common (Fig. 14-4). Calcification of the anulus fibrosus, radioulnar disc, and symphysis pubis may also be seen. Stippled calcification in bands running parallel to the subchondral bone margins may be present. Synovial fluid analysis reveals typical rhomboid-shaped crystals that exhibit weakly positive birefringence under polarized light. There are no specific

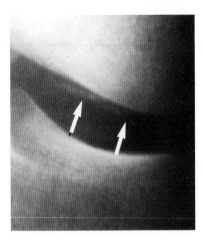

**Fig. 14–4.**
Calcification of the meniscus *(arrows)*.

changes in blood or urine. The American Rheumatism Association criteria are often used for diagnosis:

I. Demonstration of CPPD crystals (obtained by biopsy, necropsy, or aspirated synovial fluid) by definitive means (e.g., characteristic "fingerprint" by x-ray diffraction powder pattern or by chemical analysis)

II. (a) Identification of monoclinic and/or triclinic crystals showing none or a weakly positive birefringence by compensated polarized light microscopy

(b) Presence of typical calcifications in roentgenograms

III. (a) Acute arthritis, especially knees or other large joints, with or without hyperuricemia

(b) Chronic arthritis, especially knees, hips, carpus, elbow, shoulder, and metacarpophalangeal (MCP) joints, especially if accompanied by acute exacerbations. The chronic arthritis shows the following features helpful in differentiating it from osteoarthritis:

1. Uncommon site (e.g., wrist, MCP, elbow, shoulder)
2. Appearance of lesion radiologically (e.g., radiocarpal or patellofemoral joint space narrowing, especially if isolated [patella "wrapped around" the femur])
3. Subchondral cyst formation
4. Severity of degeneration is progressive, with subchondral bony collapse (microfractures) and fragmentation with formation of intraarticular radiodense bodies
5. Osteophyte formation is variable and inconstant
6. Tendon calcifications, especially Achilles, triceps, obturators

Categories: pseudogout is definitely present if criteria I or II (a) plus (b) are present; probably present if II (a) or (b) are fulfilled; and possibly present if III (a) or (b) is fulfilled.

### Treatment

Aspiration and cortisone injections are often effective in the acute phase. NSAIDs are also helpful. Structural joint damage requiring surgery is rare.

## RHEUMATOID ARTHRITIS

Rheumatoid arthritis is a systemic disorder of unknown cause characterized by chronic erosive synovitis. In contrast to many of the other arthritides, it is a potentially crippling disease. The condition is three times more common in women and the peak incidence is between the ages of 25 and 45 years. Female hormones may play a role in its pathogenesis although many factors, including genetic ones, could be involved. Pathologically, the synovium becomes thickened, inflamed, and hypertrophic. Infiltrating granulation tissue from the synovium (pannus) typically spreads over the joint cartilage. Eventually erosion and destruction of the articular surface results from the chronic inflammatory process.

### Clinical Features

The onset is usually gradual, although acute cases may occur. Weakness, fatigue, and anorexia are common prodromal symptoms. Eventually joint involvement becomes apparent, with stiffness, swelling, heat, and redness. Stiffness is most pronounced in the morning as a result of the "gelling" effect of the excess fluid. Most cases initially present with multiple symmetric joint involvement, often in the hands and feet (Table 14-3). Remissions and exacerbations are common, but the condition is chronically progressive in the majority of cases. The disease shortens life expectancy from 3 to 7 years.

The physical signs are a result of the inflammation of the synovial membrane. Joint effusions, warmth, tenderness, and restriction of motion are usually present early in the disease. Eventually characteristic deformities appear that consist of subluxations, dislocations, and joint contractures.

In addition to the joint manifestations, extraarticular findings are common. Tendon sheaths and bursae are often affected by the chronic inflammation. Tendon rupture may even occur. Rheumatoid nodules are present in 25% of cases and are most common over bony prominences such as the elbow and shaft of the ulna.

Involvement of other organ systems may lead to pulmonary fibrosis, pericarditis, and vasculitis as well as Felty's and Sjögren's syndromes.

The roentgenogram usually reveals soft-tissue swelling and osteoporosis early in the disease. Joint space narrowing, erosion, and deformity eventually become visible as the result of continued inflammation and cartilage destruction (Fig. 14-5).

The laboratory findings consist of a mild anemia, leukocytosis, and elevated sedimentation rate and C-reactive protein levels. The rheumatoid factor is positive in approximately 75% of cases. The joint fluid is usually turbid and forms a poor mucin clot. The cell count is elevated, with an increase in polymorphonuclear leukocytes.

### Treatment

Proper management requires close cooperation among primary physician, therapist, rheumatologist, and orthopedist. Patient education is of utmost importance. Rest is beneficial in reducing inflammation. When combined with an exercise program, moist heat, and splinting, joint deformities can often be prevented or corrected.

Pharmacologic management is beyond the scope of this text but NSAIDs are commonly used as the initial treatment to relieve inflammation. Aspirin remains the drug of choice for most patients although other NSAIDs may also be effective. Disease-modifying antirheumatic drugs (DMARDs) such as gold and methotrexate are used when the other drugs begin to lose their effectiveness. These are usually slow-acting and may require several weeks to become effective. Oral and intraarticular steroids are helpful as well.

Among the surgical procedures commonly used are synovectomy, soft-tissue releases, arthroplasty, and arthrodesis. The soft-tissue procedures are most beneficial early in the disease before significant fixed deformity or subluxation appears.

## Juvenile Rheumatoid Arthritis (Still's Disease)

The rheumatoid arthritis that occurs in youth differs in many respects from that which occurs in the adult. The main differences are the systemic toxicity that occurs in children and the tendency for fewer joints to be involved. The juvenile variety is often difficult to differentiate from other childhood diseases, especially rheumatic fever. It is the most common arthritis affecting children and is often called "chronic arthritis of children."

### Clinical Features

Juvenile rheumatoid arthritis is usually one of three types: (1) systemic (20%), (2) pauciarticular (30%), or

**TABLE 14–3.**

American Rheumatology Revised Classification of Rheumatoid Arthritis (American College of Rheumatology)

Rheumatoid arthritis (RA) is said to exist when four of the following conditions are present (criteria 1-4 must be present for at least 6 weeks):
1. Morning stiffness over 1 hour
2. Arthritis in three or more joints with swelling
3. Arthritis of hand joints with swelling
4. Symmetric arthritis
5. Rheumatoid nodules
6. Roentgenographic changes typical of RA
7. Positive serum rheumatoid factor

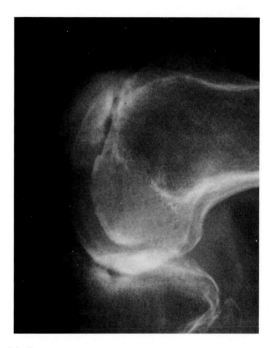

**Fig. 14–5.**
Rheumatoid arthritis of the knee. Osteoporosis and severe joint space narrowing are present. Hypertrophic spurring is typically absent.

(3) polyarticular (50%). *Systemic* or acute febrile juvenile rheumatoid arthritis is characterized by extraarticular manifestations, especially spiking fevers and a typical rash. The rash often appears in the evening and may be elicited by gently scratching the skin in susceptible areas (Koebner's phenomenon). Splenomegaly, generalized lymphadenopathy, pericarditis, and myocarditis may also occur. The articular findings are often minimal and usually are overshadowed by the systemic symptoms. The morbidity from this form is usually from chronic arthritis, however.

The *pauciarticular* or *oligoarticular* form usually involves the larger joints, such as the knees, elbows, and ankles. Girls are affected four times more often than

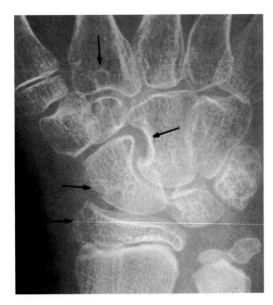

**Fig. 14–6.**
Juvenile rheumatoid arthritis. Osteoporosis is present, but joint destruction is minimal. Multiple erosions and cysts *(arrows)* are present as a result of synovial hypertrophy.

boys. Systemic features are often minimal, and only one to three joints are usually involved. The joint disease rarely causes impairment, but iridocyclitis develops in

approximately 30% of cases with this form, and permanent loss of vision will develop in a high percentage of these patients. Frequent ocular examinations, early detection, and treatment are therefore indicated. In this form of juvenile rheumatoid arthritis, accelerated growth of the affected limb from chronic hyperemia may result in a temporary leg length discrepancy. This is eventually equalized in most cases on control of the inflammation.

*Polyarticular* juvenile rheumatoid arthritis resembles the adult rheumatoid disease in its symmetric involvement of the small joints of the hands and feet. Cervical spine involvement is not uncommon and may produce marked restriction of motion. Early closure of the ossification centers of the mandible may produce a markedly receding chin, a characteristic of this form. Systemic manifestations are similar to the febrile variety but are not as dramatic.

The roentgenographic findings in juvenile rheumatoid arthritis are the same as those in the adult, except that joint destruction is less common (Fig. 14-6). The laboratory findings are also similar, except that the peripheral WBC count may be very high and the rheumatoid factor is rarely demonstrable in the serum of children.

### Treatment

The treatment is similar to that given the adult.

## NEUROARTHROPATHY

The neuropathic or Charcot's joint is one that results from a disturbance in the sensation to the joint. An underlying neurologic disorder must always be present. Diabetes mellitus with peripheral neuropathy is the most common cause. (Five percent of diabetic patients with peripheral neuropathy will develop a neuropathic foot.) Other causes are tabes dorsalis, Charcot-Marie-Tooth disease, and syringomyelia. The most widely accepted theory on the etiology is the "neurotraumatic" theory in which the impairment and loss of joint sensation decreases the protective mechanisms about the joint. This leads to rapid destruction. Chronic inflammation and repetitive effusions develop, further contributing to instability and incongruity of joints (usually the weight-bearing ones).

### Clinical Features

The foot is usually involved in diabetes; the shoulder and elbow joint in syringomyelia; and the vertebrae and lower extremities in tabes dorsalis. Gradual enlargement and instability of the affected joint is a common complaint. Pain is usually present but tends to be relatively mild when compared with the severity of the joint destruction.

The examination is characterized by swelling and hypermobility. Palpation often reveals overgrowth of bone, crepitus, and loose bodies.

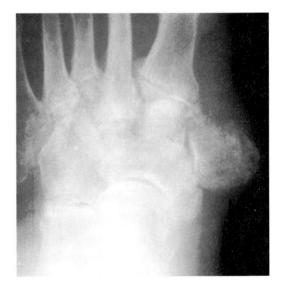

**Fig. 14–7.**
Diabetic neuroarthropathy of the midfoot. Destruction, debris, dislocation, and density (4 Ds) are usually present in neuropathic joints. The medial cuneiform is dislocated.

Variable degrees of joint destruction and disintegration with exuberant osteophyte formation are usually present on roentgenographic examination. Later, subluxation and deformity may be seen (Fig. 14-7).

In questionable cases, sepsis may need to be ruled out by aspiration, sometimes with biopsy. Usually, 2 to 3 hours of elevation will relieve the redness of neuropathy but not sepsis.

### Treatment

Once the full-blown neuropathic joint has developed, treatment can be difficult. In the lower extremity, effusions, sprains, and fractures should be well protected until all hyperemic response has subsided. Braces, special shoes with molded inserts, and elevation of the extremity are helpful. Surgery has only limited value.

## SYSTEMIC LUPUS ERYTHEMATOSUS

Systemic lupus erythematosus (SLE) is an inflammatory disease that affects the vascular and connective tissue of many organ systems, but commonly appears with joint pain and swelling similar to that seen in rheumatoid arthritis. It should always be considered in the differential diagnosis of systemic arthritis. It is most common in women in the third and fourth decades and affects the joints in 90% of patients. The joint involvement is usually accompanied by the other characteristic features of the disease: a butterfly rash on the face; and hematopoietic, renal, and cardiac involvement. Lupus erythematosus cells and antinuclear antibodies are usually present in the serum.

## OCHRONOSIS

Alkaptonuria is an uncommon inherited disorder that results from a failure to properly synthesize homogentisic acid oxidase. Homogentisic acid is thus excreted in the urine, causing it to turn black on oxidation. Ochronosis is the result of alkaptonuria and is characterized by the deposition in the soft tissue and cartilage of a pigment derived from homogentisic acid. The arthropathy of ochronosis primarily involves the spine, hips, knees, and shoulders. Typical calcifications appear in the intervertebral discs and menisci. Eventually the peripheral joint changes become indistinguishable from osteoarthritis, and the spine involvement resembles ankylosing spondylitis (see Chapter 8).

No specific treatment is available. The peripheral arthritis is treated as osteoarthritis.

## REITER'S SYNDROME

This is a disorder of unknown etiology characterized by urethritis, conjunctivitis, and arthritis. It is one of the seronegative spondyloarthropathies (see Chapter 8). Many enteric and sexually acquired agents, including Chlamydia and Shigella, appear capable of inducing the disorder. It is also commonly called *reactive arthritis*. This term denotes a sterile arthritis that develops in a joint as a result of an infection at a site distant from the inflamed joint itself.

The syndrome is often incomplete, making the diagnosis difficult. The patients are usually young and the joint symptoms generally appear within 3 to 4 weeks after the infection. The arthritis is usually oligoarticular, with large joints of the lower extremity more commonly affected. Low back pain is also common, and many patients are positive for the HLA-B27 antigen. The patient may be febrile and the joint is often warm and tender. Enthesitis (inflammation at sites of ligament and tendon insertion) is highly specific for the condition.

Symptomatic treatment including the use of NSAIDs is advised. The use of antibiotics is controversial, but many authorities recommend a tetracycline for 10 to 14 days, especially if urethritis is present. The arthritis is often self-limited and commonly resolves in a few months. The joint symptoms do not appear to be affected by the use of antibiotics.

## PSORIATIC ARTHRITIS

Psoriasis may occasionally be accompanied by a form of arthritis that is clinically similar to adult rheumatoid arthritis. Like Reiter's syndrome, it is one of the seronegative spondyloarthropathies (see Chapter 8). The skin disorder usually precedes the arthritis by several years. The arthritis is usually progressive and initially involves the distal interphalangeal joints of the fingers and toes. Its activity tends to parallel the activity of the skin disease. Severe bone destruction and ankylosis are not uncommon, especially in the hands.

# PALINDROMIC RHEUMATISM

Palindromic rheumatism is an uncommon, benign condition characterized by episodic attacks of arthritis. The small joints of the hands are typically involved. The attacks may last only a few hours or days and are usually followed by complete remission. The condition is believed by many to represent an atypical pattern of onset of rheumatoid arthritis and 20% to 40% will progress to typical rheumatoid disease.

# SJÖGREN'S SYNDROME

Sjögren's syndrome is a fairly common autoimmune disorder characterized by dry eyes (keratoconjunctivitis sicca) as a result of destruction of salivary glands and dry mouth (xerostomia) as a result of destruction of lacrimal glands. The condition may be primary or a secondary complication of preexisting connective tissue disease. Among the conditions often associated with the primary entity is a chronic arthritis, usually polyarticular in nature, which occurs in two thirds of cases. Conversely, up to 25% of patients with rheumatoid arthritis have evidence of secondary Sjögren's. The patients are typically middle-aged women.

The joint involvement resembles rheumatoid arthritis in its pathologic, clinical, and roentgenographic appearance. It commonly precedes and may be accompanied by rheumatoid nodules. The rheumatoid factor is positive in almost 100% of patients. Treatment of the arthritis is the same as for rheumatoid arthritis.

# POLYMYALGIA RHEUMATICA

This is a disorder of unknown cause affecting older adults. It is characterized by chronic inflammation that causes stiffness and aching of the shoulder and hip regions. It is sometimes called "anarthritic rheumatoid syndrome." The diagnosis is often difficult to make because there are no diagnostic criteria for the disorder.

### Clinical Features
The condition is rare before the age of 50 with an average age of 70 years at onset. Females are affected twice as often as males. Symptoms are commonly of sudden onset but have often been present for months before the diagnosis is made. Neck, shoulder, low back and thigh pain are common complaints. Morning stiffness lasting 2 to 3 hours is typical, and patients often have difficulty getting out of bed. Malaise, depression, weight loss, and a low grade fever are common constitutional symptoms and may suggest a systemic inflammation.

Physical findings are usually limited. Synovitis may be present in peripheral joints and may also be responsible for the proximal girdle symptoms in spite of the fact that they appear to be "muscular" in origin. Mild soft tissue tenderness may be present. The temporal arteries should be carefully examined as a result of the strong relation of polymyalgia rheumatica with temporal or giant cell arteritis.

Laboratory findings are usually normal except for a typically elevated erythrocyte sedimentation rate (ESR) over 45. Mild anemia may also be present. Muscle biopsies are always normal. Synovial biopsy may show mild inflammation. Some patients have a vasculitis similar to that seen in giant cell arteritis, one of the several manifestations that the two disorders have in common. (Giant cell arteritis may rarely present as a medical emergency with headache and variable degrees of blindness.)

### Treatment and Prognosis
Low doses of prednisone (10 to 20 mg per day) have traditionally been used. The response is often so dramatic that it can be used to confirm the diagnosis. Improvement is usually noted within a few days. Steroids are gradually tapered as symptoms permit but small doses (5 mg/day) may be needed for more than 2 years. NSAIDs may be effective in mild cases. Physical therapy is unnecessary.

The prognosis is usually favorable. Occasionally relapse occurs in several years but again responds well to prednisone.

# FIBROMYALGIA

This is a controversial clinical syndrome characterized by multiple trigger points and chronic (more than 3 months) diffuse pain. Similar disorders have been called fibrositis, myofascial pain syndrome, and psychogenic rheumatism.

Many physicians doubt the existence of such syndromes, partly because the patients often seem anxious and depressed. No pathologic inflammatory changes have ever been demonstrated. The diagnosis is often used in patients with vague aching near joints (especially the spine, shoulder and hip girdles) for which no other obvious cause can be found.

### Clinical Features

The female/male ratio is 9:1 and the prevalent age range is 30 to 50 years. The patient is often depressed. There may have been some recent trauma, such as a motor vehicle accident. Complaints of spinal pain are common. The patient may occasionally present with a list of other vague symptoms such as headache, stiffness, sleep disorders, chronic fatigue, and even abdominal complaints. Tender "nodules" and trigger points may be present, and when palpated, regional referral of the pain may occur. (These tender sites may simply represent normal variations in muscle density or fatty deposits.) There are never any objective physical findings. The usual roentgenographic and laboratory assessments are always normal.

Subsets of this disorder are often described if symptoms develop in conjunction with other conditions or after motor vehicle accidents, but the primary disorder is often suggested by the following criteria from the American College of Rheumatology:

1. History of widespread pain.
2. Pain in 11 of 18 selected tender spots on digital palpation. These tender spots are mainly in the spine, elbows and knees.

### Treatment

Before making this diagnosis, rule out other more likely causes for the pain. Then the treatment is mainly empiric and symptomatic. Physical therapy, NSAIDs, acupuncture, transcutaneous nerve stimulation, sympathetic blockade, muscle relaxants, trigger point injections, and antidepressants are among the many treatments used, all with varying success. An aerobic fitness program can be helpful.

Education and self-management are important. Social and environmental factors may need to be addressed, especially stress and pending litigation. Simply establishing a diagnosis can be helpful in that the patient learns that the condition is not progressive or fatal. A compassionate and reassuring approach is helpful. Support groups are also beneficial. The prognosis is uncertain. Symptoms may come and go for years in spite of an aggressive, multifaceted approach to treatment.

## HYPERTROPHIC OSTEOARTHROPATHY

This syndrome is characterized by clubbing of the fingers and toes, periosteal new bone formation (periostitis), and osteoarthritis. The periosteal reaction is usually associated with pulmonary neoplasm or long-standing suppurative disease of the lung, although a primary form has been described.

### Clinical Features

The findings are usually bilateral and symmetric. A typical clubbing of the fingers and toes usually develops first, although early pain over the shafts of the bones of the extremities is common. Joint stiffness, swelling, and pain are usually later in onset and may simulate rheumatoid arthritis.

### Roentgenographic Findings

Periosteal new bone formation is usually present. The long bones of the extremities are most often involved.

### Treatment

Treatment is strictly symptomatic. NSAIDs are helpful. The signs and symptoms usually subside when the underlying pulmonary disease is successfully treated.

## LYME ARTHRITIS

Lyme disease is a spirochetal infection (*Borrelia burgdorferi*) transmitted by deer ticks. The greatest exposure is between the months of May and November. Diagnosis can be difficult because a multitude of symptoms may develop that mimic many other conditions. It is characterized in its early stages by flu-like symptoms (fever, myalgia, headache) and a typical skin rash (erythema migrans) that often occurs at the site of the tick bite. The early stage may last up to 30 days and be accompanied by arthralgias.

Weeks to months later, recurrent skin lesions and neurologic and cardiac abnormalities may develop along with intermittent bouts of arthritis. Joint involvement is the most common late complication and occurs in more than half the cases. Usually less than two or three joints are involved, and the knee is almost always affected. Other large joints may be involved but small joint involvement is unusual. Five to ten percent of patients may develop chronic arthritis, most commonly involving the knees. Effusions are typical and erosion with cartilage destruction may even occur. Exacerbations and remissions are common.

Serologic testing is available but not always reliable, especially in early Lyme disease. Most patients with arthritis are seropositive. The diagnosis must usually be made on protean clinical findings.

### Treatment

Antibiotics (usually penicillin or tetracycline) given for the disease can prevent the chronic arthritis. Even after the arthritis is established, antibiotic therapy (for 4 weeks) may be curative. Children rarely have any long-term joint complications, and even in adults the arthritis usually resolves without any significant destruction. Chronic cases may require synovectomy.

Vaccine therapy is under investigation. If patients are active in tick-infested areas, sprays containing diethyltoluamide or permethrin may be effective in prevention. Patients should check clothing and exposed areas carefully for the tick; it takes 24 hours of attachment for infection.

## MIXED CONNECTIVE TISSUE DISEASE

This is a term used to describe a set of symptoms of connective tissue nature that sometimes overlaps with other known connective tissue diseases such as SLE, progressive systemic sclerosis, and polymyositis. Whether or not these symptoms make up a distinct, separate clinical entity remains under debate. The disorder is sometimes referred to as an "overlap syndrome" but many prefer the term "undifferentiated connective tissue disease." Initially, it was thought to be a mild variant of SLE, sometimes called "benign lupus."

### Clinical Features

The disorder is eight times more common in females. Polyarthritis, polyarthralgia, Raynaud's phenomenon, hand swelling or sclerodactyly, esophageal hypomotility, and muscle weakness are among the common initial complaints. Pericarditis, facial erythema, and psychosis are even noted in some patients. Pulmonary involvement may lead to pulmonary hypertension and even death in rare cases.

Rheumatoid factor is often demonstrated in low titers, and creatine phosphokinase (CPK) levels will be increased if myositis is present. The ESR is usually elevated and the antinuclear antibodies (ANA) may be positive with a speckled pattern. Anti-ribonucleoprotein (anti-RNP) antibodies may be present.

The response to corticosteroids is excellent in most cases except for pulmonary and scleroderma-like symptoms. Other antiinflammatory agents are used, but the best therapeutic options remain uncertain.

## ANTIINFLAMMATORY MEDICATION

Throughout this text salicylates are recommended for their antiinflammatory and analgesic effects. Like all other NSAIDs, their mode of action is unclear, but they probably act to suppress the synthesis of prostaglandins by blocking the action of cyclooxygenase-2 (COX-2), an enzyme important in their production. Unfortunately, most of the agents also inhibit the production of cyclooxygenase-1 (COX-1), an agent necessary in the production of beneficial prostaglandins.

Salicylates are effective, inexpensive, and generally well tolerated. For best results, 8 to 12 tablets (5-grain) should be taken daily. Tinnitus can occur with high doses. If it does, the dose should be decreased, but aspirin treatment should not be discontinued. If stomach intolerance is a problem, enteric-coated or buffered products are available that may lessen the gastric distress. One minor disadvantage of aspirin as compared with other NSAIDs is the common dosing regimen, although most of the prescription salicylates have more convenient dosing schedules. If salicylates are ineffective, inconvenient, or not well tolerated, a number of other drugs may be tried (Table 14-4). None of these seems clearly superior to the others, and as a general class, NSAIDs are thought by some investigators to be no better than even simple analgesics in the treatment of osteoarthritis. (If only the analgesic effect is needed, plain acetaminophen may be better because of its safety profile, especially in osteoarthritis in which inflammation plays less of a role.) These drugs are categorized by several classes, and when switching from one to another it is best to select from a different class. Patients must also be reminded that all of these drugs are most effective for chronic pain when taken routinely. Although some therapeutic effect of these drugs usually begins in a few hours, the maximum benefit may require 1 to 2 weeks. However, if the pain is mild, some are effective taken as simple analgesics on an "as needed" basis. Physicians should also be reminded that prescription NSAIDs are expensive and should not be used casually. Also, combining one NSAID with another should not be done.

The new COX-2 inhibitors may prove to be important alternatives for the patient who cannot tolerate the usual NSAIDs because of their renal and GI side effects; but their clinical effectiveness may be no better, and their cost is high.

### Side Effects

Because of their common mechanism of activity, many of these agents have similar side effects. Most of them are reversible when the drug therapy is discontinued.

**TABLE 14–4.**

Commonly Used NSAIDs

| NSAID | Usual dose | Comments |
|---|---|---|
| **Salicylates** | | |
| *Acetylated* | | |
| Aspirin | 3000 mg/d | Give in divided doses after food consumption |
| *Non-acetylated* | | |
| Diflunisal (Dolobid) | 500 mg BID | May cause marrow depression |
| Choline magnesium trisalicylate (Trilisate), salicylsalicylic acid (Disalcid, Mono-Gesic) | 3000 mg/d | Less toxic, less effective? |
| **Acetic acids** | | These may cause the most serious CNS side effects, which may limit their use (headache, depression, etc.) |
| Sulindac (Clinoril) | 150-200 mg BID | |
| Indomethacin (Indocin) | 25-50 mg TID | Indocin available in timed-release capsule |
| Tolmetin (Tolectin) | 600 mg TID | |
| Diclofenac (Voltaren) | 50 mg TID | Available in sustained-release form |
| **Propionic acids** | | Use carefully in patients with renal dysfunction |
| Ibuprofen (Motrin, etc.) | 600-800 mg TID | |
| Fenoprofen (Nalfon) | 600 mg TID | |
| Ketoprofen (Orudis) | 75 mg TID | |
| Flurbiprofen (Ansaid) | 100 mg BID | |
| Naproxen (Naprosyn) | 500 mg BID | Available over the counter and in sustained release form |
| Oxaprozin (Daypro) | 1200 mg/d | Once daily dosing |
| Ketorolac (Toradol) | 30-60 mg IM 10 mg PO q4h | Mainly for short-term (5 days) pain relief |
| **Others*** | | |
| Etodolac (Lodine) | 400 mg BID | |
| Nabumetone (Relafen) | 500 mg BID | Less GI toxicity |
| Piroxicam (Feldene) | 10-20 mg/d | Occasional photosensitivity |
| Meclofenamate (Meclomen) | 100 mg TID | Less hepatotoxic |

*Each is different chemically from all others. Diclofenac, phenylbutazone and sulindac have greatest potential for hepatotoxicity. Propionic acids occasionally can cause photosensitivity. The following side effects are common to most NSAIDs: (1) gastric irritation, (2) interference with platelet function, (3) salt and water retention, and (4) visual disturbances. These drugs should not be used in combination. When changing drugs, change from one class to a separate class. Aspirin, the most commonly used NSAID, is also available under the trade name of ZORprin. This drug is released in the small intestine rather than the stomach. The usual dose is two 800-mg tablets twice a day.
**Note**: Most of the popular NSAIDs are becoming available in sustained-release forms, often with less GI toxicity. Celocoxib, the new COX-2 inhibitor, is usually prescribed in doses of 100-200 mg once or twice each day.

**Central Nervous System.** All of these drugs can cause CNS symptoms. Most of them are minor but probably more common than appreciated. Dizziness, drowsiness, and confusion may occur. Salicylates, in particular, can cause mild lethargy. Confusion in the elderly can be especially troublesome because it is this group that usually requires the medication the most. Depression may be subtle and hard to recognize, unless the possibility that it could be drug induced is kept in mind. Low doses of amitriptyline may be needed at night. Tolmetin, sulindac, and especially indomethacin often cause such unpleasant symptoms as headache and nausea.

**Renal and Hepatic.** Ibuprofen, fenoprofen, and meclofenamate are most likely to cause renal problems, and all of the drugs can cause some loss of hepatic function. These effects do not seem related to dose or duration and are uncommon in healthy patients. Diclofenac, phenylbutazone, and sulindac seem to have the greatest potential for hepatotoxicity. The symptoms resolve in most cases when treatment with the drug is stopped. Patients with impaired function should probably avoid the drugs.

**Fluid Retention.** Salt and water retention are fairly common. Salt retention may even affect the lens and cornea and lead to blurred vision.

**Gastrointestinal.** Gastric irritation is common to all of these drugs. Elderly patients, who need these drugs the most, have three times more GI side effects than those under 60. In most cases, the discomfort can be minimized by giving the drug with food. When ulcers develop, they are usually gastric rather than duodenal. As many as 60% of patients taking NSAIDs will develop gastric erosions. Many are asymptomatic. Because prostaglandins normally protect the gastric mucosa, injury appears to be caused by the inhibition of prostaglandin production. Erosions also may be the result of some direct local irritative effect. Although these drugs may have detrimental gastrointestinal side effects, they are all that is available for the treatment of many inflammatory conditions. For those patients at greater risk of gastric ulceration (the elderly or patients with a past history of ulcer disease), misoprostol (Cytotec) may be helpful. An analogue of prostaglandin, misoprostol is effective in the *prevention* of gastric (not duodenal) ulcers caused by NSAIDs. It is recommended for use in those patients more likely to develop ulceration: (1) older (over 60 years) or debilitated patients, (2) those with a known ulceration or previous gastrointestinal bleed, and (3) patients taking oral steroids. Cotreatment with misoprostol (200 mg four times a day) has been shown to be effective during NSAID use. However, not everyone taking NSAIDs should be treated with it because the cost of the two drugs together would be prohibitive. Misoprostol also can cause diarrhea, and is contraindicated during pregnancy (it may cause spontaneous abortion) and nursing. Other drugs (such as $H_2$ antagonists and antacids) produced inferior results to misoprostol in preventing gastric ulceration, although even their use is often recommended on an empiric basis in patients at high risk.

**Others.** The antiplatelet effect of these drugs is well known, and any elective surgery may have to be postponed several days, depending on the half-life of the medication. Aspirin needs 7 to 12 days. NSAIDs are also not recommended in pregnant or nursing mothers, for whom acetaminophen remains the safest choice for analgesic purposes.

## BIBLIOGRAPHY

Aegerter E, Kirkpatrick JA: *Orthopedic diseases*, ed 3, Philadelphia, 1968, WB Saunders.

Alexander CJ Osteoarthritis: A review of old myths and current concepts, *Skeletal Radiol* 19:327-333, 1990.

Allison MC et al: Gastrointestinal damage associated with the use of nonsteroidal anti-inflammatory drugs, *N Engl J Med* 237:749-754, 1992.

Alpert SW, Koval KJ, Zuckerman JD: Neuropathic arthropathy: review of current knowledge, *J Am Acad Orthop Surg* 4:100-108, 1996.

Arnett FC et al: The American Rheumatism Association 1987 revised criteria for the classification of rheumatoid arthritis, *Arthritis Rheum* 31(3):315-324, 1988.

Bahlas S, Ramos-Remus C, Davis P: Clinical outcome of 149 patients with polymyalgia rheumatica and giant cell arteritis, *J Rheumatol* 25:99-104, 1998.

Bjelle A, Sunden G: Pyrophosphate arthropathy: a clinical study of 50 cases, *J Bone Joint Surg Br* 56:246, 1974.

Bloom BS: Risk and cost of gastrointestinal side effects associated with nonsteroidal antiinflammatory drugs, *Gastroenterology* 149:1019, 1989.

Chuang T et al: Polymyalgia rheumatica: a 10-year epidemiologic and clinical study, *Ann Intern Med* 97:672, 1982.

Decker JL, editor: Primer on the rheumatic diseases, *JAMA* 190:127-140, 425-444, 509-530, 741-751, 1964.

Edmonds MC et al: Antirheumatic drugs. A proposed new classification, *Arthritis Rheum* 36:336-339, 1993.

Flatt AE: *The care of the rheumatoid hand*, ed 2, St Louis, 1968, CV Mosby Co.

Gatter RA: *A practical handbook of joint fluid analysis*, Philadelphia, 1984, Lea & Febiger.

Graham DY: Prevention of gastroduodenal injury induced by chronic nonsteroidal anti-inflammatory drug therapy, *Gastroenterology* 96:675, 1989.

Gutman AB: Views on the pathogenesis and management of primary gout—1971, *J Bone Joint Surg Am* 54:357, 1972.

Harris C. Osteoarthritis: How to diagnose and treat the painful joint. *Geriatrics* 48:39-46, 1993.

Harris ED: Treatment of rheumatoid arthritis . . . for now and the future. In Kelly WN, Harris ED, Ruddy S, Sledge C, editors: *Textbook of rheumatology* (Update 18), New York, 1995, WB Saunders.

Hollander JL, McCarty DJ, editors: *Arthritis and allied conditions*, ed 8, Philadelphia, 1972, Lea & Febiger.

Hunder GG: The use and misuse of classification and diagnostic criteria for complex diseases, *Ann Intern Med* 129:417-418, 1998.

Hunder GG: Giant cell arteritis and polymyalgia rheumatica. In Kelley WN, Harris ED, Ruddy S, and Sledge CB, editors: *Textbook of rheumatology*, Update 20. Philadelphia, 1996, WB Saunders.

Jaffe HL: *Metabolic, degenerative, and inflammatory diseases of bones and joints*, Philadelphia, 1972, Lea & Febiger.

Katz WA: *Rheumatoid diseases, diagnosis, and management*, Philadelphia, 1977, JB Lippincott.

Kallenberg CG: Overlapping syndromes, undifferentiated connective tissue disease and other fibrosing conditions, *Curr Opin Rheumatol* 5:801-815, 1993.

King BG Jr, Galveston SN, Evans EB: Palindromic rheumatism: an unusual cause of the inflammatory joint, *J Bone Joint Surg Am* 56:142, 1974.

Laskar FH, Sargison KD: Ochronotic arthropathy, *J Bone Joint Surg Br* 52:653, 1970.

Laurin CA et al: Long-term results of synovectomy of the knee in rheumatoid patients, *J Bone Joint Surg Am* 56:521, 1974.

Lawrence SJ: Lyme disease: an orthopedic perspective, *Orthopedics* 15:1331-1342, 1992.

Loeb DS, Ahlquist DA, Talley NJ: Management of gastroduo-denopathy associated with use of nonsteroidal antiinflam-matory drugs, *Mayo Clin Proc* 67(4):354-364, 1992.

McLaughlin et al: Chronic arthritis of the knee in Lyme dis-ease, *J Bone Joint Surg Am* 68:1057, 1986.

Myerson MS, Edwards WHB: Management of neuropathic fractures in the foot and ankle, *J Am Acad Orthop Surg* 7: 8-18, 1999.

Reynolds JC: Famotidine therapy for active duodenal ulcers, *Ann Intern Med* 111:7, 1989.

Roubenoff R: Gout and hyperuricemia, *Rheum Dis Clin North Am* 16:539-550, 1990.

Sigal LH: Pitfalls in the diagnosis and management of Lyme disease, *Arthritis Rheum* 41:195-204, 1998.

Simmons BP, Nutting JT, Bernstein RA: Juvenile rheumatoid arthritis, *Hand Clinics* 12:573-589, 1996.

Steere AC et al: The overdiagnosis of Lyme disease, *JAMA* 269:1812-1816, 1993.

Steere AC et al: Successful parenteral penicillin therapy of established Lyme arthritis, *N Engl J Med* 312:869, 1985.

Tamblyn R et al: Unnecessary prescribing of NSAIDs and the management of NSAID-related gastropathy in medical practice, *Ann Intern Med* 127:429-438, 1997.

Wallace SL, Singer JZ: Therapy in gout, *Rheum Dis Clin North Am* 14:441-457, 1988.

Wolfe F et al: The American College of Rheumatology 1990 criteria for the classification of fibromyalgia: report of the multicenter criteria committee, *Arthritis Rheum* 33:160-172, 1990.

# CHAPTER 15

# Sports Medicine

Participation in athletics is both an enjoyable pastime and a part of keeping physically and mentally fit. Some individuals may be only interested in general conditioning and weight loss (Table 15-1). Others may want specific exercises for certain events. Regardless of the activity, risks are always involved, and today's physician must be able to treat not only the various injuries that arise but also to offer counsel on a wide range of interrelated subjects such as technique, training, and injury prevention.

If the participants are children, other responsibilities are also necessary. The physician should help make certain that realistic goals are set and that the activity is enjoyed by those taking part in it. Parents and coaches should be reminded that success is not necessarily measured just by winning but also by the enjoyment and the amount of effort put forth. Whenever team sports are involved, all members should be allowed to play, and attempts should be made to match size and physical maturity as closely as possible. Children should learn how to play the various games as well as how to follow their rules. They should be properly supervised and should not be encouraged to play with pain. The role of the coach should be to instruct and supervise and not to give medical treatment or advice.

Treating athletes is also somewhat different in that many of these patients, whether young or adult, are unwilling to simply give up playing when injuries arise. Many of them will accept a substitute activity that is more physically tolerable, however.

## PREVENTION OF INJURIES

The most effective means of minimizing the complications of sports injuries is by prevention, and the first step in that prevention is a complete physical examination. This is especially important in the young and should take place even before conditioning is begun. Special attention should be paid to those areas that will be most involved in the athletic activity, and all musculotendinous disorders or abnormalities should be noted and evaluated. The incidence and severity of many injuries may then be lessened by proper conditioning and preparation.

### Conditioning

Proper conditioning means the development of strength, endurance, cardiovascular fitness, power, and flexibility. It also includes the development of proper body mechanics, form, and agility. The exact skill training will depend upon the specific sport involved. Lower extremity injuries can generally be lessened if individuals with loose joints use strengthening exercises to protect against ligament damage. Individuals with tight joints can use stretching exercises to avoid muscular strains. Staying in shape during the off-season may involve running on stairs and jogging in place at home.

### Warming Up

In any sports activity, a gradual beginning will reduce the incidence of injury, especially injury to the muscle-tendon unit. Stretching is especially important to avoid strain. Flexibility is often diminished after a long period of inactivity, and stretching is particularly important when resuming a sport. The heel cord, hamstrings, and quadriceps should have special attention (Fig. 15-1).

Tissue stretches better when warm; therefore stretching is best performed after 5 minutes of slow jogging or walking. Two types of stretching exercises may be performed. *Static* stretching is a slow, gradual stretching through full movement, holding at the position of maximum stretch for 10 to 20 seconds before relaxing. A pulling sensation, not pain, should be felt. *Ballistic* stretching, which involves rapid, repetitive movements, is also occasionally used but is generally less effective and may even cause minor muscular tears. It is usually not recommended.

## Cooling Off

Proper habits after rigorous exercise permit muscles to cool off adequately and to dissipate heat. After running, it is usually advisable not to simply stand still or lie supine but to walk for 5 to 10 minutes and then rest in a sitting position. This may be especially important for the cardiac status of the individual. If the exercise is stopped abruptly, blood pooling can occur in the legs, causing syncope, hypotension, and arrhythmias.

**TABLE 15–1.**

Calories Expended in Common Activities*

| Activity | Calories per Hour |
|---|---|
| Light housework | 120 |
| Walking | 250-300 |
| Golf | 300 |
| Singles tennis | 480 |
| Bicycling | 450-500 |
| Jogging | 600 |
| Swimming | 650-700 |

*To be effective, an exercise should be performed three to five times per week for at least 30 to 60 minutes each time.

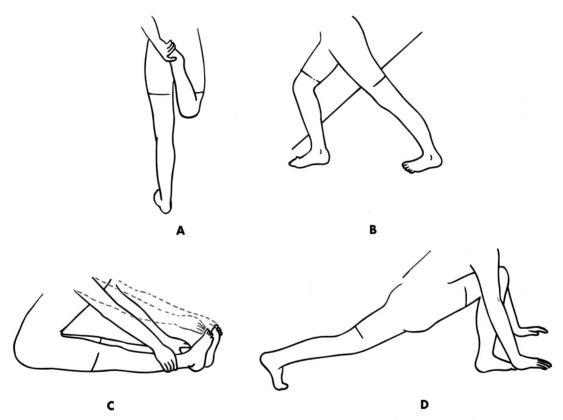

**Fig. 15–1.**
Stretching exercises. These should be performed before vigorous exercise and after warming up for a few minutes by walking. The patient should be instructed not to "bounce" or cause strain. The stretch is held for several seconds and repeated several times, and then the legs are reversed. **A**, Quadriceps stretch. **B**, Heel cord stretch. **C**, Hamstring stretch. **D**, Hamstring and quadriceps stretch.

## INJURIES TO MUSCLES

### Strains

Vigorous muscular activity can lead to three common problems: (1) muscular tears, (2) cramping during exercise, and (3) soreness after exercise.

### *Muscular Tears*

Pain that develops acutely from violent activity is usually the result of a muscle tear. This may be partial or complete and may even involve the fascia. Muscles that cross two joints (such as the hamstrings) seem to be the most vulnerable.

The diagnosis is usually not difficult, although it may not be easy to differentiate complete from incomplete ruptures. Sudden onset of pain, swelling, and marked local tenderness are characteristic. Pain is increased by stretching the affected muscle unit. Complete rupture may reveal a palpable defect on examination, but swelling often makes it difficult to diagnose a complete tear.

Ice (for 30 minutes every hour) should be applied immediately, and the injured area should be elevated. There is probably little to be gained by attempting to aspirate the hematoma. A pressure bandage is always applied, and complete bed rest may even be necessary. After 24 to 48 hours, gentle, active contraction of the muscle may be started. Ice should be continued when the exercises begin. Heat and massage should be avoided, and the extremity should be protected against further injury. Weight bearing, passive stretching, or excessive muscular activity should also be avoided until swelling is under control and the limb can be actively moved through a full range with little pain. Crutches are often needed in lower extremity injuries. Cool whirlpool baths are often helpful at this stage. A gradual return to activity is allowed when motion is painless.

Although, theoretically, complete tears should be surgically repaired, many (if not most) surgeons do not support this concept. Immediate repair is often difficult because of the poor texture of the muscle and the difficulty in making the sutures hold. The results are often poor. Late repair may occasionally be indicated, but the overall results are only fair. Therefore unless surgery is contemplated, all acute muscular strains should be treated essentially the same.

Rehabilitation is often slow, and occasionally the functional capacity of the athlete never returns to normal. Stretching exercises should be continued as strength returns. An elastic wrap is occasionally helpful when activity is resumed. If the injury has been to a hamstring muscle, strains can often be prevented by being certain that the hamstrings are at least 60% to 70% as strong as the quadriceps. This 60:40 ratio of quadriceps to hamstring strength is important to prevent strain of the hamstrings because of their relative weakness as compared with the quadriceps. Athletes may return to regular activity when full, pain-free motion is present; when muscle strength is restored; and when tenderness and swelling have subsided.

## Muscle Cramps and Soreness

Muscle cramps are common during exercise and are of unknown cause. They usually occur during the latter part of exercise and may be a result of the accumulation of waste products or of electrolyte imbalance. Any muscle may be affected, but the most common are those in the thigh, calf, and foot. Treatment is primarily by static stretching through a full range of motion and local massage. Cramps may be prevented by proper stretching exercises and warm-up and by the maintenance of adequate oral fluid and electrolyte intake. It is inappropriate to ever have an athlete "run it out."

Muscle soreness may also develop 24 to 48 hours after exertion. The etiology of this type of muscle pain is also not completely understood but may be the result of localized muscular spasm and ischemia. It is treated by rest, stretching exercises, and heat. NSAIDs may be helpful.

Nocturnal muscle cramps are also common in both adults and children. In adults, they are not usually common in the athletic individual, whereas they are common in the physically active child. In the adult, these cramps may be quite severe and cause the development of a palpable muscular knot. The acute contraction is treated by static stretching and massage. Stretching exercises during the day (especially calf-stretching) may prevent their development. Heavy blankets that keep the feet in the plantar-flexed position should be avoided. Sleeping with the feet over the edge of the bed may also prevent plantar flexion and allow more frequent changes in foot position during the night. Quinine tablets have been used before retiring, although their effectiveness is uncertain.

Children's night cramps, sometimes referred to as a cause of "growing pains," are usually not as severe as in the adult and do not cause contractions. They often occur late in the day or at night and may awaken the child. They usually occur in the thighs or calves and may be the result of fatigue. The child does not generally limp and the physical examination is normal. The disorder is treated symptomatically by heat, massage, and acetaminophen. It may be prevented by not allowing the child to become fatigued during play. Stretching exercises two or three times a day during play may also help.

## Contusions

Muscular bruises are common in all athletic events, even in the so-called "noncontact" sports. They are differentiated from ruptures and strains because function remains after the injury and the contusion usually results from direct trauma. The thigh and upper portion of the arm are most commonly involved. The diagnosis is usually not difficult: tenderness is present at the site of injury, and there is usually ecchymosis, although it may not appear until later.

Treatment is directed at avoiding the complications of myositis ossificans and contractures and returning the athlete to full, pain-free competitive activity. This is accomplished by the rapid application of ice to the affected area to control bleeding and removing the athlete from further competition. Crutches may be necessary for the lower extremity injury, and complete bed rest with elevation of the extremity may even be indicated to control swelling and pain. A compression wrapping is sometimes helpful in early stages. After 24 to 48 hours, gentle isometric muscle contractions may be started, and active, gentle range of motion is gradually added at the patient's tolerance. Passive range of motion should be avoided. Any increase in pain or swelling is an indication to resume complete bed rest and application of ice. Full strength and complete flexibility are gradually restored by exercise. Reinjury is avoided by allowing complete healing to occur before returning to activities and by appropriately protecting the injured site. A return to athletics should only follow complete recovery.

## Myositis Ossificans

This is a condition characterized by the formation of heterotopic bone in the soft tissues. It usually develops in muscle as the result of trauma (myositis ossificans circumscripta). It also occurs in the lower extremities in conjunction with severe brain injuries. A rare congenital form (myositis ossificans progressiva) may begin without trauma or shortly after birth.

The common traumatic form usually follows a single injury. The mechanism of bone formation is unknown, but interstitial hemorrhage is thought to play a role. Eventually the hematoma becomes calcified and ossified.

The most common sites of development are the quadriceps, brachialis, deltoid, and hamstrings. After the injury, a large hematoma forms. The area becomes swollen and tender, and motion is restricted. Over the next few days, increased heat may even be present locally, and some patients have a mild febrile episode. The tenderness and heat will likely persist. The erythrocyte sedimentation rate (ESR) is sometimes increased. As the swelling, pain, and heat subside, a firm mass becomes palpable in the involved area. Motion may continue to be restricted because of obstruction from the mass or from inelasticity of the muscle.

The roentgenographic diagnosis can usually be made 2 to 4 weeks after the contusion. The initial appearance is that of a poorly defined, opaque mass in the soft tissue adjacent to the bone (Fig. 15-2). As the mass matures, it becomes more clearly outlined and dense. The lesion usually stabilizes in 3 to 6 months and begins to resorb slowly, often without any disability. Eventually it transforms itself into mature bone and is partially resorbed.

Ice, elevation, and rest will control swelling. Although usually not practical, early aspiration of large,

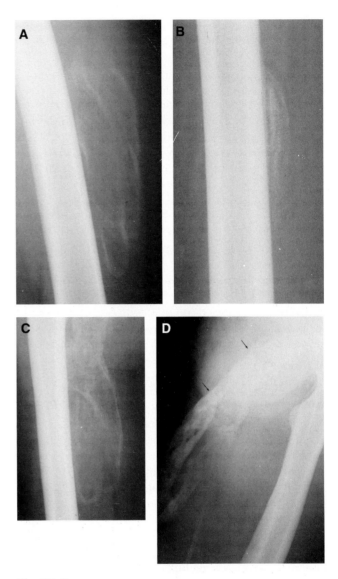

**Fig. 15–2.**
Examples of myositis ossificans (ossifying hematoma). **A**, The typical early (2½ weeks) roentgenographic appearance. **B**, A more broad-based variety. **C**, Massive involvement of the hamstring area. **D**, The same case as **C** after maturity. These injuries can occasionally be confused with malignant bone lesions, but in contrast to tumors, there is no involvement of the adjacent bone.

well-localized hematomas could prevent heterotopic bone formation. Once bone formation has developed, rest of the affected part is indicated. Gentle exercise may help prevent stiffness but vigorous physical therapy will only lead to more disability. If the heterotopic bone is locally painful or disabling it may be removed, but excision is absolutely contraindicated until complete maturity of the bony mass is reached. This may take several months. Premature removal could result in a recurrence more extensive than the original mass. It is generally recommended that athletes not resume their physical activity until the bone has completely matured, which may take 3 to 6 months. The injured area should then be protected by padding.

## Fascial Hernias

These often develop as a result of a simple contusion or small puncture wound that causes a rent in the fascia and aponeurosis that envelops each muscle. Often, however, there is no history of trauma. The defect may vary in size, the smallest being 1 cm. Hernias may also develop in weak fascial areas in patients with chronic compartment syndromes as a result of increased pressure in the compartment. They are also seen where nerves emerge from the fascia. Examination will reveal a palpable "tumor" mass, especially when the muscle is relaxed (Fig. 15-3). Muscle contraction may cause the mass to disappear, and direct pressure will also "reduce" the mass. There may be numbness in the foot if the hernia protrudes through a neural foramen.

Treatment is usually unnecessary. Good elastic support stockings may be advisable if symptoms of pain or

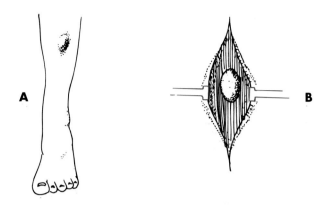

**Fig. 15–3.**
Fascial hernia. **A**, The clinical appearance. **B**, The lesion at surgery.

fatigue are present. If pain is present, surgical closure or enlargement of the hole is indicated. However, closure of the defect in a compartment syndrome is contraindicated because this could cause a further increase in the pressure inside the compartment.

## INJURIES TO RUNNERS

Millions of Americans enjoy running, and each year, more than half of these runners will sustain injuries. Many physicians from whom they seek advice are unfamiliar with their particular injuries; they may simply prescribe medication and suggest that these patients give up running for a while. Although these are good recommendations, many runners will seek more specific advice. Therefore it is important that physicians treating these patients have at least some understanding of the special problems that develop in these athletes.

## Biomechanics

The running gait pattern is a repetitive movement that consists of a support phase, when the foot is on the ground; and a nonsupport phase. It is during the support phase that most injuries develop. Distance runners usually begin this phase by landing on the heel (sprinters usually land on the forefoot). As weight is taken on the heel, the calcaneus begins to roll laterally (pronate, evert) under the talus at the subtalar joint (Fig. 15-4). This allows the heel to absorb shock and adapt to the underlying surface. The forefoot will follow this motion by pronating, and at the same time, the tibia begins to rotate internally in proportion to the amount of heel pronation. As the weight moves forward, the calcaneus begins to supinate (invert) or roll back medially under the talus, and the tibia begins to externally rotate. This allows the foot to become more rigid and gives the heel cord a strong lever upon which to act and transfer

power. There are also a number of coordinated motions that occur in the pelvis, hip, and other joints throughout the gait cycle, but an understanding of the subtalar joint mechanics is most important.

## History

An accurate history, especially of the training program, is extremely important in evaluating injuries to runners because only 40% will actually have an anatomic problem causing their disorder (James, 1978). The remaining 60% of injuries can usually be traced to errors in training. The history begins by determining whether the individual was ever treated for any childhood malalignment problem. It should be ascertained whether the individual has had any other significant

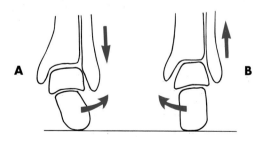

**Fig. 15–4.**
Movements of the subtalar joint. **A**, Eversion (pronation) allows for shock absorption upon impact. **B**, Inversion (supination) converts the hindfoot to a more powerful lever for push-off.

past musculoskeletal diseases. An accurate running history is then taken:

1. How often does the patient run and how many miles?
2. Has there been any recent change in the running pattern?
3. When does the pain occur?
4. What effect does running have on the pain?
5. On what sort of surface and terrain does the running take place?
6. Does the runner do stretching or other exercises to warm up?
7. What kind of shoe is used, and what is its wear pattern?

## Examination

The examination should consist of a complete evaluation of the lower extremities to determine whether any anatomic problems of extremity alignment are present as well as a local examination of the injured part. There is obviously a proper position or alignment for the foot and leg in which they function most efficiently. This is the neutral, or straightforward, position. Minor deviations from this alignment may not cause problems with normal walking or running, but because of the great accumulation of repetitive stresses applied to the lower extremities in long distance running, subtle malalignment problems may translate into major disturbances for the runner. Abnormal compensatory motions may even develop in other joints and cause them to break down. To determine whether a problem with alignment exists, a complete examination of the lower extremities is necessary. The most important aspects of the examination can be ascertained with the patient standing, lying supine, and kneeling.

With the patient standing, any gross abnormalities such as torsion, varus, or valgus of the legs; laterally directed patellae; or obvious foot deformities such as high or low arches should be noted. Any eversion of the heels as visualized from behind is especially important.

In the supine position, the true leg lengths are measured between the anterior superior iliac spines and the medial malleoli. Discrepancies of 0.5 to 1.0 cm may be significant in the runner and require correction by a shoe lift. The range of motion of the hips is then determined. Internal and external rotation should be within 30 degrees of each other. Marked external rotation may cause an out-toed gait. The knee is closely examined, especially if patellar pain is present, and the Q angle is determined (Fig. 15-5). Patients with high Q angles may develop knee pain with running. The range of motion of the ankle is then determined with the knee extended. Fifteen degrees of dorsiflexion is normal. Any tightness of the heel cord is noted.

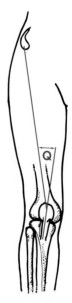

**Fig. 15–5.**
The Q angle, formed by the intersection of a line from the anterior superior iliac spine (ASIS) through the midpatella and a line from the midpatella to the tibial tubercle. The normal angle is 15 to 20 degrees. Higher angles, by causing a bowstringing effect and lateral tracking, may cause peripatellar pain.

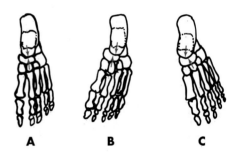

**Fig. 15–6.**
A, The neutral position of the foot. B, Inversion. C, Eversion.

The patient then kneels on the examining table, and leg-heel and heel-forefoot alignments are determined. First, the neutral position of the subtalar joint is found by everting and inverting the foot and finding the point where the head of the talus is placed in the navicular and is no longer palpable (Fig. 15-6). This may require a little practice and is often only a rough estimate. Next, leg-heel alignment is determined by drawing lines posteriorly that bisect the lower portion of the leg and calcaneus (Fig. 15-7). The lines should be parallel or have no more than 2 to 3 degrees of varus. Heel-forefoot alignment is estimated by observing the relationship of the calcaneal line to the plane of the metatarsal heads. Normally, these lines should be perpendicular.

If the alignment of the leg is not satisfactory, the knee and the foot are the most commonly affected areas. The foot may be adversely affected by too little pronation or a heel that is in too much inversion. This will not allow force to be absorbed during weight bearing. Excessive pronation may lead to strain on the medial side of the foot and ankle. This also prevents the heel from completely returning to the stable position before push-off.

The knee may also be secondarily affected because as the heel pronates, the tibia normally internally rotates and the femur externally rotates. If heel pronation is excessive, internal tibial rotation may increase and require that the knee absorb more rotation during this support phase. This may lead to strain or inflammation.

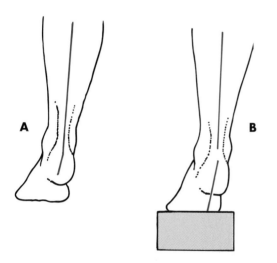

**Fig. 15–7.**
Leg-heel (**A**) and heel-forefoot (**B**) alignment. The foot and subtalar joint are held in the neutral position.

A common example of a malalignment problem is what James calls "malicious malalignment syndrome" (1978). The patient with this disorder usually has a broad pelvis, femoral anteversion, genu valgum, a high Q angle, external tibial torsion, and pronated feet.

## Back, Hip, and Thigh Pain

Back, hip, and thigh pain are relatively uncommon in long-distance runners. Back pain is especially rare but may be caused by disc disease with or without radicular symptoms. Congenital or developmental problems such as spondylolisthesis may also become symptomatic under the conditions of long-distance running. The usual early course of treatment is symptomatic, but long-distance running may aggravate the condition under treatment, and a decision may have to be made not to return to the sport.

*Trochanteric bursitis* is occasionally seen in runners and may be associated with tendinitis of the gluteus medius. The pain often radiates down the iliotibial band of the lateral aspect of the thigh and thus may be confused with disc herniation. Point tenderness is usually present. The condition may develop in the patient who has a leg length inequality or who runs on banked surfaces. The treatment is heat, antiinflammatory medication, and a local cortisone injection. A lift in the running shoe may help compensate for a leg length inequality.

*Stress fractures* occasionally occur in the pelvis and femur of the distance runner (Fig. 15-8). They should be ruled out in all cases of chronic pain that fail to respond to routine symptomatic management. The appropriate roentgenographic study should include a bone scan if the diagnosis is uncertain. As with other stress fractures,

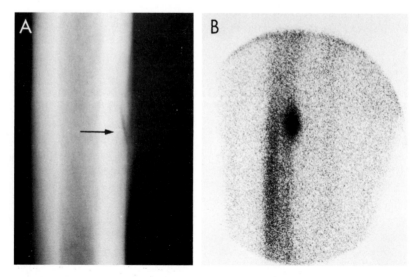

**Fig. 15–8.**
Stress fracture of the femur. **A,** Plain anteroposterior (AP) roentgenogram . **B,** Bone scan.

reduction of activity is usually curative, but fractures of the femoral neck may require internal fixation.

*Hamstring strains* are a less common cause of disability in the distance runner than in the sprinter. They are treated as previously described. Stretching exercises are important not only because they can prevent local injuries but also because tight hamstrings may cause excessive lumbar lordosis that adds strain to the back when running.

*Contractures* of the hip joint also add strain to the back and should be treated by static stretching exercises. Inflammation may also develop in the piriformis, adductor, and iliopsoas tendons and in the ischial and iliopsoas bursae. Inflammation of the symphysis pubis (osteitis pubis) and sacroiliac joints may also develop because of the repetitive shearing forces applied to these areas. The treatment for these disorders is also symptomatic.

## Knee Pain

### Overuse Syndromes

Major injuries of the meniscus or ligaments are uncommon in the knees of runners. More common are *overuse* injuries that develop because of the repetitive nature of the running activity (Fig. 15-9). Several areas are commonly affected:

1. Tenosynovitis of the popliteus tendon may develop near its insertion just above the lateral joint line and anterior to the lateral collateral ligament. This insertion is deep to the iliotibial band (ITB). The inflammation may be caused by excessive downhill running.

2. The iliotibial band friction syndrome is an inflammation of the band as it rubs over the lateral femoral condyle. A snapping sensation may be present during flexion and extension.

3. Anserine bursitis causes pain beneath the anserine tendons over the medial flare of the tibia. A stress fracture of the upper portion of the tibia should be ruled out in resistant cases.

4. *Jumper's knee* is a tendinitis of the patellar tendon, usually where it attaches to the patella. As the name implies, it is also seen in athletes whose events require jumping.

5. Tendinitis of the quadriceps mechanism may also occur over its wide insertion or over the medial or lateral retinaculum that helps support the patella.

6. Synovitis. Chronic inflammation of the joint may also develop from overuse. An effusion is usually the only physical finding, and a history will not reveal any apparent cause for the swelling except, occasionally, a history of increased mileage. Oral anti-inflammatory medication and a period of decreased mileage may be curative, but complete rest for 6 to 8 weeks may be necessary. An occasional steroid injection may be tried if all other treatments fail, but repeated injections are probably not advisable.

### Chondromalacia Patella ("Anterior Knee Pain Syndrome")

This is a condition in which pain develops beneath or, more commonly, *around* the patella, sometimes in conjunction with varying amounts of fibrillation and degeneration of its articular cartilage (see Chapter 11). Anything that adversely affects the normal "tracking" of the patella in its femoral groove may lead to pain, usually on the lateral side. The causes are often those of malalignment: (1) an increased Q angle with a bowstringing effect, (2) tightness of the lateral retinaculum with relative weakness of the vastus medialis muscle, (3) subluxing patella, (4) direct trauma, and (5) genu valgum, excessive heel pronation, and/or external tibial torsion (Fig. 15-10).

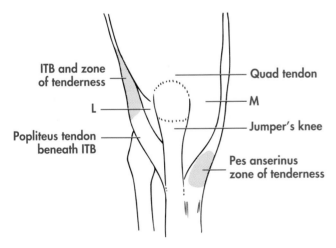

**Fig. 15–9.**
Common areas of tendinitis of the knee. The most common areas of involvement are the quadriceps tendon and its medial *(M)* and lateral *(L)* expansions.

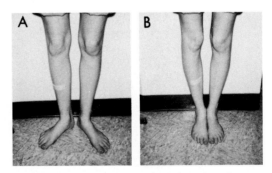

**Fig. 15–10.**
External tibial torsion. **A,** With the patella pointing straight forward, the feet are externally rotated. This may cause peripatellar pain with excessive use because of abnormal pressure. Note the high Q angles. **B,** The knees face inward with the feet pointing straight ahead.

Clinically, patellar or peripatellar pain and discomfort are present and are usually aggravated when stress is applied to the extensor mechanism by stair walking or running up and down hilly terrain. Sitting with the knee flexed for any excessive period may cause a stiff feeling to develop that is usually relieved by knee extension. An effusion is rarely present, and palpation of the undersurface of the patella may be painful. A Q angle of more than 20 degrees or other physical findings of malalignment may be present. Roentgenograms are usually not helpful unless subluxation is present.

The variety of treatments used to manage this condition attests to the difficulty in curing it. Conservative measures such as rest, antiinflammatory medication, local heat, stretching exercises, quadriceps exercises in extension, and avoiding the offending activity are useful. Patellar straps or braces seem to be of only limited benefit. Theoretically, removal of the damaged articular cartilage by shaving could relieve the symptoms. This

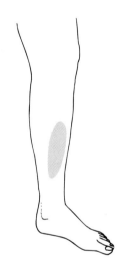

**Fig. 15–11.**
The area of tenderness and pain with posterior tibial tendinitis.

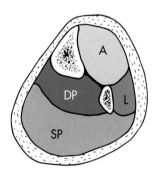

**Fig. 15–12.**
A cross section of the lower portion of the leg shows its four compartments; *A* = anterior; *L* = lateral; *DP* = deep posterior, and *SP* = superficial posterior.

can easily be done arthroscopically, but the results are often inconsistent, probably because the changes in the articular cartilage are *not* the source of pain. If a distal malalignment problem is present, an orthotic device in the shoe may occasionally be beneficial to help correct the tracking problem. As a last resort, a surgical procedure to realign the patella could eliminate the symptoms, but it would seem difficult to justify such a major operation simply to allow continued running.

## Lower Leg Pain

### Posterior Tibial Tendinitis

A common cause of leg pain is what is sometimes referred to as the *shin splint* or medial tibial stress syndrome. This is a specific overuse syndrome involving the origin of the tibialis posterior muscle and causing pain along the deep midthird of the medial border of the tibia (Fig. 15-11). It often develops in poorly conditioned athletes or runners who run on hard surfaces. There is usually tenderness to palpation along the posteromedial border of the midtibia. The roentgenogram may show some late periosteal reaction or cortical thickening in this area.

The treatment is by modification of the running schedule or complete rest. Stretching exercises, NSAIDs, and ice may help. A change to a softer running surface may be necessary. The condition usually does not become chronic.

### Compartment Syndromes

Vigorous exercise may lead to swelling and mild ischemia in any of the four natural compartments in the calf (Fig. 15-12). The anterior and lateral compartments are the two most commonly affected in runners, and the condition is usually chronic or recurrent rather than acute when it develops in runners. The disorder develops either from local arterial spasm or swelling that increases the pressure in the unyielding compartment. This compromises the local blood flow and leads to muscle ischemia and pain. Permanent muscle and nerve damage may result, but this is rare in the common chronic type seen in runners. More often, the only symptom is cramping pain during exercise that is relieved by rest and recurs after resumption of activity. Physical findings are minimal, but tenderness may be present in the affected compartment as well as slight weakness of the involved muscles. Mild paresthesias are occasionally noted.

The rare acute case is usually treated by surgical release of the affected compartment. The more common recurrent type seen in runners is treated by rest and modification of training techniques and mileage. Conservative treatment is often unsuccessful, and individuals who wish to continue competitive long-distance running may require fasciotomy to decompress the affected compartment.

### Stress Fractures

These are common injuries of the lower leg and must always be ruled out in the evaluation of pain. They usually develop in response to a sudden increase in the stress applied to a weight-bearing bone. Thus they are more likely to occur in the novice who is just beginning running or in the individual who suddenly increases mileage. Any weight-bearing bone may be affected. The proximal medial tibial border and the lower portion of the fibula are the most commonly affected areas in the lower part of the leg.

The only physical findings are local tenderness and edema. The roentgenograms are usually negative initially and begin to show healing changes in 2 to 4 weeks. The bone scan is often more sensitive.

The treatment is symptomatic by modification of activities. Casts are usually not necessary. Activity is resumed as symptoms subside. Swimming may be substituted for running during the healing phase to allow the runner to maintain fitness.

## Ankle and Foot Pain

Several overuse syndromes may affect the ankle and foot. They are all treated in the same manner: by rest (or modification of activities), antiinflammatory medication, and local heat. An occasional local steroid injection may also be helpful, but the Achilles tendon should not be injected. Rupture of this tendon is always a concern, and it is possible that this event may be hastened by local injections.

Stress fractures also occur in the foot, and the most common areas of involvement are the metatarsals, navicular, and calcaneus (Fig. 15-13). They are treated by protection.

### The Pump Bump

This is a painful thickening that develops over the lateral attachment of the Achilles tendon (Fig. 15-14). It is usually the result of friction and irritation from a poorly padded heel counter. Conservative measures including proper shoes are usually curative. The back of the shoe may have to be cut out for a time. A heel lift may also be helpful. In resistant cases, the small bump must be removed surgically.

### Blisters

Blisters are common in runners and are best treated by the following preventive means:

1. Begin workouts gradually and increase the mileage as tolerated.

2. Make certain shoes are well ventilated and socks are clean and dry.
3. Before long runs, apply powder or petroleum jelly to the areas prone to blister.
4. Use tincture of benzoin to toughen the skin before running. Once a blister does form, it should be drained with a sterile needle. The dead skin, which is a good dressing, should be left intact and a bandage applied over antibiotic ointment. Broken blisters should be trimmed and kept clean and dry.

Another common condition that develops in runners is the black toe or subungual hematoma. This often develops in a shoe that lacks sufficient room to accom-

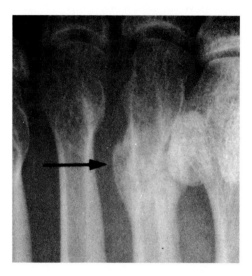

**Fig. 15–13.**
Stress fracture of the second metatarsal *(arrow)*.

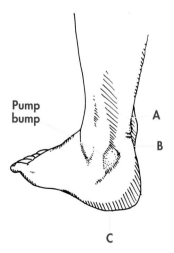

**Fig. 15–14.**
The "pump bump" and common areas of inflammation around the heel. *A* = Achilles tendon; *B* = retrocalcaneal bursa; *C* = plantar fascia.

modate the forefoot. It may be the result of repetitive shearing, which then leads to bleeding beneath the nail. Seromas develop in a similar manner. It is usually asymptomatic, but the occasional painful, tense hematoma may be evacuated by penetrating the nail with a heated paper clip or an 18-gauge needle spun between the fingertips.

## Running Shoes

A properly constructed shoe is an absolute necessity for the runner (Fig. 15-15). The running shoe functions mainly to protect the foot from the environment and to prevent overpronation. When being fitted with a new shoe, the same socks should be worn that will be used when running. There is no perfect shoe, but a good shoe should have the following:

1. A long, firm heel counter to control the hind foot, with a soft Achilles pad to prevent heel cord irritation
2. A beveled heel that is flared for stability
3. A cushioned heel lift 1.5 cm thick and a cushioned sole
4. A high and rounded toe box and a well-padded tongue
5. A last that is straight rather than adducted, with the shoes balanced (that is, not leaning to one side)
6. A midsole that is flexible and that contains a soft arch support

Shoes should be kept in good repair and replaced or resoled once they become badly worn. The most important aspect in selecting jogging shoes—or any shoes—is the fit.

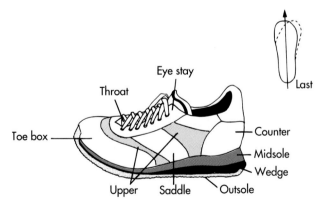

**Fig. 15–15.**
The properly constructed running shoe. Good heel fit is particularly important. The last or form from which the shoe is made should be straight and not 6 to 7 degrees inward as it is in many manufactured shoes. It should be unnecessary to "break in" good running shoes. They should be fitted at the end of the day when feet are the largest.

## Orthotics

From the previous discussion, the importance of the position and movements of the subtalar joint is apparent. The ability of this joint to absorb shock and function normally is greatest when the center of gravity passes through the joint in the neutral position. The subtalar joint absorbs shock by pronation, but excessive pronation can, at least theoretically, lead to some of the overuse syndromes that are seen in runners not only in the foot and ankle but also in the knee. This excessive pronation is one of the most common *malalignment* problems seen in runners and is the usual reason orthotic appliances are prescribed. Orthotics can be used in an attempt to support the foot, especially the heel, more near its neutral position. They are used more or less on an empiric basis as a last resort. There are no conclusive studies that show that these devices actually perform as expected, but some patients seem to benefit from their use, and they continue to be prescribed. However, they can be expensive and are best used only when more simple treatment modalities have failed.

Orthotics may be soft, semirigid, or hard; several materials can be used. Semiflexible devices seem to be preferred by most runners. Simple supports are available in sporting goods stores and are usually made from rubber. Other soft orthotics can be made from materials that are heated and applied to the individual's foot while the heel is held in a neutral position (Fig. 15-16). "Posts" may be added for additional support. Laboratories that specialize in their preparation can also make custom-fabricated, rigid orthotics from plaster molds of the feet.

## Treatment Summary

The general care of runners involves accurate diagnosis, evaluation for alignment problems, and assessment for training errors. It has been found that the majority of injuries are related to training errors, and that exces-

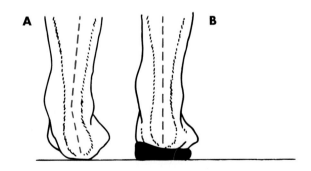

**Fig. 15–16.**
The "neutral" orthotic device. Excessive hindfoot pronation (**A**) may occasionally be corrected by the use of an orthotic device (**B**).

sive mileage accounts for many of these. In addition to excessive mileage, other causes of training problems are running on improper surfaces or terrain and abrupt increases in the intensity of the runner's routine. Therefore minor modifications in the runner's schedule may be helpful. However, complete rest is occasionally the only acceptable treatment, and a rest of 4 to 6 weeks is often necessary to allow for complete recovery. The following recommendations are often helpful:

1. Heavy workouts should alternate daily with light workouts.
2. Rest or at least reduce mileage until symptoms subside. Substitute bicycle riding or swimming temporarily.
3. Gradually return to running the previous mileage after the injury resolves.
4. Static stretching exercises for 10 to 15 minutes should precede each workout. This should be particularly directed to the hamstrings and calf muscles.
5. Proper shoes should be worn at all times and should be changed as necessary.
6. Runners who use roads should train on alternate sides because the crown of the road may create uneven stress. Training should take place on as flat a surface as possible, and slopes should be avoided. Asphalt is the favored surface.

7. Complete rest may be necessary for 6 weeks in some cases. It should also be remembered that not all individuals are able to run long distances any more than they are able to run fast. Biking, swimming, and rowing may be better activities for some.

**Running, Walking and Arthritis.** Regular exercise for many patients includes jogging or walking. The question often arises regarding potential damage to joints with such exercise. The following guidelines may be helpful:

1. There is no evidence that regular exercise such as running causes cartilage degeneration in the normal knee.
2. Regular exercise promotes better health and less disability.
3. Only the aging process is related to the onset of primary osteoarthritis.
4. Patients who may be at risk for joint problems (those with previous ligament damage, malalignment, or prior history of painful running) should be directed toward low impact or non–weight-bearing aerobic exercise. Biking, swimming, cross-country ski machines, and rowing are more appropriate than running for these patients.
5. Patients with joint replacement should also avoid high impact weight-bearing exercise.

# INJURIES TO THE UPPER EXTREMITY

## The Shoulder

### Disorders of the Rotator Cuff

The overarm throwing motion may rank second only to running as the most common factor in athletic events. The range of motion of the shoulder is the greatest of all joints and is made possible because of the relatively minimal amount of bony contact between the humeral head and the glenoid. Thus stability is sacrificed for flexibility, and this places a great burden on the capsule and rotator cuff musculature for joint stability. As a result, the soft tissue may develop overuse injuries because of repetitive strains placed on it during exercise. These strains may lead to overuse changes ranging from simple tendinitis or bursitis to rotator cuff rupture. Tissue calcification may even occur. Swelling of the rotator cuff and subacromial bursa then develops, which narrows the space between the head of the humerus and the overlying acromion and coracoacromial ligament. An abnormally-shaped (hooked) acromion may contribute to the problem. This may lead to the development of crepitus and impingement when the shoulder is abducted. Abduction further narrows the sub-

acromial space and can result in a painful catching sensation, thus the term "impingement syndrome" (see Chapter 5).

Clinically, shoulder pain is present during and after use. The pain may radiate down the deltoid muscle because of the common innervation of the deltoid and supraspinatus muscle. Crepitus is common, and there is tenderness to palpation over the rotator cuff, usually the supraspinatus tendon.

The treatment of rotator cuff tendinitis is usually conservative. Rest and avoiding the offending activity are most important. Push-ups should be avoided. Local steroid injections may relieve pain but should be used cautiously in athletes. Repetitive injections should certainly be avoided (especially in the young), and vigorous use of the shoulder after injections should not be allowed. Rest, stretching and strengthening exercises, and proper throwing or swimming mechanics should be stressed.

Surgery is occasionally helpful in resistant cases. A complete rotator cuff rupture may sometimes benefit from repair. In addition, removal of the bursa and the underneath surface of the acromion and release of the coracoacromial ligament may eliminate much of the impingement. However, surgery is somewhat unpredictable, and it may not always allow a full return to the athlete's previous competitive status.

*Little League shoulder* is a condition seen in adolescence that was previously thought to be overuse tendinitis. The presenting complaints are similar. This is now considered to be a traction irritation of the upper humeral epiphysis that causes a stress reaction around the epiphysis. Roentgenography may reveal widening of the epiphyseal plate. The disorder usually heals with rest and leaves no residuals. Pitching limits should be placed on the young athlete to prevent such injury.

### Injuries to the Acromioclavicular Joint

The acromioclavicular joint sustains a wide range of injuries. The most minor is the so-called *shoulder pointer*, which is a contusion of the deltoid, trapezius, and acromioclavicular joint. It usually heals with rest and protection.

More common is acromioclavicular separation or dislocation (see Chapter 5). The lesion often is graded 1 through 5. A grade 1 injury is simply a minor strain of the acromioclavicular ligaments. A grade 2 injury involves rupture of the acromioclavicular ligaments but preservation of the coracoclavicular ligaments. In grade 3, 4, and 5 injuries, there is complete rupture of all supports with upward displacement of the clavicle. (Grade 4 and 5 injuries are rare.)

Grade 1 and 2 incomplete injuries are usually treated symptomatically. The treatment for grade 3 injuries remains unsettled. If the injury involves the dominant shoulder of an athlete who throws, surgical repair is probably indicated. However, except for the cosmetic deformity, most individuals with chronic acromioclavicular separations are asymptomatic. Grade 4 and 5 injuries in the athlete are severely displaced and usually need repair.

### Dislocation of the Glenohumeral Joint

Most shoulder dislocations are anterior in direction and result from trauma (see Chapter 5). The usual cause is a fall on the outstretched arm. The diagnosis is suspected when there is an absence of the normal fullness beneath the deltoid. If the dislocation is anterior, the humeral head is palpable anteriorly, the arm is held externally rotated, and internal rotation is painful. Posterior dislocations characteristically have pain on external rotation, the arm is held in internal rotation, and there is flatness of the anterior shoulder contour. Both types often become recurrent.

The treatment is reduction, and this should be accomplished as soon as reasonable. Roentgenograms should always be taken before reduction to rule out other bony injury. Epiphyseal fracture of the upper portion of the humerus, especially, should be ruled out.

After reduction, the shoulder should be rested in a sling for 1 to 2 weeks. General strengthening exercises are begun, although there is little evidence that they prevent recurrence. (After a third anterior dislocation, the risk for another is almost 100%.) Surgery is often necessary upon recurrence and is usually successful in preventing dislocation, but the throwing abilities of the athlete may never return to their previous status.

Shoulder instability may also manifest itself by subluxation rather than dislocation. This is sometimes termed *anterior capsular insufficiency*. In this disorder, the anterior capsule and cartilaginous rim of the glenoid become weak from repetitive stretching, mainly from the throwing motion. The shoulder may not completely dislocate but instead slips slightly forward and downward. This causes a feeling of weakness (the *dead arm syndrome*), pain, and apprehension, especially when the arm is externally rotated and abducted. Rehabilitation exercises may help but surgery is often necessary to restore strength to the anterior shoulder capsule.

## The Elbow

### Epicondylitis

Inflammation of the tendinous origin of the forearm muscles at the epicondyles is a common disorder (see Chapter 6). The extensor origin (tennis elbow) is more commonly involved than the flexor side. The disorder is not restricted to tennis players but may be caused by any activity that involves repeated forceful gripping. Tennis players who use both hands for backhand strokes do not develop this condition as often as those who use the one-handed grip.

Physical examination will reveal point tenderness over the affected epicondyle, with the pain being aggravated by gripping against resistance.

The treatment includes rest; antiinflammatory medication; local heat, ice, or ultrasound; and local steroid injections. A tennis-elbow brace may help relieve the strain, and a gradual, progressive, controlled stretching and strengthening exercise program for the forearm and hand muscles may be helpful (Fig. 15-17). Tennis players can prevent recurrences by using proper techniques. The handle of the tennis racquet should be the proper size, and the ball should be struck in the center of the racquet face. The body rather than the arm should be used for power. In addition, a good ball should always be used, and there should be less tension on the strings for the average player. Oversized racquets seem to help by providing a larger "sweet spot."

### Little League Elbow

*Little League elbow* is a term that has been used for a variety of lesions in immature athletes. All of them are related to the repetitive act of throwing, an act that places unusual (medial tension stretching and lateral compression) stress on the elbow. Osteochondritis, avulsion fractures, loose bodies, tendinitis, and a variety of other bony and soft-tissue disorders have been reported.

The symptoms may be of acute or gradual onset. When the onset is sudden, the symptoms are usually secondary to an avulsion injury of either the lateral or the medial epicondyle (Fig. 15-18). More commonly the process is chronic, and the symptoms are usually those of persistent discomfort and stiffness that are aggravated by use of the extremity.

The physical findings are dependent on the specific lesion. There is usually point tenderness to palpation over the affected area. The range of motion may be restricted, and a chronic joint effusion is not uncommon.

Treatment is usually conservative, with rest and the elimination of the offending activity being all that is necessary. If osteochondritis dissecans is present, the joint may have to be protected for several months to allow healing to occur and to prevent the formation of a loose body. If a loose body is present, surgical removal is usually indicated.

Prevention is the key. To protect the elbow from developing these disorders, most authorities believe that no more than 6 innings of baseball should be pitched per week by the immature player. In addition, at least 3 or 4 days of rest should be allowed between pitching. (Both games and practices count.) If enough irritation and swelling is present that a flexion contracture of 20 to 30 degrees exists, the adolescent should not be allowed to pitch again until normal motion has returned. Young pitchers should never "pitch through" their pain. Permanent growth disturbances and arthritis could be the end result.

## The Hand

The anatomy of the hand and finger is complex, and injuries to the bones and soft tissues are common in sports (Fig. 15-19). The joint may simply be referred to as *jammed*, and the injury is therefore often not fully appreciated or properly treated. Permanent loss of function may be the end result.

### *Mallet Finger (Baseball Finger)*

Avulsion of the insertion of the extensor tendon at the base of the distal phalanx is a common injury. It occurs secondary to sudden forceful flexion of the distal phalanx, often from a blow to the tip of the extended finger. A fragment of bone may be avulsed along with the tendon. Active extension of the distal phalanx is lost. Tenderness and swelling are noted on the dorsum of the distal interphalangeal (DIP) joint, and the distal phalanx rests in the position of moderate flexion. Long-

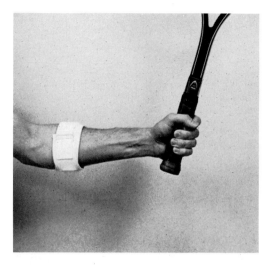

**Fig. 15–17.**
Tennis-elbow brace. The brace should be applied approximately 2.5 cm below the epicondyle and fit snugly enough to partially relieve the strain on the affected muscles. A variety of other devices are available.

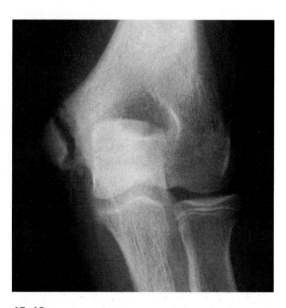

**Fig. 15–18.**
Avulsion of the medial epicondyle in association with a throwing injury in an adolescent.

standing cases occasionally develop a mild hyperextension deformity of the proximal interphalangeal joint (Fig. 15-20). Roentgenographic examination may reveal an avulsion fracture of the distal phalanx.

If no fracture is present, or if the fracture is small, the joint is immobilized in slight hyperextension for 5 weeks (Fig. 15-21). Vigilance is the key. The splint should not be removed by the patient until the treatment is complete. If the fracture fragment is large (more

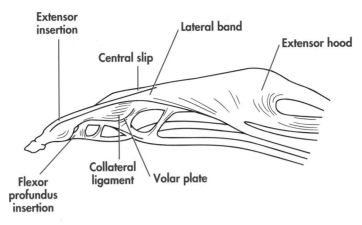

**Fig. 15–19.**
Structures often involved in soft-tissue injuries to the finger. Local tenderness or instability will usually assist in establishing the diagnosis.

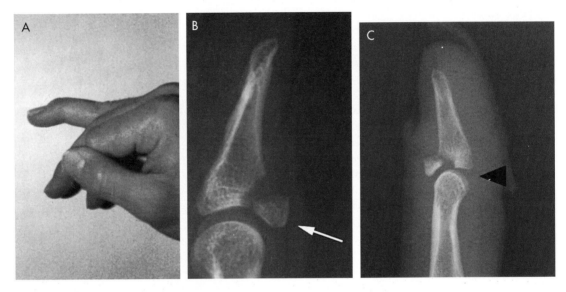

**Fig. 15–20.**
**A,** Mallet finger. A mild hyperextension deformity is present at the proximal interphalangeal joint. After avulsion of the extensor insertion distally, overpull of the central slip mechanism at the middle phalanx will often result in recurvatum at the middle joint, producing a "swan-neck" deformity. **B,** Roentgenogram of a mallet finger with a large avulsion fracture. **C,** Volar opening of the DIP joint indicative of instability.

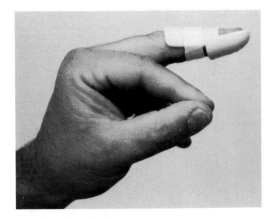

**Fig. 15–21.**
Mallet finger splint maintaining the distal interphalangeal (DIP) joint in slight extension.

than 25% of the joint surface) and displaced, the joint should be tested for stability (Fig. 15-22). If the joint is stable, the same treatment is recommended (that is, treatment in hyperextension). If the joint is unstable or the fragment is quite large, surgical repair may be necessary. Some residual lack of extension may persist regardless of treatment, but the functional result is usually excellent.

Cases diagnosed after 4 to 6 weeks may still be helped by splinting for 3 or 4 weeks. If a major fragment has been avulsed, surgical repair is often beneficial. If no fracture is present, the amount of actual functional loss that the injury represents to the patient should be assessed. If the impairment is minimal, which is often the case, then no treatment is indicated. Otherwise, surgical reconstruction is necessary.

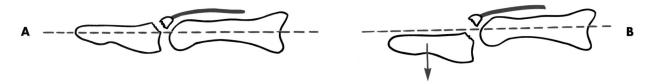

**Fig. 15–22.**
Testing for subluxation of the distal phalanx. The phalanx is grasped, and volar pressure is applied (**A**). If instability is present, the distal phalanx will sublux (**B**).

### Flexor Digitorum Profundus Avulsion (Jersey Finger)

The deep flexor may be avulsed from its attachment by sudden distal interphalangeal (DIP) hyperextension. The ring finger is most often involved. The injury commonly occurs in football when a tackler grabs the jersey of the opponent who pulls away. The tendon eventually retracts proximally into its sheath (Fig. 15-23). If bone is avulsed, it may be evident, but otherwise, roentgenograms are not revealing. Clinically, the volar aspect of the distal interphalangeal (DIP) joint is tender, and the patient is unable to flex the distal phalanx. The end of the tendon with its bony fragment may be palpable.

Treatment is surgical repair. Early recognition is important because direct repair produces the best clinical results. Late cases may require tendon-grafting procedures.

### Proximal Interphalangeal (PIP) Joint Injuries

This joint is one of the most commonly called *jammed*. Several different areas may be injured. A careful physical examination should always be performed to establish the diagnosis.

**Central Slip Injuries.** Damage to the central slip attachment to the middle phalanx is easily missed. The PIP joint is usually swollen, and if injury to the slip is present, there will be point tenderness on the dorsum of the joint. If the slip is completely avulsed, Elson's test is usually positive (Fig. 15-24).

The diagnosis may be difficult. The injury often occurs in conjunction with the rare volar PIP dislocation. If untreated, the lateral bands may gradually migrate into a volar position, anterior to the axis of the PIP joint (Fig. 15-25). The lateral bands then become flexors of the PIP joint and hyperextend the DIP joint to produce the typical boutonnierre deformity. Late loss of DIP flexion is the most disabling problem.

Roentgenograms are usually normal, although on rare occasions a fragment of bone may be avulsed (Fig. 15-26).

These cases should probably be referred whenever this injury is suspected, especially if there has been a straight volar dislocation. The PIP joint must be splinted

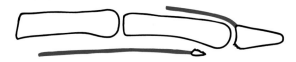

**Fig. 15–23.**
Flexor digitorum profundus avulsion.

in extension for 4 to 6 weeks to allow healing. The DIP and metacarpophalangeal (MCP) joints are allowed movement. Chronic injuries may require reconstructive surgery, but the results are never as good as with acute care.

**Volar Plate Injuries.** The volar plate normally acts to protect the PIP joint and prevent hyperextension. It can be avulsed (with or without a bony fragment) in conjunction with the common dorsal PIP dislocation or by a forced hyperextension to the joint (Fig. 15-27).

Clinically, there is usually local volar tenderness, and passive joint extension may be increased and painful. If untreated, hyperextension of the PIP joint may occur and produce a "swan-neck" deformity.

The injury is treated by splinting both interphalangeal (IP) joints in 20 degrees of flexion or buddy-taping for 3 or 4 weeks if no instability is present. Large fragments may need surgical repair.

**Collateral Ligament Injuries.** Rupture of either collateral ligament is usually the result of a dislocation but may occur with other injuries. Stress testing usually reveals the diagnosis. Incomplete ruptures are treated by buddy-taping to the adjacent finger for 3 to 4 weeks. Complete ruptures (mainly the radial collateral ligament of the index) are sometimes treated surgically, but good results are also obtained by splinting at 30 degrees for 3 weeks and buddy-taping for an additional 3 weeks.

### Interphalangeal Dislocations

These common injuries are almost always dorsal in direction and usually involve the PIP joint (Fig. 15-28). They are usually easily reduced. Although the volar plate may be damaged, these injuries are generally sta-

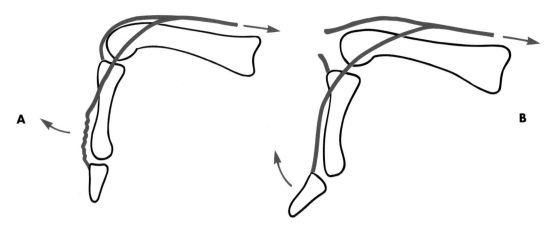

**Fig. 15–24.**
Elson's test. The PIP joint is held firmly flexed over the edge of a table, and the patient is asked to extend the finger. If the central slip is intact, pressure will be felt against the middle phalanx, and the distal phalanx will remain flail (**A**). If the central slip is ruptured (**B**), the pressure will be felt at the distal phalanx, which will extend via the lateral bands.

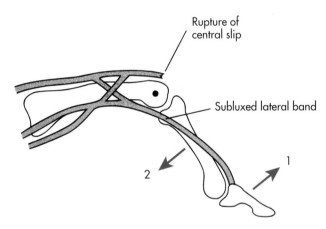

**Fig. 15–25.**
Central slip rupture with boutonnierre deformity. As the attempt to extend the finger is made *(1)*, the subluxed lateral bands, which are now volar to the axis of PIP joint motion, cause PIP flexion *(2)* rather than extension.

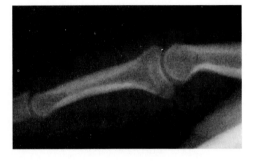

**Fig. 15–27.**
Avulsion fracture of the volar plate *(arrow)*.

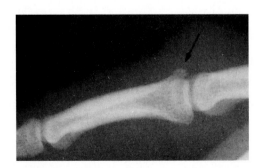

**Fig. 15–26.**
Avulsion fracture of the central slip *(arrow)*. Also note the dorsal soft-tissue swelling.

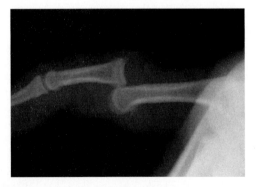

**Fig. 15–28.**
Proximal IP dislocation. Simple traction will usually reduce most IP dislocations. Occasionally, the joint must be hyperextended and the reduction accomplished by digital pressure.

ble after reduction, and may be treated by taping the finger to the adjacent finger for 3 to 4 weeks. Collateral ligament stability should always be evaluated. Unstable injuries should be referred. Volar PIP dislocations have the potential for central slip rupture and should probably be referred after reduction.

### Proximal Interphalangeal Fracture-Dislocations

Many minor IP joint injuries are accompanied by small *chip fractures*. If the joint is stable, the fracture can usually be ignored and the joint injury treated conservatively by splinting for 4 weeks. A more serious injury is the fracture-dislocation or subluxation of the PIP joint (Fig. 15-29). This injury should be suspected if any volar instability is present when the finger is tested in extension or if the volar fracture fragment is greater than 30% of the joint surface. Special splinting is usually necessary, and surgery may even be indicated.

### Metacarpophalangeal (MCP) Dislocations

These injuries are sometimes difficult to recognize. The index finger and thumb are more commonly involved. The proximal phalanx is usually displaced dorsally (Fig. 15-30). This injury often requires surgical reduction because the metacarpal head may buttonhole through the volar soft tissue. The more vigorous the attempt at reduction, the more the tissue tightens around the metacarpal neck. Closed reduction should be attempted, however, by hyperextending the joint and gradually reducing the phalanx. If the joint is stable, buddy taping for 3 weeks is sufficient. As after any reduction, the joint should "feel" reduced, and motion should be free. If the joint does not feel reduced, soft-tissue interposition or an incomplete reduction should be suspected. Open reduction is then required. Referral is indicated if the joint is unstable.

### Bowler's Thumb

This is a traumatic digital neuroma that develops from the irritation of the bowling ball against the digital nerve on the web side of the thumb. Pain and tenderness are present over the affected nerve, and paresthesias may be present along the course of the nerve. A tender mass is usually present, and Tinel's sign may be positive. Rest and avoiding the offending activity are often curative. Changing the grip on the ball may also help, and protective devices are available to prevent recurrent irritation.

### Gamekeeper's Thumb, Skier's Thumb (Ruptured Ulnar Collateral Ligament)

The radial and ulnar collateral ligaments of the metacarpophalangeal joint of the thumb prevent subluxation of the proximal phalanx and provide the stability that is necessary for normal function. Either ligament may be chronically or acutely injured, but injury to the ulnar col-

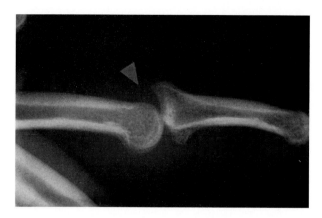

**Fig. 15–29.**
Proximal interphalangeal fracture-dislocation *(arrow)*.

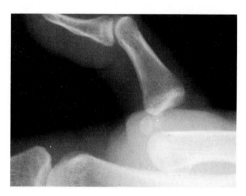

**Fig. 15–30.**
Metacarpophalangeal dislocation of the thumb. The sesamoid may seem to remain in the joint after an unsuccessful attempt at reduction.

lateral ligament is more common and potentially more serious because of its importance in pinch and grip.

The patient usually has a history of a sprained thumb, often from a fall on the hand. Chronic cases of ulnar collateral ligament (UCL) injury (called gamekeeper's thumb) may have a history of instability, weakness with pinch, and recurrent effusions of the metacarpophalangeal joint. Local tenderness over the ligament and a joint effusion are usually present on physical examination. The ligamentous laxity is usually manifested clinically and may be confirmed by stress roentgenograms (Fig. 15-31).

Surgical repair is usually indicated in acute cases of complete rupture of the UCL. Partial ruptures are treated by immobilization for 5 weeks in a cast that includes the thumb. Chronic cases without traumatic arthritis are treated by ligamentous reconstruction. If the disorder has progressed to the point where degenerative arthritis is present, arthrodesis of the metacarpophalangeal joint is usually necessary. Complete radial collateral ligament (RCL) injuries are safely treated with a thumb spica cast.

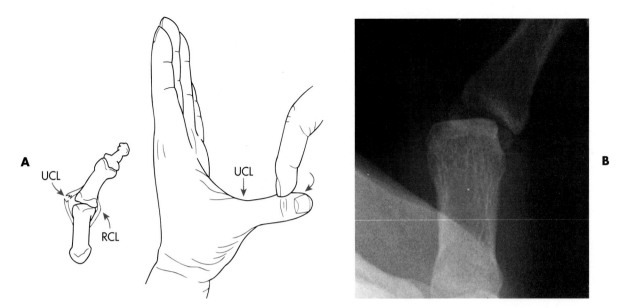

**Fig. 15–31.**
The ulnar collateral ligament (UCL) maintains stability of the thumb when pinching. Injury to this ligament may cause significant loss of strength of the thumb (**A**). Rupture of this ligament may require repair. (**B**), Stress roentgenogram of the thumb with complete UCL rupture. Injury to the radial collateral ligament (RCL) is less serious and can generally be treated with casting.

# INJURIES TO THE LOWER EXTREMITY

## The Knee

### Injuries to Ligaments

Along with fractures, these are the most important injuries to diagnose immediately. The first individual on the sideline has the best chance to evaluate the knee before spasm and swelling develop. As previously described (see Chapter 11), the knee should first be palpated for specific areas of tenderness. With the knee flexed 30 degrees, the collateral ligaments are evaluated, and Lachman's test is performed. If possible, the cruciate ligaments are then tested with the knee flexed 90 degrees. Any acute rapid swelling suggests an anterior cruciate ligament rupture, especially if a "pop" is felt at the time of injury. If only a minor strain is present, it may be possible for the athlete to return to activity, but any more severe injury should have a compression dressing and ice applied, and the activity should be ceased pending further evaluation.

Plain roentgenograms should always be performed. Stress films may be especially helpful in the adolescent with open growth plates. In this age group, epiphyseal fractures are more common than ligamentous injuries because the growth plate is weaker than the ligaments (Fig. 15-32).

### Injuries to the Meniscus

These are the most common of all knee injuries. They usually result from a twisting force applied to the knee with the extremity bearing weight. The athlete will experience sudden pain and is often unable to continue playing. Swelling develops gradually, in contrast to ligament injury, and may not be noticed until the following day. The pain may be localized to one joint line. The knee may actually lock if the meniscus is sufficiently torn and catches across the joint surface.

Suspected meniscus injuries are initially treated conservatively with a Robert Jones dressing, ice, quadriceps exercises, and elevation. Over the next several weeks, the response to rest and time will determine whether or not surgery will be necessary to repair or remove the torn meniscus.

### Rehabilitation

A program of progressively increasing exercises to improve strength and endurance is begun as soon as tolerated on all athletes with injured knees (see Chapter 11). Specific exercises to strengthen the quadriceps, hamstrings, and calf muscles are begun. Progressive range-of-motion exercises are added as tolerated, and the athlete is allowed to return to activities only when the effusion and pain have completely subsided and

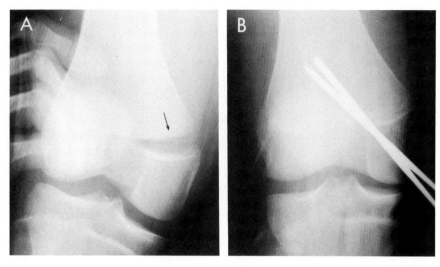

**Fig. 15–32.**
**A**, Stress roentgenogram of an epiphyseal fracture of the lower portion of the femur that easily simulates ligamentous disruption *(arrow)*. **B**, The same injury reduced and pinned.

strength, range of motion, and thigh circumference have returned to normal.

## The Ankle and Foot

### Ankle Sprains

The ankle sprain may be the most common of all athletic injuries. The lateral ligaments are the most commonly involved as a result of an inversion force (see Chapter 12). Mild to moderate sprains are best treated by early gentle motion (avoiding inversion) and exercise starting the day after the injury when pain begins to subside. Ice should be continued. Heat is never used. Peroneal muscle exercises are added and progressed against resistance as tolerated. More strenuous activity is allowed when the athlete is able to perform more vigorous activities such as hopping. Limited workouts may be resumed at this stage, but the ankle should always be taped. Return to full activity should not be allowed until there is full, pain-free motion and equal strength and the athlete is able to change direction quickly and jump without discomfort.

Treatment of severe sprains remains controversial. Although surgery, casting, and simple symptomatic treatment have all been recommended with good results, functional rehabilitation without surgery is the preferred treatment regardless of severity. Lace-up ankle stabilizers and taping are helpful.

### Wrapping and Taping

To prevent ankle injury, many physicians and trainers advise wrapping the uninjured ankle (Fig. 15-33). A reusable dressing may be applied by the athlete over a sock.

Although half of the support of tape loosens in 10 minutes, the athlete who has had previous injury will benefit from taping when activity is resumed. For this individual, wrapping is probably not adequate, and applying adhesive tape is necessary to prevent reinjury. Adhesive taping is more beneficial because it can be applied tighter and extended as high on the leg as necessary for protection.

Several taping techniques are commonly used. Each physician should become familiar with a single method and learn to apply it easily. The closed basket weave described by Gibney is commonly used (Fig. 15-34). The open basket weave is the same except that the tape does not overlap in front. The open method may be used in acute sprains with excessive swelling because the tape is not circumferential and allows for swelling and ankle motion. An elastic wrap is applied over the open taping method.

The closed basket weave may be supplemented by a heel lock taping system for added medial or lateral support (Fig. 15-35). With any method, the ankle is first prepared by shaving and spraying with adhesive spray or tincture of benzoin. Either 1- or 1½-inch tape is normally used. Many modifications of these techniques are used (Figs. 15-36 and 15-37). Sensitivity to benzoin is possible; it must be used with caution.

### Athlete's Foot

Many varieties of fungus affect the foot. The most common areas of involvement are between the toes and under the arch. Moisture and warmth predispose feet to the development of athlete's foot. Itching, redness, and burning are present. Allergy to stockings or shoe materials should be ruled out. Treatment is with one of the many commercial or prescription medicated powders available. The foot should be kept dry, and stockings may need to be changed often.

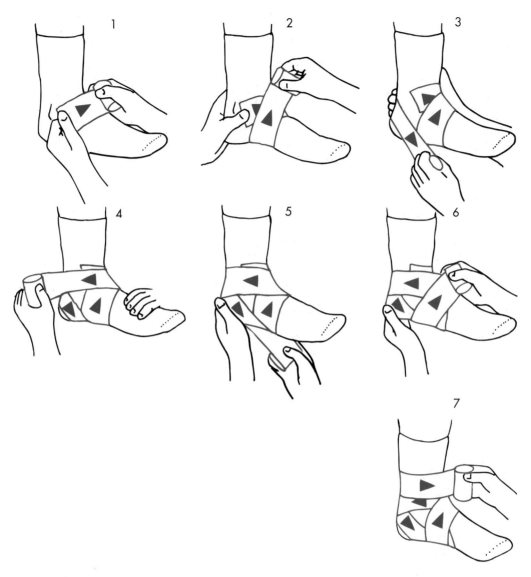

**Fig. 15–33.**
The "Louisiana" ankle wrap. Approximately 100 inches of webbed bandage is used. The patient sits on the table, holding the ankle at 90 degrees. The wrap may be applied over a stocking. Steps 1 and 2 secure the wrap; steps 3, 4, and 5 are the lateral and medial "heel locks" that prevent eversion and inversion, respectively. After step 6, the procedure is repeated. The wrap is then spiraled up over the ankle, as shown in step 7, and secured with tape. This technique may prevent needless ankle taping.

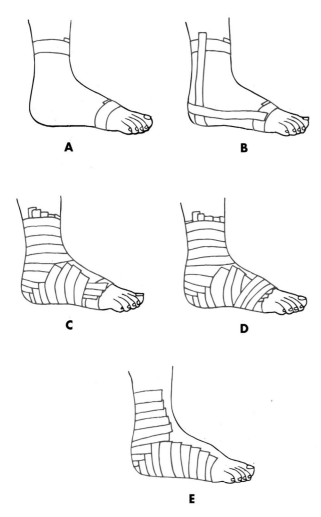

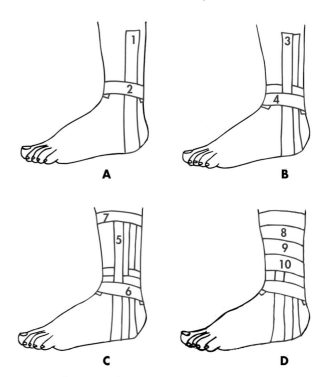

**Fig. 15–36.**
The modified Gibney technique. **A,** The circular strip completely encircles the leg, and the vertical strips may extend as high as necessary. **B,** Additional vertical and circular strips are added. **C,** A top circular strip (7) anchors the vertical strips. After the rest of the circular strips have been applied (**D**), heel locks should be added.

**Fig. 15–34.**
The closed basket weave taping technique. **A,** Two anchor strips are applied, one at the base of the gastrocnemius and one below the midfoot. **B,** The first stirrup and horizontal strips are applied. **C,** The finished weave. Close the strapping by alternating strips with stirrups. Overlap half the width of the tape. **D,** Apply three circular anchoring strips distally and add a set of medial and lateral heel locks (not shown). **E,** The open Gibney method. No heel lock system is used. Whatever method is used, avoid taping too low and avoid wrinkles.

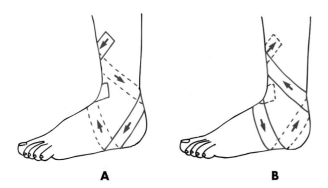

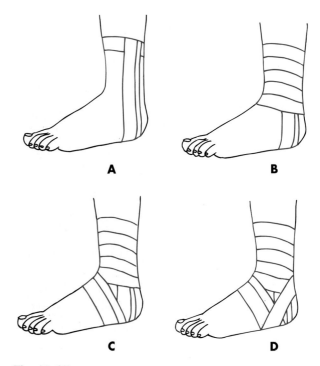

**Fig. 15–35.**
The heel lock system. **A,** The lateral heel lock that prevents eversion. **B,** The medial heel lock that prevents inversion. Both may be applied together in a continuous wrap.

**Fig. 15–37.**
A slightly quicker method than the Gibney technique uses an anchor and two stirrups (**A**), five or six circular strips (**B**), two or three arch strips (**C**), and a heel lock system (**D**).

## MISCELLANEOUS PROBLEMS

### Avulsion Fractures

Avulsions of the bony origin of muscles are common injuries in young athletes. The areas most commonly affected are: (1) the coracoid process, (2) the greater tuberosity of the humerus, (3) the lesser and greater trochanters, (4) the iliac apophysis, (5) the ischial tuberosity, (6) the anterior superior iliac spine, and (7) the transverse and spinous processes of the vertebrae (Fig. 15-38).

These injuries usually result from sudden muscular contraction or strain that causes the muscle to pull a portion of its bony attachment away from the main body of the bone. This causes sudden pain, and roentgenography usually reveals the injury.

Treatment will depend on the athlete and the area involved. The professional athlete may require open reduction and reattachment of the avulsed tendon. The recreational athlete is usually treated nonsurgically. Enough soft-tissue healing will occur to restore function. In spite of surgical repair, the skills of the professional athlete are sometimes diminished.

### Brachial Plexus Injuries

An injury that is common in American football players is sometimes referred to as the *burner* or *stinger*. This results from the vulnerability of the brachial plexus or cervical roots to trauma during contact sports. Two mechanisms of injury are described. The most common is a

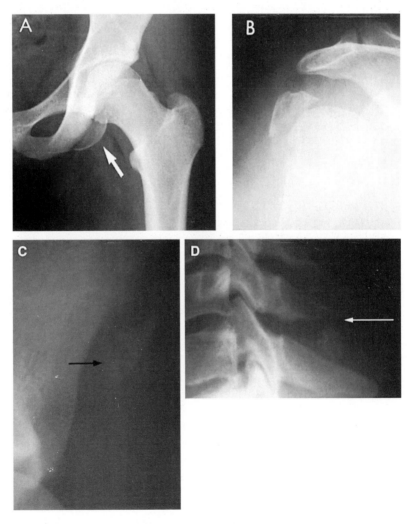

**Fig. 15–38.**
Avulsion fractures. **A**, The ischial tuberosity. **B**, The greater tuberosity of the humerus. **C**, The anterior superior iliac spine. **D**, The spinous process of C6 (clay-shoveler's fracture).

stretch or traction injury of the upper brachial plexus caused by sudden depression of the shoulder with extension or lateral deviation of the neck to the opposite side (Fig. 15-39). The upper plexus is usually involved. It is characterized by sudden unilateral burning pain originating in the neck and radiating to the shoulder, arm, and hand. It does not usually follow a specific dermatome. It may be accompanied by weakness of the affected area, especially the deltoid, rotator cuff, and biceps.

The second mechanism of injury is compression of cervical nerve roots at the foramen, resulting from extension and lateral bending of the neck toward the shoulder. This injury is more common in older athletes (college, professional), especially those whose intervertebral foramen may already be compromised as a result of degenerative disc disease. Cervical stenosis may also predispose the athlete to this problem.

The injury is sometimes graded according to resolution of symptoms. Grade I (neuropraxia) injuries are most common. Typically, there is transient pain and motor loss that resolves within minutes or hours without any anatomic damage. Grade II (axonotmesis) and III (neurotmesis) injuries are more severe, with evidence of nerve damage lasting for weeks or months.

### Evaluation

The player often comes off the field unable to move the arm. These symptoms are usually *unilateral*. Bilateral symptoms such as "burning hands syndrome" or symptoms involving the legs should cause concern for a *neck* injury. There is usually no neck pain with the burner. (Any patient with neck pain or symptoms of spine injury should not be moved without proper immobilization on a spine board.)

It is important to determine whether the injury is *outside* or *inside* the cervical spine. On-the-field screening should include an evaluation of: (1) the location of pain and tenderness; (2) the amount of pain with isometric contraction of neck muscles, (3) deltoid, biceps, and triceps strength, and (4) range of neck motion. The last should be evaluated carefully. Range of motion should not be tested if spine injury is suspected. When cervical spine injury has been ruled out, stretching the brachial plexus by pulling down the arm may elicit symptoms if the injury is the result of traction. There may also be tenderness in the supraclavicular fossa. Spurling's test (see Chapter 3) may be positive in the patient with a compression injury.

If there are any signs of neck injury, cervical spine films are taken. CT and MRI may be needed to rule out cord or cervical root involvement. If one or more cervical roots are involved, MRI studies may be helpful to determine if there are related disc changes. If not, a plexus injury is probably the cause, and clinical progress can be used to determine when there can be a return to sports. EMG is not helpful.

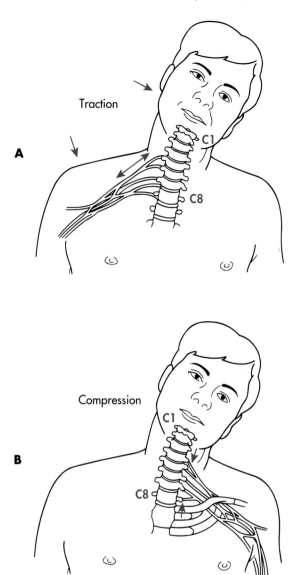

**Fig. 15–39.**
Traction of the brachial plexus (**A**) may cause symptoms of the stinger when the shoulder is depressed and the neck is bent laterally. A blow can also compress cervical nerve roots at the foramen (**B**), especially in older athletes whose foramina may be already narrowed by degenerative disc narrowing with osteophyte formation.

### Treatment

If the neck examination is negative and complete recovery (full strength and motion with no pain or tenderness) occurs in 1 to 2 minutes, the athlete may return to play. Stretching the plexus should not reproduce symptoms. In most cases, the symptoms from burners subside quickly; often they are not reported at all. A protective collar worn inside the shoulder pads may prevent further injury. Strengthening and range-of-motion exercises are recommended. Reinjury can be avoided with proper technique and good equipment.

### *Prognosis*

Most brachial plexus injuries are minor and recover in a short time without residuals. Athletes with disc degeneration or stenosis, however, are at greater risk of serious neurologic injury and may have to be excluded from further participation in contact sports.

### Turf Toe

This is a sprain of the volar plate and plantar capsule of the metatarsophalangeal joint (MPJ) of the great toe that is often caused by hyperextension. The incidence has increased with greater use of artificial playing surfaces. The capsular structures are stretched and cause painful swelling. The plantar surface is tender on palpation and extension. The injury may take several weeks to heal. The disorder is initially treated with ice and rest. A stiffer, solid shoe that inhibits movement of the forefoot may be tried, and figure-8 taping to limit motion is usually helpful. Some permanent loss of motion may result.

### The "Loose-Jointed" Athlete

During the physical examination of the athlete, especially the adolescent one, it is important to note any characteristics or physical problems that might predispose the individual to injury. One determination that should always be made is whether the athlete is vulnerable to ligamentous or musculotendinous injury. It is possible to make some predictions in this regard if the athlete has loose or tight ligaments. The value of this determination is that the loose-jointed athlete is at higher risk for ligamentous injuries. The "tight-jointed" athlete is more vulnerable to muscular injuries. Some of the criteria used to determine whether an athlete is loose-jointed are as follows:

1. Greater than 100 degrees of MPJ hyperextension
2. Greater than 30 degrees of ankle dorsiflexion with the knees straight
3. The ability to touch the thumb to the forearm (Fig. 15-40)
4. Greater than 15 to 20 degrees of knee or elbow hyperextension
5. The ability to touch the palms flat to the floor with the knees locked
6. The ability to stand with the feet turned out 180 degrees

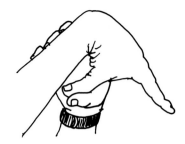
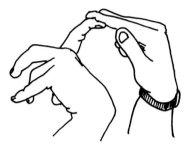

**Fig. 15–40.**
Tests for loose-jointedness.

Loose-jointedness is often familial and affects the female athlete more often than the male. Laxity often diminishes during the late teenage years, but before that time the athlete is vulnerable to injury, especially at the knee. This is commonly the result of a subluxing patella or ligament damage.

The goal of treatment is prevention of injury. Tight joints withstand stress better but often suffer more severe muscular injuries. These athletes require stretching exercises to increase flexibility and avoid muscular strain. The athlete with loose joints, however, needs strengthening exercises to avoid ligamentous injury and sprain.

### The Hip Pointer

This injury is a contusion of the iliac crest and is often seen in football players. It can be extremely painful, and a large hematoma often develops. Activities are allowed as tolerated, and a protective pad should be worn over the involved iliac crest for the remainder of the season.

## BIBLIOGRAPHY

Adams JE: Bone injuries in very young athletes, *Clin Orthop* 58:129, 1969.

Albright JP et al: Nonfatal cervical spine injuries in interscholastic football, *JAMA* 236:1243, 1976.

Clanton TO, Coupe KJ: Hamstring strains in athletes: diagnosis and treatment, *J Am Acad Orthop Surg* 6:237-248, 1998.

Cofield RH, Simonet WT: The shoulder in sports, *Mayo Clin Proc* 59:157-164, 1984.

Dimsdale JE et al: Postexercise peril: plasma catecholamines and exercise, *JAMA* 251(5):630-632, 1984.

Dobyns JH et al: Bowler's thumb: diagnosis and treatment, *J Bone Joint Surg Am* 54:751-755, 1972.

Elson RA: Rupture of the central slip of the extensor tendon of the finger. A test for early diagnosis, *J Bone Joint Surg Br* 68:229, 1986.

Fries JF et al: Relationship of running to musculoskeletal pain with age: a six-year longitudinal study, *Arthritis Rheum* 39:64-72, 1996.

Goldfarb SJ, Kaeding CC: Bilateral acute-on-chronic exertional lateral compartment syndrome of the leg: a case report and review of the literature, *Clin J Sports Med* 7:59-62, 1997.

Heyman P: Injuries to the ulnar collateral ligament of the thumb metacarpophalangeal joint, *J Am Acad Orthop Surg* 5:224-229, 1997.

Ireland ML, Hutchinson MR: Upper extremity injuries in young athletes, *Clin Sports Med* 14:533-569, 1995.

Jackson DW, Feagin JA: Quadriceps contusions in young athletes, *J Bone Joint Surg Am* 55:95-105, 1973.

James SL: Running injuries to the knee, *J Am Acad Orthop Surg* 3:309-318, 1995.

James SL, Bates BT, Osternig LR: Injuries to runners, *Am J Sports Med* 6:40-50, 1978.

Levitz CL, Reilly PJ, Torg JS: The pathomechanics of chronic, recurrent cervical nerve root neuropraxia, the chronic burner syndrome, *Am J Sports Med* 25:73-76, 1997.

Light TR: Buttress pinning techniques, *Orthop Rev* 10:49-55, 1981.

Maffulli N et al: Acute haemarthrosis of the knee in athletes, *J Bone Joint Surg Br* 75:945-949, 1993.

Martin SD, Martin TL: Running injuries. In Kelly WN et al, editors: *Textbook of rheumatology* (Update 22), New York, 1996, WB Saunders.

Manfroy PP, Ashton-Miller JA, Wojtys EM: The effect of exercise, prewrap, and athletic tape on the maximal active and passive ankle resistance to ankle inversion, *Am J Sports Med* 25:156-163, 1997.

Mannarino F, Sexson S: The significance of intracompartmental pressures in the diagnosis of chronic exertional compartment syndrome, *Orthopedics* 12:1415, 1989.

O'Donoghue DH: *Treatment of injuries of athletes*, ed 3, Philadelphia, 1976, WB Saunders.

Teitz CC, Hu SS, Arendt EA: The female athlete: evaluation and treatment of sports-related problems, *J Am Acad Orthop Surg* 5:87-96, 1997.

Torg JS put bkc europraxia of the cervical spinal cord with transient quadriplegia, *J Bone Joint Surg Am* 68:1354, 1986.

Torg JS, Glasgow SG: Criteria for return to contact activities after cervical spine injury, *Clin J Sport Med* 1:12-26, 1991.

Tullos HS, King JW: Lesions of the pitching arm in adolescents, *JAMA* 220:264, 1972.

# CHAPTER 16

# Radiologic Aspects of Orthopedic Diseases

Dean F. Tamisiea, M.D.

This chapter contains a radiologist's viewpoints and suggestions regarding the interpretation of bone roentgenograms. It is hoped this will serve as a useful and practical guide for the busy family practitioner. Principles concerning roentgenographic positioning, anatomy, and pathology will be presented by utilizing a regional anatomic approach.

Additionally, the musculoskeletal applications of specialized radiologic modalities are discussed. This includes comments on nuclear medicine procedures, diagnostic ultrasound, arthrography, xerography, angiography, and standard radiographic tomography. Importantly, the more advanced imaging technologies of computed tomography (CT) and magnetic resonance imaging (MRI) as they pertain to the evaluation of orthopedic problems are detailed.

## GENERAL CONSIDERATIONS OF ROENTGENOGRAPHIC BONE ANATOMY

Before beginning a detailed discussion of regional roentgenographic anatomy and pathology, a consideration of pertinent radiologic bone anatomy is important. A bone can be evaluated according to its various components (Fig. 16-1).

### Epiphysis

The primary growth center of a bone is termed the *epiphysis*. It contributes to the growth in length of the bone. It, as well as the following components, can be affected and changed in appearance by congenital, metabolic, nutritional, traumatic, and other disease processes.

### Physis

The radiolucent band between the epiphysis and metaphysis constitutes the *physis*, or epiphyseal cartilage plate. It is formed in part by the zone of provisional calcification.

### Metaphysis

The *metaphysis* is characteristically splayed or funnel shaped. It is a common site for the development of benign and malignant lesions.

### Diaphysis

The longer tubular segment of bone forms the *diaphysis*. The constituent parts include the central medullary cavity and spongiosa; and the dense cortex, lined internally by the endosteum and covered externally by periosteum.

### Apophysis

There are several *apophyses* found throughout the skeletal system, the best example being the greater trochanter of the proximal portion of the femur. They do not contribute to bone growth but are considered accessory ossification centers. They tend to appear

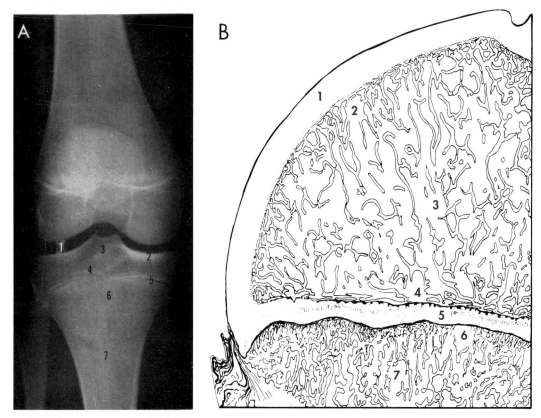

**Fig. 16–1.**

Anatomy of a bone. **A**, Radiologic terms: *(1)* articular cartilage does not show in the film; *(2)* white outline of the subarticular margin of the epiphysis; *(3)* epiphysis; *(4)* increased density of the terminal plate, inner bone margin of the epiphysis; *(5)* epiphyseal line, strip of lesser density, epiphyseal plate, diaphyseal-epiphyseal gap (roentgenographically, these terms exclude the recently calcified cartilage, which appears as part of the metaphysis); *(6)* metaphysis, including both calcified cartilage and newly formed bone, *(7)* diaphysis or shaft. **B**, Histologic terms: *(1)* articular cartilage; *(2)* compact bone of subarticular margin; *(3)* epiphysis, spongy bone; *(4)* terminal plate; *(5)* physis, epiphyseal disc, growth cartilage (histologically, these terms include the calcified cartilage); *(6)* metaphysis, including only newly formed bone of primary ossification; *(7)* spongy bone of diaphysis. (From Pyle SI, Hoerr NL: *Radiographic atlas of skeletal development of the knee*, Springfield, Ill, 1955, Charles C Thomas Publishers. Used by permission.)

later than the epiphyses in normal bone development and form protrusions to which ligaments and tendons attach.

Epiphyses and apophyses occasionally fail to unite to the parent bone, and this results in unfused ossicles or accessory bones that are often misinterpreted as fractures. Most of these will be discussed under regional anatomic variations. When confronted with such problems as accessory bones, *An Atlas of Normal Roentgen Variants That May Simulate Disease* (Keats, 1992) and *Borderlands of the Normal and Early Pathologic in Skeletal Roentgenology* (Kohler and Zimmer, 1993) are excellent reference sources.

In addition to the status of nonfusion, epiphyseal and apophyseal centers can be divided before they unite, causing further confusion with fractures. Sesa-

moid bones, as seen in the hands and feet, can also be divided.

## Bone Vessels

Roentgenograms provide only indirect evidence of the presence of blood vessels in bone: the nutrient canals and foramina. They enter the medullary cavity by way of foramina, most often near the midshaft of a long bone, and result in radiolucent channels. When viewed on the roentgenogram, these channels can be confused with a fracture. Prominent nutrient canals are often seen in the diaphyses of the femur and tibia. Y-shaped nutrient canals occur in the midportion of the iliac bones of the pelvis and in the subspinous region of the scapulae.

# ANALYTIC APPROACH TO BONE CHANGES

## General Considerations

This section discusses some basic fundamentals and principles related to bone roentgenograms, rather than going into a great deal of confusing anatomic and pathologic detail. The first and foremost rule is that every roentgenogram is abnormal until it is proved, after thorough examination, that everything is normal. It may not work all of the time, but it encourages as complete a search of the film as possible. This results in two important objectives: first, it eliminates the method of instantaneous pattern recognition; second, it prods the physician to search for even the slightest, most subtle change in bone roentgenographic patterns.

It is important to avoid tunnel vision: one should look at the "whole picture," from the corners of the film to the center. This involves evaluating separately the soft tissues, joints, bone density, architecture, and trabecular patterns. Scrutinizing the medullary cavity and spongiosa as well as the cortex, periosteum, and endosteum is also necessary to get the overall picture.

In other words, an analytic approach should be attempted by evaluating each specific feature of bone. Each detail must be visualized separately. An obvious fracture catches one's attention, and the tendency is to forget the remainder of the picture, possible missing an associated but unsuspected dislocation or even an early destructive tumor.

Taking two views of a bone at right angles is an important law in radiology. Diagnostic interpretations should never be made on the basis of one view. The physician should not hesitate to obtain additional projections of the suspicious area if he is convinced that something is wrong. Comparative films of the opposite side are also often helpful, especially in younger patients whose growth centers cause more than enough confusion. And if the roentgenograms remain normal to the eye, but clinical suspicion persists, the patient must return in 7 to 10 days for repeated films, because it is not uncommon for a stress fracture, radial head fracture, or early osteomyelitis to have delayed appearances roentgenographically.

Once a bone lesion is discovered on an x-ray film, the physician is in the challenging position of forming a differential diagnosis. At first, the spectrum of possibilities might be quite broad, but by correlating historical, physical, and laboratory findings with the roentgenographic discovery, the spectrum can be narrowed to a few diseases and will, in most instances, lead to the correct diagnosis.

To permit the most accurate diagnosis, the differential list should be based on certain specific bone responses that are most characteristic of the disease process. There are various distinctive, visible reactions that bone may have to singular disease entities. These include the pattern of bone destruction or production, the type of periosteal reaction, and soft tissue involvement (if any).

Unfortunately, there are more diseases affecting bone than there are responses that bone can create. Consequently, there are more roentgenographic similarities than differences among the various bony lesions. For example, the periosteal reaction usually associated with Ewing's sarcoma, characteristically described as "onion skin," quite often occurs with osteomyelitis.

Conversely, there are specific disease processes that produce more than one kind of predictable bone reaction. Such is the case with osteomyelitis, which has a periosteal response that can appear benign but can also mimic malignant changes.

Any office or clinic that performs diagnostic x-ray film studies should have appropriate references available for proper positioning of the patient. Several technical books may be found to assist the nurse or technician when examining the various skeletal regions. A three-volume set by Ballinger, *Merrill's Atlas of Roentgenographic Positions* (1995), is highly recommended.

## Specific Parameters

There are certain specific parameters of bone that need careful attention. A systematic approach, employed in the process of evaluating these parameters, can lead to a logical conclusion. Among the criteria to be analyzed are an increase or decrease in bone density, alterations in osseous texture (trabecular pattern), periosteal reactions, and the conditions of the cortex, endosteum, and medullary spongiosa.

If any of these changes is observed, then the abnormality should be studied in terms of its size and configuration and the sharpness of its margins (transition zone). The specific bone involved and the position of the lesion within that bone (epiphysis, metaphysis, or diaphysis) should also be noted. For example, leukemia, metastatic neuroblastoma, a benign simple cyst, and Brodie's abscess all have a predilection for the metaphysis, whereas a chondroblastoma typically involves the epiphysis.

This is a simple, general outline, and many more particulars come into play. But by developing this type of approach, the many clues offered will help determine the nature of the pathologic process and place the lesion into a certain category (e.g., benign, malignant, infectious, traumatic, or metabolic). Table 16-1 lists some of the specific characteristics of different bone lesions.

There are two parameters that require more expanded discussion: types of bone destruction and periosteal reaction.

**TABLE 16–1.**

General Characteristics of Different Bone Lesions

*Characteristics of benign bone lesions*
Sclerotic margins (narrow transition zone)
Homogeneous periosteal reaction
Expansion of an intact cortex

*Characteristics of solitary malignant bone lesions*
Permeative or moth-eaten destruction (wide transition zone)
Irregular, sometimes spiculated periosteal reaction
Preferential metaphyseal location
Extraosseous extension with soft-tissue mass and occasional fluffy
    calcifications

*Characteristics of metastatic lesions*
Absence of periosteal reaction
Moth-eaten destruction of medulla and cortex
Preferential diaphyseal location
Pathologic fractures
Multiple bone involvement

*Characteristics of infection*
Often irregular periosteal reaction, no spiculation
Bone destruction variable
Diaphyseal involvement, often involving long segments
Destruction of adjacent cartilage, crossing joints (majority of
    malignant neoplasms lack this ability)
Sequestration and involucrum formation

## Patterns of Bone Destruction

Three roentgenographic patterns of bone destruction have been described, according to Lodwick: geographic, moth-eaten, and permeative (1971).

1. Geographic bone destruction is distinguished by single or multiple sharply marginated, relatively large, punched-out holes. Multiple myeloma and histiocytosis X (eosinophilic granuloma, Letterer-Siwe disease, and Hand-Schüller-Christian disease) tend to fit this pattern.
2. Moth-eaten bone destruction involves a lesion containing multiple coalescing holes of moderate size that suggests a somewhat aggressive process. Osteomyelitis and less pathogenic tumors may exhibit this form of destruction.
3. Permeative bone destruction is seen when the bony alterations are characterized by multiple tiny holes that become smaller and fewer in number near the periphery of the lesion; as a result there is a wide transition zone from abnormal to normal bone. This will be seen in aggressive tumors and poorly localized infections.

No matter what type of osseous resorption is taking place, as much as 50% of the bone must be destroyed before becoming evident roentgenographi-

cally. Radionuclide bone scans constitute a much more sensitive examination for determining the presence of bone replacement by the tumor or infection. The more advanced nuclear technology of single proton emission computed tomography (SPECT) imaging further enhances this lesion detection sensitivity. In one comparative study, the accuracy of isotope imaging with technetium $^{99m}$Tc phosphate complexes for skeletal lesion detection was 98%, as compared with 28% for standard roentgenography (Siberstein, Saenger, Tofe, 1973). Because of this fact, the use of skeletal roentgenographic surveys has declined in favor of nuclear scans. Nevertheless, although the sensitivity of scanning is high, its specificity is low, and therefore roentgenographic studies of the abnormal isotope areas are mandatory. MRI can be a helpful adjunct in the determination of the presence of marrow replacement by metastatic lesions.

## Types of Periosteal Reactions

When the outer periosteal membrane of bone is irritated, its constituent osteoblastic cells react by producing new bone. This new bone can take on either a solid or an interrupted appearance, and the specific form can assist in identifying the inciting cause (Table 16-2).

Solid periosteal reactions are usually indicative of a benign process. The new bone is consistently uniform in density. As seen in Table 16-2, the thickness and marginal characteristics vary according to the precipitating factor.

The interrupted forms of periosteal reactions are more commonly found in malignant disease, although benign lesions are occasionally responsible. The classic spiculated or sunburst pattern of osteogenic sarcoma and the lamellated or "onion skin" periosteal reaction of Ewing's sarcoma come under this heading (see Table 16-2).

Of the various types of periosteal reactions, Codman's triangle is of special interest. This form is produced by a lifting of the periosteum, which causes a break in its continuity and forms an angle. Thought to be pathognomonic of malignancy at one time, it is now known to develop in benign diseases as well. The sign can be induced by underlying infiltrating tumor cells, pus, or hemorrhage.

One other interesting periosteal condition is hypertrophic pulmonary osteoarthropathy. The uniform, thin but solid, undulating new bone, often associated with bone pain, is a relatively uncommon roentgenographic finding. It is seen in individuals suffering from benign and malignant thoracic tumors, chronic obstructive pulmonary disease, and chronic lung infections. The exact mechanism is uncertain, but it may be related either to decreased arterial oxygen tension or to an unrecog-

**TABLE 16–2.**

Roentgenographic Types of Periosteal Reactions*

| Types | Examples |
| --- | --- |
| *Solid periosteal reaction* | |
| Thin | Eosinophilic granuloma, osteoid osteoma |
| Thin undulating | Hypertrophic pulmonary osteoarthropathy |
| Dense undulating | Vascular |
| Dense elliptical (with destruction) | Osteoid osteoma |
| Cloaking | Long-standing malignancy |
| Chronic infection | |
| | |
| *Interrupted periosteal reaction* | |
| Perpendicular (spiculated or sunburst) | Osteosarcoma, Ewing's sarcoma, infection |
| Lamellated (onion skin) | Osteosarcoma, Ewing's sarcoma, infection |
| Amorphous | Malignant tumors |
| Codman's triangle | Malignant tumors, infection, hemorrhage |

*From Edeiken J, Hodes PJH: *Roentgen diagnosis of diseases of bone*, Baltimore, 1967, Williams & Wilkins. Used by permission.

nized humoral substance that mediates connective tissue proliferation. The long bones of the forearms and lower extremities and the distal ends of the metacarpal and metatarsal bones are most commonly involved. Clubbing of the fingers and toes may occur, and arthritic symptoms may be manifested.

# REGIONAL ANATOMIC AND PATHOLOGIC ROENTGENOGRAPHY

## Cervical Spine

### Roentgenographic Examination

The standard roentgenographic views of the cervical spine include anteroposterior, lateral, and both posterior oblique views as well as an open-mouth anteroposterior projection of the odontoid process and the first two cervical vertebral segments (Fig. 16-2). The majority of cervical spine studies are performed for the evaluation of trauma. In the more severely injured individual, the most important views are a cross-table horizontal beam lateral image and an anteroposterior supine film. By keeping patient movement to a minimum, potentially fatal spinal cord injury is prevented.

On the lateral exposure, C7 and occasionally C6 will often be excluded, especially in heavy, short-necked individuals. In such instances it becomes necessary to depress the shoulders by gentle but firm downward traction of the arms. If the cervicothoracic junction still has not been adequately visualized and severe injury to the neck has been excluded, a so-called "swimmer's view" may be obtained. The patient lies in a prone-oblique position with the higher tube-side arm above the head and the lower table-side arm beside the body. The x-ray tube is angled 15 to 20 degrees toward the feet.

There are occasions when other special projections can be of assistance. Flexion and extension lateral views will often reveal minor degrees of subluxations resulting from damage to ligaments.

Dr. Don Weir of St. Louis University developed the "pillar view" for better evaluation of the lateral articulating masses, the superior and inferior articulating facets, and their intervening joints. Moreover, this view brings into focus the anterior and posterior margins of the lamina (Fig. 16-3). The film is produced with the patient supine. Each side is done separately. The head is turned slightly to one side, with the x-ray tube angled toward the feet 35 to 45 degrees and centered over the middle to lower vertebrae. The opposite side is then examined in a similar manner.

### Roentgenographic Anatomy

To properly evaluate the cervical spine, a thorough understanding of its roentgenographic anatomy is an absolute prerequisite. Each component of the individual vertebrae should be appraised separately on all views.

**Odontoid View.**   Of the seven cervical vertebrae, the first two are anatomically distinct. The odontoid represents a superior extension of the body of C2 and is actually the vestigial body of C1. On the anteroposterior open-mouth film, the odontoid should be analyzed in terms of its position between the two lateral articulating masses of C1 (see Fig. 16-2, *D*). The spaces between the lateral edges of the odontoid and the medial borders of the C1 articulating masses should be equal. However, minor degrees of rotation can produce spurious inequality of these interval distances. How can one determine this? The alignment of the densities of the

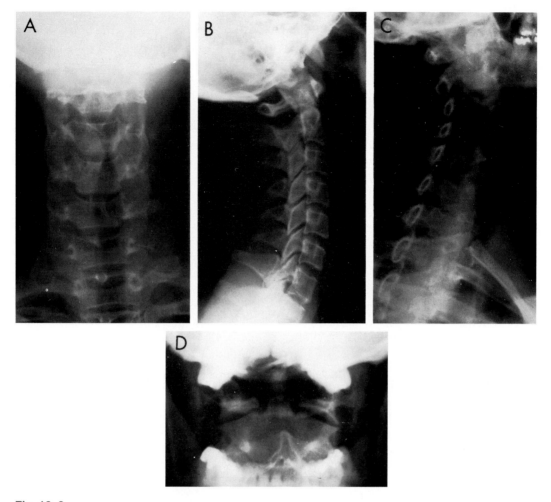

**Fig. 16–2.**
Normal roentgenographic study of the cervical spine. **A,** Anteroposterior view. **B,** Lateral view. **C,** Right oblique view. **D,** Odontoid view.

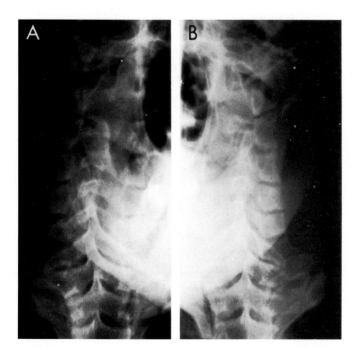

**Fig. 16–3.**
Pillar views of the cervical spine. Right (**A**) and left (**B**) projections.

spinous processes of C1 and C2 can be seen. If the C2 spinous process is to one side or the other, then rotation is present.

Also on viewing the odontoid film, the transverse processes and lateral borders of the articulating masses of C1 and C2 should not be overlooked. The horizontal joints between the atlantoaxial articulating masses should be symmetric (see Fig. 16-2, *D*).

Confusing artifacts superimposed on the odontoid can be misleading and can result in misinterpretation of fractures of this structure. The inferior margin of the posterior arch of C1 can overlie the base of the odontoid and create a "Mach" effect, a radiolucent line produced by overlap of the edges of two bones. In a similar fashion, the space between the two incisor teeth may lay over the odontoid and yield an artifactual vertical cleft (Fig. 16-4).

It is not unusual for the odontoid process to be completely obscured by the base of the occipital bone if the head is held too far in extension. In such circumstances, have the view repeated with the patient's head slightly more flexed.

**Anteroposterior View.** The straight anteroposterior film of the cervical spine demonstrates several specific structures. The vertical alignment of the spinous processes as well as the lateral margins of the articulating masses should be followed. The uncinate processes are the small triangular projections arising from the posterolateral margins of the vertebral bodies that by their apposition form the uncovertebral joints (also termed joints of Luschka). These establish the anterior boundaries of the intervertebral foramina. As synovial joints, they can be involved by degenerative osteoarthritis and produce the spurs that encroach on and narrow the foramina so as to result in impingement of the cervical nerve roots. In addition, being lined with synovium, they are subject to the alteration of rheumatoid arthritis and rheumatoid spondylitis. However, the foramina are best evaluated on the oblique films.

**Lateral View.** Several important points must be remembered when viewing the lateral projection of the cervical spine (see Fig. 16-2, *B*). Alignments of the anterior and posterior borders of the vertebral bodies, alignment of the lateral articulating masses, and alignment of the spinolaminar line are studied. The latter is formed by the anterior margins of the spinous processes, which also describe the posterior surface of the spinal canal. The superior extension of this line is in direct alignment with the posterior margin of the foramen magnum.

The distance between a line drawn through the posterior borders of the vertebral bodies and the spinolaminar line will provide the anteroposterior width of the spinal canal. This should measure no less than 13 mm from C3 through C7, being normally wider above C3. Any measurement less than this suggests the possibility of spinal stenosis.

The clivus, which is a dense line at the base of the skull continuous with the dorsum sella, is a helpful indicator for confirming normal craniovertebral alignment and should be included, at least in part, on all lateral studies of the cervical spine. A line drawn along its margin will pass through the posterior third of the odontoid.

The superior and inferior articulating facets will ordinarily be well visualized on the lateral film. The posterior borders of the lateral articulating masses should form a straight line (see Fig. 16-2, *B*). If there is a slight offset, a facetal dislocation must be considered, although slight rotation can give a similar appearance. The view should be repeated if there is any confusion, and tomography should be considered if the problem persists.

Measurement of the space between the anterior border of the odontoid and the posterior margin of the anterior arch of C1 is mandatory. This is an indicator of a possible transverse ligament tear and should measure no more than 5 mm in children and 3 mm in adults in neutral, flexion, and extension positions.

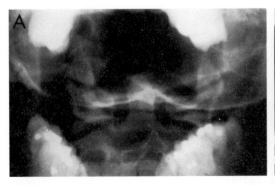 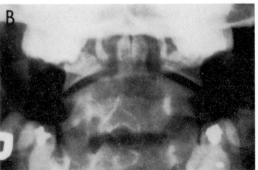

**Fig. 16–4.**
Artifacts over the odontoid process simulating fractures. **A**, Anterior arch of C1. **B**, Cleft of the incisor teeth.

Finally, evaluation of the lateral cervical spine film is incomplete without an analysis of the prevertebral soft tissues. There are minor differences in this measurement from physician to physician and from patient to patient, but the width of the soft tissues at the level of the inferior margin of the C3 body should not exceed 5 to 7 mm. Any increase in this measurement indicates swelling from hemorrhage or infection.

**Oblique Views.** The intervertebral foramina and surrounding elements, including the pedicles and uncinate processes, are the most important components demonstrated on the oblique views. The foramina on the right side are visualized on the left posterior oblique projection; those on the left are visualized on the right posterior oblique film (see Fig. 16-2, *C*).

### Trauma

Recognition of an abnormal cervical spine should be a relatively simple task once normal roentgenographic anatomy has been mastered. The primary objective, after a traumatic lesion has been identified, will be the establishment of whether or not the condition is stable. The stability of a fracture is best determined by grouping the type of injury according to the mechanisms of trauma, which are outlined in Table 16-3. From this classification, a statement of the instability of the injury can be made (Table 16-4).

**Flexion Injuries.** There are a variety of flexion injuries, and these are described below:

*Subluxation.* The roentgenographic findings in this stable lesion may be minimal, often requiring flexion and extension lateral views for confirmation. The body and posterior elements remain intact (that is, show no fracture). However, there is major soft-tissue involvement. The interspinous and posterior longitudinal ligaments as well as the interfacetal joint capsules are disrupted at the affected level. This allows the involved vertebral body to rotate anteriorly about its anterior and inferior corner, along with upward and forward displacement of its inferior articular facet on the lower adjacent vertebra's superior articular facet. The interspinous distance widens, and the inferior intervertebral disc space narrows anteriorly and widens posteriorly. These alterations are accentuated on the flexion film (Fig. 16-5). In children under 8 years of age, with the head held in flexion, the second cervical vertebra will normally be displaced anteriorly over C3. This malalignment must not be mistaken for subluxation.

*Bilateral Interfacetal Dislocation.* A more severe form of subluxation, bilateral interfacetal dislocation represents a truly unstable situation. The inferior articular

**TABLE 16–3.**

Classification of Cervical Spine Injuries According to the Mechanisms of Injury*

*Flexion*
Subluxation
Bilateral interfacetal dislocation
Simple wedge fracture
Flexion teardrop fractures
Clay-shoveler's fracture

*Flexion-rotation*
Unilateral interfacetal dislocation
Vertical compression
Bursting fractures
    Jefferson's C1
    Bursting fractures, other levels

*Extension*
 Posterior neural arch fracture
Extension teardrop fracture
Hangman's fracture

*From Harris JH Jr: *Semin Roentgenol* 13:53-68, 1978. Used by permission.

**TABLE 16–4.**

Classification of Cervical Spine Injuries Based on Stability*

*Stable*
Subluxation
Simple wedge fracture
Unilateral interfacetal dislocation
Bursting fracture, except Jefferson's fracture of C1
Clay-shoveler's fracture

*Unstable*
Bilateral interfacetal dislocation
Flexion teardrop fracture
Jefferson's bursting fracture of C1
Hangman's fracture
Extension teardrop fracture, unstable in extension but stable in
    flexion

*From Harris JH Jr: *Semin Roentgenol* 13:53-68, 1978. Used by permission.

facets of the involved vertebra move not only up and forward but also over the superior articular facet of the distal vertebra and come to rest within the intervertebral foramina. Oblique projections will be necessary to establish the diagnosis, but these have to be done with extreme caution. The changes on the x-ray film are related to a force sufficient to rupture all of the surrounding supporting ligaments at the level of the displaced vertebra. Occasionally, there will be an associated avulsion fracture.

*Compression Fractures.* Forceful flexion of the neck can result in an uncomplicated, wedge-shaped compression fracture of one and sometimes two or three vertebral bodies. Because they are stable, extension and flexion films are permissible.

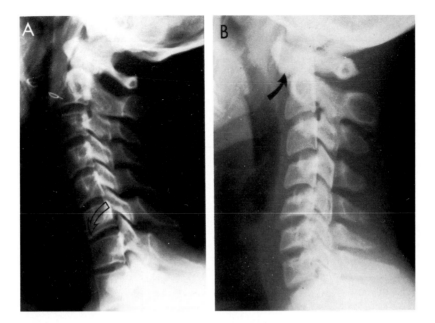

**Fig. 16–5.**
Subluxation injuries of the cervical spine. **A**, Mild subluxation of C6 and C7. **B**, Atlantoaxial subluxation. Note the increased width of space between the odontoid and the anterior arch of C1 in **B**.

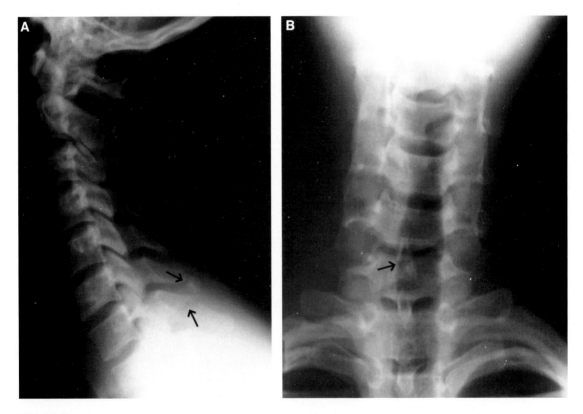

**Fig. 16–6.**
Clay-shoveler's fracture of the cervical spine. **A**, A lateral view defines spinous process fractures of C6 and C7 *(arrows)*. **B**, An AP projection demonstrates a "double" spinous process of C6, suggesting a fracture *(arrow)*.

***Flexion Teardrop Fracture.*** Considered the most dangerous and unstable of all cervical spine injuries, flexion teardrop fractures are diagnosed on the cross-table lateral film only, with no indications or justification for acquiring further studies. The name of the lesion is derived from the fact that there is a fracture through the inferior and anterior corner of the body, but the major component is comminution of the body. The posterior fragments become displaced backward into the spinal cord, with consequential acute and severe neurologic deficits. Often the posterior neural arch is also fractured.

***Clay-Shoveler's Fracture.*** This lesion is named for the injury acquired by people in occupations that require heavy lifting. This injury consists of a fracture through the spinous process of either C6 or C7 (Fig. 16-6). There is no significant ligamentous damage, and therefore a stable condition exists. Because C7 is sometimes difficult to project on the lateral film, the fracture can be missed. A clue might be apparent on the frontal film, where an extraspinous process fragment is sometimes evident as the result of inferior displacement. An unfused apophysis of a spinous process must not be misinterpreted as a fracture (Fig. 16-7).

**Flexion-Rotation Injuries.** When the cervical spine is subjected to a rotational force in addition to flexion, a unilateral interfacetal dislocation may be observed (Fig. 16-8). An inferior articular facet of one body is displaced over the adjacent superior articular facet of the next inferior vertebra on one side only. The dislocated facet is more or less locked in place, but because of associated ligament damage the lesion may be unstable; therefore, flexion and extension views are contraindicated. Oblique projections are most productive in identifying the displaced facet, but it may be suggested on the lateral film when the margins of the facets of a single vertebra do not superimpose on one another as the result of rotation. Additionally, a line drawn through the posterior borders of the bodies is offset at the level of the suspected injury.

**Extension Injuries.** Various extension injuries are described as follows:

***Posterior Neural Arch Fractures.*** The neural arch of one vertebra may be compressed between the posterior elements of the two adjoining vertebrae during

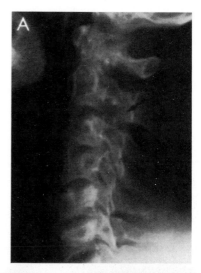

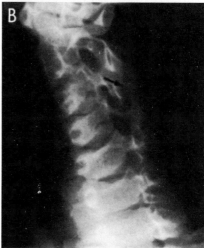

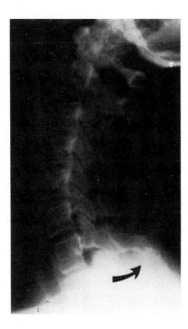

**Fig. 16–7.**
An unfused apophysis of the spinous process of C7 simulates a fracture *(arrow).*

**Fig. 16–8.**
Unilateral interfacetal dislocation. **A**, Lateral view. **B**, Oblique view.

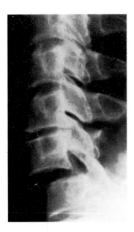

**Fig. 16–9.**
Posterior neural arch fracture.

maximal forced extension. A unilateral or bilateral fracture may be sustained. If bilateral, the fragment can be displaced posteriorly, yet there will be no encroachment on the neural canal; thus the situation is a stable one (Fig. 16-9).

***Extension Teardrop Fracture.*** Similar to the flexion variety, an extension teardrop fracture demonstrates a triangular-shaped fragment at the anterior-inferior margin of the body, most often involving C2, although other levels are affected (Fig. 16-10). However, the injury is not quite as severe because there is no posterior involvement. When the neck is held in flexion, there is stability of the spine because the posterior ligament complex is intact. However, instability occurs during extension since the minor fragment remains attached to the anterior longitudinal ligament but not to the parent body.

***Hangman's Fracture-Dislocation of C2.*** This lesion consists of vertical disruption of both pedicles of C2 and is created by flexion forces against the extended vertebrae. The body of C2 is thrust forward over C3, with concomitant rupture of both the anterior and the posterior longitudinal ligaments, giving rise to an unstable injury (Fig. 16-11).

**Vertical Compression Fractures.** A considerable force directed through the vertical axis of the spine (such as a large object falling on top of the head or a diving injury) can produce the so-called bursting fractures of the cervical vertebrae. The least common type is the Jefferson fracture of C1. The anterior and posterior aspects of the ring are fractured on both sides, with bilateral lateral displacement of the fragments. This unstable injury can be apparent on the open-mouth anteroposterior film, but more reliably is distinguished on

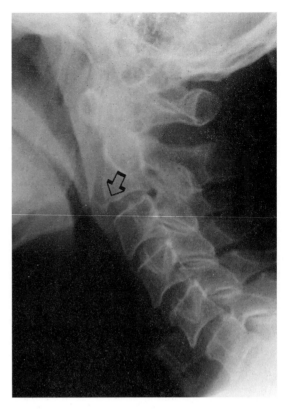

**Fig. 16–10.**
Extension teardrop fracture of C-2 *(arrow).*

the lateral roentgenogram where the fractures are seen to extend through the posterior arches.

Vertical compression or bursting fractures more often involve the middle and lower cervical vertebral segments. The longitudinally oriented pressures cause the intervertebral discs to impact against the end plates of the bodies. Ordinarily, there is no instability because the posterior elements remain intact. When viewed on the anteroposterior film, a vertical fracture line is identified within the involved body.

Although vertebra plana is not usually related to trauma, it might be mistaken for a compression fracture. This rare condition, in most instances related to eosinophilic granuloma (histiocytosis X), has the appearance of a pancake with extreme, uniform flattening of the body but with preservation of the posterior elements. Some other possible causes for this unusual finding are metastasis, multiple myeloma, osteochondritis of the primary ossification center of the body (Calvé's disease), and postradiation osteitis.

## Thoracic and Lumbar Spine

### *Roentgenographic Examination*

The thoracic spine is ordinarily examined by means of anteroposterior and lateral films. However, because of

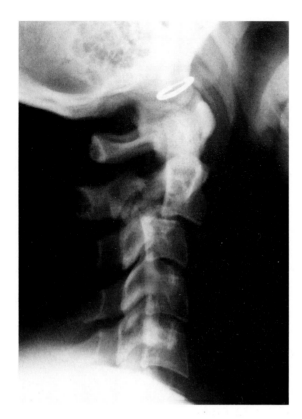

**Fig. 16–11.**
Hangman's fracture-dislocation of the second cervical vertebra.

the superimposition of the shoulders, the upper three or four vertebrae will be omitted from the lateral view, and if clinical symptoms point to this region, an oblique swimmer's projection should be obtained.

It is generally agreed that the above films will offer optimum information about the anatomy of the thoracic vertebrae. However, either or both oblique views of no more than 10 to 20 degrees can be obtained and provide a different aspect of a questionable or subtle change in the vertebral bodies or articulating facets.

Routine roentgenographic examination of the lumbar spine must be composed of anteroposterior, lateral, and both oblique projections as well as a cone-down lateral film of the lumbosacral joint.

### Roentgenographic Anatomy

**Anteroposterior View.** On the anteroposterior study, the 12 thoracic and 5 lumbar bodies will show a slight increase in size from top to bottom. The height, width, and alignment of the bodies and their cortical margins, trabecular architecture, and density need to be scrutinized carefully.

Subsequently, the round-to-oval pedicles should be evaluated separately. They overlie the superolateral corner of each body and, like them, become progressively larger inferiorly. The density and sclerotic cortical mar-

gins should be noted for any alterations, because they are involved in a number of pathologic processes.

The interpedicular distance, a line drawn between the inner boundaries of a vertebral body's pedicles, is an important observation throughout the spine. It affords an indirect evaluation of the size of the neural canal.

The transverse processes in the thoracic spine become smaller from superior to inferior, are oriented posterolaterally, and are located behind the intervertebral foramina. The normal articulations of the ribs should not be overlooked. In the lumbar spine the transverse processes are more laterally oriented and are much larger, the processes of the third vertebra usually being the largest.

On the anteroposterior projection, the spinous processes provide another guide for the evaluation of alignment. Rarely, they may be absent because of aplasia or malignant or infectious destruction.

Additionally, on the anteroposterior view, the paravertebral soft tissues should be studied. An increase in the width of the soft tissues will alert the clinician to a possible fracture, neoplasm, or infection in the spine, the result of hematoma, infiltrating tumor cells, or bacterial extension, respectively. The psoas margins in the paralumbar region are fairly sensitive indicators to similar changes when they become obliterated. This abnormal change can also reflect lymphadenopathy or urinary lesions such as a perirenal abscess. In fact, when viewing the lumbar spine, the clinician should always attempt to delineate the psoas and renal margins as well as search for urinary tract calculi as causes of back pain.

**Lateral View.** One of the goals for studying lateral views of the thoracolumbar spine is to ensure normal alignment of the anterior and posterior borders of the vertebral bodies. Furthermore, the cortical outlines and the internal structure of the bodies must be mentally recorded. Any narrowing of the intervertebral disc spaces can be established. In the thoracic spine, the intervertebral foramina can be seen on end but require oblique views for their proper visualization in the lumbar area.

The inferiorly directed spinous processes, as seen on the lateral film, may require a "hot" light to be adequately seen but should not be neglected, for reasons mentioned previously.

**Oblique Views.** Important anatomic features are introduced on the oblique views of the lumbar spine. These details are covered more extensively in Chapter 8. On the left posterior oblique film (left side down against the film), the left half of the posterior neural arch elements, including the intervertebral foramina, are identified, whereas the right half of these components are viewed on the opposite projection. In the cervical spine, the reverse condition exists.

### Developmental Variations and Congenital Abnormalities

Confusing anatomic variations are seen in the developing and mature spine. In infancy the vertebral bodies are egg shaped on lateral view. The upper and lower anterior corners are beveled until the apophyseal vertebral rings appear about each end plate. They fuse with the body by the fifteenth year, but occasionally they remain ununited and, except for the presence of a complete sclerotic border, often are confused with a corner fracture (Fig. 16-12). These are sometimes referred to as *limbus* vertebrae.

On the anteroposterior film, a vertical radiolucent cleft is seen superimposing on the vertebral bodies (Fig. 16-13). This represents the normal uncalcified portion of the posterior neural arch and spinous process and is not to be confused with spina bifida. At approximately 3 to 5 years of age, these will ossify and fuse. When they do fail to fuse completely, the cleft persists as a spina bifida occulta. This can occur anywhere in the spine, but is most common at L5. These are of no clinical importance.

True spina bifida is the result of a wide defect in the posterior neural arch, usually involving multiple vertebrae and commonly found in the lumbar region. The widened spinal neural canal is evidenced by an increased interpedicular distance. These may be associated with a meningocele that produces a prominent posterior soft-tissue density on the roentgenogram.

This wide gap of the dorsal arch and increased interpedicular width should also bring to mind the possibility of diastematomyelia, a condition in which the cord is divided by an intraspinal cartilaginous, fibrous, or bony spur. This has a predilection for the thoracolumbar junction. Syringomyelia can produce a similar appearance in the cervical spine where there is cystic dilation of the cord. The same type of appearance can also be seen with intraspinal tumors such as lipomas or dermoids.

Vascular channels may give rise to confusing appearances. Blood vessels perforate the anterior cortical borders of each body and form a radiolucent line, termed the *clefts of Hahn*. A similar vascular defect that becomes more apparent in adulthood may exist along the posterior margin of the body.

Hypoplasia of the vertebrae, fusion or block vertebrae, and hemivertebrae constitute a few of the other possible spinal anomalies (Fig. 16-14).

### Trauma

The focus of attention will now shift to some of the traumatic lesions involving the thoracolumbar spine. The majority of injuries disturb the muscular and ligamentous structures surrounding the spine. Just as in the cervical spine, the only visible roentgenographic findings may be scoliosis and/or straightening of the normal curvatures, which indicates muscle spasms.

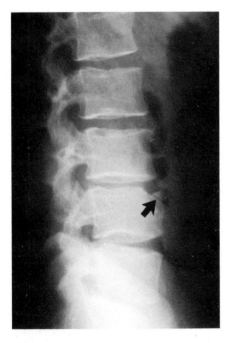

**Fig. 16–12.**
An unfused ring apophysis of a lumbar vertebra as seen here can be confused with a fracture.

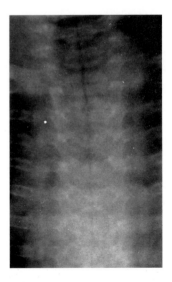

**Fig. 16–13.**
Normal thoracic spine of an infant. Note the vertical cleft of the neural arch.

When a fracture is present, the usual appearance is a wedge-shaped compression deformity, the result of hyperflexion forces. The avulsion-type corner fracture of the anterosuperior body results from extension forces. It appears as a sharp, nonsclerotic fragment, as opposed to an unfused apophysis.

Quite often, the dilemma of determining the age of a fracture presents itself. In long-standing compression fractures, degenerative changes with hypertrophic spurs arise along the articular margins, and there may be an unpredictable degree of eburnation. Yet at times these changes are absent and the determination of age may be difficult, if not impossible. Radioisotopic bone scans that utilize technetium $^{99m}$Tc phosphate complexes then become a valuable aid. Within 2 to 5 days of the injury, a recent collapse will show an increased uptake of the isotope, whereas older lesions will show no activity. However, the abnormal uptake may remain detectable for 18 to 24 months or longer, depending in part on the extent of the fracture and its location.

Wedge-shaped deformities of the vertebral bodies necessitate differentiation from other causative processes such as Scheuermann's disease. This represents a form of osteochondritis or aseptic necrosis that involves the end-plate ring apophyses and is seen in adolescents. Described as juvenile kyphosis, it predominates in the thoracic region. Schmorl's nodes commonly accompany this spinal affliction. These are round-to-oval protrusions of the anterior margins of the end plates and develop from focal intrabody herniation of the nucleus pulposus.

Biconcave deformities of the bodies (so-called fish vertebrae) have a predisposition for the thoracic and lumbar location. They represent a chronic progressive form of compression characteristically seen in postmenopausal patients with osteoporosis. Vertebral body compression fractures with a history of minimal or no trauma should alert the physician to the possibility of a metastatic or primary malignant process.

Another important traumatic lesion (particularly of the lumbar spine) that can be easily overlooked is the transverse process fracture (Fig. 16-15). The importance of its recognition rests with the fact of commonly related renal injury. It is important not to mistakenly call the unfused apophysis of the transverse process a fracture.

A seldom-seen injury to the lumbar vertebrae is the *Chance fracture* (Fig. 16-16). An extreme flexion force, often related to seat belt injuries, causes a fracture through the spinous process, across the neural arch or lamina, and into the posterosuperior aspect of the vertebral body. An isolated fracture of the spinous process is uncommon in the thoracic and lumbar regions.

One more pitfall to watch for in the assessment of spinal trauma is the unfused ossification center of the articular facets, which can resemble a fracture (Fig. 16-17). In evaluating the posterior elements, it is important to keep in mind the entities of spondylolysis and spondylolisthesis (see Chapter 8).

### Tumors

Except for metastatic neoplasms to the spine, tumors—both benign and primary malignant lesions—are uncommon. The vertebrae are the most commonly affected portion of the skeleton for metastasis and account for approximately 40% of all secondary tumors of bone. A few of the common and not-so-common tumors will be discussed.

**Hemangioma.** Hemangioma of the vertebral body may be the most common benign tumor, although few have been documented pathologically. Typically, their appearance is that of increased vertical trabeculations producing a somewhat striated pattern (Fig. 16-18). They should not be confused with Paget's disease or osteoblastic metastasis.

**Aneurysmal Bone Cyst.** Of the benign tumors of the spine, aneurysmal bone cysts are possibly the next most common after hemangiomas. Of course, they are more commonly found in the extremities, especially the distal portion of the femur. In the spine they tend to involve the posterior elements as well as the body. Possessing a thin shell of peripheral bone, they are expansile and cystic in nature. Roentgenographically, a malignant appearance can be seen with a predominant cystic pattern.

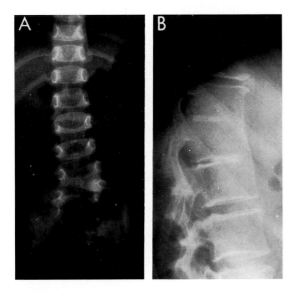

**Fig. 16–14.**
Anomalies of the spine. **A**, Hemivertebra of the lumbar spine. **B**, Fusion or block vertebrae.

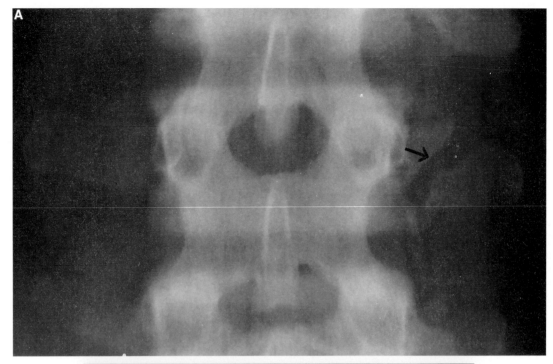

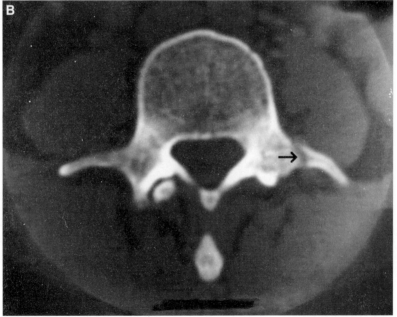

**Fig. 16–15.**
Transverse process fractures of the lumbar spine in two different patients. **A**, Fracture of L4 on the left on plain film *(arrow)*. **B**, CT in another trauma patient demonstrating a fracture of the transverse process *(arrow)*.

Unlike other tumors, benign and malignant alike, aneurysmal bone cysts have the unique capability of crossing over the cartilaginous disc space to involve adjacent vertebrae. A malignant chordoma also has this potential.

**Osteoid Osteoma.**   The osteoid osteoma is a benign tumor that can produce significant and disabling pain.

It is most often found in the extremities, but on rare occasions this tumor can involve the spine and so must be considered in the differential diagnosis of back pain. It is one of many causes of scoliosis, most likely the result of muscle splinting secondary to pain. The lesion is almost always limited to the neural arch, a position that often prevents its detection on conventional roentgeno-

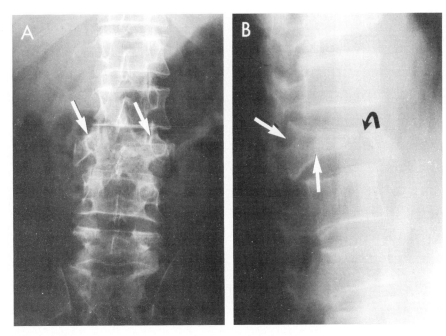

**Fig. 16–16.**
Chance fracture of the lumbar spine that extends through the body into the posterior neural elements and can be seen in individuals wearing seat belts. **A,** Anteroposterior view demonstrating lateral displacement of the pedicles *(arrows).* **B,** Lateral view showing a fracture extending through the body *(curved arrow)* and involvement of the neural arch *(straight arrows).*

graphs. Tomography and isotopic SPECT bone scanning may be required for its recognition. The lesion is composed of a small radiolucent nidus sometimes containing calcifications. A dense reactive sclerosis surrounds the central nidus and often obscures it.

**Osteoblastoma.** An osteoblastoma is a benign lesion that classically involves the spine, primarily the dorsal elements. Because of its varied histologic appearances, it has been described as a giant osteoid osteoma, and certain cases may even mimic osteogenic sarcoma.

A variety of primary malignant tumors may involve the spine, only a few of which are mentioned. Such tumors may be seen anywhere in the spine but have a preference for the sacrococcygeal region.

**Multiple Myeloma.** The most common primary malignant tumor of bone is multiple myeloma. The classic picture of "punched-out" lesions, particularly evident in the skull, is characteristic but not that common. The usual presentation is diffuse demineralization. Multiple vertebral compression deformities form in a progressive nature.

**Sarcoma.** Osteosarcoma, fibrosarcoma, and chondrosarcoma involve the spine only rarely and then usually are found in the sacrum. These tumors may arise in

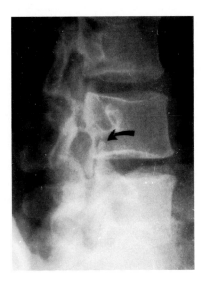

**Fig. 16–17.**
Unfused apophysis of the superior articular facet of L5 *(arrow).*

an area of previous irradiation, Paget's disease, or fibrous dysplasia.

**Round-Cell Tumors.** Ewing's sarcoma and reticulum cell sarcoma are rarely encountered in the vertebral column, having more of a predilection for the appendicu-

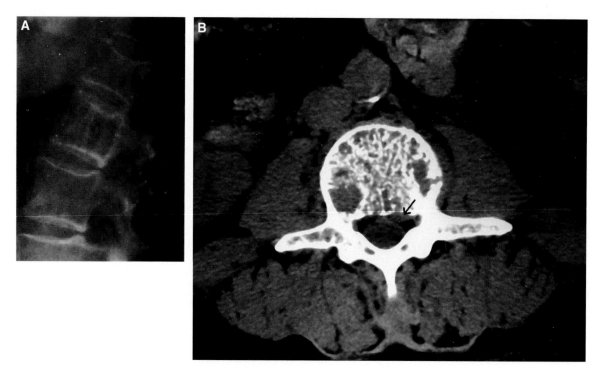

**Fig. 16–18.**
Hemangioma of a lumbar vertebra. **A,** Plain film. **B,** CT image. Note incidental finding of a herniated disc *(arrow).*

lar skeleton. However, they must be included in the differential diagnosis of destructive lesions.

**Hodgkin's Lymphoma.**   Hodgkin's disease can occasionally be seen within the bony spine and may present as an osteolytic alteration, osteoblastic alteration, or a combination of the two. More commonly, however, paraaortic lymph node involvement with lymphoma will produce erosive changes of the vertebral cortical margins.

In the same way and as an interesting sidelight, an aortic aneurysm can cause pressure destruction of the vertebra. A massively enlarged heart such as that in mitral stenosis can produce extrinsic changes of the thoracic spine. It is of interest that elderly individuals who ordinarily demonstrate degenerative spurs of the thoracic spine will only show them to any extent on the right side; apparently, the pulsating aorta prevents their formation on the left.

**Chordoma and Sacrococcygeal Teratoma.**   There are two primary malignant tumors of the spine that are classified as developmental. A chordoma is an invasive lesion arising from remnants of the primitive notochord. Therefore it can, presumably, occur anywhere along the vertebral column, although there are no reported cases of its occurrence in the thoracic region. The sacrum is the most common site and accounts for approximately

50% of cases. An intracranial chordoma located along the clivus represents about 30% of cases, and the remaining 20% originate in the cervical and lumbar areas.

Roentgenographically, the tumor presents as an expansile, lytic process with moderate soft-tissue extension. As noted previously, it may cross the disc space cartilage, an occurrence uncommon in any tumor but typical of infections. In one third of the tumors, calcifications are observed. The second type of developmental primary malignant tumor is a sacrococcygeal teratoma. However, 60% of these lesions are benign but exhibit some degree of localized infiltration. They are found in infants, within the pelvis, and around the parasacral region. Malformation of the spine can be an associated finding. They appear roentgenographically as variable-sized soft-tissue masses, often with calcifications or ossifications within them. The rectosigmoid colon is extrinsically displaced forward. Destructive changes will be present to some extent within the sacrococcygeal bony structure.

### Infection

Infections involving the spine have decreased in incidence over the years. Nevertheless, this must be considered in the differential diagnosis of a painful back and abnormal roentgenographic findings.

Acute bacterial infections or pyogenic spondylitis can involve either the disc space, the vertebral body, or both. The former condition, termed pyogenic discitis, is more common in the younger population, apparently on the basis of a healthy vascularization of the cartilage and, therefore, easy access by blood-borne bacteria. This results in a closed-space infection that can secondarily extend into the bodies.

On the other hand, infection of the vertebral body, particularly its anterior two thirds, is more commonly identified in the adult. Originating in the substance of the body, the infection may then secondarily involve the interspace by extension.

An important principle in pathophysiology should be reemphasized at this point. Cartilage serves as no barrier to the extension of infection and thereby is vulnerable to destruction. Conversely, the disc cartilage is resistant to malignant cellular infiltration, so tumors tend to remain confined to the body.

In both pyogenic discitis and vertebral osteomyelitis, the earliest roentgenographic findings may be joint space narrowing. Depending on the aggressiveness of the offending bacteria and the time of institution of therapy, the surrounding bone will show varying degrees of demineralization brought on by hyperemia. The end plates will then demonstrate progressive loss of continuity with irregular destruction and focal areas of subchondral reactive sclerosis. Extension into the posterior third of the body, then into the dorsal appendages as well as into the adjoining vertebrae, may occur. The body may eventually collapse. Some degree of surrounding soft-tissue swelling is invariably present and detectable on roentgenograms and exquisitely corroborated on MRI (Fig. 16-19).

Tuberculosis of the spine, or Pott's disease, is an extreme rarity among today's abnormal spine studies. The vertebral column remains the most common skeletal site for this chronic infection. The midthoracic and thoracolumbar junctions constitute the most prevalent sites of involvement. Because of its insidious and chronic nature, the spinal lesions are usually advanced when first examined roentgenographically, although this is not always the situation. An occasionally prominent feature is a large paravertebral soft-tissue mass that constitutes the abscess. In later phases, there may be extensive calcification within this mass (Fig. 16-20). The bony structures will show a decrease in density, and there will be narrowing of one or more of the disc spaces. The margins of the end plates will manifest irregular destruction, and a mottled sclerotic and lytic appearance will extend into the bodies, which display varying degrees of compression.

### Spinal Arthritis

Arthropathy or spondylosis of the spinal column most commonly is degenerative in nature with the formation of hypertrophic bony spurs. These osteophytes are formed by recurrent stimulation of wear and tear factors and are predominantly located along the end-plate margins of the vertebral bodies. When they bridge the interspaces and fuse, such spurs are described as syndesmophytes, which can more often be identified in specific forms of arthritis such as diffuse idiopathic skeletal hyperostosis (DISH) (Fig. 16-21).

Ossification of the anterior longitudinal ligament of the spine is characteristic of ankylosing spondylitis (Marie-Strümpell disease). Psoriatic arthritis, Reiter's disease, and other autoimmune diseases (including inflammatory bowel diseases) may lead to exuberant osteophyte formation.

Degenerative findings of the facet joints, particularly those of the lumbar spine, can result in various degrees of spinal stenosis. This is the result of bone spurs and soft tissue hypertrophy, primarily the ligamentum flavum. These produce narrowing of the central neural canal and can compromise the cord. Extension into the subarticular recesses and neuroforamina will encroach on the descending and exiting nerve roots, resulting in radiculopathy.

Degenerative disc disease is a commonly associated manifestation of arthritis. The aging process as well as trauma (either acute or related to chronic recurrent and repetitive injury) leads to eventual deterioration, dehydration, and protrusion or herniation of the nucleus pulposus through the annulus fibrosis. Broad-based posterior protrusion of disc material, along with degenerative hypertrophic spurs and thickened soft tissue elements, combine to initiate symptoms of spinal stenosis.

### Paget's Disease

One of the distinctive roentgenographic characteristics of spinal Paget's disease is that the disorder involves the entire vertebra—the body and all of the posterior elements, including the transverse and spinous processes (Fig. 16-22). Generally, there is an increase in density produced by a thickened trabeculae. A picture frame appearance can be imparted to the body, the result of a dense peripheral margin of thickened cortex. Furthermore, there is an actual increase in volume of the entire vertebra. This finding, along with total vertebral involvement, distinguishes Paget's disease from an osteoblastic metastasis.

## The Shoulder

### Roentgenographic Examination

In the majority of cases, a complete and optimal roentgenographic study of the shoulder girdle need only include upright (standing or sitting) anteroposterior views with the humerus in internal and external rotation. These two projections will usually permit adequate evaluation of the bony structures constituting

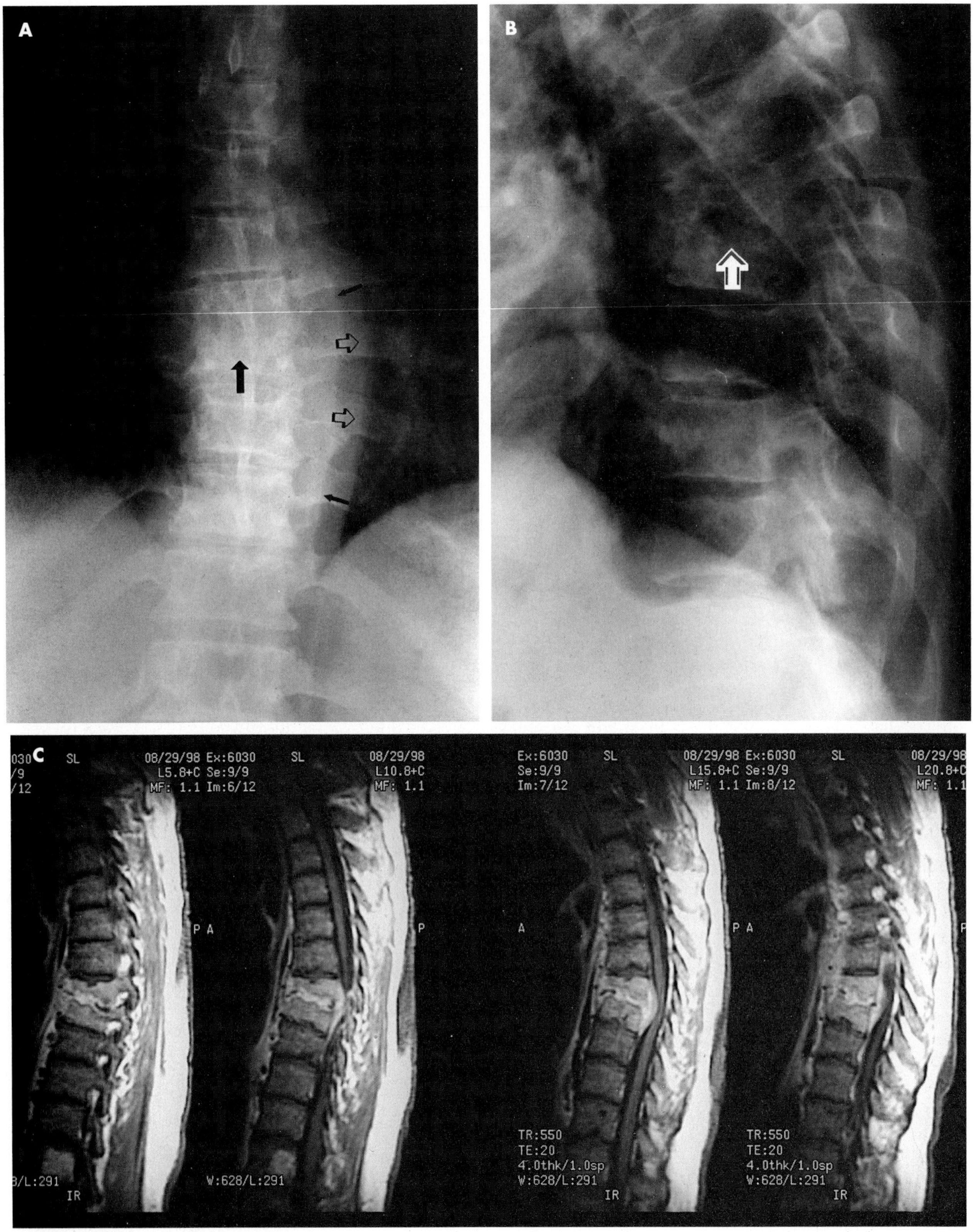

**Fig. 16–19.**
Pyogenic discitis. **A**, Anteroposterior and **B**, lateral views of the thoracic spine demonstrating pyogenic discitis *(large arrows)*. The disc space has been destroyed with extension of the infection into the vertebral bodies with trabecular compression and reactive sclerosis. An associated paravertebral soft-tissue mass *(open arrows)* indicates expansion of the inflammatory process. Note aorta *(small arrows)*. **C**, Corresponding sagittal T-1 post-gadolinium MRI images exhibit the infection extending through the posterior neural elements (pedicles and lamina) into the epidural space and producing cord compression.

the shoulder. In the uncooperative child or severely traumatized patient, these films may be obtained while the patient is in the supine position.

On these roentgenograms the complete clavicle should be visualized as well as the entirety of the scapula and at least the proximal third of the humerus. Special attention should be given to the alignments of the gleno-

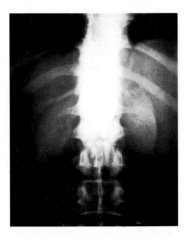

**Fig. 16–20.**
Pott's disease of the spine. The chronic tuberculous process has resulted in calcified paravertebral psoas abscesses.

humeral, acromioclavicular, coracoclavicular, and sternoclavicular joints. The tuberosities of the humeral head and its articular surface should be specifically scrutinized. The acromion and coracoid processes, in addition to the borders and flat surfaces of the scapula, require attention.

The standard examination, of course, may require modification because there are certain situations when special views must be obtained for better delineation of specific structures. In an acutely injured shoulder in which immobilization of the shoulder is required, the humerus will ordinarily be held in internal rotation. To obtain roentgenograms of the humerus in external rotation without moving the arm, patients can be positioned by rotating them 40 degrees posteriorly with the affected side toward the film. Because of pain, this requires that patients be sitting or standing.

Upright exposures are also beneficial in demonstrating fat-fluid levels. This occurs when a fracture has extended into the joint through the articular cortex, most often with fractures of the greater tuberosity. Such information is useful since articular cartilage damage is certain, and the patient should be informed that degenerative osteoarthritis in time is a possibility.

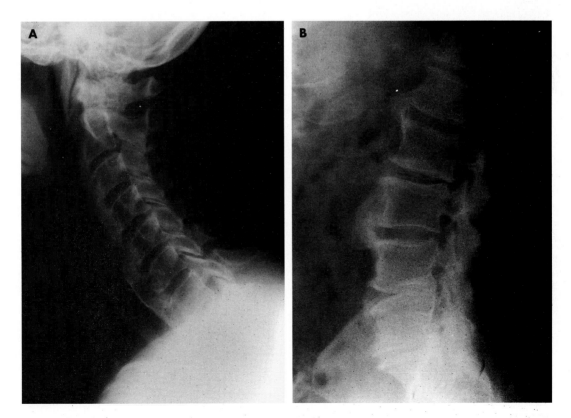

**Fig. 16–21.**
DISH (diffuse idiopathic skeletal hyperostosis). **A**, Cervical spine and **B**, lumbar spine x-rays with large bridging osteophytes (syndesmophytes).

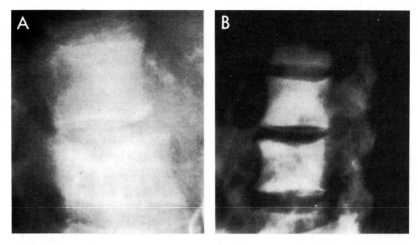

**Fig. 16–22.**
Spinal Paget's disease and osteoblastic metastasis. **A,** Paget's disease demonstrates increased trabeculations, a bone-within-bone appearance, and increased volume including the pedicles. **B,** Osteoblastic metastasis.

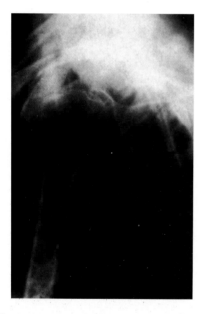

**Fig. 16–23.**
Transthoracic view of the shoulder.

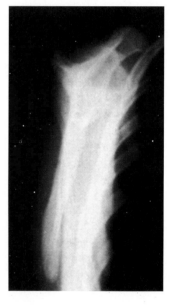

**Fig. 16–24.**
Transscapular view of the shoulder.

When there is suspicion of a fracture involving the shaft of the humerus below the neck, in addition to an anteroposterior view, a transthoracic lateral projection is necessary for evaluation of alignment (Fig. 16-23). The glenohumeral relationship can also be accessed with proper exposure, but because of superimposed ribs, fractures above the neck are difficult to see. Instead, a transscapular study will be more helpful (Fig. 16-24). This view is obtained by having the patient face the film at an angle of 45 degrees with the affected side toward the film holder. The resultant picture forms a Y where the acromion, coracoid, and scapular body intersect.

The humeral head will be superimposed on the Y. This is useful not only for fractures but also for posterior dislocations. This transscapular examination is always utilized when studying the scapula in addition to the routine anteroposterior roentgenogram. CT or MRI (particularly the latter) can give additional valuable information, especially regarding soft-tissue involvement. The multiplanar capabilities of these imaging modalities augments visualization of gross pathologic findings.

Posterior shoulder dislocations are notorious for their ability to avoid detection on the standard anteroposterior views. They are often associated with seizure dis-

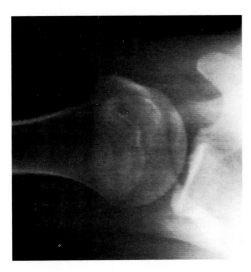

**Fig. 16–25.**
Axillary view of the shoulder. Note the glenohumeral relationship, the hooklike coracoid process, and the acromion behind the head of the humerus.

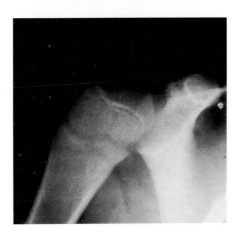

**Fig. 16–26.**
Normal proximal humeral epiphysis in a child.

orders. The tangential projection is an excellent means for detecting the abnormality. This is performed by angling the x-ray tube approximately 30 degrees so that the central ray passes tangentially across the glenoid articular surface. In this manner the glenohumeral relationship is much better defined than on the conventional straight anteroposterior view.

The axillary film also provides another perspective of the shoulder anatomy (Fig. 16-25). The acromion, coracoid, glenohumeral joint, and humeral head are viewed in a different plane. By holding the film against the top of the shoulder, the picture is produced by abducting the arm and centering the x-ray tube through the axilla. The study requires a special "grid" cassette for the film. It is helpful in determining the presence of a humeral head displacement, but it is not recommended when a dislocation has just been reduced because the required abduction may reluxate the joint.

The clavicle itself requires two projections in the anteroposterior plane to evaluate it properly. One film should be made perpendicular to the plane of the body, whereas the other exposure is made with a 15- to 20-degree cephalad angulation.

The acromioclavicular joints are best inspected with an anteroposterior film and by tilting the x-ray tube 15 degrees toward the head. Comparative films are necessary to determine the presence of a separation, and this should be performed with and without weight bearing.

A more difficult area to examine roentgenographically is the sternoclavicular joint. As a result of bony superimposition, tomography may be required, but because this is not universally available, both oblique and lateral views may suffice. However, if these attempts are unsuccessful, the patient can be positioned prone. The x-ray tube is then centered through the sternoclavicular joints and angled toward the head at a 35-degree tilt.

### Roentgenographic Anatomy and Developmental Variations

A considerable degree of confusion can be created by the ossification centers of the shoulder. The proximal humeral epiphysis does not become visible, as a rule, until the fourth to eighth month of life. There are two, and occasionally three, separate centers. By the twentieth year, the proximal epiphysis fuses to the shaft of the humerus. Before complete closure of the epiphyseal suture, the lucent line has a peculiar angulated appearance (Fig. 16-26). Overlap of the suture line occurs no matter what projection is employed and consequently produces an image simulating a fracture.

A deceptive appearance of the proximal humeral shaft is the *deltoid tuberosity,* which, incidentally, receives the tendinous attachment of the deltoid muscle. The thickened cortex in this area may bring to mind the periosteal reaction of infection or tumor.

On a congenital basis, there may be a complete absence of the clavicle or at least partial underdevelopment of its lateral end. This represents hereditary *cleidocranial dysplasia,* a disease that also affects the skull, pelvis, hips, and other skeletal regions.

The outer end of the clavicle appears less dense than the middle and sternal aspects, the result of a lesser thickness of overlying soft tissue. Soft tissues are also responsible for a discrete line density paralleling the superior border of the clavicle that measures no more than 4 mm in width and is described as the "accompanying shadow." This shadow may be thickened in cases of subtle fractures.

The *rhomboid fossa* is a common anatomic variation of the clavicle and is a notch-like depression found

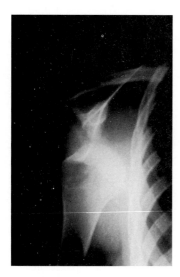

**Fig. 16–27.**
Anterior dislocation of the shoulder, subglenoid in type.

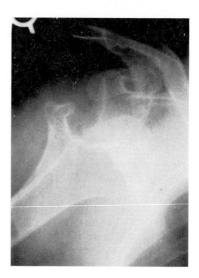

**Fig. 16–28.**
Hill-Sachs deformity in chronic recurring anterior shoulder dislocation.

along the inferior border at its medial aspect. This represents the location of the insertion of the costoclavicular (rhomboid) ligament, which secures the first rib to the clavicle. Its irregular appearance has been misinterpreted as a destructive process.

### Trauma

Of all the joints in the body, the shoulder is the most common site of dislocations. More than 97% are anterior and can be described as subglenoid or subcoracoid, depending on the location of the humeral head. Invariably this form of dislocation can be visualized by a single anteroposterior roentgenogram (Fig. 16-27).

When dislocation occurs, it is not unusual to have an associated fracture; this should be searched for on the film. With an anterior dislocation, a fracture of the greater tuberosity may exist; the lesser tuberosity is vulnerable in posterior dislocations. The lower glenoid margin is also susceptible in either type of dislocation. An infraction of the articular cartilage without a visible fracture is also possible in dislocations and may require arthrography to demonstrate.

With intraarticular extension of a fracture in the absence of true dislocation, an intact joint capsule may become progressively distended with blood. If enough blood accumulates, there will be inferior displacement of the humeral head away from the glenoid. This condition is termed *pseudosubluxation*, or "hanging shoulder."

With chronic recurring anterior dislocations, a defect becomes apparent along the superolateral aspect of the humeral head. This cortical infraction, present because of impaction against the anteroinferior rim of the glenoid, is commonly referred to as *Hill-Sachs deformity*.

This abnormality is usually best demonstrated on an internally rotated anteroposterior view (Fig. 16-28).

The less common posterior dislocation is much more difficult to visualize roentgenographically. The problem arises because the humeral head on the standard anteroposterior projections shows no apparent separation from the glenoid fossa when, in fact, it is separated. The posterolateral orientation of the glenoid articular surface accounts for this to some extent. In the normal shoulder, the head of the humerus ordinarily overlaps about three fourths of the glenoid fossa. When it becomes posteriorly dislocated because of lateral displacement of the head, this overlap is less, but the change may be subtle. This perplexing situation can usually be solved by employing the 30-degree tangential view, the axillary projection, or the transscapular film (Fig. 16-29). With recurrent posterior dislocations of the shoulder, a defect of the inferoposterior cartilaginous labrum may not be visible by standard radiography. This is termed a *Bankart lesion*, which can be diagnosed by MRI or CT arthrography.

A rare form of dislocation of the shoulder joint is *luxatio erecta*, a condition where the humeral head is located under the glenoid rim and the humeral shaft is directed above the head in fixed abduction (Fig. 16-30). A lateral fall on an elevated arm will produce such an abnormality. The acromion process of the scapula acts as a fulcrum, pushing the head of the humerus down and out of the glenohumeral joint. The dynamics of the applied forces can result in a fracture of the acromion, the lower lip of the glenoid, or the greater tuberosity of the humerus. Often there is an associated tear of the rotator cuff.

Fractures involving the proximal portion of the humerus are classified according to involvement of the

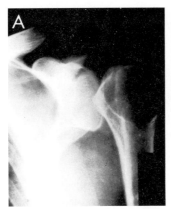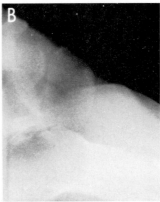

**Fig. 16–29.**
Posterior shoulder dislocation. **A,** Anteroposterior view showing some discrepancy in the glenohumeral joint. **B,** Axillary view demonstrating posterior displacement of humeral head from the glenoid fossa (see Fig. 16-25 for a normal axillary film).

head, either tuberosity, or the surgical or anatomic neck. Additionally, a fracture-displacement of the yet-unfused epiphysis may occur.

For descriptive purposes, anatomists describe the surgical neck as that portion of the humerus just inferior to the tuberosities where there is a normal narrowing. The constriction or shallow groove at the articular margin of the head of the humerus is referred to as the anatomic neck.

Fractures of the proximal portion of the humerus must be evaluated by at least two views at right angles to one another. An anteroposterior view alone with a transthoracic lateral projection will fulfill these criteria, but obliquely directed x-ray films may be necessary to best demonstrate displacement and/or angular deformity.

Transverse subcapital fractures of the surgical neck along with avulsions of the greater tuberosity are the most commonly encountered injuries to the shoulder. A fracture-displacement of the ununited epiphysis creates a more difficult diagnostic challenge. The normal epiphyseal line itself, as already alluded to, makes interpretation troublesome. The normal epiphysis has a uniform width and dense margins, whereas a fracture will demonstrate varying thickness with a sharp, nonsclerotic edge. Often there is impaction or distraction of the fragments causing some degree of overlapping, which makes the diagnosis somewhat simpler. Of course, if the presence of an abnormality is uncertain or indeterminate, an accurate comparison with the opposite uninjured shoulder should be performed.

The infraglenoid area of the scapula is the most common location of fractures of this bone. The normal lucent nutrient canal in this region with its dense margins

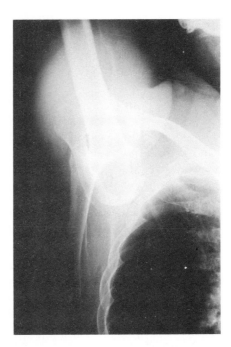

**Fig. 16–30.**
Luxatio erecta of the shoulder. Note the superior orientation of the humeral shaft and the head of the bone locked under the glenoid.

should not offer much concern. Instead of a discrete fracture line, only a zone of increased density will offer any clue to the injury. The clinician should also search for underlying rib fractures.

In most circumstances, a complete fracture of the clavicle will exhibit overriding of the fragments when they involve its midportion. Because of the forces applied by the pectoralis minor muscle, as well as the weight of the arm, the lateral fragment is displaced in-

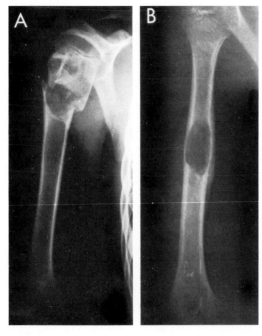

**Fig. 16–31.**
Benign cysts of the humerus. **A,** A multiloculated cyst in the meta-physis shows a fresh pathologic fracture. **B,** A simple solitary cyst in the midshaft demonstrates a healing fracture.

feriorly in most cases. An incomplete or nondisplaced fracture may be so subtle as to avoid detection initially, but the two standard views, including straight antero-posterior and cranially angulated projections, will in most instances reveal the fracture.

### Tumor

The proximal aspect of the humerus is a relatively common location for a benign solitary cyst, which may appear as either simple or multiloculated (Fig. 16-31). Such cysts are found within the metaphysis and exhibit destruction of the medullary spongiosa with more or less expansion of the bone. Thinning of the cortex can attain paper thickness, and pathologic fractures are a common event even in the absence of significant trauma. When initially discovered, the cysts extend to the epiphyseal line but do not involve the growth center itself. When followed serially until fusion of the epi-physis, the cyst appears to "migrate" toward the middle of the shaft as growth of the bone ends progresses.

Primary malignant tumors of the shoulder are a rar-ity and are often of the sarcomatous variety. Osteogenic sarcoma—as well as the round-cell tumors, Ewing's sar-coma, and reticulum cell sarcoma—has already been described.

Secondary metastatic disease is much more prevalent than primary lesions, particularly disease of the proxi-mal aspect of the humerus. As with cysts, pathologic fractures often accompany these malignant changes.

### Arthritis

The roentgenographic alterations of osteoarthritis of the shoulder are similar to those seen in the knee and are described in the section about the knee. However, the process more often has a posttraumatic relationship.

Rheumatoid arthritis of the shoulder, as in other joints, will demonstrate articular erosions without much bone production or osteophyte formation as is seen in osteoarthritis. However, unique to this area, erosions of the lateral ends of the clavicles may be present. This pathologic change, nevertheless, is not specific for rheumatoid arthritis and may be seen in hyperparathy-roidism and other less common diseases.

### Calcific Tendinitis

Calcific tendinitis represents a disease entity that is par-ticularly prone to develop in the shoulder. The majority of roentgenographic examinations performed for this disease are negative for abnormal changes. The radi-ographic diagnosis is made by the identification of calci-fications involving the tendinous insertions of the rotator cuff muscles into the head of the humerus. This most commonly affects the supraspinatus tendon as it crosses over the superior articular surface of the humeral head and inserts into the greater tuberosity. Pathogenically, the presence of calcium infers organization of a focal hematoma resulting from tearing of some of the tendon's fibers. The subacromial bursa overlies and is in contact with the supraspinatus tendon and, because of this close relationship, may become secondarily inflamed. In fact, rupture of the puttylike calcifications into the bursa her-alds the onset of subacromial bursitis. The density of the calcium can be seen to extend along the lateral aspect of the humeral head as it finds its way into the subdeltoid extension of the subacromial bursa.

## The Elbow

### Roentgenographic Examination

Standard examination of the elbow includes a straight anteroposterior film with the forearm fully extended and supinated, as well as a true lateral view with the joint flexed 90 degrees and the forearm supinated. Not uncommonly, particularly with trauma, the patient is unable or unwilling to extend or flex the elbow. To de-lineate the distal humeral articulating surface when the elbow is held in flexion, the anteroposterior view can be obtained by orienting the central beam of the x-ray tube perpendicular to the distal humeral shaft. In the same way, the proximal radial and ulnar details and re-lationships can be observed by pointing the tube per-pendicular to their shafts. Medial and lateral oblique ex-posures may become necessary to better analyze the radial head and shaft, the humeral condyles, or the coronoid process of the ulna.

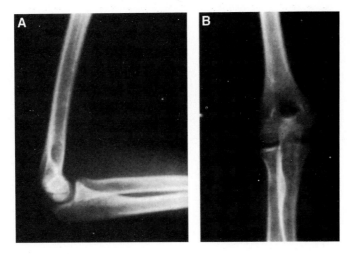

**Fig. 16–32.**
Normal elbow of a 9-year-old child. **A**, Lateral view. **B**, Anteroposterior view.

### Roentgenographic Anatomy

Before considering specific elbow lesions, pertinent roentgenographic anatomy of the elbow must be considered. Evaluating the different bony landmarks and their relationships can prove extremely useful.

In children a great deal of confusion arises because of the ossification sequence of the growth centers. The capitellum, trochlea, and the medial and lateral epicondyles compose the centers of the distal portion of the humerus. In addition, the elbow contains the olecranon apophysis and the radial head epiphysis (Fig. 16-32).

The first of the distal humeral epiphyses to appear is the capitellum, which develops by the age of 2 years. At about 6 years of age the medial epicondylar center becomes visible; the trochlea next becomes evident at 10 years of age; and finally the lateral epicondyle appears near the twelfth year of life.

The radial head epiphysis calcifies at about the same time as the medial epicondyle, in the vicinity of the sixth year. Before the age of 10 years, the olecranon ossification center is not visible.

The ossification centers normally fuse between the ages of 14 and 16 years, although union of the medial epicondyle may not occur until the eighteenth year of life.

After their union, the medial and lateral epicondyles form the flared segment of the distal third of the humerus. Between the condyles on both the ventral and dorsal surfaces are indentations identified as the coronoid and olecranon fossae, respectively, as they relate to the anatomic segments of the ulna. This area may be very thin and appear as a zone of rounded rarefaction on the anteroposterior film. In fact an actual opening, termed the *supratrochlear foramen*, is occasionally present.

Contained within these recesses are the fat pads, fairly sensitive indicators of the presence of a distended joint capsule. In the normal elbow, assuming a true lateral flexion film is obtained, the posterior fat pad is not visible. The anterior fat pad forms a slim, triangular lucency adjacent to the anterior humeral cortex. With the presence of joint fluid, such as blood resulting from an intraarticular fracture, one or both of these fat pads will be elevated. The so-called fat-pad sign is not specific and may be seen in conditions other than trauma, such as pyarthrosis or rheumatoid arthritis. In cases of injury, a positive fat-pad sign should be searched for from the beginning and, if found, should initiate further investigation for an occult fracture, particularly of the radial head (Fig. 16-33). Oblique views may be required and, if necessary, a repeat examination may be done in 7 to 10 days, at which time a fracture should be apparent. On occasion no fracture will be found, and the joint may be distended on the basis of a cartilage infraction or capsular tear. In adults an intraarticular fracture may be present in the absence of fat-pad elevation, but in children it is a more reliable indicator, being found in approximately 90% of elbow fractures (Rogers, 1978).

Two other helpful relationships will be of assistance when evaluating normal elbow anatomy. The first is the anterior humeral line. On the lateral film, a line is drawn along the anterior margin of the humeral shaft and extended through the joint. If the capitellum is divided into equal thirds, this line normally passes through the middle third. It is a simple and useful index in analyzing the normal 140-degree angle that the articular structures form with the shaft of the humerus. This easy maneuver often will alert the physician to a subtle transcondylar fracture in children: the line will be seen to extend through or anterior to the anterior third division of the capitellum (Fig. 16-34).

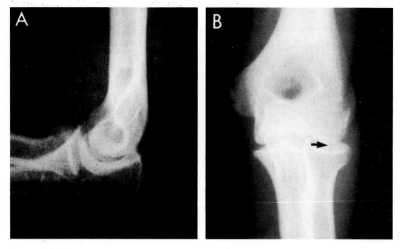

**Fig. 16–33.**
Radial head fracture with a positive fat-pad sign. **A**, Lateral view showing elevation of both anterior and posterior fat pads *(arrows)*. **B**, A fracture line through the radial head *(arrow)* is well delineated on the anteroposterior projection.

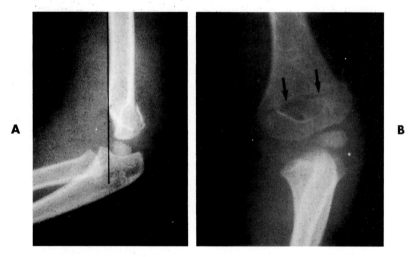

**Fig. 16–34.**
Transcondylar fracture of the humerus. **A**, Lateral view revealing anterior and posterior fat-pad elevation. An obvious fracture is identified, but note how the anterior humeral line extends anterior to the capitellum. **B**, Anteroposterior view clearly outlining the fracture *(arrows)*.

The second practical indicator is the radiocapitellar line, denoted by a line drawn through the longitudinal axis of the radius. This line will always pass through the capitellum, no matter what projection is being viewed. When the radial head is dislocated, this relationship no longer exists. Whenever there is a fracture of the ulnar shaft, this procedure should be utilized, because the radial head is often dislocated in what constitutes a *Monteggia fracture*.

### Trauma

Sixty percent of all elbow fractures in children are supracondylar. The lateral epicondyle is involved about 15% of the time, and the medial epicondyle accounts for 10% of all fractures. The radial and olecranon ossification centers are not commonly traumatized.

In adults the radial head or neck marks the most common elbow area for fractures. Unlike the pediatric age group, adults seldom suffer fractures of the distal third of the humerus.

A supracondylar fracture should more aptly be called a *transcondylar fracture* because it extends across the condyles and is seen through the coronoid and olecranon fossae (see Fig. 16-34). The anterior humeral line will indicate posterior displacement of the distal fragment when the fracture is complete, something seen in 75% of cases. The remainder, however, are incomplete, and visualizing the fracture line may be impossible. Almost always the posterior fat pad will be elevated.

When the lateral epicondylar epiphysis is traumatized, it usually contains a fragment of metaphyseal bone. Because it serves for the attachment of forearm extensor tendons, the fragment becomes displaced posteriorly and inferiorly.

Little League elbow, discussed in Chapter 15, describes an injury in which the medial epicondyle is separated. Ordinarily, the avulsed center is best identified on the anteroposterior film, often lying adjacent to the capitellum. In rare instances the fragment may become displaced into the medial joint space, where it can simulate the trochlear ossification center before its actual appearance.

The coronoid process is often avulsed in posterior dislocations of the elbow and is impacted against the trochlea. When an elbow dislocation occurs, the radius and ulna are displaced lateral and posterior to the humerus in almost all instances. In children, when the radius and ulna are medial to the humerus, there is not a dislocation but rather a fracture through the entire distal humeral epiphysis. This is extremely important to recognize because treatment of the two conditions is entirely different.

## The Wrist and Hand

### Roentgenographic Examination

Routine roentgenographic study of the wrist consists of posteroanterior, oblique, and lateral projections. The oblique film is achieved by orienting the wrist at a 45-degree angle to the plane of the film with the ulnar side down.

There are several special wrist views that are necessary for the evaluation of specific anatomic features. One of the more commonly employed studies is that for the carpal navicular bone. A fracture of this bone may easily escape detection. When clinical symptoms point to a navicular injury, yet the routine study appears normal, this view becomes mandatory. The palm is placed against the film holder with the thumb and index finger spread apart. The tube is angled 45 degrees toward the elbow. This results in an elongated appearance of the navicular, but the distortion is minimal, and it is projected free of superimposition from the other carpal bones (Fig. 16-35). The midportion of the navicular, where the majority of fractures occur, is clearly outlined.

Roentgenographic examination of the phalanges and metacarpals is performed with posteroanterior and oblique films. When the fingers are evaluated, the individual digits should also be examined with true lateral views.

### Roentgenographic Anatomy, Developmental Variations, and Pathology of the Individual Bones

In this section, anatomy, variations, and abnormalities (especially those of the individual carpal bones) of the hand and wrist will be considered together.

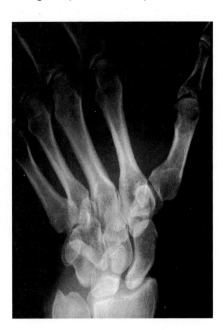

**Fig. 16–35.**
Angulated navicular view.

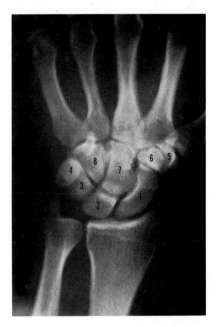

**Fig. 16–36.**
Normal carpal bones: *(1)* navicular; *(2)* lunate; *(3)* triquetrum; *(4)* pisiform; *(5)* greater multangular (trapezium); *(6)* lesser multangular (trapezoid); *(7)* capitate; *(8)* hamate.

The carpus is composed of a proximal and distal row of four bones each. To remember their names, the infamous mnemonic of ". . . Tilly's pants . . ." still applies, but a picture is sometimes more than words can describe (Fig. 16-36).

The proximal row is concave in alignment toward the hand, whereas the distal row is more or less convex in the same direction as seen on the anteroposterior

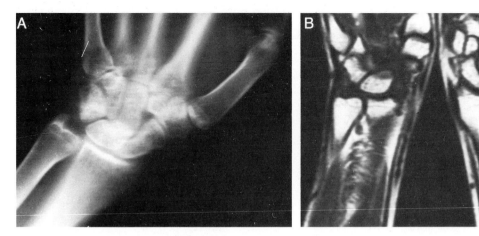

**Fig. 16–37.**
**A**, A standard linear x-ray tomogram of the wrist shows the faint sclerotic line of a healing fracture. **B**, MRI of both wrists in the same patient confirms the clinically suspected avascular necrosis of the proximal carpal navicular fragment (arrow).

film. The navicular, lunate, triquetral, and pisiform bones constitute the proximal column; the distal row is made up by the greater multangular (trapezium), lesser multangular (trapezoid), capitate, and hamate bones. For proper interpretation, each bone should be identified and scrutinized separately.

Throughout the skeleton, constitutional disease such as congenital hypothyroidism (*cretinism*) and other endocrine and metabolic diseases affect and alter the time of appearance and growth rate of ossification centers. But taken together, the wrist and hand provide one of the most sensitive indicators of growth retardation of bone age. A handbook describing the normal growth and development of the hand and wrist is found in most radiology departments (Greulich and Pyle).

A few uncommonly described congenital abnormalities affect the carpus. Agenesis or hypoplasia of one or more of the bones may be found. Fusion anomalies or synostoses also are occasionally seen.

Anatomic variations occur with such incidence that some of the more common ones will be described to permit differentiation from pathologic conditions.

Accessory bones do appear about the carpal bones, but are uncommon. They are mentioned merely to make one aware of their existence, and they need to be recalled when considering the possibility of an avulsion fragment.

Small, well-defined, round-to-oval areas of increased density are often identified in any of the carpal bones, metacarpals, and phalanges. They represent clinically insignificant bone islands.

Tiny, rounded lucencies with well-delineated sclerotic margins coincide with vascular channels, but cyst-like areas are also often encountered within or along the cortical borders of any of the hand or wrist bones,

especially the carpal bones. These may be the result of medullary fibrosis or hemorrhagic cysts. When related to the articular cortex, these cysts are the result of synovial herniation in osteoarthritis when the other classic signs of this disease are present. Erosive cysts at the juxtaarticular margins are diagnostic of rheumatoid arthritis.

In the following discussion, all of the individual wrist and hand bones are considered separately.

**Navicular.**   The navicular bone becomes visible somewhat late, usually by the fifth to sixth year. This bone may be entirely absent (agenesis), or it may become assimilated (fused) with the radial epiphysis. A small hypoplastic navicular may result in a malformed radial-carpal joint. Quite often a tubercle arises from the distal and lateral corner of the bone. A partial division of the navicular resulting from incomplete fusion of two ossification centers can simulate a fracture. This condition will require follow-up studies to determine healing, but the same may be found in the contralateral wrist.

Serial examinations of a fractured carpal navicular bone at about 3- to 4-week intervals are imperative in view of the possible complications. These include malunion, nonunion, and avascular necrosis. The latter presents as a progressively increasing sclerosis of the proximal fragment as a result of vascular interruption to this segment (Fig. 16-37).

Transverse fractures of the navicular most often involve the midportion, but any segment can be involved, including avulsions of the lateral tubercle. Dislocations of the navicular will be discussed in the following section on the lunate bone. In recent years these posttraumatic findings of navicular fractures have been readily assessed by means of MRI.

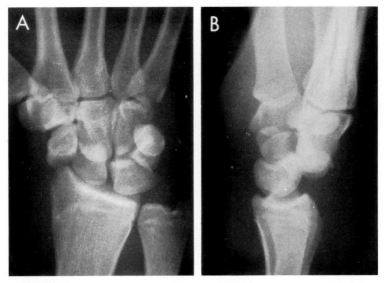

**Fig. 16–38.**
Transnavicular perilunate dislocation. **A**, Posteroanterior view. Note the obvious displaced fracture of the navicular and the overlap of the proximal pole fragment and the capitate, which should alert one to the presence of more than just a simple fracture. **B**, Lateral view showing typical posterior displacement, particularly of the capitate, with the lunate maintaining its normal position.

**Lunate.** Around the fourth to fifth year of life, the lunate bone becomes visible by ossification. Like the navicular, it may develop from two separate centers. If these centers fail to fuse, complete or partial fracturelike lines result.

One of the most notable pathologic changes affecting the carpal lunate is *Kienböck's* aseptic necrosis. This form of osteochondritis is described in more detail in Chapter 7. The carpal lunate is not commonly fractured, but is involved in one of the more important traumatic lesions of the wrist: dislocations. Three important types of wrist dislocations have been described. The first is a transnavicular perilunate dislocation (Fig. 16-38). In this condition, there is a fracture at the midnavicular. The proximal pole fragment and the lunate maintain their normal relationship with the radial articulation, but the distal pole segment of the navicular bone and the remaining carpal bones become displaced posteriorly.

In a perilunate dislocation, the navicular is intact and it, along with the carpus, becomes dorsally dislocated. The lunate remains in normal position.

The third type of carpal displacement is a pure lunate dislocation (Fig. 16-39). The articular relationship between the lunate and the capitate is disrupted. The lunate rotates anteriorly, which is best appreciated on the lateral view. On the anteroposterior film, the lunate takes on a somewhat triangular appearance, which should alert the clinician to this abnormality.

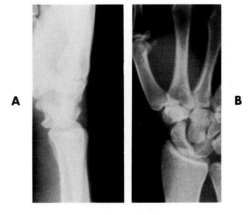

**Fig. 16–39.**
Pure lunate dislocation. **A**, The lateral view reveals the semilunar articular margin of the lunate faces forward. **B**, On the frontal view note the abnormal relation of the lunate to the navicular, capitate, and triquetrum.

**Triquetrum.** The triquetrum, or triangular bone, appears between the second and third year. It is probably the second most commonly fractured bone of the carpus. This usually consists of a posterior chip fracture, identified on the lateral roentgenogram, and is usually of no clinical importance.

**Pisiform.** The pisiform is the smallest bone of the carpus and the last to ossify (usually in the ninth or tenth year of life). Because it often develops from multiple centers, its early appearance has often been misinterpreted as a fracture or aseptic necrosis. Traumatic lesions of the pisiform are almost nonexistent, although fractures and dislocations have been reported in the literature.

**Greater Multangular.**   Moving on to the distal row, the first bone to be considered is the greater multangular, or trapezium. Appearing at approximately the fifth year, this carpal bone should be observed for its concave articulation with the base of the first metacarpal bone. A fusion between the two is not uncommon. In addition, the trapezium exhibits a tendency for fusion with the navicular. This bone, along with the lesser multangular, is somewhat difficult to evaluate because of the superimposition of the two.

Degenerative osteoarthritic alterations are common at the greater multangular joint at the first metacarpal bone. Joint narrowing, subarticular sclerosis, and spurring are characteristic findings of this process.

**Lesser Multangular.**   The lesser multangular, or trapezoid, makes its appearance some time after the navicular is visualized. It is rarely involved in pathologic processes, including trauma. Synostosis between it and the adjoining capitate has been observed.

**Capitate.**   The first carpal bone to ossify, and the largest of the eight, is the capitate. Cystlike lesions seem to predominate in the capitate bone. Its position appears to protect it from trauma.

**Hamate.**   The last carpal bone to be visualized is the hamate. To the inexperienced observer the uncinate process or hamulus (the bony protuberance of the hamate extending toward the palm) will appear as a lucent lesion with a sclerotic border when seen *en face* in the anteroposterior projection. Because avulsion fractures of this hooklike process may occur, it is helpful to obtain an oblique view of the wrist with the posterior surface of the small finger resting against the film. This will project the hamulus free of overlapping bones.

**Distal Radius and Ulna.**   When analyzing the wrist roentgenogram, the distal radius and ulna can hardly escape attention. We are all aware of what constitutes a *Colles' fracture* and its reverse, a *Smith fracture*; but subtle impaction fractures of the distal third of the radius may evade detection. A helpful rule to follow is to measure the anterior angle of the tilt of the distal articular margin of the radius, which normally measures 15 degrees on the lateral view. The only indication of a fracture may be straightening or reversal of this tilt.

A transverse fracture of the radial styloid may be an isolated finding and constitutes the so-called chauffeur's fracture. A styloid fracture of the ulna usually accompanies another fracture, but it may be an isolated finding.

Dislocations of either or both the distal radius and ulna must not be overlooked, and this is easily done if a true lateral roentgenogram is not performed. The displacement is invariably posterior.

**Metacarpals and Phalanges.**   When describing the individual fingers, the term *ray* is employed. Each of the five rays is composed of a metacarpal and its three associated phalanges (proximal, middle, and distal).

A number of congenital abnormalities exist at birth. These include fusion of two or more of the digital rays, a condition referred to as syndactyly. Duplicative anomalies, or polydactyly, can involve any of the rays. Arachnodactyly of the fingers occurs in the generalized skeletal disorder of *Marfan's syndrome*; here the digits are elongated and very thin.

When assessing the metacarpal bones, there are several important anatomic features to be considered (Fig. 16-40). The epiphysis of the first metacarpal bone (the thumb) is located proximally, whereas the growth center occupies the distal aspect of the remaining four metacarpals. This property is consequential in terms of an examination made for assessing the presence of fractures in the growing patient. But, as is usual, there is always some variation to confuse the issue. On occasion the clinician

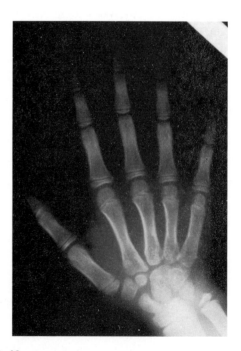

**Fig. 16–40.**
Normal hand bones of a 9-year-old child. Note the position of the epiphyses of the metacarpal bones.

may see what appear to be epiphyses involving the distal first metacarpal or the proximal second metacarpal; these are appropriately termed *pseudoepiphyses.*

Sesamoid bones located about the hand and wrist deserve mention because of their incidence and their occasional misidentification as fractures. They typically overlap the heads of the metacarpal bones. A fracture of a sesamoid is rare, being more commonly found in the foot.

The appearance of the phalanges, particularly the terminal ones, is extremely variable, and the variants, for all practical purposes, should be considered normal. The ungual tuberosity or tuft of the distal phalanx can have many shapes and sizes, yet a number of disease processes may alter them considerably. Deformity and erosive changes of the tufts are seen in scleroderma, sarcoidosis, psoriasis, and leprosy.

Cystlike or erosive changes in the tufts can be ascribed to glomus tumors, which produce pressure erosion of bone and are accompanied by severe pain. Enchondromas can involve any of the phalanges and are prone to pathologic fracture.

Of all of the fractures involving the fingers, those of the tuft are probably the most common. These may be avulsion types or comminuted. When analyzing the injured finger, the importance of obtaining a true lateral view, in addition to anteroposterior and oblique projections, cannot be stressed too much (Fig. 16-41). This becomes particularly apparent in cases of volar plate in-

juries. A fragment of bone is avulsed from the palmar aspect at the base of the middle phalanx and involves the proximal interphalangeal joint. The result of hyperextension forces, the fragment may be obscured on all but the lateral film.

Degenerative osteoarthritis is a relatively common disorder of the terminal interphalangeal joints of the elderly. The deformity is characterized by joint space narrowing, irregularity of the articular margins, subarticular sclerosis, and hypertrophic spurs. Clinically, palpable *Heberden's nodes* are a distinctive, characteristic finding of this disease.

Rheumatoid arthritis produces distinctive transformations in the joints of the hand and wrist (Fig. 16-42). The earlier roentgenographic finding may be periarticular soft-tissue swelling. Later demineralization around the joint with slight widening of the joint space will be noted, the result of inflammatory hyperemia with intraarticular fluid and synovial thickening. This progresses to juxtaarticular cortical erosions, which are related to synovial hypertrophy and pannus formation. Eventually the joint space becomes narrowed, and classic ulnar subluxations occur. Unlike degenerative osteoarthritis, there is no reactive spur production in rheumatoid arthritis.

Hyperparathyroidism produces a pathognomonic change in the hands. Typically, there is subperiosteal resorption along the radial aspect of the middle phalanges.

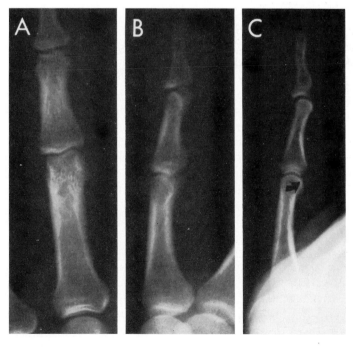

**Fig. 16–41.**
Volar plate fracture of the finger. **A,** Posteroanterior view. **B,** Oblique view. **C,** Lateral view. Note that the fragment is identified only on the lateral film *(arrow).*

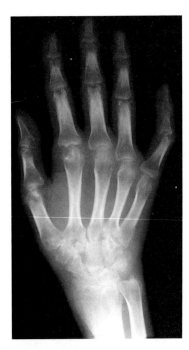

**Fig. 16–42.**
Typical radiographic findings of rheumatoid arthritis of the hands.

## The Pelvis and Hips

### Roentgenographic Examination

The anteroposterior view is the only standard projection required for roentgenographic examination of the pelvis. This film should include the entirety of the body pelvis, from iliac crests to the ischial tuberosities, which inherently encompasses the sacrococcyx and sacroiliac joint. Furthermore, both hips will be imaged on the film, and this should include the femur to the subtrochanteric region (below the lesser trochanter) whenever possible.

There are special projections that will aid the analyses of certain pelvic segments and clarify suspected regions. Films performed in the anteroposterior direction with the x-ray tube angled 30 degrees toward the head (cephalad) and 30 degrees toward the feet (caudad) are practical under certain circumstances. These will give a different perspective of the sacroiliac joints, sacrococcyx, the iliac wings, and the anterior pelvic arch (the ischiopubic rami). Nondisplaced fractures of the rami may initially go undetected on the straight anteroposterior exposure but can be clearly delineated on these angled projections.

The anteroposterior views may suffice for complete preliminary pelvic assessment in cases of trauma. Minimal motion of the patient is the best policy to prevent possible compromise to already injured soft tissues (e.g., blood vessels and urinary bladder). However, oblique films can be helpful adjuncts on follow-up stud-

ies. The supine patient is first rotated 45 degrees with the right hip down against the film (right posterior oblique) and then to the left 45 degrees (left posterior oblique). Because of the outward orientation of the sacroiliac joints, oblique films allow the viewer to look straight down the joints without confusing overlap of the free edges. Moreover, the ischiopubic rami and the margins of the obturator foramen will be visualized in a different manner. The posterior margin of the acetabulum can also lend itself to more direct inspection. Acetabular fractures, a topic that is discussed later in this chapter, require not only oblique roentgenograms but also lateral films for proper evaluation. However, computerized tomography has become essential for the evaluation of complex acetabular fractures identified on plain film, and with the new spiral technology, 3-D reconstruction images can be performed (see Fig. 16-83).

When the focus of attention is the hip, it is useful to include both sides on a single film for reasons of comparison. The straight anteroposterior roentgenogram of the pelvis and hips is an appropriate examination, but it is imperative to view the hip from the lateral aspect when at all possible. This can be achieved in one of two ways: (1) a frog-like position with the femur maximally rotated externally, or (2) a horizontally directed roentgenogram with the tube placed along the inner aspect of the thigh and directed through the hip to a grid film placed alongside the hip. This latter method is generally the desired technique in cases of fracture because the patient usually will not tolerate rotation of the leg and hip, and little or no motion of the injured part is preferred.

### Roentgenographic Anatomy and Developmental Variations

The pelvis is formed by two innominate bones, each consisting of an ilium, an ischium, and the pubis. These are distinct entities in youth but fuse to form a single, solid structure in the adult. The sacrum serves as a posterior bridge between the two by way of the essentially nonmobile sacroiliac joints.

The epiphyses and apophyses of the pelvis and hips ordinarily do not unite until the second decade of life. The apophyses of the iliac crest normally make their appearance by the twelfth to fifteenth year and fuse by 21 to 25 years of age. They are separated from the body of the ilium by no more than 2 to 3 mm, often have an irregular rippled appearance, and may show segmentation into two or more parts.

Small centers of ossification arise from the anterior inferior iliac spines by the thirteenth year and fuse 2 to 3 years later. Athletes are prone to avulsion of these centers, and this should be looked for when there is localized pain in a sports-related injury. Oblique films are most useful in such situations, and

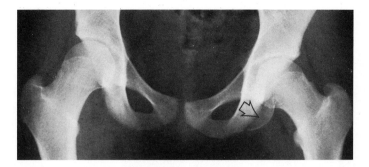

**Fig. 16–43.**
Avulsion fracture *(arrow)* of the ischial tuberosity on the left side.

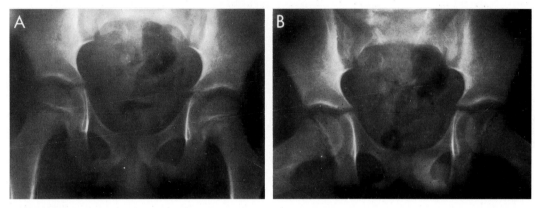

**Fig. 16–44.**
Normal pelvis and hips of a 10-year-old child. **A**, Anteroposterior view with the hips in the neutral position. **B**, Anteroposterior view with the hips in the froglike lateral position. Note the triradiate cartilage and the bulbous appearance of the ischiopubic synchondroses of the inferior rami.

a view of the opposite side is almost always needed to make the diagnosis.

Cheerleader's "splits" can create a similar avulsion of the ischial tuberosity apophysis on one or both sides (Fig. 16-43). The time of appearance and fusion of these ossification centers parallels those of the iliac crest.

Until the tenth or eleventh year of life, a radiolucent cartilage separates the ischium and pubis along the inferior ramus (Fig. 16-44). This area of normal development is often misjudged as a fracture. During the process of union, this region appears more dense and expanded so as to give the impression of callus formation or tumor. The bilateral appearances are often asymmetric.

The triradiate cartilage forms a Y-shaped configuration at the acetabulum and constitutes the junctures of the pubis, ischium, and ilium (see Fig. 16-44). This will become completely filled in with bone about the time of puberty. There have been many occasions when this, too, has been called a pelvic fracture.

In evaluating the symphysis pubis, it is more important for the inferior margins to align, whereas the superior borders are commonly and normally offset. Ordinarily, the width of the symphysis pubis joint measures no more than 8 mm in adults and 10 mm in children. Widening of the joint is characteristic of late pregnancy.

The posterior margin of the acetabulum, somewhat obscured by the femoral head and requiring an oblique view to see adequately, may arise from a separate ossification center and easily simulate a fracture because of its linear appearance. This variation is often a bilateral finding. A variable-sized ununited center, the *os acetabuli*, may persist throughout life. It is located along the superolateral margin of the acetabulum (Fig. 16-45).

The developmental features are of utmost importance in consideration of the anatomy of the hip. The femoral capital epiphysis appears during the first year. Synostosis of the head with the femoral neck is completed by the eighteenth year, but a cartilaginous fissure may persist. A central indentation along the articular margin of the femoral head corresponds to the fovea centralis, where the ligamentum teres is embedded.

The greater trochanter apophysis becomes visible by the fifth year and unites at the same time as the femoral capital epiphysis, namely, 18 years of age. The line of fusion may also persist for a long time and result in confusion.

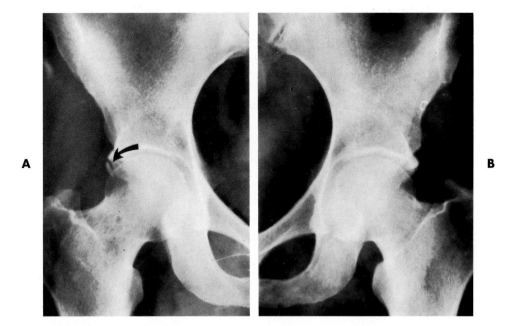

**Fig. 16–45.**
Os acetabuli. The right side (**A**) demonstrates this normal variant *(arrow)*. None is seen on the left (**B**).

In addition to the bones themselves, there are certain soft-tissue densities about the hips and pelvis that demand attention. The shadows of the obturator internus, the iliopsoas, and gluteus medius muscles are ordinarily outlined by radiolucent adipose tissue. Because of their close approximation to the joint capsule, blood or pus that distends the joint will be reflected on the roentgenogram by displacement of these fat stripes.

### Trauma

A rather significant degree of correlation exists between the presence of an extracapsular subtrochanteric hip fracture and a pathologic process. In other words, do not take for granted that such a fracture is related purely to trauma, because this is a favorable site for metastasis.

Hip dislocations are discussed in Chapter 10. From a radiologist's point of view, it is useful to comment on some of the roentgenographic changes seen in this type of injury. First of all, hip dislocations are classified as anterior, posterior, and central. In posterior dislocation, the most common form, the injury may not always be readily apparent on the anteroposterior film. There may be a slight difference in the size of the femoral heads as a result of slight rotation of the displaced hip. Shenton's line may be askew. This is a continuous, smooth line formed along the sweep of the inner margin of the femoral neck, and it normally follows the inferior boundary of the arched contour of the superior ischiopubic ramus. Any disruption of this line would in-

dicate a dislocation. The posterior lip of the acetabulum may be fractured, but as previously noted, a persistent unfused apophysis is sometimes located here.

When an anterior dislocation is present, the femoral head may lie medial and below the acetabulum, sometimes superimposed on the obturator foramen. Uncommonly, however, the head may overlie the acetabular roof and simulate a posterior dislocation. This will require a horizontal groin lateral roentgenogram for differentiation.

When either a posterior or an anterior dislocation has been reduced, postreduction roentgenograms should be inspected for associated fractures. Also, the width of the hip joint space requires measurement. A difference of more than 2 mm should make one suspect the possibility of interposed tissue (such as a portion of the torn capsule), which will necessitate surgical removal. Short of surgical exploration, the diagnosis may need tomography or even hip arthrography with radiopaque material.

A central dislocation of the hip is always associated with an acetabular fracture; hence, the condition where the femoral head intrudes into the pelvis is termed a *central fracture-dislocation*. However, a central acetabular fracture may exist without a dislocated hip. There are four basic types of acetabular fractures, but the central form constitutes the most common.

As seen in Fig. 16-46, a central acetabular fracture may be transverse or oblique. The transverse type extends from the anterior acetabular margin backward

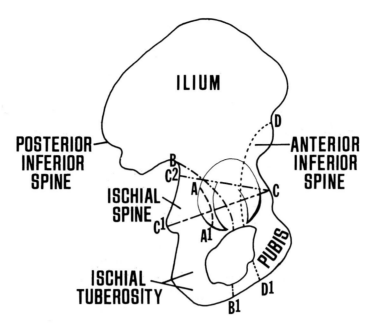

**Fig. 16–46.**
Types of acetabular fractures. This drawing of a lateral view of the pelvis describes the basic fractures that can involve the acetabulum: $A-A^1$ = posterior rim fracture; $B-B^1$ = posterior column fracture (ilioischial); $C-C^1$ = central transverse fracture; $C-C^2$ = central oblique fracture; $D-D^1$ = anterior column fracture (iliopubic). (From Thaggard A, Harle TS, Carlson V: *Semin Roentgenol* 13:117-133, 1978. Used by permission.)

through the ischial spine, whereas the oblique form is directed more superiorly to the greater sacrosciatic notch. Both actually divide the innominate bone into superior and inferior segments.

The second variety of acetabular fracture, as discussed previously, involves the posterior rim. Most often, this is produced by a posteriorly dislocated hip.

Two other categories of acetabular fractures are depicted in the schematic drawing of Fig. 16-46: anterior (iliopubic) and posterior (ilioischial) column fractures. Oblique films will be required for their proper interpretation.

In addition to acetabular fractures, the remainder of the pelvis can be fractured in various ways. It is best to classify these fractures as either stable or unstable.

Stable fractures can be categorized as avulsions, ischiopubic rami fractures, iliac wing fractures, and fractures of the sacrococcyx. Avulsions of the anterior superior and inferior iliac spines, as well as the ischial tuberosities, have already been discussed.

The most common pelvic fractures are those involving the ischiopubic rami. Occasionally, these may be stress-type infractions. Their visualization may call for cephalic and caudal tilt films.

A fracture of the iliac wing often results from a direct lateral blow to the pelvis. These are best depicted with an oblique roentgenogram.

Anteroposterior and lateral exposures of the sacrococcyx are required for the assessment of fractures, but it is often useful to include an anteroposterior cephalic (upward) tilt projection. Overlying intestinal content can obscure a fracture in this area, and linear tomography may be required.

A variety of fractures and/or dislocations result in unstable conditions of the pelvis. Among the more common types that might be encountered is the straddle fracture (Fig. 16-47, *A*). This situation exists when there are vertical fractures involving the superior and inferior ischiopubic rami on both sides. Less often, the fractures are unilateral but with separation of the symphysis pubis. Approximately 30% of such injuries will have associated urethral or bladder trauma.

More serious forms of unstable fractures are classified as double vertical fracture-dislocations (see Fig. 16-47). There are three such types; all have in common a double component involving the pelvic ring, anterior and posterior to the acetabulum.

When there are unilateral vertical fractures of the ischiopubic rami, or a dislocation of the symphysis pubis in combination with a fracture about the ipsilateral sacroiliac joint or a dislocation of that joint, the condition is termed *Malgaigne's fracture* (Fig. 16-47, *B* and *C*). The hemipelvis on the involved side may become displaced up or down and create a true unstable situation.

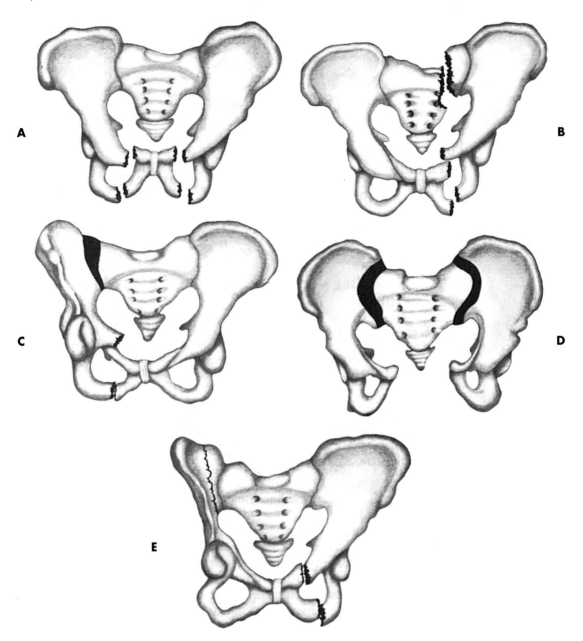

**Fig. 16–47.**
Types of unstable pelvic fractures. **A**, Straddle fracture. **B**, Malgaigne's fracture with an ipsilateral double vertical fracture. **C**, Malgaigne's fracture with dislocation of the sacroiliac joint. **D**, Sprung pelvis. **E**, Bucket-handle fracture. (From Dunn AW, Morris HD: *Bone Joint Surg* 50:1639-1648, 1968. Used by permission.)

A "sprung pelvis" is another form of an unstable double vertical injury. Here, there is separation of one or both sacroiliac joints and a disjunction of the symphysis pubis (Fig. 16-47, *D*). Careful inspection of the sacroiliac joints should be made in any patient with displacement of the pubis.

The third type of double vertical pelvic injury is the so-called bucket-handle fracture (Fig. 16-47, *E*). There will be fractures through the upper and lower rami of the anterior pelvic ring. The opposite or contralateral

sacroiliac joint will be separated or will demonstrate a juxtaarticular fracture.

CT has revolutionized the radiologist's ability to evaluate fractures of the pelvis. The transverse images provide greater anatomic detail. This allows one to distinguish important relationships and significant fragment displacements not readily apparent on the standard x-ray films. Alterations in the soft tissues, such as the development of associated hematoma formation, can be better determined. Totally unsuspected fractures that

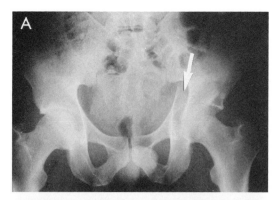

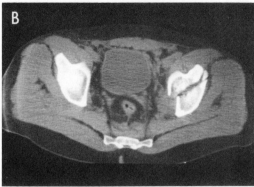

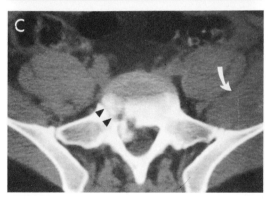

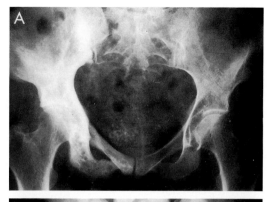

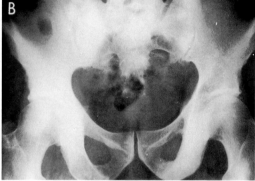

**Fig. 16–49.**
Increased bone density in the pelvis. **A,** Paget's disease. **B,** Osteoblastic metastasis.

**Fig. 16–48.**
These CT images of the pelvis dramatically disclose the extent of fractures not apparent on a routine x-ray film. Note also the unsuspected displaced fragment at S1 that extends into the central neural canal. Additionally, a fracture of the right transverse process of L5 was documented on the CT films that was not appreciated on the standard x-ray films (not shown). **A,** Routine pelvic x-ray film showing an obvious fracture of the left hemipelvis *(arrow).* **B,** Comminuted fracture of the acetabulum. **C,** Unsuspected fracture of S1 *(arrowheads).* Note the large hematoma *(curved arrow).*

are not apparent on routine films often are visualized by CT. Furthermore, the sacroiliac joints are much better depicted (Fig. 16-48).

## Tumor

Our attention is now directed to neoplastic disease of the pelvis. Primary tumors are seldom seen and usually present no diagnostic dilemmas. Most of these are similar to those described in the discussion of the spine.

On the other hand, metastatic disease is quite common in the pelvis, which constitutes approximately 12% of all bone metastatic sites. Difficulty in distinguishing minimal involvement may be related to confusing overlying intestinal gas and fecal material. The sensitivity of nuclear bone scanning will help to solve these difficult situations.

Often a pelvic roentgenogram that shows a marked increase in density is seen. The majority of these cases will represent either diffuse osteoblastic metastasis or *Paget's disease.* The differentiation, as already observed, can often be made by utilizing basic characteristics of each (Fig. 16-49). Notably, Paget's disease will disclose increased volume of bone and a greatly thickened trabecular pattern. Moreover, it may be confined to one side of the pelvis, a less likely occurrence in metastasis. In a small percentage of individuals (fewer than 1%), Paget's disease may transform to osteogenic sarcoma.

## Infection

Infections that involve the hips and pelvis, such as acute pyogenic arthritis and tuberculous osteomyelitis, are extremely rare today. Secondary seeding of infection, either directly from pelvic inflammation or through the blood stream, can take place and result in either an infected joint or osteomyelitis.

## Sacroiliac Joints

There are a number of conditions that can alter the sacroiliac joints in characteristic roentgenographic patterns and distributions. A frontal projection of the pelvis usually does not afford an adequate view of the sacroiliac joints, and it becomes necessary to perform a 45-degree oblique x-ray film as a result of their posterolateral oblique orientation. However, the addition of an anteroposterior film with the tube angled 20 to 35 degrees toward the head can project the joints' articular surfaces to better advantage.

Anatomically, the sacroiliac joints are true synovial joints with restricted mobility. The joint spaces themselves occupy only the lower half to two thirds of the joints, the upper portion being formed by interosseous ligaments. In adults, the spaces normally measure 2 to 5 mm in width.

In older individuals, the joints quite often reveal the changes of degenerative arthritis. This most often is bilateral and symmetric in distribution. The joint spaces narrow, and a thin line of sclerosis forms along the iliac aspect. Osteophytes or spurs commonly accompany the process, particularly along the anterior aspect. These can be focal and sclerotic and may be confused with an osteoblastic metastasis when seen on the frontal film. The spurs can extend inferiorly from the joints as well.

Excluding infection, a variety of inflammatory diseases may produce sacroiliitis. Listed among these are rheumatoid arthritis, rheumatoid spondylitis, psoriasis, *Reiter's syndrome*, and inflammatory intestinal disorders such as ulcerative colitis, regional enteritis (*Crohn's disease*), and *Whipple's disease*. Although there may be subtle differences among these, differentiation is often impossible and requires correlation with clinical and laboratory findings.

Because they are lined with synovium, the sacroiliac joints, like other synovial joints, may be involved with rheumatoid arthritis, but only in advanced cases. The alterations may involve only one side, but both are usually included and almost always in an asymmetric fashion. Demineralization about the joints is seen along with distinctive subarticular erosions that eventuate in narrowing of the spaces. Spurring and ankylosis (fusion) are not features of rheumatoid arthritis in the sacroiliac joints.

On the other hand, ankylosing spondylitis (*Marie-Strümpell disease*) is often bilaterally symmetric. The roentgenographic changes are distinctly different from those of rheumatoid arthritis. However, the sacroiliac

joint alterations of rheumatoid arthritis and the other noninfectious inflammatory lesions can be similar and preclude a differentiation in some cases. The fundamental findings of ankylosing spondylitis initially involve the ilium and consist of irregular deossification, articular erosions, indistinct subchondral line density, and spotty sclerosis. Subsequent reactive new bone formation often bridges the joint space and can eventuate in actual ossification and obliteration of the joints. Another distinguishing peculiarity of rheumatoid spondylitis as it pertains to the pelvis is a fine-to-coarse spiculated or "whiskering" appearance that may develop along the inferior margins of the ischial tuberosities.

The distribution and pattern of involvement caused by the sacroiliitis of intestinal diseases may be similar to that of rheumatoid spondylitis. But psoriasis and Reiter's syndrome are more often unilateral, or show asymmetry of each side, and lack any bony bridging. The separation of these entities might be facilitated by moving up to the lumbar spine where the classic changes of rheumatoid spondylitis, the "bamboo spine," may be identified. The bony bridges or syndesmophytes between the vertebral bodies (as seen in ankylosing spondylitis and bowel disease spondylitis) are smooth, uniform, thin, and symmetric. Those found in psoriasis and rheumatoid arthritis present as irregular, asymmetric, and thick outgrowths.

Gouty arthritis involving the sacroiliac joints occurs in long-standing and severe cases in a minority of individuals with this affliction. One or both joints may exhibit involvement. The most striking features are those seen in other skeletal regions: irregular, often large, subarticular erosions and related sclerosis.

An uncommonly recognized source of back pain in elderly individuals suffering from osteoporosis is the stress or *insufficiency fracture* of the sacroiliac joints. This entity can be readily diagnosed on radionuclide bone scans with a characteristic H-shaped uptake of the isotope (Fig. 16-50).

## The Knee

### Roentgenographic Examination

The basic minimum examination of the knee consists of supine anteroposterior and flexed lateral views. The latter film should be obtained with the knee bent at least 45 degrees, although this may be impossible in an acutely injured, fluid-filled joint or in a severely osteoarthritic knee.

Certain situations will call for other views. Internal and external oblique films may help visualize otherwise nonvisible subtle fractures of the tibial plateaus or femoral condyles. These features, as well as the intercondylar space and the tibial spine (intercondylar crest), can also be evaluated with a tunnel film (Fig. 16-51).

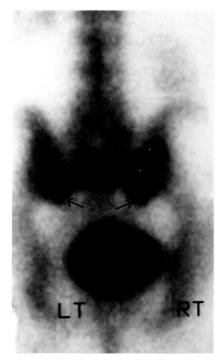

**Fig. 16–50.**
Insufficiency stress fracture of the sacrum in an elderly patient with osteoporosis, who presented with low back pain. Note the somewhat H-shaped configuration of the abnormal isotope uptake *(arrows).*

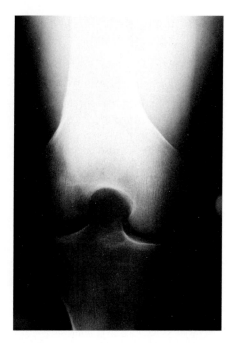

**Fig. 16–51.**
"Tunnel" view of the knee.

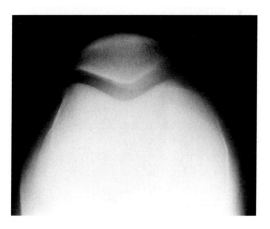

**Fig. 16–52.**
"Sunrise" view of the knee.

The tangential or "sunrise" projection affords another perspective of the patella and the femoropatellar joint (Fig. 16-52).

Stress films, including valgus and varus manual forces, can bring out ligamentous injuries or laxity. Standing anteroposterior weight-bearing studies give information related to subtle joint space narrowing in degenerative osteoarthritis. Occasionally, tomography will elucidate abnormalities not identifiable on standard films. With the advent of better fluoroscopic equipment, intraarticular changes of the invisible cartilaginous menisci, articular cartilage, and ligaments can be successfully evaluated by means of double air-contrast arthrography.

### Roentgenographic Anatomy and Developmental Variations

The distal femoral epiphysis normally appears in the ninth month of gestation and therefore is utilized in determining fetal maturity. At birth it measures approximately 5 mm. The distal femoral epiphysis normally fuses at 20 years of age. As in other areas of the skeleton, the epiphyseal line may persist as a faint track.

The intercondylar fossa, best evaluated on the tunnel film, forms a smooth arch. It serves primarily as a compartment for the proximal origins of the anterior and posterior cruciate ligaments.

The joint space, which is divided into medial and lateral compartments, normally measures 3 to 5 mm in height. It represents the thickness of the articular cartilages of the femur and tibia as well as the medial and lateral semilunar cartilages (menisci).

The proximal tibial epiphysis becomes visible by ossification in the last 2 months of fetal life. Like the femoral epiphysis, it fuses to the shaft by the twentieth year. Between the ages of 7 and 15 years, the tongue-shaped anterior and inferior extension of the epiphysis is visible and forms the anterior tibial tuberosity or spine (Fig. 16-53, *A*). The tuberosity is an extremely variable structure that develops in an irregular fashion

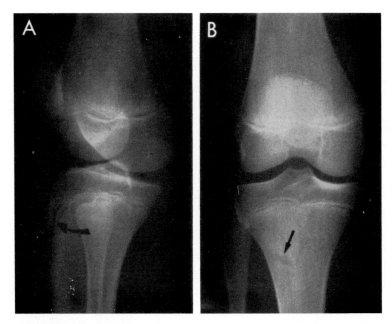

**Fig. 16–53.**
Normal appearance of the anterior tibial tuberosity in a 12-year-old. **A**, Lateral view. **B**, Anteroposterior view. Note the radiolucent line *(arrow)* superimposing the tibial metaphysis.

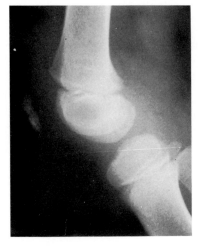

**Fig. 16–54.**
Normal appearance of the patella in an 8-year-old. Note the irregular, fragmented, and sclerotic character simulating osteochondritis.

and often has a fragmented appearance. This should not be confused with a fracture or *Osgood-Schlatter disease*. Its features on the anteroposterior view can be particularly bewildering (Fig. 16-53, *B*). On the frontal view, a radiolucent cleft often appears over the proximal tibial shaft.

The articular surfaces of the proximal third of the tibia present a varied number of appearances, and this is especially true of the intercondylar eminence of the tibial spine. There are two major crests, lateral and me-

dial. Occasionally, the clinician may identify an anteromedial tubercle, to which the anterior cruciate ligament attaches. A similar but less commonly found posterolateral tubercle marks the insertion of the posterior cruciate ligament. The "tunnel" view of the knee usually demonstrates this anatomy to the best advantage. Small avulsion fragments arising from the crests and presenting as loose intraarticular bodies will be best projected on this x-ray film view.

The patella is considered a large sesamoid bone embedded in the quadriceps tendon. It should always be examined with a tangential film in addition to the lateral and frontal roentgenograms. On the anteroposterior projection, the details of the patella may become completely lost in the shadow of the distal portion of the femur, and hence pathologic changes may be overlooked. Tangential, lateral, and sometimes oblique views are therefore required.

Ossification of the patella is irregular in nature and arises from multiple foci. In the young it may be divided into several segments. It often has a granular appearance with irregular borders. Before complete fusion of the patellar ossification centers, there can be confusion with fractures, or its irregular outline may suggest osteochondritis (Fig. 16-54).

One of the more difficult problems associated with roentgenographic appraisal of the patella is the commonly observed anomaly of patella partita. This condition is usually bilateral but must be differentiated from fractures. A bipartite status is the most prevalent form,

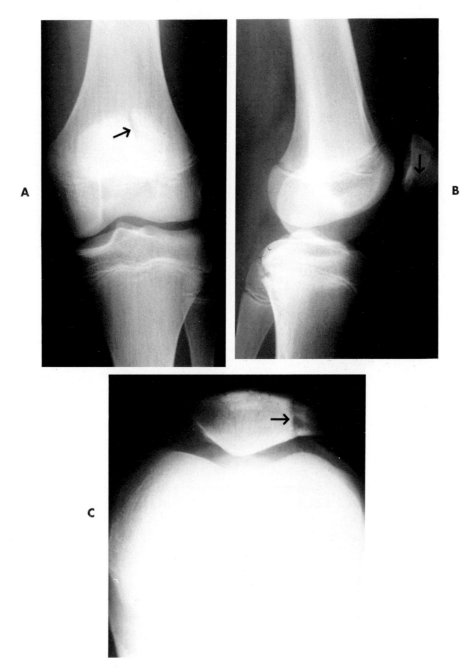

**Fig. 16–55.**
Bipartite patella. **A**, Anteroposterior. **B**, Lateral. **C**, Sunrise view. Note the upper outer position of the separate bone, the sclerosis of the line, and its curvilinear course, whereas a fracture would be sharp and straight. This is an unusual case of unilateral involvement.

but multipartite patellae also exist, and as many as six different segments have been reported. In the usual bipartite state, a radiolucent line separates a smaller segment that almost always occupies the upper-outer quadrant, although many other rare variations are found (Fig. 16-55). There have been cases described for patellar partition into anterior and posterior portions.

A somewhat distracting osseous shadow, the *fabella*, is seen along the posterior aspect in 10% to 20% of knees (Fig. 16-56). A small sesamoid bone of varying size and shape, it lies within the lateral head of the gastrocnemius muscle and is best seen on the lateral view. Many times it overlies the border of the lateral femoral condyle and appears as an avulsion fragment on the an-

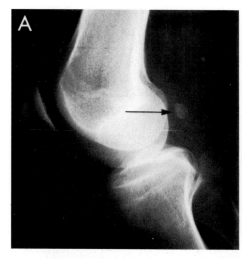 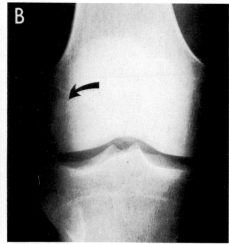

**Fig. 16–56.**
The fabella *(arrows)*. **A**, Lateral view. **B**, Anteroposterior view.

teroposterior film. The bone is most often a bilateral finding and is seen more often in males. It must be differentiated from a fracture, loose joint body, foreign body, and phlebolith.

The soft tissues about the knee deserve particular attention and must not be overlooked on the knee roentgenogram. The fundamental observation in the presence of joint effusions is an anterior displacement of the patella and an elongated oval area of increased density above the patella that represents fluid in the suprapatellar bursa. A small amount of fluid may not produce these changes.

Not uncommonly, short slivers of ossification immediately above and below the patella—and usually attached to it—represent the tendons of the quadriceps muscle and the patellar ligament, respectively. They can be misleading shadows to the unwary and probably represent the end result of tendinitis, much like that seen in the rotator cuff tendons of the shoulder.

It is not too surprising to visualize a radiolucent slit within the knee joint and, more commonly, within the hip and shoulder joints of children. This phenomenon is linked to a vacuum effect and is caused by pulling on the extremity or by producing forced adduction or abduction. It is important that this not be interpreted as abnormal. Nevertheless, in the elderly population it is a pathologic observation and may be seen in severe arthritis with degeneration of the cartilage. The finding may be seen in a vertebral spine with advanced degenerative disc disease.

### Trauma

The majority of roentgenograms done because of trauma to the knee will be normal. At times a joint effusion will be demonstrated with soft tissue fullness of the suprapatellar bursa, but visualized fractures are un-common. With fractures extending into the joint, a fluid-fluid level can be demonstrated on cross-table lateral views resulting from blood layering with marrow fat (lipohemarthrosis) (Fig. 16-57). Fractures can involve one or both femoral condyles, the tibial tuberosity, or the proximal third of the fibula as well as the patella. As many views as are necessary should be utilized to evaluate these injuries. Stress fractures about the knee, especially the proximal tibia, are not uncommon and occasionally show a dense line of compacted trabeculae but may require a radionuclide bone scan or MRI to document.

Femorotibial dislocations are rare. These can be anterior or posterior, and are often associated with a fracture. The major concerns in such situations are tearing of the collateral and cruciate ligaments and, more acutely important, severing of the popliteal artery, which will require angiography for proper assessment.

### Tumor

Of the many benign tumors involving the knee region, osteochondroma is probably one of the most common, with the exception of benign cortical defects (Fig. 16-58). The latter are peripherally located, round-to-oval radiolucencies that often measure no more than 2 cm. They have a sharply defined sclerotic margin and are common in the metaphyseal areas of the distal portion of the femur and the proximal and distal thirds of the tibia. They are asymptomatic and are usually discovered incidentally on roentgenograms performed for other reasons. With advancing age they tend to disappear.

The *osteochondroma* is seen as a bony protuberance of variable size, contiguous with the femoral or tibial metaphyseal or diaphyseal bone marrow and extending away from the joint in the direction of the tendons and muscles (Fig. 16-59). Osteochondromas have an invisi-

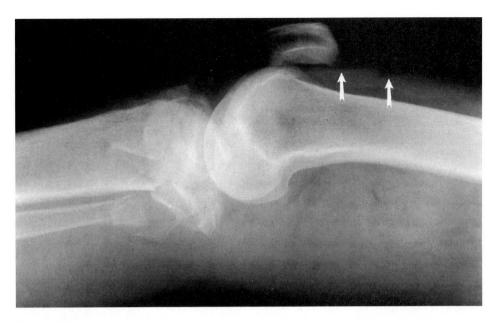

**Fig. 16–57.**
Cross-table lateral view of knee demonstrating a fluid-fluid level of a lipohemarthrosis indicating an intraarticular fracture.

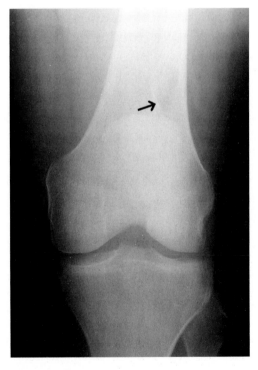

**Fig. 16–58.**
Benign cortical defect of the distal femur *(arrow).*

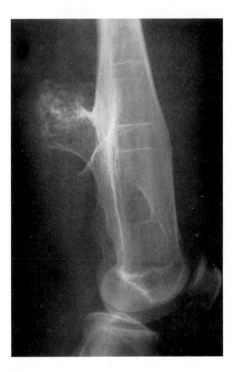

**Fig. 16–59.**
Osteochondroma of the knee.

ble cap of cartilage. Solitary osteochondromas are less often demonstrated about other joints of the body. When these exostoses are multiple, they constitute a hereditary bone dysplasia designated as diaphyseal aclasis.

Aneurysmal bone cysts are found in the neural arches of the vertebrae; in the ends of long bones; and,

most often, in the distal third of the femur. They become very expansive but are confined by a thin layer of cortical bone and contain many septa of bone.

A giant-cell tumor characteristically involves the distal portion of the femur. It is considered a benign vascular lesion, but occasionally it transforms into a locally invasive malignant process. There is a gradual,

**A**   **B**   **C**

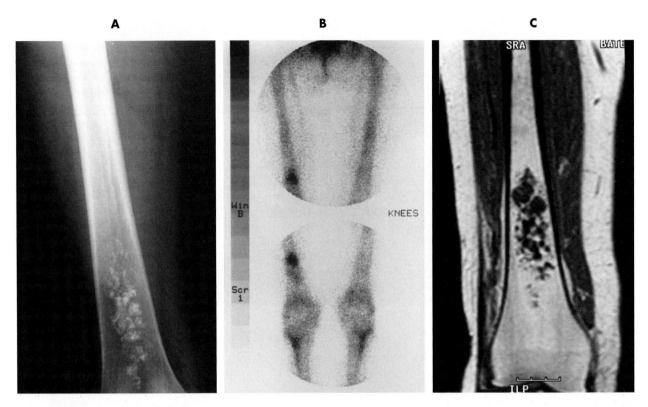

**Fig. 16–60.**
Bone infarct of the distal third of the femur. **A**, X-ray. **B**, Radionuclide bone scan. **C**, Coronal T-1 weighted spin echo magnetic resonance image.

eccentric expansion of a thinned cortex, but not to the same extent as an aneurysmal bone cyst. A "soap-bubble" appearance is characteristic. The lesion involves the closed epiphysis and metaphysis and extends to the subarticular cortex but not into the joint (see Fig. 16-99).

Although not ordinarily considered under the topic of tumors, *bone infarcts*, often located in the distal third of the femur, can create confusing roentgenographic changes. They occur in caisson disease, pancreatitis, and various vascular disorders. Any segment of bone, epiphysis, metaphysis, or diaphysis can be involved, but the alterations are confined to the medullary cavity. They appear as irregular sclerotic longitudinal streaks, occasionally with fine cystic patterns resembling a corkscrew. If relatively recent in onset, infarcts can display new bone turnover with increased uptake on a diphosphonate nuclide scan. Although rarely required, MRI may support the diagnosis of a benign lesion in confusing cases (Fig. 16-60).

The knee has the dubious distinction of being the most common site for the development of osteosarcoma. The metaphysis of the distal portion of the femur accounts for approximately 75% of all osteogenic sarcomas. This primary bone malignancy tends to occur during puberty, with boys being more commonly affected than girls. The roentgenographic changes take many forms, either being purely osteolytic or showing a mixed destructive and osteosclerotic pattern (Fig. 16-61). Extensive soft-tissue involvement is the rule. Periosteal reaction can be exuberant, eventually forming the typical spiculated "sunburst" appearance, although this is not always present (Fig. 16-62).

Under the heading of round-cell tumors, *Ewing's sarcoma* is manifested as a solitary lesion arising in the diaphyses and metaphyses of long bones, particularly the femur. However, it has been observed with relative frequency in the humerus and ulna as well as the pelvis. Originating in the bone marrow, it produces a characteristic layered periosteal thickening resembling an "onion skin." A variable patchy dissolution without significant expansion is imparted to the osseous architecture. Unfortunately, the symptoms of fever and pain and the sarcoma's roentgenographic manifestations can resemble those of osteomyelitis in the child and adolescent, and indeed the distinction may be extremely difficult to make.

### Arthritis

Osteoarthritis is a common affliction of the knee (Fig. 16-63). Degenerative wear and tear produce the

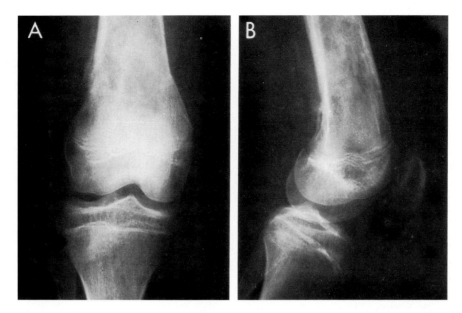

**Fig. 16–61.**
Osteosarcoma of the knee. **A**, Anteroposterior view; **B**, Lateral view. Note the mottled bone destruction with interrupted periosteal reaction and soft-tissue extension.

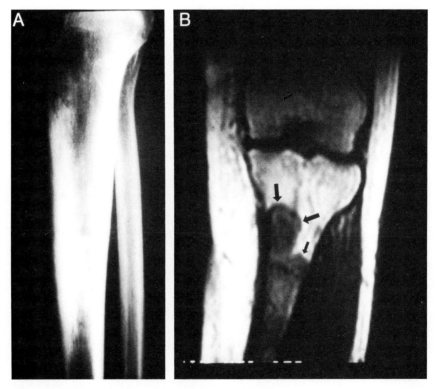

**Fig. 16–62.**
Osteosarcoma. **A**, Lateral roentgenogram of the proximal third of the tibia. **B**, Coronal MRI of the same area. The medullary extent of the disease *(arrows)* is easily identified by MRI.

changes with progressing age, but secondary posttraumatic arthrosis is also a leading offender. Minimal joint space narrowing will be one of the earliest roentgenographic changes, reflecting wearing and thinning of the articular cartilage. Standing weight-bearing films might be required to demonstrate this finding. The decreased height of the joint space may be accompanied by increasing sclerosis of the subarticular region of the tibia, quite often the medial condyle. The femoropatellar joint will undergo similar alterations of narrowing and associated sclerosis of the articular surface of the patella. Eventually the process leads to bony spurs arising from the articular margins of the femur, tibia, and patella. These osteophytes may become so significantly large that function is impaired.

Subchondral cysts, which are not always evident, are a unique feature of osteoarthritis, even in joints other than the knee. They are well-defined, round-to-oval lucencies, one or more in number. They measure anywhere from a few millimeters to 3 to 4 cm. One proposed theory for their evolution states that, because they are lined with synovium, they represent protrusions of the membrane through a defect in the articular cartilage. A small channel forms a direct communication between the cysts and the joint space, and this has been proved on pathologic dissections. The mechanism for their formation is thought to be a change in the intraarticular fluid and pressure dynamics of the disorganized joint.

The actual size of the intercondylar fossa, as seen on the tunnel view, may enlarge somewhat in osteoarthritis. However, this feature is more pronounced in rheumatoid arthritis and the arthrosis of hemophilia with repeated intraarticular hemorrhages.

Other types of arthropathies that can involve the knee, but are seen in other joints as well, have characteristic radiologic appearances. Opaque crystalline material can be deposited within the articular cartilage and periarticular tissues in several distinct diseases. Monosodium urate crystals are distinctive of gouty arthritis and give rise to the typical radiographic findings of gouty tophi. Another form of crystalline arthropathy is pseudogout or calcium pyrophosphate dihydrate deposition disease (CPPD), which has also been described as chondrocalcinosis. Seventy-five percent of patients with CPPD are asymptomatic but a few individuals will have a progressive debilitating joint disorder that can have all of the characteristics of typical degenerative osteoarthritis (Fig. 16-64). Another sporadic form of chondrocalcinosis is termed calcium hydroxyapatite crystal deposition disease. This may be connected to renal osteodystrophy or collagen vascular diseases.

### Osteochondritis

Several disease entities classified as osteochondritis or aseptic necrosis involve the knee. The abnormalities of osteochondritis dissecans have already been described. Osgood-Schlatter disease is another form involving the anterior tibial tubercle. As mentioned previously, there is a significant variation in the roentgenographic appearance of the normal tuberosity, and the diagnosis is primarily a clinical one. Although there may be sclerosis and/or fragmentation, this does not necessarily constitute Osgood-Schlatter disease. The only roentgenographic abnormality, almost universally present in the acute phase, is overlying soft-tissue swelling. The prin-

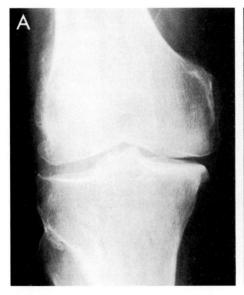
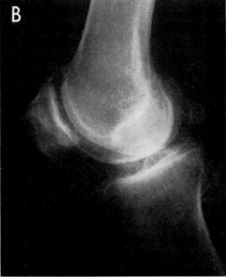

**Fig. 16–63.**
Osteoarthritis of the knee. **A**, Anteroposterior view. **B**, Lateral view.

cipal purpose for obtaining the films is to exclude some other lesion, such as tumor or infection.

One other type of osteochondritis that might be encountered in the knee is Blount's disease, or tibia vara. For some unknown reason, possibly stress, a localized growth disturbance occurs along the medial-posterior aspect of the tibial metaphysis. The changes may ap-

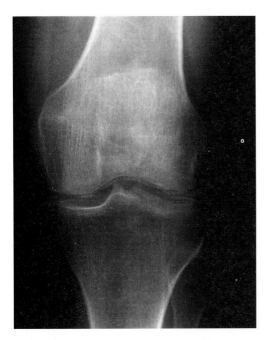

**Fig. 16–64.**
Pseudogout. Calcium pyrophosphate dihydrate has been deposited in the articular hyaline cartilage as well as the menisci.

pear between the ages of 1 and 12 years and culminate in outward bowing of one or both legs. Roentgenographically, the medial tibial metaphysis is widened and forms a broad spur that extends both medially and posteriorly. The medial surface of the tibial epiphysis becomes flattened and produces a slope of concavity where this growth center is normally convex. Without correction, the fully developed knee may exhibit a persistent downward slope of the medial tibial articular surface. The medial femoral condyle hypertrophies to compensate for the tibial deformity.

## The Ankle and Foot

### Roentgenographic Examination
Three views are mandatory for proper evaluation of the ankle, and three projections are necessary for the foot examination. As elsewhere in the skeleton, modified and special films can clarify suspicious areas.

For the ankle, the three films include anteroposterior, lateral, and oblique projections. The oblique study, or mortise view, is obtained by rotating the foot internally 10 to 15 degrees (Fig. 16-65). Although the calcaneus, tarsal bones, and bases of the metatarsal bones are not considered anatomically a part of the ankle, they should be included because associated or isolated injuries to these structures may be found when symptoms point only to the ankle. A good example of this is a fracture of the base of the fifth metatarsal bone.

An external oblique view might be requested when there is still a question of an abnormality in the absence of findings on the three standard x-ray films. A subtle fracture of either malleoli may be brought out in this way.

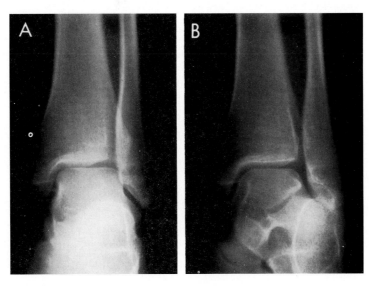

**Fig. 16–65.**
Normal ankle films. **A**, Anteroposterior view; **B**, Oblique (mortise) view.

In the presence of soft-tissue swelling after trauma—but without an associated fracture—ligamentous damage must be considered. Stress anteroposterior filming utilizing manual abduction and adduction of the heel may be indicated. Widening of the ankle mortise strongly suggests a tear in either or both the medial deltoid and lateral collateral ligaments. Because of pain, maneuvering the ankle for stress views may require local anesthesia.

The standard roentgenographic study of the foot should include anteroposterior, internally rotated oblique, and lateral projections. Because of superimposition, the metatarsal and phalangeal bones cannot be evaluated to any extent on the lateral film, but the talus, calcaneus, and tarsal bones are relatively clearly outlined. Additionally, the talocalcaneal, talonavicular, and calcaneocuboid joints are well depicted. On the anteroposterior film, the cuboid and lateral cuneiform bones are superimposed, and the bases of the metatarsals tend to be obscured by overlap. These bones are projected into profile with internal oblique films. An externally rotated oblique view will delineate the first metatarsal and medial cuneiform bones.

The toes should be examined with anteroposterior and internal and external oblique films. An individual toe that causes concern requires a lateral view. This may be performed by having the patient hold the toe in extension with a pencil while the other toes are held in flexion, a maneuver that also is utilized for finger roentgenograms.

The heel is best demonstrated with lateral and axial (tangential) films. However, as is pointed out later in this chapter, oblique exposures sometimes aid in the study of this bone.

### Roentgenographic Anatomy, Variants, and Pathology

**Ankle.**    The ankle mortise is formed by the distal third of the fibula (lateral malleolus), styloid process of the tibia (medial malleolus), the horizontal articular plate of the tibia (plafond), and the dome-shaped articular surface of the talus (tenon).

On the lateral view, the width of the joint space between the tibia and talus narrows from anterior to posterior in the normal subject. Because of this, most ankle dislocations are anterior, except where there is a disruptive fracture of the mortise.

As has been mentioned previously with other growth centers, a linear sclerotic zone of bone condensation or a lucent line of incomplete union may persist in the distal portion of the tibia where the epiphyseal line existed. Additionally, just as in the distal thirds of the radius or femur, a variable number of regular transverse bands of increased bone density may be observed in the tibial metaphysis. These so-called growth lines are normal; they tend to disappear with age and should not be confused with evidence of a pathologic process such as the lines of lead poisoning.

Often, the tip of the medial or the lateral malleoli arises from separate ossification centers that fail to fuse. The resultant os subtibiale and os subfibulare can be variable in size, but like all accessory bones, will have a well-defined thin cortical margin throughout their circumference. This will differentiate them from recent fractures.

Because of the high incidence of accessory bones in the ankle and foot, comparative views are recommended. The findings are usually, but not always, bilateral. If the distinction between fracture and an accessory ossicle is difficult, the clinician should consider one of several textbooks dealing with normal variants (Birkner, 1978; Keats, 1992; Kohler and Zimmer, 1993).

One of the best-known accessory skeletal elements of the ankle—in addition to the os subtibiale and os subfibiale—is the os trigonum (Fig. 16-66). Situated behind the talus near the posterior aspect of the talocalcaneal joint, it is best viewed on the lateral roentgenogram. Its shape and size are variable, and it may measure 1 cm or more. Despite its incidence, it still is commonly misinterpreted as a fracture.

Rarely, the os trigonum may be mimicked by a fracture of the posterior tubercle of the talus. This may occur when the posterior talar process becomes wedged between the posterior articular rim of the tibia and the calcaneus with severe forced plantar flexion.

On the anteroposterior projection of the ankle, the Achilles tendon is seen as a thick band of slightly increased density behind the tibia. The resultant shadow can create a bewildering roentgenogram. On the mortise film, the clinician may see a horizontal V-shaped lu-

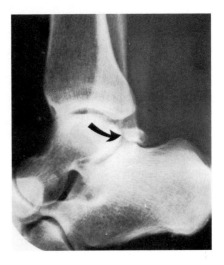

**Fig. 16–66.**
Os trigonum *(arrow).*

cency through the medial margin of the talus. This corresponds to the inner margin of the talus, which corresponds to the inner margin of the talocalcaneal joint.

Overlap of the cortical margins of the fibula and tibia occurs in most views of the ankle (except a correctly positioned mortise film). This overlap results in an apparent radiolucent defect termed a *"Mach"* effect and often leads to fracture misinterpretation.

On the lateral view of the ankle, distention of the joint capsule with blood can be discerned in either or both the anterior or posterior soft-tissue compartments. Such a finding is often indicative of a fracture of the distal portion of the tibia or talus, but not the lateral malleolus. This is because the synovial membrane of the capsule invests only the talus and tibia, but not the distal third of the fibula.

Benign cortical defects are a relatively common finding in the distal portion of the tibia in children. These defects are just as common in the femur and tibia about the knee. Their characteristics have been described under the section of the knee. On roentgenograms they are easily distinguishable from more serious lesions (Fig. 16-67).

The distal third of the tibia is a common site for the development of Brodie's abscess. This lesion results from a sharply localized pyogenic infection of low virulence. This isolated form of osteomyelitis, seen primarily in children, quite often involves the metaphysis.

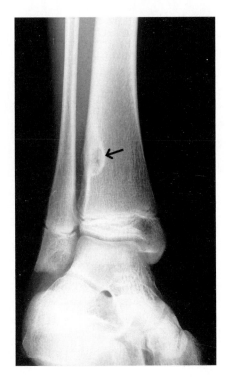

**Fig. 16–67.**
Benign cortical defect *(arrow)* of distal tibia.

Its intramedullary location is usually eccentric. It is seen on roentgenograms as a central irregular lucency surrounded by a thick capsule of sclerotic bone.

Osteochondritis dissecans, discussed elsewhere, is most commonly found involving the knee. This form of avascular necrosis, which is thought to be related to trauma, occurs in other areas as well (including the elbow and ankle). An osteochondral fragment of varying size, but usually small (less than 5 mm), can retain its position in relation to the articular margin or become displaced into the joint as a loose body. Rarely, the abnormality may not be identified on standard radiographs. CT or MRI may be required to detect the defect in the clinical setting of persistent pain and disability and a normal x-ray study (Fig. 16-68).

**Foot.**   Overlap of the individual bony elements of the foot tends to make evaluation of the roentgenographic anatomy somewhat difficult. Anatomically, the bones of the foot include the phalanges, metatarsals, cuboid, the three cuneiforms, navicular, and the calcaneus, as well as the talus, although the latter is also considered a component of the ankle.

Of the tarsal bones, the talus is second only to the calcaneus as the most common bone to be fractured. The majority of these injuries are chip and avulsion types. They may occur along the anteroposterior surface of the neck, and therefore a lateral film is required. Such fractures have also been described along the medial, lateral, and posterior processes. A fragment of the posterior eminence may simulate the os trigonum. Less commonly, the talus is fractured through the neck.

The talus is more susceptible to dislocation than the other tarsal bones because it is the only bone in the lower extremity not having direct muscle attachments. Furthermore, because of its tenuous vascular supply, posttraumatic aseptic necrosis of the talus may eventually take place.

The calcaneus anatomically consists of a body and a large posterior tuberosity. The *sustentaculum tali* forms a platform of bone along the inner superior surface of the body and provides support to the anterior portion of the talus. The posterior facet, behind the sustentaculum tali, is that portion of the talocalcaneal (subtalar) joint that slopes downward, as seen on the lateral roentgenogram, and into which the lateral triangular process of the talus projects (Fig. 16-69).

The apophysis of the posterior calcaneal tuberosity appears early in life and fuses in or about the seventeenth year. The margins of the apophysis and the posterior tuberosity can look quite irregular and ragged. The apophysis itself may exhibit fragmentation and varying degrees of sclerosis. *Sever's disease*, a form of osteochondritis or aseptic necrosis (discussed in a previous section), has been ascribed to this ossification

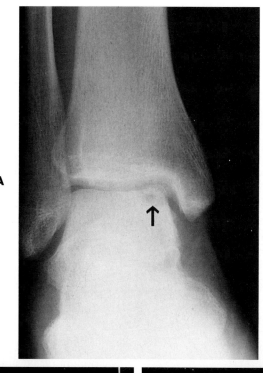

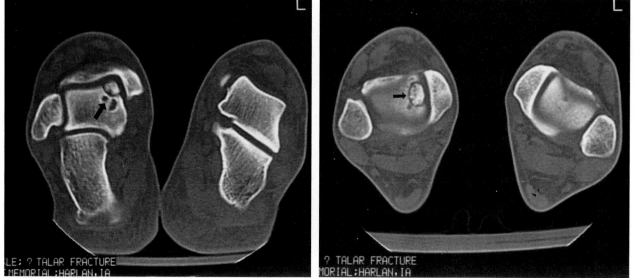

**Fig. 16–68.**
Osteochondritis dessicans of the talus. **A**, Articular defect *(arrow)*. **B**, Axial and **C**, coronal CT images of the ankle display the osteo-chondral bone nidus *(arrows)*.

center; but much like Osgood-Schlatter's disease of the knee, the diagnosis is principally clinical because the normal x-ray film appearance is extremely inconstant. Once fused, the area may show multiple irregular striations and some irregularity of the margins. It is of interest that in rheumatoid spondylitis the posterior surface of the tuberosity may display typical "whiskering" or fraying of its margins much like that seen in the ischial tuberosities of the pelvis.

To properly evaluate the heel, especially in cases of trauma, a tangential (axial) projection and both oblique views are required in addition to the lateral film. To obtain the axial exposure, the patient is seated on the table with the heel against the film. A towel or long piece of gauze is placed around the ball and toes of the foot, and the individual is instructed to flex the foot by pulling on the cloth. The tube is angled 40 degrees toward the head and centered over the heel. Multiple ax-

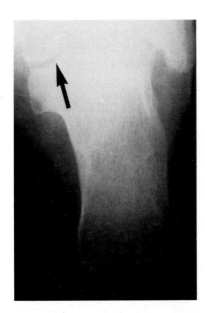

**Fig. 16–69.**
Axial view of the os calcis. Note the sustentaculum tali *(arrow).*

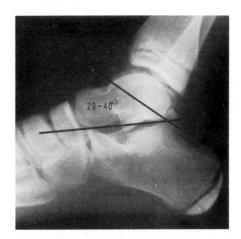

**Fig. 16–70.**
This lateral film of an ankle demonstrates Boehler's angle. Normal measurement is 20 to 40 degrees.

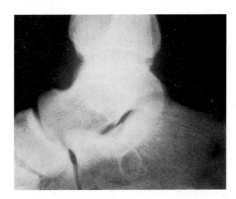

**Fig. 16–71.**
Normal lucency within the os calcis simulates a cyst.

ial films from angles of 20 to 40 degrees may be necessary to properly demonstrate the location and extent of a fracture.

Fractures of the os calcis are often the result of a feet-first fall from a height, producing crushing injuries with compression and comminution. In 10% of such cases, the fractures are bilateral, and in a similar percentage there will be an associated injury of the lumbar or thoracic spine as a result of the vertical compression forces dispersed into the back.

The lateral convex and medial concave surfaces of the calcaneus should be well delineated on the axial view. If the film is accurately exposed, the sustentaculum tali along the medial aspect will also be identified.

When viewing the os calcis on the lateral examination, it is mandatory that *Boehler's angle* be measured. This is formed by the intersection of (1) a line drawn from the dome of the os calcis at the talocalcaneal joint to the anterior process of this same bone and (2) a line extending from the posterior tubercle to the dome of the calcaneus (Fig. 16-70). Normally this measures between 20 and 40 degrees. With compression fractures, this angle will be reduced. Subtle compression fractures may be overlooked if this angle is not measured.

Stress fractures of the os calcis, as in some other bones of the body, are not manifested immediately after injury. It may take 10 or more days before a line of sclerotic endosteal new bone is detected that parallels the posterior border of the heel. Often, no abnormal changes occur. A bone scan or even MRI may be necessary in the clinical setting of unexplained, persistent pain.

Exostoses or spurs are a common finding in the heel. They can arise from the posterior or inferior margin of

the tuberosity. The posterior bony outgrowths extend in the direction of the Achilles tendon. Inferior or plantar spurs grow toward the sole of the foot within the plantar fascia. These excrescences may lead to local irritation and subsequent pain.

A somewhat round-to-triangular area of lucency that is relatively well circumscribed will occasionally be observed in the body of the calcaneus on the lateral roentgenogram (Fig. 16-71). This finding can create interpretive difficulties because it simulates a cyst. This has been proved anatomically to represent a normal area of thinned, deficient trabeculae. This is usually an incidental finding and can be worrisome when seen.

When considering the tarsal navicular bone roentgenographically, there are several lesions that deserve discussion because of their relatively common occurrence. Traumatic injuries to the tarsal navicular are uncommon. Avulsion fractures along the dorsal surface may be found near the talonavicular joint and require differentiation from an os supranaviculare. The medial tuberosity that serves for the insertion of the posterior tibial tendon may be subjected to forces resulting in fracture. Importantly, such a fracture may be associated with a fracture of the cuboid bone, often with dorsal subluxation of the navicular. An accessory bone, the *os tibiale externum*, is located behind the tuberosity. It is more common than tuberosity fractures and may be confused with one (Fig. 16-72).

Of all of the tarsal bones, the cuboid initially has the most striking features because of its multifragmented appearance. After a short interval, the fragments become united into one solid structure.

Rarely encountered, cuboid anomalies are synostoses to the calcaneus, talus, navicular, or metatarsals. Accessory bones closely related to the cuboid are the relatively common os peroneum and less common os vesalianum. Their distinction from avulsion fractures is not always simple.

It is a rare occasion for the cuboid to exhibit an isolated fracture. Ordinarily, there are associated tarsal injuries, usually the tuberosity of the navicular or anterior process of the calcaneus.

The three cuneiform bones are anatomically labeled and numbered as follows: (1) medial or internal, (2) middle, and (3) lateral or external. Like the navicular and cuboid bones, the internal cuneiform may demonstrate multicentric ossification. A not-so-uncommon finding is division of the first cuneiform into dorsal and plantar segments representing a true bipartite condition. An isolated fracture of any of the three cuneiforms is definitely an uncommon situation.

With the correct roentgenographic projection on the internal oblique film, the joint space between the first and second cuneiform bones can appear quite wide and might lead the clinician to a false impression of a separation. The middle and external cuneiforms often elude appropriate inspection because of their inconspicuous positions within the framework of the bony arch.

In the growing foot, the epiphyseal centers of the metatarsal bones are essentially similar in location to those of the hand. They appear in the third year and normally fuse at about 15 years of age. Each of the metatarsals contains one epiphysis, but the fifth metatarsal also possesses an apophysis at its proximal end. The epiphyses of the second through fifth metatarsals are distal, whereas that of the great toe is proximal. On rare instances the clinician may encounter pseudoepiphyses at the bases of the lateral four metatarsals (particularly the third) and also at the head or distal aspect of the first metatarsal. Occasionally, a cleft divides the epiphysis of the great toe metatarsal bone and should not be misconstrued as a fracture.

Several interpretive challenges are presented by the appearance of the base of the fifth metatarsal bone. The longitudinally oriented, shell-like apophysis can be roentgenographically dissimilar in the feet of the same individual and vary in size and shape. Furthermore, it may persist unfused throughout life, but this is an uncommon event. Ordinarily, the distinction between the apophysis and a fracture is relatively simple because the growth line is oriented to the axis of the shaft, whereas a fracture is transverse in almost all instances (Fig. 16-73). An acces-

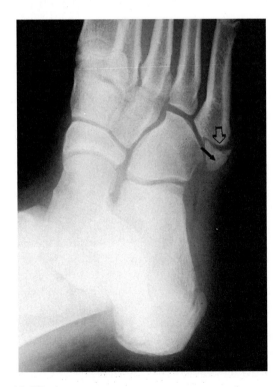

**Fig. 16–73.**
Transverse fracture *(large arrow)* through the base of the fifth metatarsal bone. Note the normal apophysis *(small arrow)*.

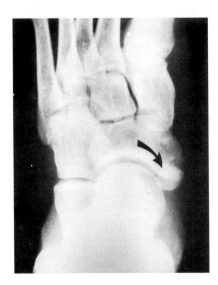

**Fig. 16–72.**
Os tibiale externum *(arrow)*.

sory bone, the os vesalianum, alluded to previously, is located near the junction of the proximal metatarsal tuberosity and the cuboid. This fact should be remembered when evaluating trauma to this area.

A moderate degree of overlap of the bases of the metatarsal bones is noted to a greater or lesser degree on all views, but more so on anteroposterior projections. With the "Mach" effect in mind, this has led to many erroneous diagnoses of fractures. The internal oblique film tends to reduce this problem to some extent.

When viewing the foot, the tarsometatarsal joints form a somewhat curvilinear line convex toward the toes. This is disrupted only by the recessed base of the second metatarsal bone, which results from a relatively short middle cuneiform. The base of this metatarsal is therefore wedged between the first and third cuneiform bones. Furthermore, the medial margins of the base of the second metatarsal and the middle cuneiform are always in line.

In the proximal space between the bases of the first and second metatarsal bones may be found the os in-termetatarseum. It is located along the dorsal surface and, like most accessory ossicles, can assume various sizes and shapes. Radiopacities in the form of arteriosclerotic vascular plaques can also be seen in this same interdigital space. Both of these can simulate avulsion fractures.

There is one traumatic lesion involving the metatarsal area that deserves special attention but that, fortunately, is uncommon. *Lisfranc's fracture-dislocation* involves the tarsometatarsal junction and consists essentially of dorsal displacement of the metatarsal bases. Two basic forms exist: homolateral and divergent. In the homolateral type, the lateral four metatarsals are dislocated posteriorly and laterally, often with associated fractures at the bases. The divergent type exists when the first metatarsal is displaced medially and the others are dislocated laterally. The disfigurations may be subtle, and the normal straight alignment of the second metatarsal and middle cuneiform bones should be utilized (Fig. 16-74).

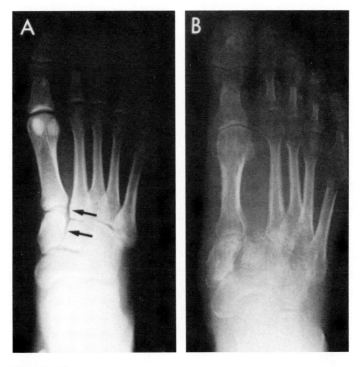

**Fig. 16–74.**
**A**, Normal alignment of the second metatarsal and middle cuneiform bones *(arrows)*. **B**, Lateral dislocation of the three middle metatarsal bones (a divergent form of a Lisfranc type of injury).

## SPECIALIZED RADIOLOGIC STUDIES OF THE MUSCULOSKELETAL SYSTEM

### Nuclear Medicine Procedures

The use of radioactive isotopes in the evaluation of certain bone disorders has been touched upon in previous sections. For some time now it has been known that phosphorus compounds will be metabolized in bone at a rapid rate, and this assimilation can be readily detected by a scintillation camera when the substance is tagged by the radiotracer technetium $^{99m}$Tc phosphate (Fig. 16-75). Areas of rapid bone turnover (such as those seen in healing fractures, aggressive tumors, and infections) can readily be detected by bone scanning.

There are occasions when fractures are extremely subtle or undetectable on standard roentgenograms, such as fractures that may be seen in the hip. Two to 5 days are required after the injury before scans demonstrate the fracture optimally. Abnormal increased activity may persist for up to 2 years or longer, depending on the severity of the injury. Nuclear scans can be particularly helpful in determining the age of compression deformities of the vertebral bodies.

In recent years, single proton emission computed tomography (SPECT) imaging has provided an even more sensitive nuclear method for detecting bone abnormalities. The technology is not unlike computerized x-ray tomography in that the detector heads (up to three) rotate about the patient. The digital information derived from the amount of isotope activity from bone can be reconstructed by a computer into tomographic slices in all planes (sagittal, coronal, and axial). In effect, thin slices of anatomic and physiologic data can be displayed (Fig. 16-76).

Staging of tumors for therapeutic protocols has been greatly enhanced by the improved quality of bone scans over the past few years. Skeletal scintigrams are extremely sensitive to the presence of metastatic lesions, although their specificity is not as good as routine x-ray films. All patients with diagnoses of bronchogenic carcinoma, breast carcinoma, carcinoma of the prostate, and hypernephroma, in addition to those who have a number of other tumors known to metastasize to the osseous system, should have a baseline bone scan for staging purposes.

Benign tumors are less often evaluated by radionuclide bone scans. One exception is the osteoid osteoma, a painful lesion that can affect the spine as well as the extremities and go undetected by the usual methods of examination. This tumor will take up the isotope intensely and thus reveal its location.

The presence and progress of osteomyelitis and its response to therapy can be adequately documented by bone scintigraphy. Gallium-133 can also be utilized because of its affinity for inflammatory and neoplastic processes. It is seldom used in the study of bone infections, but it can quantitate soft-tissue involvement.

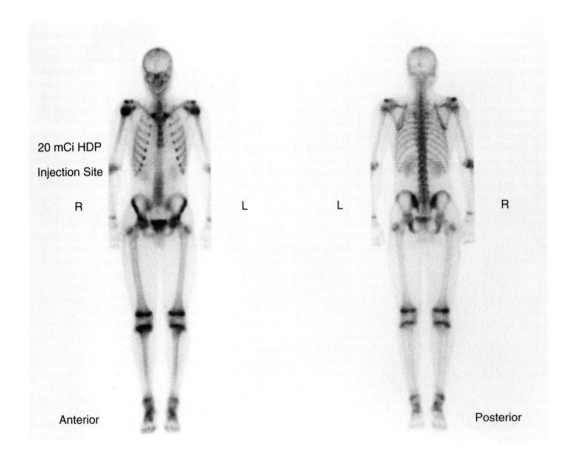

**Fig. 16–75.**
Normal whole body static scintiphotos of a radionuclide bone scan in the anterior and posterior projections.

The value of the radionuclide *three-phase bone scan* in differentiating osteomyelitis from cellulitis is depicted in Fig. 16-77. In the majority of cases, a limited three-phase study over the area of interest can distinguish between the two processes. This examination consists of an initial dynamic, or vascular, phase performed at the time of isotope injection followed by an immediate second phase, or soft-tissue uptake stage. Standard 2-hour delay images are then obtained for bone uptake. If the results are inconclusive, an Indium-111 leukocyte or serotec technetium $^{99m}$Tc phosphate white blood cell study can be performed in which the patient's own white blood cells are tagged and reinjected. This often will help identify bone versus soft-tissue inflammatory infectious disease.

Reflex sympathetic dystrophy, described more extensively in Chapter 18, often can be followed by serial bone scans to determine whether it is quiescent, progressing, or improving.

## Diagnostic Ultrasound

Exquisite image resolution and anatomic detail are possible with state-of-the-art, real-time diagnostic ultrasound systems. High-precision, small-parts transducers in the range of 7.5 to 10 mHz are now available. These afford excellent structural delineation of the thyroid gland, testicles, and breast lesions, as well as vascular studies combined with Doppler flow measurements. Both venous and arterial vascular assessments can be performed by Doppler ultrasound methods to evaluate for deep venous thrombosis and arterial occlusive disease. Bone cannot be imaged with ultrasound: that, along with its inability to be transmitted through air, is

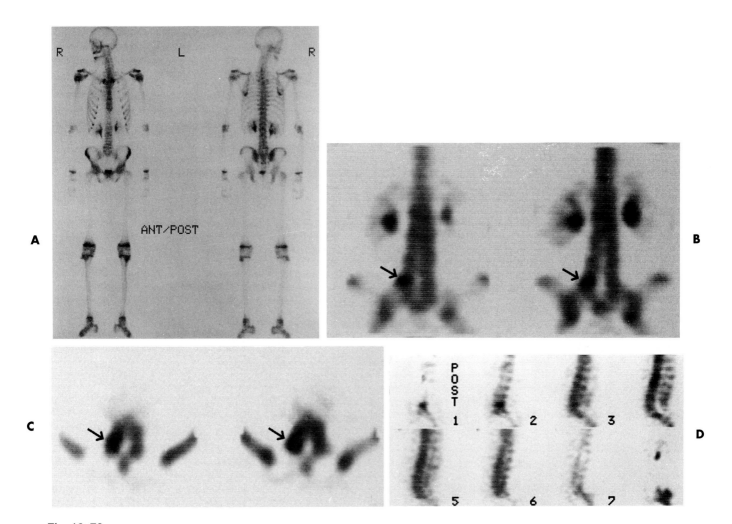

**Fig. 16–76.**
Value of SPECT imaging. **A,** Normal appearing anterior and posterior whole-body static bone scans in a young patient with posttraumatic back pain. **B, C,** and **D,** SPECT images in the coronal, axial and sagittal planes, respectively, demonstrate an intense focus of abnormal uptake of the pedicle of L-5 on the right *(arrows)*, which represents an occult fracture. (Courtesy of Sam Mehr, M.D., Omaha.)

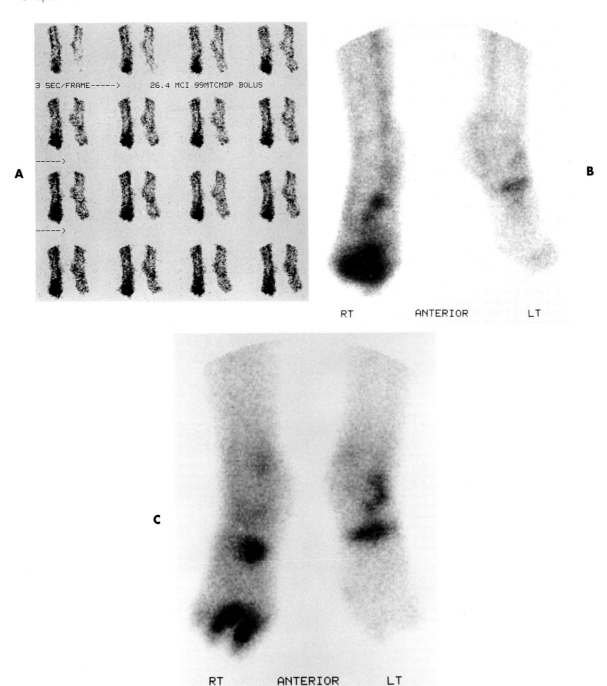

**Fig. 16–77.**
Three-phase bone scan demonstrating osteomyelitis of the second and third toes of the right foot in the absence of x-ray findings. **A**, Dynamic, or angiographic, phase shows definite focal hyperemia to the sites of infection. **B**, The second, blood-pool, phase depicts persistent focal uptake. **C**, The final delayed images document localized isotope activity in the region of bone infection.

a distinct disadvantage. However, soft tissues provide an excellent medium for evaluation by sonography. The muscles of the extremities, in particular, can be examined easily and without discomfort to the patient.

Although uncommon, unresectable soft-tissue tumors can be followed by sequential sonographic studies, with their response to therapy recorded. Invasive

characteristics such as osseous, neural, or vascular involvement cannot be depicted as well with ultrasound as with CT or MRI, however. Biopsies of such masses are easily performed under the guidance of ultrasound.

Sonography offers one of the best approaches to the detection of abscesses in the soft tissues. The location and extent can be adequately shown. Furthermore, ultrasonically guided needle aspiration of inflammatory masses (for culture and sensitivity as well as for drainage) adds another dimension to the procedure.

## Arthrography

Many joints in the body are accessible to needle entry and can be opacified for radiographic visualization by the introduction of iodinated contrast media, air, or both (double-contrast arthrography). Fluoroscopic spot films or overhead roentgenograms can then be obtained in multiple projections to delineate the intrinsic intraarticular anatomy.

The knee and shoulder are the most commonly examined joints, but the wrist, elbow, hip, and ankle—as well as the temporomandibular joints—may be studied by arthrography. The greater availability of the arthroscope and increased surgical expertise in its use have led to a decline in the number of knee studies, but the orthopedic surgeon occasionally will request the examination in difficult diagnostic cases.

Arthrographic procedures carry a low morbidity, are easily tolerated as an outpatient examination, and are quite simple to perform. Sterile technique is required in all cases, along with local lidocaine (Xylocaine) anesthesia. Shoulder arthrography has its greatest application in the study of rotator cuff tears (Fig. 16-78). It is also useful in the analysis of adhesive capsulitis (frozen shoulder), arthritis, synovitis, and capsular integrity, besides being helpful in the detection of loose bodies and abnormalities of the biceps tendon. The cartilaginous rim of the glenohumeral joint, the glenoid labrum, can be depicted and examined for tears and degeneration similar to examination of the knee menisci (Fig. 16-79).

Adequately performed arthrography of the knee will define pathologic conditions of the medial and lateral meniscal cartilages, cruciate ligaments, collateral ligaments, articular cartilage, synovium (e.g., Baker's cyst), and joint capsule.

## Xerography

The physical principles relating to x-ray xerography need not be detailed here, other than to state that the resultant images are imprinted upon a special form of paper and that soft-tissue detail is much greater than that obtained with standard roentgenograms (Fig. 16-80). However, by itself it offers no great advantage over x-ray films in the interpretation of bone.

Xerography can provide information regarding the soft tissues that is not available on x-ray film images. It can be particularly helpful in detecting relatively nonopaque foreign bodies such as glass and wood. On occasion, the process will reveal anatomic data about primary soft-tissue tumors that are not visible otherwise, such as microcalcifications. Extension of tumors or

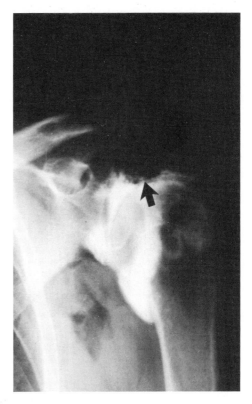

**Fig. 16–78.**
An example of a double air-contrast arthrogram of the shoulder demonstrates a tear of the rotator cuff *(arrow)*.

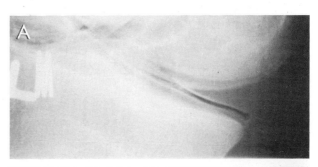

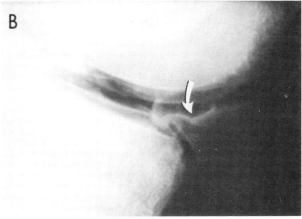

**Fig. 16–79.**
These images demonstrate a normal-appearing medial meniscus (**A**) and a tear of the meniscus (**B**, *arrow*) as seen on arthrography.

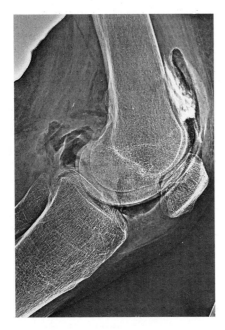

**Fig. 16–80.**
Xerogram of a knee arthrogram. Soft tissue detail is better delineated than on standard radiographs. Also note bone trabecular detail.

inflammatory lesions of the muscles into bone may be better depicted by xerograms than by radiographs. However, xerography has essentially been supplanted by CT and MRI in the appraisal of musculoskeletal abnormalities.

Rarely, subtle fractures will be identified or seem more apparent than on routine x-ray films. The fine periosteal reaction related to stress fractures may be detected more readily on xerograms.

## Angiography

Angiography has a somewhat limited role in orthopedics. Its principal contribution is in the area of trauma, when fractures of the extremities are uncommonly complicated by vascular injury (Fig. 16-81).

Less often, the evaluation of primary osseous or soft-tissue neoplasms can be aided by employing angiograms (Fig. 16-82). Preoperative assessment of the degree of vascularity of the lesion, in addition to its major blood supply, can be invaluable to the surgeon's approach.

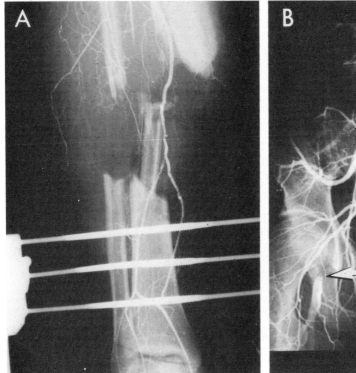
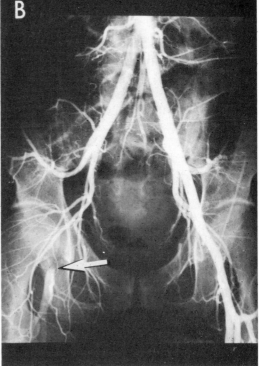

**Fig. 16–81.**
Both of these angiograms are examples of the importance of angiography in cases of trauma in which arterial injury is suspected. **A**, A lower extremity study shows extensive vascular damage with complete disruption of the anterior and peroneal arteries and severe irregularity of the posterior tibial artery. **B**, This young man received blunt trauma to the pelvis. A routine x-ray film failed to reveal a fracture, but angiography demonstrates complete severance of the external iliac artery *(arrow)* with loss of all pulses to the extremity.

## Standard Radiographic Tomography

There is a limited, potentially rewarding number of applications of standard x-ray tomography in the assessment of the skeleton. Simple linear tomography or more sophisticated pluridirectional tomographic systems can be indicated in certain instances of traumatic, neoplastic, or infectious processes involving the peripheral skeleton or the spine. Subtle but clinically important fractures may be outside the limits of visibility on plain radiographs. But if symptoms warrant, tomography may be indicated to be certain of the presence or absence of pathology, such as in a suspected carpal navicular fracture, a possible subcapital fracture of the hip, or a case in which a vascular groove needs to be differentiated from a true fracture (e.g., in the scapula). Questionable fractures involving the spine, particularly the odontoid or posterior neural arch elements, may require tomographic study.

The early changes of osteomyelitis or an osteogenic sarcoma may not be detected on plain films, yet may be clearly delineated by the use of tomograms. Benign osteoid osteomas will give a characteristic appearance of a central lucent nidus surrounded by dense sclerosis, and this usually requires sectional filming to be seen.

Tomography obviously improves image detail over standard x-ray films. Although it is much less expensive than CT, it has some major practical disadvantages. It cannot define the intricate intrinsic bone detail, nor can it demonstrate the exquisite soft-tissue anatomy that CT or MRI scanning is capable of showing.

## Computed Tomography

Detailed cross-sectional depiction of musculoskeletal anatomy and pathology has clearly established CT as a secondary diagnostic modality in the evaluation of bone, joint, and soft-tissue abnormalities. It is the imaging procedure that can clarify findings on conventional roentgenograms, standard tomography, and bone scans. The CT scan demonstrates greater sensitivity and specificity than do these other methods. Additionally, CT has a definite position in assessment of the spine, particularly the lumbar region, and this is most applicable in complex fractures and lesions (such as herniated discs) that affect the spinal canal.

The accuracy of CT in defining individual muscles, vessels, and nerves depends on the presence of fat in the surrounding soft tissues. In cases in which there is a paucity of fat, CT has a limited role. Such is the case in the distal parts of extremities, in infants, and in thin or emaciated patients.

In primary bone tumors, CT can accurately describe marrow and soft-tissue extent, including vascular and nerve involvement. Conventional roentgenograms cannot identify such details, which can influence the surgeon's approach or help in the selection of radiation ports.

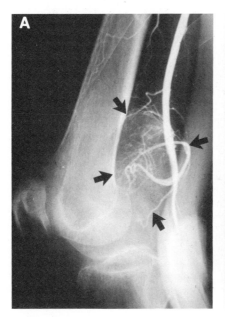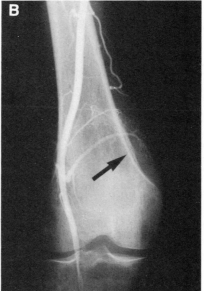

**Fig. 16–82.**
An angiogram of a lower extremity in an elderly male with a large soft-tissue mass above the knee. The study delineates the neovascularity and mass displacement of the tumor (**A**, *arrows*) with secondary erosion of the adjacent bone (**B**, *arrow*). Pathologic findings disclosed this to be a fibrosarcoma.

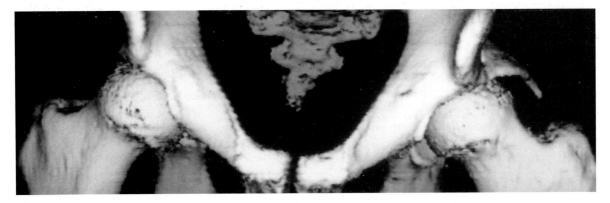

**Fig. 16–83.**
3-D reconstruction spiral CT of the hips. By computer manipulation, the image can be turned on its axis and viewed on the CT monitor to evaluate the hips in all directions.

Evaluation of metastatic bone disease is more appropriately performed by standard filming and radionuclide bone scanning. However, CT may be extremely helpful in areas of complex anatomy, such as in the spine or pelvic regions. Often, a person with known cancer demonstrates a single abnormal focus on a nuclear bone scan. It has been found that nearly 40% of these individuals eventually are proved to have bone metastasis. CT or MRI can be invaluable in the workup of these solitary bone scan abnormalities.

Distinguishing between benign and malignant soft-tissue tumors in certain cases can be accomplished by CT. Benign lesions can be sharply demarcated and uniformly homogeneous, and are confined to a single muscle or compartment. They may compress or displace vessels and nerves but, of course, do not invade them, and this can be identified by CT. Conversely, malignant soft-tissue masses have no well-defined margins because of their infiltrative nature, and naturally invade and distort adjacent nerves and vessels. Extension into adjoining bone is also well demonstrated by CT. Furthermore, malignant tumors often involve multiple muscle groups and compartments.

With the advent of spiral technology to CT, 3-D computer reconstruction of bony anatomy is available and provides yet another advancement in imaging capabilities (Fig. 16-83). CT can be useful in selected trauma cases, particularly those involving complex anatomic areas such as the spine, pelvis, hips, shoulders, and knees (Fig. 16-84). The cross-sectional image display of CT eliminates the overlapping structures and depicts the spatial relationship of fracture fragments to joints, muscles, nerves, and vessels. In addition, it can detect and define the extent of associated hemorrhage and hematoma formation.

On occasion, infectious processes involving bone, joints, and soft tissues can be best demonstrated by CT. However, osteomyelitis of long bones and infections of the spine and intervertebral discs usually do not require CT, except when the diagnosis is in doubt with the more conventional means. Soft-tissue abscesses may at times be difficult to distinguish from tumor and hematoma. Early in the process, an abscess may have the same density as surrounding muscles, but it eventually undergoes central necrosis with liquefaction and acquires a low-density center with an irregular peripheral high-density wall. The presence of air within an abscess suggests communication with the skin surface or air-forming bacteria.

## Magnetic Resonance Imaging

Clinical indications for MRI are becoming well established. Applications of this newest diagnostic modality are well known and increasingly utilized, particularly in the central nervous system. However, the development and usefulness of MRI in musculoskeletal disorders has become overwhelming, to say the least. Recent developments in computer software and techniques have led to an increased usage of MRI in evaluation of the spine and extremities, and it has replaced CT in a number of areas.

MRI has multiplanar capabilities: that is, it can image in the sagittal, coronal, and the axial (transverse) planes in addition to oblique variations of these. It thus provides more useful information than does CT, which is limited to the axial plane. Furthermore, unlike CT, it possesses greater contrast resolution and better delineates muscles, tendons, ligaments, fat, and fluids. Because it does not utilize ionizing radiation, MRI has no harmful effects and, indeed, is thought to be risk free for most patients. MRI contraindications include pregnancy (unknown teratogenic effects), those patients with pacemakers and neuroelectrostimulating devices, and individuals with intracranial ferromagnetic metal clips and metallic foreign bodies in close proximity to vital structures. These metal

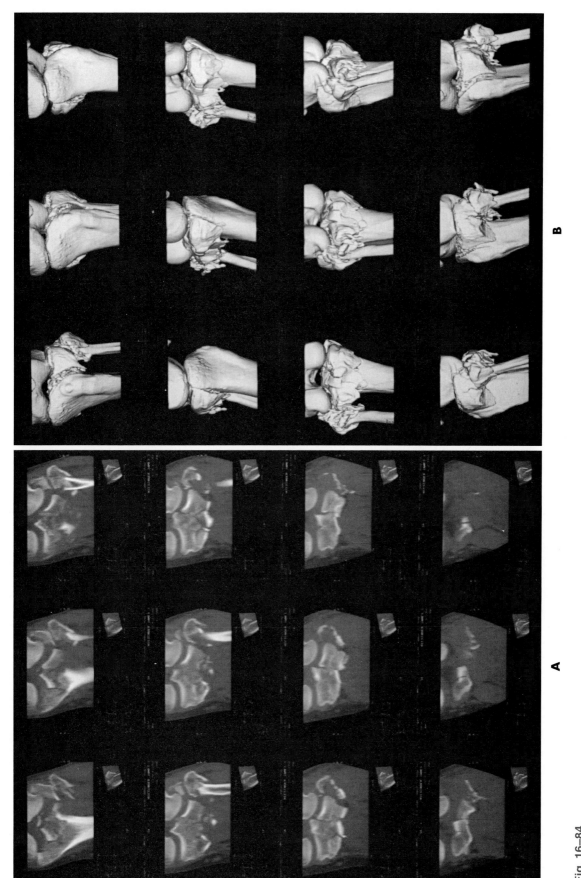

**Fig. 16–84.**
Comminuted intraarticular fracture of the tibia. **A,** 2-D and **B,** 3-D reconstruction computerized tomographic images delineate the complexity and extent of the injury providing detailed information for the orthopedic surgeon's approach to reconstruction.

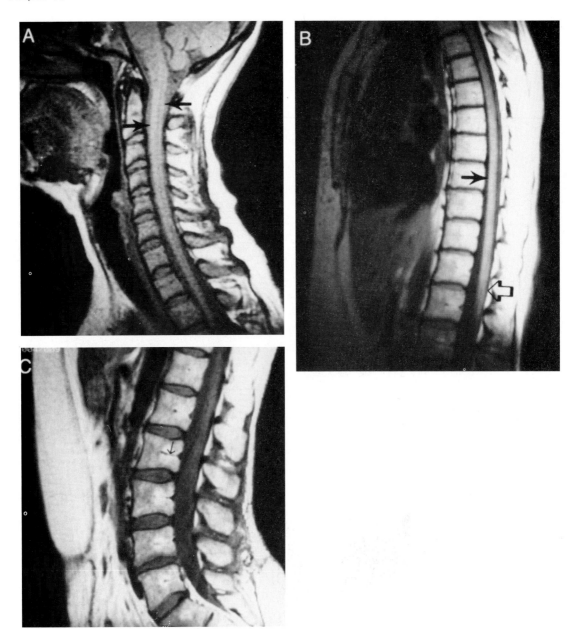

**Fig. 16–85.**
Normal midline sagittal MRI of the entire spine. **A**, Cervical spine. **B**, Thoracic spine. **C**, Lumbar spine. Note in detail the cord *(closed arrows)*, the conus medullaris *(open arrow)*, and the bones and intervertebral discs. Also note the vascular channels in the posterior aspects of the vertebral bodies *(vertical arrow).*

bodies can be displaced by the strong magnetic force. Most prosthetic devices and surgical clips today are non-ferromagnetic and do not cause significant problems to the patient or degrade the images.

In general physical terms, MRI employs a strong, uniform, magnetic field into which the patient is placed. Specially designed surface conduction coils are placed near or around the region to be examined. Somewhat like a compass in the earth's magnetic field, the person's cellular hydrogen nuclei (protons) will align themselves appropriately. The polarized nuclei are in an elevated energy state. A specified radio wave is transmitted through them via the coils, and a complex physical change produces the release of energy that is tissue characteristic. This energy, in the form of radio waves, is then detected and amplified and the data collected by a computer, where it is processed into an image.

A number of disease entities that affect the spine and the soft tissues, bones, and joints of the extremities can be exquisitely demonstrated by MRI. These include musculoskeletal infections, bone and soft-tissue tumors, and various traumatic lesions. Also adequately evaluated are a long list of miscellaneous conditions such as congenital abnormalities, osteonecrosis, myopathies, arthritides, and bone marrow disorders. The discussions that follow will touch on a few of these and illustrate when MRI can be helpful in certain clinical situations.

### MRI of the Spine

The vertebral bodies and their posterior neural arch components, as well as the surrounding muscles, can be well demonstrated with MRI. Additionally, the intervertebral discs are optimally visualized. MRI also depicts the contents of the central neural canal, including the cord, nerve roots, dura, and ligamentum flavum. The neural foramina and associated exiting nerve roots can be identified on sagittal and axial views. Fig. 16-85 illustrates the normal midline sagittal appearance of the cervical, thoracic, and lumbosacral spine. Standard MRI protocol consists of 3- to 5-mm contiguous sagittal images from the neural foramina from one side to the other (Fig. 16-86). Selected axial images through the intervertebral disc spaces are also performed (Fig. 16-87). Occasionally, coronal views are obtained that simulate x-ray contrast myelography.

**Congenital Malformations.** In some instances, MRI of congenital malformations of the spine may be the only means of delineating the abnormality. Sagittal cervical spine films clearly depict the *Arnold-Chiari malformation* with herniation of the cerebellar tonsils through the foramen magnum. There may be an associated syringomyelia dissecting the cord, and this can be extremely well seen on MRI studies (Fig. 16-88). MRI provides a noninvasive way to evaluate meningoceles and meningomyeloceles. With these entities, a tethered cord and associated lipoma are well appreciated below the conus medullaris.

**Spinal Trauma.** Because of the increased examination times, and the limitation on the use of life-support equipment that is affected by the magnet, acute trauma of the spine is best evaluated by plane x-ray films and CT rather than MRI. An MRI study of the cervical spine, for example, may take 30 minutes or more to perform, whereas a modified or limited CT examination can take as little as 10 minutes. However, delayed posttraumatic complications can be extremely well depicted by MRI. The site and extent of fractures and the displacement of fragments are probably best defined on CT, but can be properly accessed by magnetic imaging. The direct effect of displaced fragments on the cord and nerve roots may be determined by MRI. It also clearly identifies the integrity of the cord and the presence of intramedullary hemorrhage. Epidural and subdural hematomas around the cord are also visibly documented.

**Disc Disease.** The role of MRI in the assessment of disc herniation, degenerative disc disease, and spondylitis

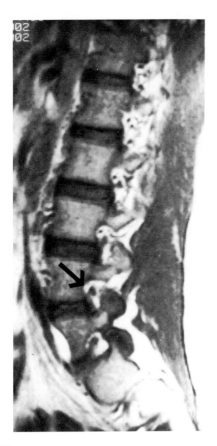

**Fig. 16–86.**
Off-midline sagittal MRI of the lumbar spine demonstrates the neural foramina and their exiting nerve roots *(arrow)*.

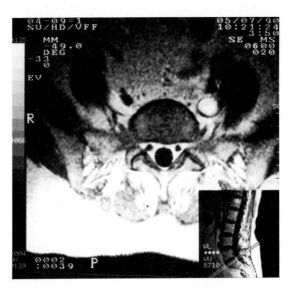

**Fig. 16–87.**
Selected axial image of the L5, S1 disc space *(see the sagittal inset with the cursor)*. Note the dural sac and two descending nerve roots *(black)* surrounded by the epidural fat *(white)*.

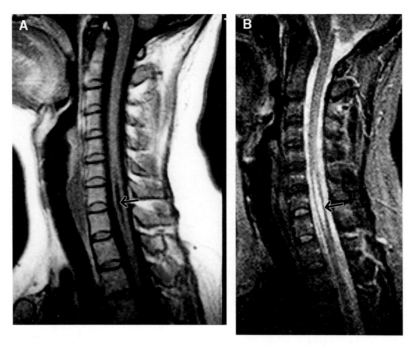

**Fig. 16–88.**
**A** and **B**, Syringomyelia of the cervical cord *(arrows)* without cerebellar herniation on T1 and T2 weighted spin-echo images.

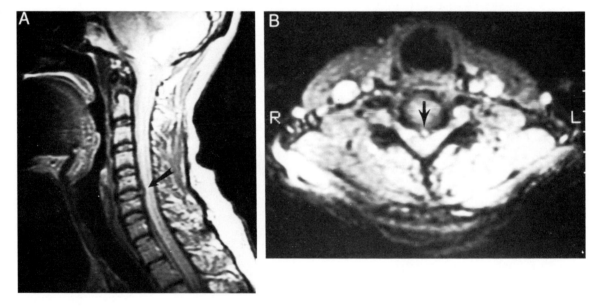

**Fig. 16–89.**
Herniated disc of the cervical spine at the C5-C6 level *(arrows)*. **A**, Sagittal, and **B**, axial views. Note on the lateral image an appearance simulating paste being squeezed from a tube. Also note deformity of the dural sac.

with osteophyte formation—as compared with CT and contrast myelography—is currently undergoing considerable scrutiny in clinical practice. Most studies agree that the accuracy of the three modalities in these disease states is relatively equal in lumbar spine evaluations; however, the diagnostic sensitivity in the cervical and thoracic regions seems to favor MRI. CT at these spinal levels is limited unless intrathecal contrast is used, because the cord and dural sac are not well demonstrated. MRI shows these structures well. Contrast myelography is equally sensitive in detecting abnormalities, but the fact that MRI is essentially noninvasive favors its use.

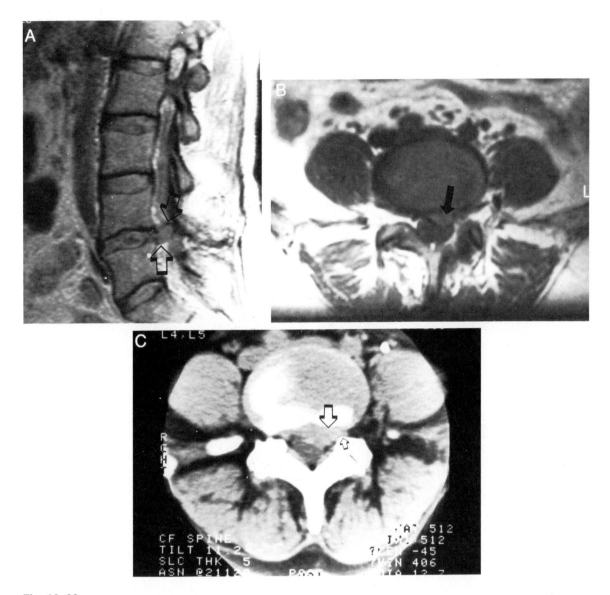

**Fig. 16–90.**
Herniated disc of the lumbar spine at the L4-L5 level *(arrows)*. **A**, Sagittal, and **B**, axial MRI images. Note the deformity of the dural sac and the encroachment on the left neural foramen. **C**, CT image of the same disc.

The clinical diagnosis of a herniated intervertebral nucleus pulposus can be dramatic, but on occasion it also can be subtle. After following a conservative clinical approach for a time without improvement of symptoms, the clinician may elect to evaluate the patient by some type of imaging procedure to diagnose and document the presence or absence of a herniated disc. By any method, graphic visualization of a herniated disc can be an imaging challenge. In the cervical region, bulging, protruding, and herniated discs lend themselves readily to MRI evaluation (Fig. 16-89), although the distinction between bulging and herniation may at times be impossible. However, lumbar spine disc herniation continues to be accessed equally by CT or MRI

(Fig. 16-90). The choice of procedure will depend on availability, economic considerations, and, to some extent, patient selection. An equivocal CT study may require MRI to best delineate the lesion, but less often the opposite is true.

One area of difficult clinical management is the postoperative spine. Contrast myelography or CT seldom can distinguish between postsurgical scar tissue and a recurrent herniated disc. With the introduction of an intravenously administered "contrast" agent, MRI is capable of making the distinction between the two. Gadolinium is a stable paramagnetic metal ion that is combined with diethylenetriamine pentaacetic acid (DTPA). When injected, the substance can enhance tissues with adequate vascularity by changing their magnetic field. Disc material, being essentially nonvascular, will not enhance, whereas scar tissue, which possesses a vascular supply, will (Fig. 16-91).

**Spondylitis.** Early degeneration of the intervertebral disc material can be identified by MRI even before changes occur on x-ray films and CT. These changes include disc space narrowing and spur formation. A change in signal intensity (brightness) of the disc on the MRI sagittal images heralds the beginning of the pathologic process (Fig. 16-92). As the disease progresses, with disc space compression and production of osteophytes, MRI aids in defining the degree of spinal stenosis that can occur on the central neural canal and the neural foramina in both the axial and sagittal planes. The encroachment of degenerative spurs on the dural sac, their displacement of nerve roots, and their effect on the cord are all adequately assessed by MRI (Fig. 16-93).

**Infection.** MRI of infectious processes in and about the spine can be rewarding. Fig. 16-94 demonstrates an unsuspected epidural abscess of the lumbar spine in an individual presenting with a relatively sudden onset of lower extremity neurologic symptoms including back pain, fever, and elevated white blood cell count. A lung infection was thought to be the source for this hematogenously introduced infection.

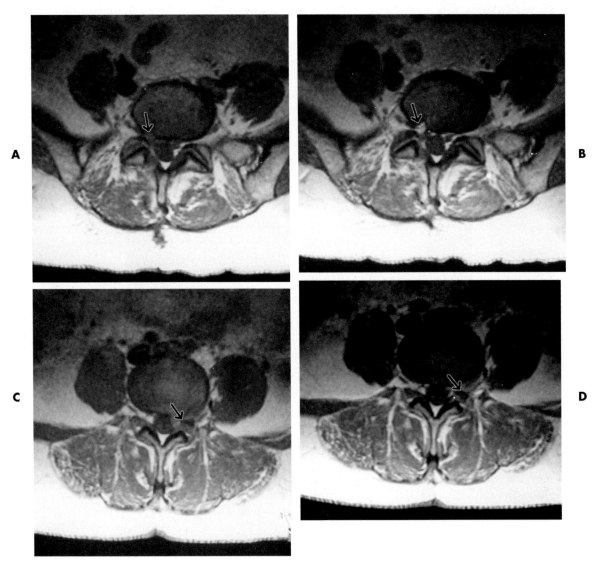

**Fig. 16–91.**
Distinguishing between postoperative scar and recurrent herniated disc by MRI utilizing gadolinium. **A** and **B**, Pre- and postcontrast images demonstrating enhancing scar *(brighter)* at L5, S1 *(arrows)*. **C** and **D**, Pre- and postcontrast films depicting a herniated disc *(arrows)* with no enhancement at L4, L5 in the same patient.

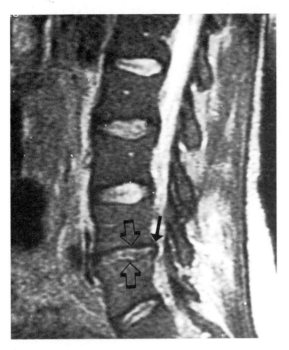

**Fig. 16–92.**
Degenerative disc disease of the lumbar spine at the L4-L5 level. Narrowing of the interspace is evident, and osteophyte formation is noted *(open arrows)*. Also note the decreased signal intensity *(darkness)*, greatest at L4-L5 but involving all discs; this indicates the decreased water content of the degenerating nucleus pulposus. Posterior osteophyte *(closed arrow)* resulting in some degree of spinal stenosis.

More common but still rare are spinal infections occurring after surgery to the spine. Osteomyelitis of the bony vertebrae, with extension into the discs and eventual advancement into the epidural space, can be easily pictured by MRI. The use of gadolinium can even further improve the ability to detect infections of the spine.

**Tumor.**    MRI has been found to be highly sensitive for the detection and characterization of tumors involving the spine. Gadolinium plays an important role in the evaluation of these lesions.

Secondary or metastatic neoplasms are the most commonly encountered tumors that involve the spine (Fig. 16-95). These may be hematogenous, such as from lung or breast cancer; lymphatic, such as that from the prostate; or by direct extension from a contiguous lesion. Better definition of the margins of these tumors is afforded by the use of gadolinium, which distinguishes the tumor from surrounding edema and thereby better establishes radiation ports.

Primary spinal tumors are divided into intradural intramedullary, intradural extramedullary, and extradural lesions. Intramedullary neoplasms may not be optimally visualized on unenhanced MRI because of extensive infiltration, associated edema, or intratumor necrosis or hemorrhage. Ependymomas and astrocytomas constitute the most common intramedullary tumors. A less

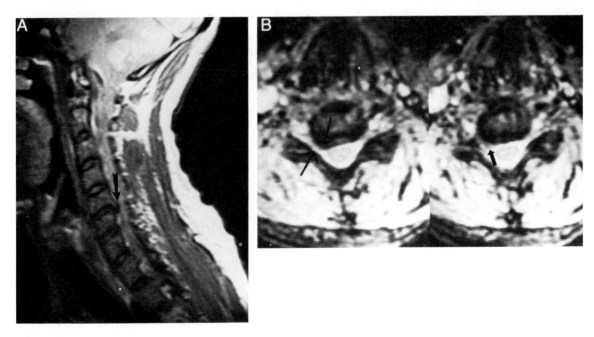

**Fig. 16–93.**
Degenerative disc disease of the cervical spine at the C5-C6 level. **A**, Sagittal, and **B**, axial images. A large posterior spur *(arrows)* deforms the dural sac extending to the right and is creating stenosis of the neural foramen and subarticular recess.

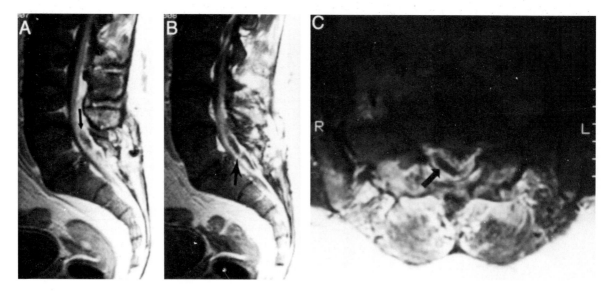

**Fig. 16–94.**
**A** and **B**, Sagittal lumbar spine images at two different planes, and **C**, axial image at the L5, S1 level. An irregular dark (low signal intensity) area *(arrows)* signifies an epidural abscess.

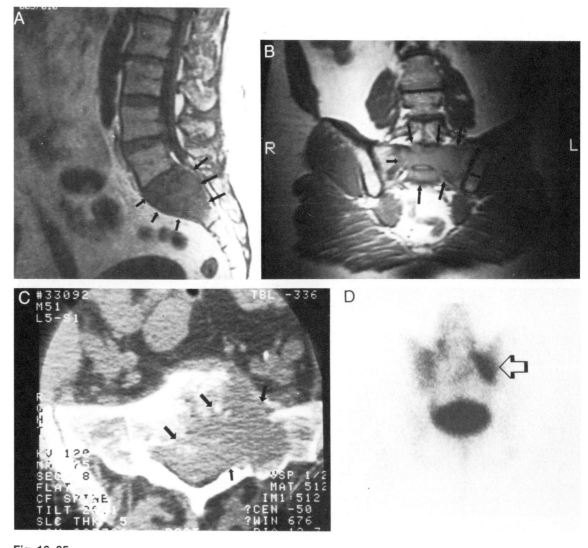

**Fig. 16–95.**
Metastasis *(arrows)* to the sacrum from an occult lung cancer. **A**, Sagittal, and **B**, coronal MRI. **C**, CT image. **D**, Nuclear bone scan of the pelvis. All three modalities show sensitivity to the process, but MRI provides more anatomic information.

common lesion is the hemangioblastoma. All three are best evaluated by MRI after gadolinium injection.

Intradural extramedullary tumors are commonly found to be meningiomas, neurofibromas, or schwannomas (Fig. 16-96). These may be difficult or impossible to identify on conventional unenhanced MRI studies, especially if they are less than 5 mm. Larger lesions can displace the dural contents, and are more easily detected by these indirect signs.

Metastases constitute the majority of extradural tumors and, as noted, are best evaluated by magnetic imaging. However, one area where MRI has an obvious advantage over any other imaging procedure is in the presence of diffuse leptomeningeal spread of tumor. There is a marked increase in signal arising from the thickened leptomeninges after gadolinium administration.

**Miscellaneous Spinal Lesions.** Demyelinating diseases, of which multiple sclerosis is the most common, are characteristically sensitive to magnetic imaging detection. Histopathologically, the lesions are multifocal destructive myelin zones of as-yet-unknown etiology that can involve the optic nerves, brain, and spinal cord. They present as areas of increased signal intensity (bright), are of variable size and distribution, range from a few millimeters to several centimeters, and are scattered throughout the white matter. There appears to be a direct relationship between the number and size of these "plaques" and the severity of the symptoms. In addition, as the symptoms wax and wane, so does the appearance of the lesions seen on MRI.

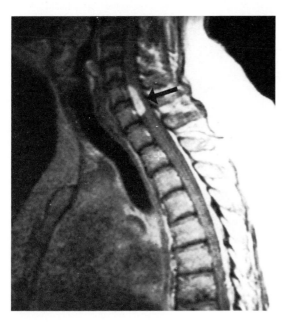

**Fig. 16–96.**
Meningioma of the cervical spine *(arrow)* displays high signal intensity (bright).

Involvement of the spinal cord by multiple sclerosis is uncommon; but when discovered, the lesions tend to be elongated or linear rather than round or oval as seen in the brain, where they are typically periventricular in location. Lesions in the thoracic and lumbar cord are identified less often than those in the cervical cord. Symptoms are variable and can range from weakness and/or paraesthesias in one or more limbs to gait disturbances and problems with micturition.

Although a rare event today, postradiation transverse myelitis is also susceptible to MRI detection. In addition to signal derangements in the cord, radiation also causes changes within the marrow of the vertebrae that can be easily identified only by magnetic imaging.

### Musculoskeletal MRI

Diagnostic orthopedic applications of MRI for disorders of the bones, joints, and soft tissues of the extremities are rapidly gaining acceptance. Although MRI will not totally replace the use of CT, nuclear imaging, or even conventional x-ray films in evaluation of the musculoskeletal system, there are certain areas and specific abnormalities that are best examined by the magnet.

Because of its excellent inherent contrast resolution, MRI can superbly delineate the separate soft-tissue components of the extremities (Fig. 16-97). Muscles, tendons, ligaments, fat, cartilage, and fibrous tissues are all excellently displayed. Although the calcium of cortical and trabecular bone possesses no magnetic signal, it can be defined by the adjoining marrow and surrounding muscles and tendons. However, this property of magnetism prevents MRI from defining cortical stress fractures. Tumoral calcifications and ossifications, as well as early cortical destruction and endosteal and periosteal reaction, are all adequately seen on CT but cannot be optimally identified by MRI. This gives it a distinct disadvantage in such situations. Despite these limitations, MRI has become the diagnostic modality of choice for the evaluation of bone and soft-tissue trauma such as cartilage, ligament, tendon, or muscular damage.

With the development of newer software, the role of MRI has expanded in the area of vascular anatomy. MRI angiography is able to depict brachiocephalic and cerebral vessels and is showing promise in peripheral angiography as well. Without the use of contrast material, arterial and venous structures can be displayed utilizing appropriate phase sequences. As technologic research in this area progresses, it is hoped that MRI angiography may someday replace conventional invasive angiographic procedures.

**Tumor.** Today the surgical approach for the treatment of malignant bone and soft-tissue tumors is a conservative one. The objective is limb salvage and restricting resections to a limited degree, thereby providing as

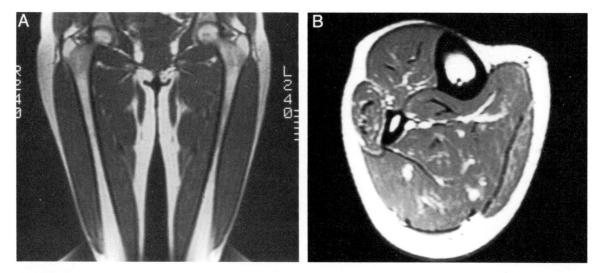

**Fig. 16–97.**
**A,** Coronal MRI of the femur and thigh. **B,** Axial image of the tibia and fibula and associated soft-tissue detail.

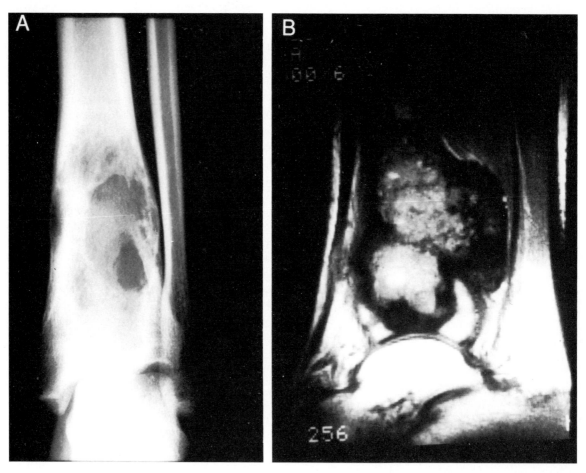

**Fig. 16–98.**
Chondrosarcoma. **A,** Anteroposterior roentgenogram of the distal third of the tibia. **B,** Sagittal MRI of the same area.

much functional capability as possible. The multiplanar display of MRI and its excellent contrast resolution aid greatly in defining the size, location, and extent of a tumor. It can adequately assess marrow involvement, skip lesions, and invasion of adjoining muscles, compartments, blood vessels, and nerves (Fig. 16-98). Of great importance is establishment of the integrity of adjacent joints and articular surfaces.

Unfortunately, MRI cannot differentiate between benign or malignant tissue characteristics in the majority of cases. There are a few exceptions: giant cell tumor of bone, for example, will give rise to characteristic fluid-fluid levels within a multi-septated lesion, a unique feature for these neoplasms (Fig. 16-99). Certain types of tissues (such as fat, or the vessels of a hemangioma) have distinctive appearances (Fig. 16-100). Fluid-filled cystic lesions can be separated from solid masses with MRI, and this can aid in appropriate assessment such as needle aspiration or biopsy.

**Infection.** The diagnosis and treatment of osteomyelitis, pyogenic arthritis, and soft-tissue infections of the extremities can be challenging. The earlier the detection, and the better the process is delimited by imaging, the more precise will be medical and surgical approaches and the better will be the outcomes. Evaluations by standard x-ray films, conventional tomography, radionuclide bone scans, and CT all have a place, but each has its limitations and may delay appropriate therapy.

Bone infections may not become evident on x-ray films and tomography until up to 40% to 50% of the bone is destroyed; this may take up to 10 or 14 days after the onset. As previously discussed, nuclear bone scans are sensitive but nonspecific. They may not differentiate tumor from infection, nor can they adequately define the anatomic extent of the disease. Gallium 67–labeled and indium 111–labeled leukocytes are radioisotopes that are more specific for infection than are technetium $^{99m}$Tc phosphate complexes; but again, they provide poor resolution.

CT is helpful in determining cortical bone and periosteal findings but is less sensitive to marrow or surrounding soft-tissue changes. Because it is limited to transverse planes, the true upper and lower margins of the infection may be missed. Also, in cases of infections involving internal metallic fixation devices, the artifacts produced by CT prevent delineation of the abnormalities. The MRI artifacts produced by such devices are much less marked.

Hematogenous osteomyelitis, seen most often in children, commonly begins in the bone marrow of long bones in the lower extremities. On MRI studies, the intramedullary tissues will demonstrate signal changes of inflammation at an early stage. Furthermore, the

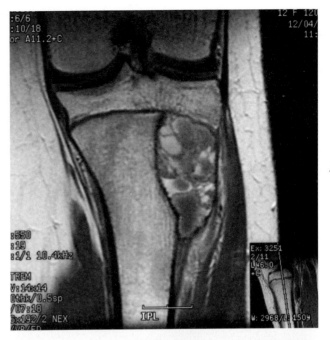

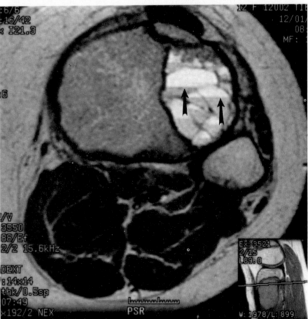

**Fig. 16–99.**
Giant cell tumor of the tibia. **A**, Coronal T-1 spin echo and **B**, axial T-2 weighted images demonstrate a sharply demarcated multiseptated lesion. Note fluid-fluid levels *(arrows)* on the axial film, a finding that can be seen in benign tumors.

anatomic extent of the process can be clearly demonstrated to include soft-tissue extension, joint involvement, and skip areas. If unresponsive to medical management, this can be valuable in planning surgical debridement.

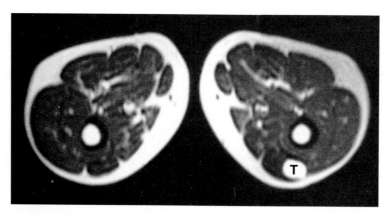

**Fig. 16–100.**
Benign lipoma. Axial MRI of the thighs demonstrates a sharply marginated lesion
*(T)* with high signal intensity.

MRI has been found to be of value in the evaluation of postsurgical bone, joint, and soft-tissue infections. Most metal fixation appliances today are nonferromagnetic and cause only minimal distracting image artifacts on MRI. This property is a significant problem with CT. However, subtle bone changes immediately adjacent to metal implants may be obscured by the minimal artifacts seen on MRI, and early infectious changes may be missed.

**Trauma.** The primary diagnostic modality for the study of skeletal injuries does not include magnetic imaging. These are reserved, of course, for standard roentgenologic procedures. However, an evaluation of soft-tissue injury (especially in deep tissues) becomes more difficult with conventional tests. MRI, because of its multiplanar ability and its exquisite soft-tissue contrast and resolution, is gaining greater acceptance for elucidating extraosseous injuries.

Contusions of soft tissue that result in hemorrhage, edema, inflammation, or hematoma formation can be depicted by MRI. The location and size of the process and, importantly, the involvement of adjacent muscles, tendons, ligaments, blood vessels, and nerves, is easily assessed. This can serve as a guide to excision and evacuation procedures when required.

Muscles, ligaments, and tendons can be torn or ruptured as a result of severe muscle contraction or direct trauma. Such findings—especially in the shoulder, knee, and ankle but also in other locations—will be directly visualized by magnetic scanning, something that up to now was difficult to do even with arthrography and might be surmised only clinically or by direct surgical exposure.

Evaluation of the knee joint is presently approached by direct visualization via arthroscopy, which has essentially supplanted arthrography. However, orthopedic surgeons are beginning to rely more often on the non-invasive, accurate diagnostic images provided by MRI. The menisci, cruciate and collateral ligaments, articular cartilage, synovial capsule, and surrounding muscles and tendons are extremely well depicted on MRI scans (Fig. 16-101). Recent studies have shown MRI to have an accuracy of 90% for meniscal tears and 95% for cruciate ligament tears (Fig. 16-102). Magnetic imaging can define early degeneration of menisci and cartilage, and even intrameniscal tears not visible by endoscopy. MRI also easily detects loose intraarticular osteochondral bodies.

The diagnostic capabilities of MRI in examining the shoulder have only recently been realized. This is a result of the development of better-designed, dedicated surface coils and updated computer software programs. Although arthrography is still being utilized (and, in some instances, combined with CT), MRI appears to be taking the same direction it did in knee evaluations and is becoming more commonly utilized. Coronal oblique, sagittal oblique, and axial planes of imaging of the shoulder offer a tremendous advantage over other modalities. So also does the use of variable-pulse sequencing protocols, which can be modified to bring out or accentuate subtle findings. Degenerative changes as well as partial or complete tears of the rotator cuff are sensitive to MRI detection (Fig. 16-103).

Impingement of the supraspinatus tendon, as caused by an abnormal acromion process or osteophyte formation of the acromioclavicular joint, can lead to early degenerative changes and make the tendon more susceptible to tears. Tendinitis, bursitis, rupture of the biceps tendon, or determination of the integrity of the cartilaginous glenoid labrum also lend themselves to identification by MRI.

MRI is also helpful for assessing injuries to other regions of the musculoskeletal system. As will be men-

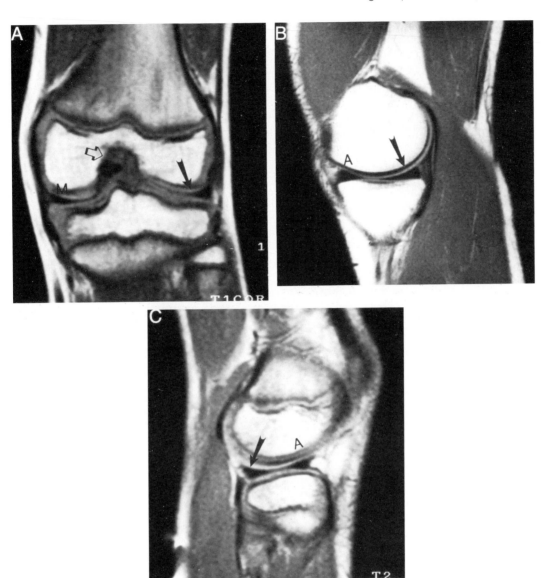

**Fig. 16–101.**
Normal knee anatomy. **A,** Coronal MRI shows the intercondylar notch *(open arrow)*, the medial meniscus *(M)*, and the lateral meniscus *(closed arrow)*. **B,** Sagittal MRI shows the normal anterior *(A)* and posterior horns of the medial meniscus *(arrow)*. **C,** Sagittal MRI demonstrates the normal anterior *(A)* and posterior horns of the lateral meniscus *(arrow)*.

tioned later, aseptic or avascular necrosis of the navicular bone of the wrist is receptive to MRI detection. There are several studies available that indicate the value of MRI in assessing carpal tunnel syndrome. In this condition, magnetic imaging can define thickening of the tendon sheaths and distortion in the outline of the median nerve.

The elbow and ankle can be appropriately analyzed for traumatic abnormalities by MRI (Fig. 16-104). Tears of the Achilles tendon are a prime example, and the severity and extent of the lesion can be properly deter-

mined by the magnet. On occasion, loose bone or cartilaginous bodies can be appreciated within joints.

Examination of the temporomandibular joints is facilitated with the use of MRI. Tears and dislocations of the meniscus and whether it reduces with opening or closing of the jaw are discerned.

Acute trauma, chronic stress tenosynovitis, or bursitis often lead to the production of synovial fluid as a result of inflammation. Traumatic hemorrhage into joints or bursae can also occur. These abnormal fluid collections are well demonstrated by MRI.

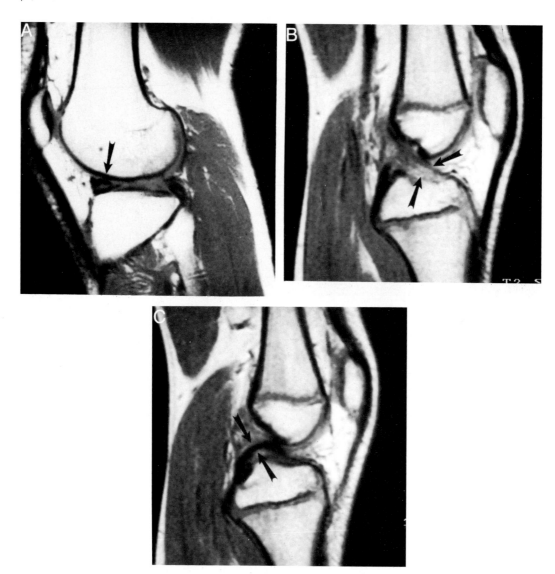

**Fig. 16–102.**
**A**, Tear in the lateral meniscus of a sagittal image of the knee *(arrows)*. **B**, Disruption of the anterior cruciate ligament *(arrows)*. **C**, Normal-appearing posterior cruciate ligament, albeit slightly kinked as a result of the tear in the anterior cruciate ligament *(arrows)*.

**Osteonecrosis.**   There are numerous causes of aseptic necrosis or avascular osteonecrosis of bone, the most common being trauma that results in disruption of the regional vascular supply. Nontraumatic etiologies include vascular thrombosis secondary to hemoglobinopathies such as sickle cell anemia. A commonly encountered reason for aseptic necrosis is exogenous steroids. Less commonly found diseases accounting for osteonecrosis are barotrauma, irradiation, collagen vascular diseases (vasculitis), lymphoproliferative diseases (Hodgkin's lymphoma), pancreatitis, and even some cases of gout.

The common denominator in the pathogenesis of both traumatic and nontraumatic aseptic necrosis is vascular compromise. The resultant marrow ischemia, which

most often occurs in the growth centers or metaphyseal regions of long bones, provokes an inflammatory response with vascular congestion and edema of the bone marrow.

This pathophysiologic response can be detected by conventional radiographs on a delayed basis, or earlier by the sensitive but nonspecific and poorly resolved images of a nuclear bone scan. CT can also detect the changes of avascular necrosis relatively early, but the findings are also nonspecific, and CT of the distal parts of extremities has been found to be limited.

MRI of osteonecrosis has been determined to be sensitive and specific early in the disease process. In the femoral head (Fig. 16-105), the images will delineate

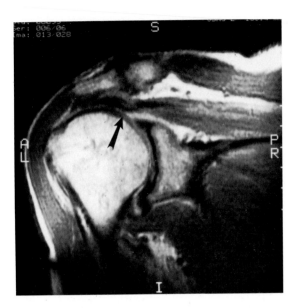

**Fig. 16–103.**
Coronal oblique MRI of the shoulder demonstrates a rotator cuff tear *(arrow).*

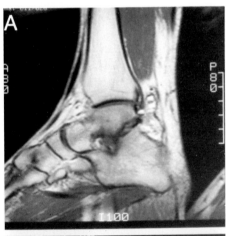

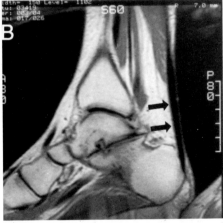

**Fig. 16–104.**
**A** and **B**, Normal sagittal images of the ankle. Note the Achilles tendon *(arrows).*

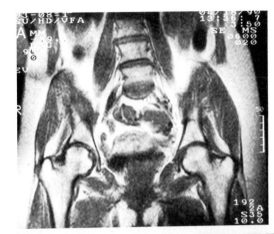

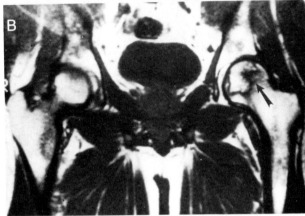

**Fig. 16–105.**
**A**, Normal coronal MRI of the hips. **B**, A coronal view of the hips demonstrates avascular necrosis on the left *(arrow).*

subarticular areas of decreased signal intensity (dark). As pointed out previously, injuries to the carpal navicular bone can defy detection by standard imaging. Appreciation of the process of aseptic necrosis of the proximal navicular fracture fragment requires early detection for best results, and MRI provides an accurate means to determine this abnormality. Other regions vulnerable to osteonecrosis (such as the humeral head [Fig. 16-106], knee [Fig. 16-107], mandibular condyle, and spine) are easily examined by magnetic imaging.

**Kinematic MRI.** With the introduction of open-design MRI systems, which allow for greater patient flexibility, joint motion can now be assessed. Dynamic evaluation of the knee, shoulder, elbow and wrist joints is possible. Static MRI images of a joint are acquired during progressive movement of a joint in flexion/extension, adduction/abduction, or rotation. Specially designed stabilizing and support hardware permits precise incremental positioning of a joint. The multiple images are then displayed on a cine loop video, simulating a joint's tracking movements.

The primary purpose of kinematics is to access joint instability (such as glenohumeral and patellofemoral dysfunction and malalignment) that can be surgically corrected before complications (such as chondromalacia and osteoarthritis) develop. The abnormal dynamics of wrist and elbow movements (such as radioulnar ligament and scapholunate ligament tears) can also be identified. The application of this technique can be particularly helpful in the surgical approach to correcting abnormal joint motion in athletes.

## Dual Energy X-ray Absorptiometry (DEXA Scan) and Osteoporosis

Osteoporosis now has and will continue to have a significant socioeconomic impact on health care. The morbidity and mortality related to osteoporotic fractures in the post-menopausal patient have not received appropriate attention until the last few decades. A satisfactory and low-cost method of calculating bone mineral density (BMD) had to be developed that would adequately diagnose the disease and precisely quantify and predict those individuals who are at increased risk for insufficiency fractures of the spine, hips and other skeletal locations. Accurate BMD measurements could also be used for therapeutic response.

A number of techniques have been developed over the past few years, the majority of them linked in some way to the computation of the attenuation of ionizing radiation through bone. The first commercially available DEXA (dual energy x-ray absorptiometer) scanner was introduced in 1987, and has since undergone considerable refinement and improvement.

BMD values are expressed as gm/cm². Measurements are made over the upper four lumbar vertebrae and the left hip (Fig. 16-108). The results are then given as standard deviations or percentile scores. A Z-score is a measure of the difference of the patient's BMD and the mean BMD for individuals matched by age and sex. A T-score measures the difference in standard deviations of the patient's BMD and the mean BMD of normal young persons. A fracture risk profile then can be established and appropriate therapeutic measures instituted.

Conditions and factors that can lead to imprecise calculations of BMD include severe degenerative disease of the spine or hip resulting in osteophytes and eburnation of bone. Compression fractures involving vertebrae also result in erroneous values secondary to the sclerosis that occurs with healing. Other considerations that cause inaccurate readings are Paget's disease, diffuse osteoblastic metastases, extensive calcified plaque of the abdominal aorta overlying the spine, and scoliotic curvatures. Metal artifacts related to the field of data acquisition of measurements including x-ray contrast media (barium) and orthopedic devices such as Harrington rods must be considered. Recent radionuclide studies can even interfere and give spurious results.

A number of indications have been established for acquiring BMD measurements. Probably the most important is the estrogen-deficient woman (see Chapter 8). In addition to the post-menopausal female, this can be seen in malabsorption syndromes (celiac disease), poor diet

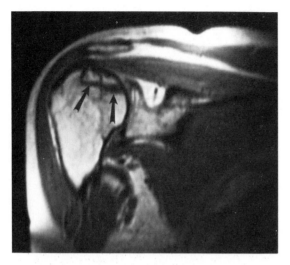

**Fig. 16–106.**
Coronal oblique MRI shoulder image demonstrates osteonecrosis of the humeral head in a steroid user *(arrows)*.

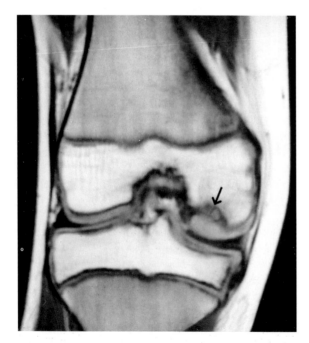

**Fig. 16–107.**
A coronal MRI image of the knee delineates the typical defect of osteochondritis dissecans *(arrow)*, which was also well demonstrated on the sagittal views (not shown).

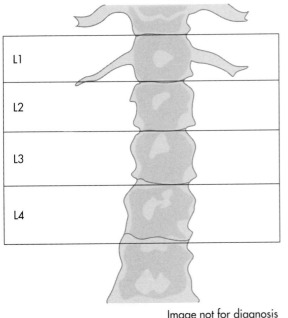

Image not for diagnosis
3.00ma:Hi-Res Fast  DPXIQ  0.6×1.2mm  1.68mm
677148:393029  274.69:204.25:146.01
%Fat = 7.0 (1.379)

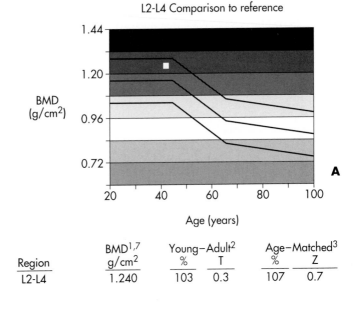

L2-L4 Comparison to reference

| Region | BMD[1,7] g/cm² | Young–Adult[2] % | T | Age–Matched[3] % | Z |
|--------|----------------|------------------|-----|------------------|-----|
| L2-L4  | 1.240          | 103              | 0.3 | 107              | 0.7 |

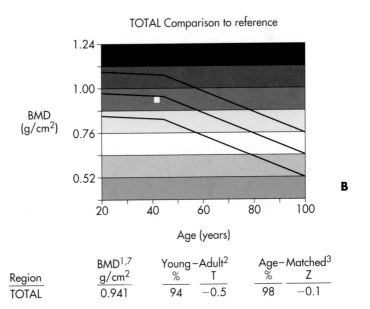

TOTAL Comparison to reference

| Region | BMD[1,7] g/cm² | Young–Adult[2] % | T | Age–Matched[3] % | Z |
|--------|----------------|------------------|------|------------------|------|
| TOTAL  | 0.941          | 94               | −0.5 | 98               | −0.1 |

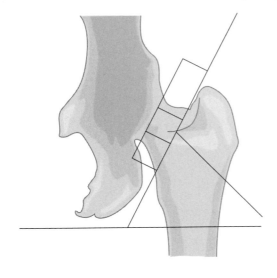

Image not for diagnosis
3.00ma:Hi-Res Fast  DPXIQ  0.6×1.2mm  1.68mm
677148:393029  274.69:204.25:146.01
%Fat = 32.9 (1.326)  Neck angle = 63

**Fig. 16–108.**
Standard DEXA scan charts for the evaluation of osteoporosis. **A**, Lumbar spine and **B**, the hip.

and anorexia, disorders of menstruation, and premature ovarian failure. Illnesses such as Cushing's disease, hyperparathyroidism, renal osteodystrophy, and rheumatoid arthritis can lead to osteoporosis. Decreased BMD is also associated with certain drugs such as cortico-steroids, anticoagulants, and anti-neoplastic medications. Also those with radiographic evidence suggesting osteoporosis (namely, osteopenia with or without spine and hip fractures) are candidates for BMD assessment. Finally, any person being monitored who is on preventive and therapeutic prescription (such as estrogen, alendronate, and raloxifene or calcitonin) meets the criteria for DEXA evaluation of bone mineral density.

DEXA techniques have also been utilized in the evaluation of the postoperative hip, especially with the newer prosthetic materials. After placement of an uncemented prosthesis, the degree of bone remodeling and healing can be accessed. A decrease in BMD can serve as a predictor for prosthetic failure.

## BIBLIOGRAPHY

Aegerter E: Diagnostic radiology and the pathology of bone disease, *Radiol Clin North Am* 8:215, 1970.

Aerts P, Disler DG: Abnormalities of the foot and ankle: MR findings, *AJR* 165:119, 1995.

Alazraaki NP: Radionuclide imaging in the evaluation of infections and inflammatory disease, *Radiol Clin North Am* 31:783, 1993.

Anderson RE: Practical aspects of CT imaging of the spine, *Curr Probl Diagn Radiol* 11:2, 1982.

Bassett LW, Grover JS, Seeger LL: Magnetic resonance imaging of knee trauma, *Skel Rad* 19:401, 1990.

Bates D, Ruggieri P: Imaging modalities for evaluation of the spine, *Radiol Clin North Am* 29:675, 1991.

Beabout JW, McLeod RA, Dahlin DC: Benign tumors of the spine, *Semin Roentgenol* 5:419, 1970.

Berquist TH: *Magnetic resonance of the musculoskeletal system*, New York, 1987, Raven Press.

Berquist TH: Magnetic resonance imaging of primary skeletal neoplasms, *Radiol Clin North Am* 31:411, 1993.

Birkner R: *Normal radiologic patterns and variations of the human skeleton*, Baltimore, 1978, Urban Schwarzenberg.

Bisese JH: *Orthopaedic MRI: a teaching file approach*, New York, 1990, McGraw-Hill.

Blaser SI, Berns DH: Disks, degeneration and MRI, *MRI Decisions* 2:23, 1988.

Brodeur AE: *Radiologic diagnosis in infants and children*, St Louis, 1965, CV Mosby Co.

Brodeur AE et al: The basic tenets for appropriate evaluation of the elbow in pediatrics, *Curr Probl Diagn Radiol* 12:5, 1983.

Brown M: Bone scintigraphy in benign and malignant tumors, *Radiol Clin North Am* 31:731, 1993.

Brown SM, Bradley WG Jr.: Kinematic MR imaging of the knee, *MRI Clin North Am* 2:441, 1994.

Burk DL, Mitchell DG, Rifkin MD: Recent advances in magnetic resonance imaging of the knee, *Radiol Clin North Am* 28:379, 1990.

Caffey J: *Pediatric x-ray diagnosis*, ed 9, Chicago, 1993, Year Book Medical Publishers, Inc.

Chhem RK et al: Ultrasonography of the musculoskeletal system, *Radiol Clin North Am* 32:275, 1994.

Christenson PC: The radiologic study of the normal spine: cervical, thoracic, lumbar and sacral, *Radiol Clin North Am* 15:133, 1977.

Crim JR et al: Diagnosis of soft-tissue masses with MRI: Can benign masses be differentiated from malignant ones? *Radiology* 185:581, 1992.

Cummings SR et al: Bone density at various sites for prediction of hip fractures, *Lancet* 341:72, 1993.

Daffner RH: Ankle trauma, *Radiol Clin North Am* 28:395, 1990.

Dahlin DC: *Bone tumors: general aspects and data on 3,987 cases*, ed 2, Springfield, Ill, 1967, Charles C Thomas Publishers.

Dalinka MK et al: The use of magnetic resonance imaging in the evaluation of bone and soft-tissue tumors, *Radiol Clin North Am* 28:461, 1990.

De Smet AA et al: Osteochondritis dissecans of the knee: Value of MR imaging in determining lesion stability and the presence of articular cartilage defects, *AJR* 155:549, 1990.

Deutsch AL, Mink JH: Magnetic resonance imaging of musculoskeletal injuries, *Radiol Clin North Am* 27:983, 1989.

Djukic S et al: Magnetic resonance imaging of the postoperative lumbar spine, *Radiol Clin North Am* 28:341, 1990.

Donovan-Post MJ, Green BA: The use of computed tomography in spinal trauma, *Radiol Clin North Am* 21:327, 1983.

Dunn AW, Morris HD: Fractures and dislocations of the pelvis, *J Bone Joint Surg* 50:1639, 1968.

Edeiken J, Cotler JM: Ankle trauma, *Semin Roentgenol* 13:145, 1978.

Edeiken J, Hodes PJ: *Roentgen diagnosis of diseases of bone*, Baltimore, 1989, Williams & Wilkins Co.

Edelman RR, Siegel JB: Advances in musculoskeletal MRI, *MRI Decisions* 2:27, 1988.

Epstein BS: *Atlas of tumor radiology: the vertebral column*, Chicago, 1974, Year Book Medical Publishers Inc.

Forrester DM, Brown JC, Nesson JW: *The radiology of joint disease*, ed 2, Philadelphia, 1978, WB Saunders.

Forrester DM, Kerr R: Trauma to the foot, *Radiol Clin North Am* 28:423, 1990.

Foster SC, Foster RR: Lisfranc's tarsometatarsal fracture dislocation, *Radiology* 120:79, 1976.

Frank JA et al: Detection of malignant bone tumors: MRI vs. scintigraphy, *AJR* 155:1043, 1990.

Freedman GS: Radionuclide imaging of the injured patient, *Radiol Clin North Am* 11:472, 1973.

Freiberger RH: *Bone disease syllabus*, Set 9, American College of Radiology Self-evaluation and Continuing Education Program, Baltimore, 1976, Waverly Press, Inc.

Gabriel J et al: MR imaging of hip disorders, *RadioGraphics* 14:763, 1994.

Gaskill MF et al: Lumbar disc disease and stenosis, *Radiol Clin North Am* 29:753, 1991.

Gelman MD: *Radiology of orthopedic procedures, problems and complications*, Philadelphia, 1984, WB Saunders.

Gold RI et al: An integrated approach to the evaluation of metastatic bone disease, *Radiol Clin North Am* 28:471, 1990.

Goldman AB, Freiberger RH: Localized infections and neuropathic diseases of the spine, *Semin Roentgenol* 14:19, 1979.

Greenfield GB: *Radiology of bone diseases*, ed 2, Philadelphia, 1975, JB Lippincott Co.

Greulich WW, Pyle SI: *Radiographic atlas of skeletal development of the hand and wrist*, Stanford, Calif, 1959, Oxford University Press.

Harris JH Jr: Acute injuries of the spine, *Semin Roentgenol* 13:53, 1978.

Harris JH Jr, Edeiken J: Acute cervical spine trauma, *Radiol Sci Update Series No 17*, 1976.

Harris JH, Jr, Harris WH: *The radiology of emergency medicine*, ed 3, Baltimore, 1993, Williams & Wilkins.

Hill HA, Sachs MD: The grooved defect of the humeral head: a frequently unrecognized complication of dislocations of the shoulder joint, *Radiology* 35:690, 1940.

Holder LE: Bone scintigraphy in skeletal trauma, *Radiol Clin North Am* 31:739, 1993.

Jacobson HG: *Bone disease syllabus: disorders of the skeleton*, Set 2, American College of Radiology Professional Self-evaluation and Continuing Education Program, Baltimore, 1972, Waverly Press, Inc.

Jahnke RW, Hart BL: Cervical stenosis, spondylosis, and herniated disc disease, *Radiol Clin North Am* 29:777, 1991.

Kaye J: Fractures and dislocations of the hand and wrist, *Semin Roentgenol* 13:109, 1978.

Kaye JJ, Nance EP: Thoracic and lumbar spine trauma, *Radiol Clin North Am* 28:361, 1990.

Keats TE: *An atlas of normal roentgen variants that may simulate disease*, ed 5, Chicago, 1992, Year Book Medical Publishers Inc.

Kohler A, Zimmer EA: *Borderlands of the normal and early pathologic in skeletal roentgenology*, ed 4, New York, 1993, Thieme.

Kransdorf MJ et al: Imaging of soft tissue tumors, *Radiol Clin North Am* 31:359, 1993.

Kricun R, Kricun ME, Dalinka MK: Advances in spinal imaging, *Radiol Clin North Am* 28:321, 1990.

Kursonoglu-Brahme S, Gundry CR, Resnick D: Advanced imaging of the wrist, *Radiol Clin North Am* 28:307, 1990.

Lee JH et al: Lipohemarthrosis of the knee: A review of recent experiences, *Radiology* 173:189, 1989.

Lee JKT, Sagel SS, Stanley RJ: *Computed body tomography*, ed 2, New York, 1989, Raven Press.

Lichtenstein L: Bone tumors, ed 5, St Louis, 1977, Mosby Year Book.

Littleton JT: Tomography: a current assessment, *Curr Probl Diagn Radiol* 4:3, 1974.

Lodwick GS: *Atlas of tumor radiology: the bones and joints*, Chicago, 1971, Year Book Medical Publishers, Inc.

Ma LD et al: Differentiation of benign and malignant musculoskeletal tumors: potential pitfalls with MR imaging, *RadioGraphics* 15:349, 1995.

Magid D: Computed tomographic imaging of the musculoskeletal system: current status, *Radiol Clin North Am* 32:255, 1994.

Maravilla KR, Hartling RP: Imaging decisions in degenerative spinal disease, *MRI Decisions* 2:3, 1988.

Magid D: Two-dimensional and three-dimensional computed tomographic imaging in musculoskeletal tumors, *Radiol Clin North Am* 31:425, 1993.

Mark AS, Atlas SW: MRI of the cervical spine and cord, *MRI Decisions* 2:23, 1988.

Masaryk TJ: Neoplastic disease of the spine, *Radiol Clin North Am* 29(4):829-845, 1991.

McLeod RA et al: Computed tomography of the skeletal system, *Semin Roentgenol* 13(3):235-247, 1978.

Merrill V: *Atlas of roentgenographic positions and standard radiologic procedures*, ed 4, St Louis, 1995, Mosby Year Book.

Meschan I: *Roentgen signs in clinical practice*, vol 1, Philadelphia, 1966, WB Saunders.

Mirvis SE, Wolf A: Emerging MRI Role: assessing cervical spine trauma, *MRI Decisions* 4:21, 1990.

Modic MT, Maszryk TJ, Ross JS: *Magnetic resonance imaging of the spine*, ed 2, St Louis, 1995, Mosby Year Book.

Moss AA, Gamsu G, Jenant HK: *Computed tomography of the body*, Philadelphia, 1983, WB Saunders.

Munk PL, Helms CA, Holt RG: Immature bone infarct: findings on plain radiographs and MR scans, *AJR* 152:547, 1989.

Moulton JS, Braley SE: MRI of soft tissue tumors, *Contemporary Diagnostic Radiology* 17(12):1-6, 1994.

Mounts RJ, Schloss CD: Injuries to the bony pelvis and hip, *Radiol Clin North Am* 4:307, 1966.

Murphey MD: Imaging aspects of new techniques in orthopedic surgery, *Radiol Clin North Am* 32:201, 1994.

Murray RO, Jacobson HG: *The radiology of skeletal disorders*, Baltimore, 1971, Williams & Wilkins.

Nelson DW, DiPaola J, Colville M: Osteochondritis dissecans of the talus and knee: prospective comparison of MR and arthroscopic classifications, *J Comput Assist Tomogr* 14:804, 1990.

Nelson SW: Some important diagnostic and technical fundamentals in the radiology of trauma with particular emphasis on skeletal trauma, *Radiol Clin North Am* 4:241, 1966.

Newberg AH: Computed tomography of joint injuries, *Radiol Clin North Am* 28:445, 1990.

Pathria MN, Petersilge CA: Spinal trauma, *Radiol Clin North Am* 29:847, 1991.

Patten RM: Musculoskeletal neoplasms: imaging approach, *MRI Decisions* 3:13, 1989.

Patten RM, Shuman WP: MRI of osteonecrosis, *MRI Decisions* 4:2, 1990.

Paul LW, Juhl JH: *Essentials of roentgen diagnosis of the skeletal system*, ed 6, New York, 1993, Harper & Row.

Pavlov H, Freiberger RH: Fractures and dislocations about the shoulder, *Semin Roentgenol* 13:85, 1978.

Peh WC et al: Imaging of pelvic insufficiency fractures, *Radiographics* 16:335, 1996.

Peterfy CG et al: Recent advances in magnetic resonance imaging of the musculoskeletal system, *Radiol Clin North Am* 32:291, 1994.

Petterson H, Gillespy T III, Hamlin DJ: Primary musculoskeletal tumors: examination with MR imaging compared with conventional modalities, *Radiology* 164:237, 1987.

Pitt MJ, Speer DP: Imaging of the elbow with an emphasis on trauma, *Radiol Clin North Am* 28:293, 1990.

Pyle SI, Hoerr NL: *Radiographic atlas of skeletal development of the knee*, Springfield, Ill, 1955, Charles C Thomas Publishers.

Richardson ML: Magnetic resonance imaging of the musculoskeletal system, *Radiol Clin North Am* 24:2, 1986.

Rogers LF: Fractures and dislocations of the elbow, *Semin Roentgenol* 13:97, 1978.

Rogers LF: The radiology of sports injuries, *Curr Probl Diagn Radiol* 12:1, 1983.

Rogers LF, Campbell RE: Fractures and dislocations of the foot, *Semin Roentgenol* 13:157, 1978.

Rogers LF, Lowell JD: Occult central fractures of the acetabulum, *AJR* 124:96, 1975.

Ross J et al: Imaging decisions in low back pain, *MRI Decisions* 1:16, 1987.

Ross JS: Magnetic resonance assessment of the postoperative spine: degenerative disc disease, *Radiol Clin North Am* 29:793, 1991.

Ruff C et al: Imaging patterns of displaced meniscus injuries of the knee, *AJR* 170:63, 1998.

Runge VM et al: The clinical utility of IV gadopentetate dimeglumine for MRI of the head and spine, *MRI Decisions* 3:2, 1989.

Sans N, Richardi G, Railhac J: Kinematic MR imaging of the shoulder, *AJR* 167:1517, 1996.

Scott JA, Rosenthal DI, Brady TJ: The evaluation of musculoskeletal disease with magnetic resonance imaging, *Radiol Clin North Am* 22:4, 1984.

Sherman RS: General principles of the radiologic diagnosis of bone disorders, *Radiol Clin North Am* 8:173, 1970.

Sherman RS: The nature of radiologic diagnosis in diseases of bone, *Radiol Clin North Am* 8:227, 1970.

Shiwei Y et al: Magnetic resonance imaging and anatomy of the spine, *Radiol Clin North Am* 29:691, 1991.

Siberstein EB, Saenger E, Tofe AJ: Imaging of bone metastasis with Tc-99m EHDP and skeletal radiography, *Radiology* 107:551, 1973.

Simeone FA, Rothman RH: Clinical usefulness of CT scanning in the diagnosis and treatment of lumbar spine disease, *Radiol Clin North Am* 21:197, 1983.

Smith AS, Blaser SI: Infectious and inflammatory processes of the spine, *Radiol Clin North Am* 29:809, 1991.

Smith GR, Loop JW: Radiologic classification of posterior dislocations of the hip: refinements and pitfalls, *Radiology* 119:569, 1976.

Sonin AH, Fitzgerald SW, Hoff FL: MR imaging of the posterior cruciate ligament: normal, abnormal and associated injury patterns, *RadioGraphics* 15:551, 1995.

Steiner RM, Mitchell DG: Magnetic resonance imaging of diffuse bone marrow disease, *Radiol Clin North Am* 31:383, 1993.

Subbarzo K, Jacobson HG: Fractures and dislocations around the adult knee, *Semin Roentgenol* 13:135, 1978.

Subbarzo K, Jacobson HG: Primary malignant neoplasms of the spine, *Semin Roentgenol* 14:44, 1979.

Sze G: MRI of tumor metastases to the leptomeninges, *MRI Decisions* 2:2, 1988.

Teplick JG, Hakin ME: CT and lumbar disc herniation, *Radiol Clin North Am* 21:259, 1983.

Thaggard A, Harle TS, Carlson V: Fractures and dislocations of the bony pelvis and hip, *Semin Roentgenol* 13:117, 1978.

Tehranzadeh J et al: Comparison of CT and MR imaging in musculoskeletal neoplasms, *JCAT* 13:466, 1989.

Theros, EG: *Bone disease syllabus,* Set 16, American College of Radiology Self-evaluation and Continuing Education Program, Baltimore, 1980, Waverly Press Inc.

Vahey TN et al: MRI imaging of anterior cruciate ligament injuries, *MRI Clin of NA* 2:451, 1994.

Vande Streek PR et al: Nuclear medicine approaches to musculoskeletal disease: current status, *Radiol Clin North Am* 32:227, 1994.

Vanel D, Verstraete KL, Shapeero LG: Primary tumors of the musculoskeletal system, *Radiol Clin North Am* 35:213, 1997.

Vix VA, Ryu CY: The adult symphysis pubis: normal and abnormal, *AJR* 112:517, 1971.

Wahner HW, Fogelman I: *The evaluation of osteoporosis: dual-energy x-ray absorptiometry in clinical practice*, London, 1994, Martin Dunitz Pub.

White EM: MRI in synovial disorders and arthropathy of the knee, *MRI Clin North Am* 2:451, 1994.

Wilkinson RH, Kirkpatrick JA: Pediatric skeletal trauma, *Curr Probl Diagn Radiol* 6:3, 1976.

Wilkinson RH, Strand RD: Congenital anomalies and normal variants of the spine, *Semin Roentgenol* 14:7, 1979.

Wiot JF, Dorst JP: Less common fractures and dislocations of the wrist, *Radiol Clin North Am* 4:261, 1966.

Yiu-Chiu VS, Chiu LC: Complementary values of ultrasound and computed tomography in the evaluation of musculoskeletal masses, *Radiographics* 3:1, 1983.

Zlatkin HR: Trauma to the foot, *Semin Roentgenol* 5:419, 1970.

Zlatkin MB, Dalinka MK, Kressel HY: Magnetic resonance imaging of the shoulder, *Magn Reson Q* 5:3, 1989.

# CHAPTER 17

# Maxillofacial Injuries

John J. Heieck, M.D.

Increasing violence in today's society, combined with the development of local hospital emergency rooms as trauma centers, has placed many emergency and primary-care physicians in the position of initial responsibility for the isolated or multicomplex-injured patient. These physicians are usually able to recognize potential thoracic or abdominal injuries more easily than maxillofacial defects. Of course, the ability to identify maxillofacial injuries is necessary for the complete evaluation of any trauma patient. Although not lethal *per se*, undiagnosed facial fractures may have potential lethal complications or may produce contour deformities with or without functional disabilities.

Automobile accidents are the most common cause of maxillofacial injuries and represent a high velocity type of injury. Other modes of injury include motorcycle accidents, fistfights, sports, falls, bicycle accidents, and convulsive disorders. Identification of the cause is important because one third of patients with maxillofacial injuries caused by motor vehicle accidents will have associated life-threatening cranial, pulmonary, or intraabdominal injuries. About one third will also be accompanied by nonlethal injuries such as extremity fractures or eye loss. On the other hand, patients with maxillofacial injuries secondary to low-velocity causes (assaults or falls) have a markedly decreased incidence of associated injuries, both life-threatening (4%) and nonlethal (10%).

## ASSOCIATED INJURIES

The primary physician's initial introduction to the maxillofacially injured patient may be as an isolated injury or as part of a multisystem involvement. However, the principles of treatment are similar in either case. Establishment of a patent airway should be the most immediate concern. Control of hemorrhage from open wounds or bleeding orifices by pressure dressing or packing should be accomplished next. If shock does exist, treatment should include rapid infusion of intravenous lactated Ringer's solution followed by blood administration as soon as possible. Investigation for possible cranial, thoracic, or intraabdominal injuries should be completed before identifying the maxillofacial abnormalities.

Airway obstruction with subsequent hypoxemia can easily develop in the patient with a maxillofacial fracture. Blood clots, broken teeth or dentures, and foreign bodies such as dirt or glass can physically obstruct the airway. The posterior displacement of the tongue secondary to the patient's position or to a mandibular fracture may occlude the airway. Other potential causes include glossopharyngeal edema and expanding hematoma. In all situations, a patent airway must take immediate priority. Sweeping debris from the oropharynx and mouth by using one's finger may be a lifesaving technique. Suction, if available, is helpful. Simple traction on a posteriorly displaced tongue by suture or towel clip may alleviate obstruction. If these methods fail, oral intubation must be instituted. If facial edema, facial fractures, or cervical spine fractures prevent oral or nasal intubation, a cricothyroidotomy can be performed through the membrane between the thyroid and cricoid cartilages. This site is a bloodless field, and the procedure can easily be done in the emergency room with only a scalpel. Later, an elective lower tracheotomy can be performed under controlled circumstances in the operating room. A low tracheotomy performed in the emergency room may be hazardous and should be avoided.

Hemorrhage from open wounds can be controlled most easily by pressure dressings consisting of layers of gauze (Kerlix) and elastic bandages. Occasionally, an active bleeder in a facial wound can be easily clamped and ligated. However, blind clamping of possible bleeding sites is condemned because of the high incidence of iatrogenic complications such as facial nerve dysfunction. Nasal hemorrhage may require packing. Shock seldom occurs from an isolated maxillofacial injury and most commonly results from a thoracic or abdominal injury.

All patients should be considered candidates for cervical spine fractures, which occur in 4% to 7% of maxillofacial injuries. The initial examiner should palpate the neck for tenderness over the cervical spine and evaluate grip strength and motion in all extremities. Before other roentgenograms are taken, a cross-table lateral view of the cervical spine with all seven vertebrae visible should be examined for fracture or dislocation.

Other associated injuries in the maxillofacial patient may involve one or more systems. Subdural, epidural, or intracerebral hematoma may be present in a comatose or semilucid patient, indicating the need for skull roentgenograms and axial computerized axial tomographic scan. Possible chest injuries include rib fractures, pneumothorax or hemothorax, flail chest, aortic rupture, and pulmonary or cardiac contusion. Chest films and arterial gas studies may be indicated. Intraabdominal injuries, of course, would include a ruptured spleen, transected liver, major vessel injuries, and/or perforated intestine. A pregnant woman may suffer an abortion as a result of such an injury. Single or multiple extremity fractures may also be present.

All associated life-threatening injuries must receive first priority in the treatment of the multiinjured patient. After repair and/or stabilization of the associated injuries has been accomplished, reduction of the maxillofacial fractures may be performed.

## EXAMINATION AND DIAGNOSIS

An accurate history should be obtained whenever possible from the patient and/or witnesses at the scene of the accident. The type of accident, the patient's position in the car, the use of safety belts, the mode of impact, and the patient's condition at the time of injury are all important considerations in the initial assessment. Because alcohol is involved in 50% of automobile accidents, a blood alcohol sample should be drawn. Ingestion of other drugs should be considered by an appropriate drug screen analysis.

A review of the patient's past history should include other illnesses, previous surgery, allergies, and all current medications.

A diagnosis of facial bone injury can be established by three methods: observation, palpation, and roentgenographic evaluation. Moderate to severe facial edema may mask bony irregularities and asymmetries (Fig. 17-1). However, facial asymmetry after resolution of the edema is suggestive of an underlying fracture. Light manual palpation is important in making the initial diagnosis.

A systematic approach should be used routinely in examining all potential facial fracture patients. The clinician should palpate the boundaries of the orbit, the projection of the malar eminences and zygomatic arches, the maxillary and mandibular arches, and the nasal bones. During palpation, the physician should assess possible asymmetry by noting any depressions or step deformities as well as any tenderness observed in areas of potential fracture.

Evaluation of the function of the extraocular muscles may demonstrate superior gaze impairment with

subsequent diplopia. Orbital ridge or floor fractures will commonly result in infraorbital nerve numbness of the cheek and the maxillary gingiva on the side of the fracture. Crepitus to light touch suggests fracture extension through the nasal airways or paranasal si-

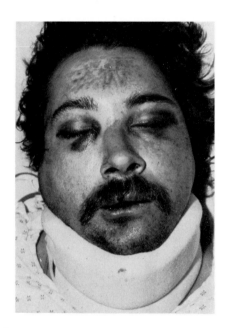

**Fig. 17–1.**
This 32-year-old man suffered a Le Fort III maxillary fracture, nasal fractures, a displaced mandibular fracture, and an undisplaced fracture of the seventh cervical vertebra. The nasal deformity is easily recognized, but the remaining deformities are masked by facial edema.

nuses. Rhinorrhea confirms the involvement of the fracture through the cribriform plate. The presence of trismus may indicate a hematoma or contusion in the muscles of mastication or could suggest either zygomatic arch or mandibular fractures. A complete examination for possible facial injuries includes a thorough evaluation of dental occlusion for any abnormality.

Roentgenographic assessment is extremely important in the evaluation of facial fractures. The studies available in most emergency rooms should be considered a preliminary evaluation that will be supplemented by more sophisticated techniques at a later date. Before any x-rays of the facial bones are undertaken, an evaluation of the cervical spine should be completed. Initially a cross-table portable view of the cervical spine should be obtained to rule out the possibility of neck fracture. If this film is negative, a complete cervical spine series should be done. When this study shows no abnormality, then specific views of the facial bones can be done.

Radiologically, the Waters' view is the single most informative roentgenogram in evaluation of the maxillofacial patient in the emergency room (Fig. 17-2). This study visualizes the floors and rims of the orbits, the walls of the sinuses, the zygomatic bones, the zygomatic arches, and the nasal septum with minimal interference of other bony structures. Opacity of a maxillary sinus suggests hemorrhage as a result of an orbital ridge and/or floor fracture. However, the Waters' view requires the cooperation of the patient and a normal cervical spine because the patient must be in the prone position during the examination. If the patient is comatose, uncooperative, or suspected of having a cervical fracture, a reverse Waters' view with the patient in the supine position is a satisfactory substitute because it gives almost the same level of detailed information. Other films worth consideration in the emergency room are the submental vertex view of the zygomatic arches and a mandible series. More sophisticated and detailed studies can be obtained later during the hospitalization or as an outpatient for isolated facial fractures.

Since the development of computerized tomography, CT scanning has become essential for the diagnosis of facial trauma. The CT scan is a more accurate diagnostic study and allows an evaluation of complicated facial fractures before the resolution of edema. Additionally, injuries to the soft-tissue structures in the area of trauma can be better evaluated (e.g., the optic nerve or orbital herniation of the orbit) (Fig. 17-3).

Reformatting the data from both axial and coronal views of the CT scan allows the development of a three-dimensional picture of the facial bone structures. The cost/benefit ratio of such a study does not justify the routine use of three-dimensional CT scanning except in complex facial fracture patients.

The only disadvantage to the use of the CT scan is seen when artifacts occur, caused by either dental fillings or metal appliances. Radiation is not considered a disadvantage; CT exposes the patient to a radiation

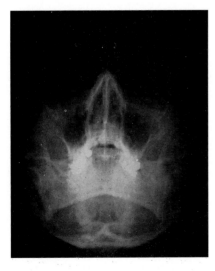

**Fig. 17–2.**
The Waters' view is the best single roentgenographic study of the facial bones. It most clearly visualizes the rims of the orbits, the zygomatic bones and arches, and the maxilla. Note the clarity of the maxillary sinuses.

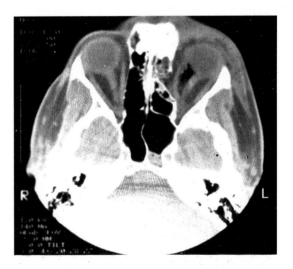

**Fig. 17–3.**
Axial CT of the orbits clearly demonstrates the optic nerve and the medial and lateral rectus extraocular muscles.

dosage equal to the amount from linear tomography. Studies suggest that the amount of radiation from either study is less than the amount needed to cause cataracts.

The role of magnetic resonance imaging (MRI) in the craniofacial injury patient is primarily confined to evaluation of soft-tissue trauma. When injuries to the ocular structure are noted, and disturbances of vision are present, the MRI may help localize the site of the injury (Fig. 17-4).

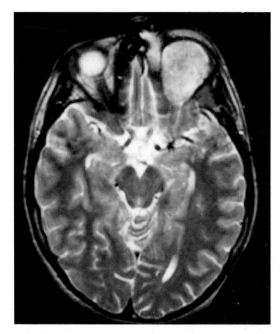

**Fig. 17–4.**
MRI of the orbits shows a large hematoma along the roof of the left side, which displaces the globe inferiorly. The eye was blind on initial examination.

# FRACTURES OF THE MANDIBLE

Although it is the thickest and heaviest of the facial bones, the mandible is the second-most commonly fractured (after nasal bones). Mandibular fractures may occur as isolated injuries or as components of complex maxillary and mandibular fractures.

The most common causes of mandibular fractures are acts of violence that may range from simple falls to motor vehicle accidents. Occasionally, systemic diseases such as hyperparathyroidism and osteomalacia may predispose to mandibular fractures. Uncommonly, benign or malignant tumors, cysts, or osteomyelitis may precipitate such fractures.

Factors influencing the severity of the displacement of the fracture segments are multiple and interrelated. Variations in the direction and intensity of the force of injury will cause different fractures. High-velocity injuries cause a fracture at the site of impact, whereas a slow, less violent force not only causes a fracture at the impact site but also may fracture the opposite condylar neck. A blow to the area of the symphysis may cause fractures of both condylar necks. Second, the site of the fracture may influence the amount of displacement of the segments, depending on the direction of the fracture line and the direction of the different muscle movements in the area. A fracture line that runs downward and forward from the molar area has less displacement than does a line that runs downward and backward.

The muscle groups that operate the mandible include the anterior (depressor-retractor) group and the posterior (elevator) group. The anterior muscle group will displace fragments in a downward, posterior, and medial direction, whereas the posterior group displaces fragments in an upward, forward, and medial direction. Consequently, a fracture through the angle of the mandible in a downward and backward direction will have a far greater displacement because of the distracting forces of the posterior muscle group. However, if the fracture line is in the downward and forward direction, the muscle pull of the posterior group will tend to keep the fracture segments in an anatomic position. Third, the presence or absence of teeth will influence displacement of the fractures. Teeth on the proximal segment may decrease the displacement of the fractures by meeting the corresponding teeth of the maxilla. Finally, the presence and extent of soft-tissue wounds will result in a larger displacement with larger defects.

Clinically, patients may present with varying degrees of malocclusion. They may simply admit, "My teeth don't feel right," or physical examination may demonstrate gross malocclusion. Anesthesia of the lower lip is common in fractures of the body of the mandible. Edema and ecchymosis may mask mandibular asymmetry. On examination, tenderness to palpation over the fracture site and pain with movement will be observed.

Crepitation may be seen with motion. Oral excursion will be decreased. However, the principal physical abnormality will be malocclusion.

Although the clinical examination most often establishes the diagnosis of mandibular fractures, roentgenographic studies more clearly define the direction of the fracture line, the relationship of the teeth to the fracture, and the degree of displacement. Posteroanterior and oblique lateral views of the mandible will demonstrate fractures of the body and the angle without difficulty. If available, a Panorex view of the mandible is an excellent and necessary study that will show fractures at any site. However, fractures of the temporomandibular joint and condylar area are sometimes difficult to demonstrate on routine mandibular roentgenograms and may require tomograms for the final diagnosis (Fig. 17-5).

The most common fracture of the mandible is in the neck of the condyle (36%). The incidence of fractures in this site is closely followed by that of fractures in the angle of the mandible (20%), the body (21%), and the area of the symphysis (14%). Other sites are much less commonly involved.

The principles of treatment for mandibular fracture include early anatomic reduction of the fracture, immobilization, and control of infection. An isolated mandibular fracture should be reduced at the time of injury. However, if other life-threatening injuries are present, treatment of the mandibular injury may be postponed for 7 to 10 days. All mandibular fractures are considered compound if the slightest displacement is present; consequently, preoperative and postoperative antibiotics are recommended. Immobilization will require at least the application of arch bars and intermaxillary fixation

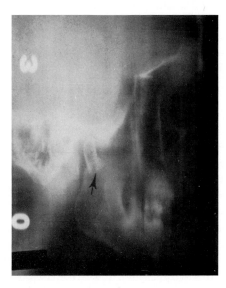

**Fig. 17–5.**
Tomograms of the condylar process are sometimes required to establish a fracture of the condylar neck *(arrow).*

(IMF) with rubber bands or wires for a minimum of 5 weeks.

Specific treatment for each mandibular fracture will vary with the site of the fracture, the degree of displacement, and the presence or absence of teeth. Whenever possible, closed reduction of the mandibular fracture with application of arch bars and intermaxillary fixation is the treatment of choice.

In the last 10 years, significant changes have occurred in the open reduction techniques of mandibular fractures. The acceptance of rigid fixation with either compression plates or lag screws has produced better, more accurate reductions of difficult fractures and lessened the postoperative morbidity of the procedure. Because IMF is not usually required after rigid stabilization, patients are able to begin a soft diet almost immediately after open reduction. Consequently, the weight loss and compromised oral hygiene present in patients with IMF is markedly reduced.

Fractures in the region of symphysis or the angle of the mandible commonly require open reduction and internal fixation with compression plates and lag screws. An arch bar will be placed on the alveolar ridge of the mandible to act as a tension band. However, IMF is not usually needed, and the patient can return to oral intake as soon as the recovery from surgery allows. Similarly, fractures in the body of the mandible, with teeth absent on the proximal side or no teeth present on either side of the fracture, will require open reduction and internal fixation with plates (Fig. 17-6).

The use of compression plates has made the treatment of edentulous patients with mandible fractures much simpler. Instead of using the patient's dentures for the application of arch bars and then suspending the dentures from the zygomatic arches, open reduction and internal fixation with compression plates is used.

Postoperatively, the care of the patient with a mandibular fracture will depend on the type of treatment. If open reduction with internal fixation using compression plates or lag screws has been the method of treatment, the postoperative course is markedly simple. The patient is allowed a liquid to soft diet beginning almost immediately. A soft diet is continued for approximately 5 or 6 weeks postreduction. Consequently, the patient's nutritional status is maintained and the problem of possible weight loss does not normally become a matter of concern.

On the other hand, if closed reduction using arch bars and IMF with rubber bands or wires has been the treatment, a 5-week period of immobilization will be needed for solid union to develop at the fracture site, even though roentgenograms will not demonstrate healing at that time. The use of the Water-Pik™ is highly recommended to maintain good oral hygiene during the

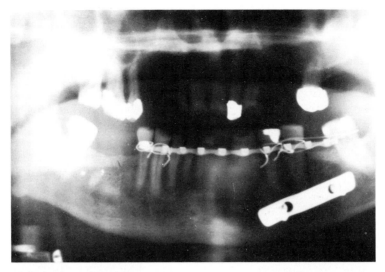

**Fig. 17–6.**
A postoperative Panorex film of a mandibular fracture demonstrates the use of the compression plate in an open reduction and internal fixation of a mandible fracture. No IMF was needed. The arch bar acts as a tension band.

period of mobilization. Nutrition is maintained by simply blenderizing a regular diet. To maintain immobilization, the patient should be seen weekly to check dental occlusion and to replace broken rubber bands. Dental wax may be applied to irritating wires. At the end of 5 weeks, the rubber bands are removed and the patient is allowed to eat for a week. If the patient experiences no pain with oral ingestion, the arch bars are removed with the patient under intravenous sedation. However, if pain or movement at the fracture site can be elicited with eating, the rubber bands are reapplied for another 7 to 10 days of immobilization.

Occasionally, after removing the arch bars, the patient experiences a transient period of trismus because of the prolonged contraction of the muscles of mastication during the period of immobilization. By sliding a gradually increasing number of tongue blades between the teeth, it should be possible to forcibly open the mouth over time.

Early complications of mandibular fracture may include infection, avascular necrosis, osteitis, and osteomyelitis. Factors predisposing to infection are poor oral hygiene, multiple caries, and a compound fracture. Diabetic patients are more susceptible to infections. Acute infection will be manifested as an abscess and is reflected by pain, swelling, and erythema in the area of the abscess. Incision, drainage, and systemic antibiotics constitute the treatment of choice. Chronic infections such as osteitis and osteomyelitis usually occur when a comminuted fracture with an avascular bone segment has occurred. Pain and roentgenographic changes suggestive of osteomyelitis are usually evident. Late complications may also include malocclusion or nonunion and require further corrective surgery.

## FRACTURES OF THE MAXILLA

Fractures of the maxilla or midface are most commonly the result of a high-velocity–type injury. Their incidence in recent years has decreased, primarily because of the increased use of seat belts. The presence of force necessary to cause fractures of the maxilla also increases the likelihood of severe injuries to other organ systems. Associated injuries of various degrees of severity more often involve the head, but occur in the chest and abdomen as well. Skeletal injuries may be present in approximately one third of the patients, whereas blindness is observed in one tenth. Additionally, the incidence of cervical spine injury is much higher than other types of facial fractures and is a result of the effects of sudden cervical hyperflexion.

Maxillary fractures can be divided into two groups: vertical and horizontal. Vertical fractures will split the palate on either side of the septum. However, the three classic fractures of the maxilla are those horizontal defects described by Le Fort. The *Le Fort I (transverse) fracture* is a horizontal fracture immediately above the level of the teeth. The *Le Fort II fracture* has the configuration of a pyramid, with the apex being across the nasal bridge. It extends through the nasal bones, the frontal processes of the maxilla, the lacrimal bones, the inferior

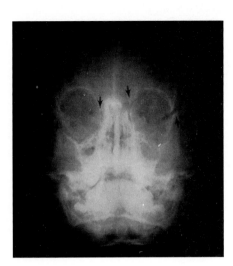

**Fig. 17–7.**
A Le Fort III craniofacial separation *(arrows)* is evident in a Waters' view of an 8-year-old patient. The opacity of the left maxillary sinus is more severe than the right.

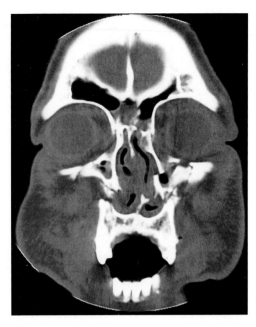

**Fig. 17–8.**
Coronal CT scan of multiple facial fractures shows obvious injuries to the nasoethmoid complex, horizontal maxilla (Le Fort I) and orbital rims.

rim and floor of both orbits, and the maxillozygomatic suture line. From this last point, the fracture continues posteriorly through the lateral wall of the maxilla and the pterygoid plates into the pterygoid maxillary fossa. The *Le Fort III fracture* separates the craniofacial complex and extends through the zygomaticofrontal, maxillofrontal, and nasofrontal suture lines; the floors of the orbit; and the ethmoid and sphenoid bones (Fig. 17-7).

Clinically, the patient may be comatose and may require immediate neurosurgical consultation. If conscious, there may be complaints of the inability to "match" the teeth properly. Infraorbital nerve numbness may be present. In Le Fort II or III fractures, nasal hemorrhage is usually evident. On physical examination, facial deformities may be masked by edema and ecchymosis. Bimanual palpation along the orbital ridges may detect steplike deformities or separations and tenderness. Forward movement of the maxilla will be elicited with all three types of Le Fort fractures; in the Le Fort III fracture, the entire midthird of the face may move. Occasionally, however, these fractures may be impacted and no movement will be evident. Malocclusion can be an initial sign and should suggest a maxillary fracture if the mandible is intact. Extraocular muscle dysfunction may be manifested by diplopia with superior gaze. Blindness is uncommon but may occur.

With extension of the maxillary fractures into the cribriform plate, rhinorrhea mixed with blood will be detected as a result of the dural defect. The patient may mention a salty taste in the back of the mouth. Any clear fluid from

the nose should be tested for glucose. Glucose levels greater than 30 mg/100 cc confirm the presence of cerebrospinal fluid (CSF), and a tear in the dura has occurred. Consequently, the patient's nose should not be packed despite the possible presence of depressed nasal fractures, and the patient should be instructed not to blow the nose. Prophylactic antibiotics that cross the blood-brain barrier should be instituted to decrease the possibility that a retrograde infection will develop. When meningitis has occurred in this type of injury, the most common organism isolated has been *Pneumococcus*, sensitive to penicillin.

Roentgenographically, the Waters' view is the most reliable in demonstrating maxillary fractures in the emergency room. For vertical or alveolar fractures, occlusal views are more suitable. CT scans of the facial bones will detail more accurately the full extent of the fractures. The study is usually done in the coronal view and will show the amount of the comminution, the degree of rotation, and the extent of displacement of the fracture segments (Figs. 17-8, 17-9). Additionally, injury to the optic nerve or fat herniation may be visible.

In those cases where the presence of rhinorrhea has persisted for more than 2 to 3 weeks after the injury or after reduction of the facial bone fractures, an intrathecal injection of metrizamide contrast by lumbar puncture before CT scanning will localize the cranial defect for the neurosurgeon. Radionuclear scans are no longer indicated for the evaluation of CSF leak.

Initially, the airway may be compromised by the posterior displacement of the maxillary fractures or by the

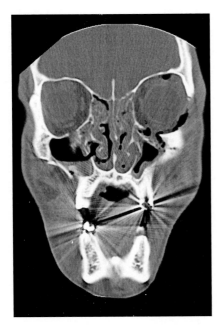

**Fig. 17–9.**
A more posterior CT scan view of the fractures in Fig. 17-8 reveals extensive orbital floor fractures.

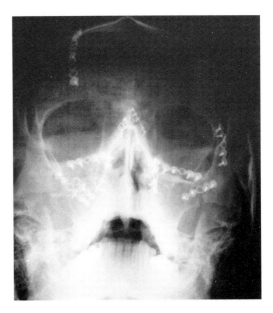

**Fig. 17–10.**
Postreduction x-ray of Le Fort I, nasoethmoid complex and left zygoma fractures treated by rigid fixation. A split cranial bone graft was necessary to reconstruct the left orbital floor. No IMF was required.

combination with mandibular fractures. An endotracheal tube is the preferred treatment, although a cricothyroidotomy occasionally may be necessary.

Over the last 10 years the management of maxillofacial fractures has undergone a complete evolution. No longer is surgical repair delayed until facial edema has resolved. Wire fixation of the fractured segments combined with prolonged intermaxillary fixation has been replaced by an aggressive approach based on concepts adopted from the correction of congenital craniofacial deformities. Currently, wide exposure of all fracture segments, precise anatomic reduction with rigid internal fixation, and intermediate bone grafting are the standards for appropriate treatment of maxillofacial injuries. Exposure of the entire facial skeleton can be obtained through four incisions that are aesthetically acceptable.

Rigid fixation devices include compression plates, stabilization plates, and lag screws. Primary bone grafting at the time of initial reduction of facial fractures has also become an important component of the treatment (Fig. 17-10). Bone grafting is required to replace missing or damaged bone as well as to correct contour deformities secondary to the original traumatic insult. As a consequence, secondary soft-tissue scarring and contraction is minimized. The types of bone graft available include the outer table of the cranium as well as split rib grafts. Fixation with either mini-plates or lag screws is necessary to decrease the rate of reabsorption of the grafts.

For the treatment of maxillary injuries, plates are placed across the fracture sites and give good stability. IMF is usually not required, although in areas of severe

complex fractures elastics may be required for several weeks instead of wire fixation. The orbital floors are explored in Le Fort II or III fractures, and defects are reconstructed with either synthetic implants or cranial bone grafts. Preoperative and postoperative antibiotics are recommended.

Rarely is a tracheotomy required in the isolated midface fracture. Maxillary fractures combined with pulmonary or thoracic injuries may require a tracheotomy to ensure proper ventilation and adequate pulmonary toilet postoperatively.

In the edentulous patient with minimal displacement of the midface, correction of the anatomic defect may be maintained by adjustment with new dentures. Any significant displacement will require open reduction and internal fixation with rigid stabilization.

Occasionally, the patient with extensive maxillary fractures will also suffer a severe head injury with resultant coma. After stabilization of the neurologic status and with the approval of the neurosurgeon, correction of the maxillary fractures is recommended. If treated within 3 weeks of injury, adequate reduction and fixation of the fracture can be accomplished. Otherwise, months may elapse before some degree of consciousness occurs, and surgical intervention then will be markedly more difficult; will probably require osteotomies with bone grafting; and will have less satisfying postoperative results.

Usually, the presence of rhinorrhea will spontaneously cease about 5 days after injury. Alternatively, the CSF leak will cease with adequate reduction of the maxillary fractures. If rhinorrhea continues 3 weeks after injury or after reduction, a craniotomy will be required to close the dural defect.

The use of compression plates allows the airway to be easily managed and lessens the patient's stay in the intensive care unit. Postoperatively, improved oral hygiene and food intake result in the patient's quicker rehabilitation. And finally, the use of plates avoids the possible midfacial shortening and/or midfacial retrusion sometimes seen with wire fixation and craniomandibular suspension.

Late complications of maxillary fractures include nasal obstruction, chronic sinusitis, and lacrimal duct dysfunction. Anesthesia or hypoesthesia of the infraorbital nerve may persist. Malunion of the fracture may occur and will require planned osteotomies with bone grafting for correction. Malocclusion after treatment may occur about 20% of the time. Orthodontics usually can correct this problem; only in severe cases will reconstructive osteotomies be required.

## FRACTURES OF THE ZYGOMA

The zygoma, or malar bone, forms the prominence of the cheek and, consequently, is often injured. The usual cause of a zygoma fracture is the low-intensity, less violent type of injury: fistfights, falls, and collisions.

The zygoma articulates with the maxilla, frontal, and temporal bones. Injury to it may cause a separation at the suture lines (in an isolated injury) or may be combined with fractures of the middle third of the face. If displaced, the zygoma will be depressed in the direction of the traumatic force, which most commonly is in the posterior, downward, and medial direction. Although six different groups of malar fractures have been described, fractures of the zygoma are basically either an isolated zygomatic arch fracture (Fig. 17-11) or the "tripod" fracture (Fig. 17-12).

Clinically, the patient may complain of pain in the area of the zygomatic arch when attempting to open his mouth. Infraorbital nerve anesthesia may be present in both the ipsilateral cheek and the maxillary gingiva (gingival numbness suggests orbital floor and rim fractures). The patient may also admit to diplopia with upward gaze.

On initial examination, the anatomic abnormalities may be masked by significant edema. Ecchymosis may involve the conjunctiva and sclera as well as the eyelids. Bimanual palpation of both the orbital rims and the zygomatic arches should be done simultaneously and may elicit tenderness at the fracture site.

Ocular injury occurs in 25% of facial bone fractures, and complete blindness develops in 14% of these cases. The incidence of ocular injury was greatest when the fractures involved the bones of the orbit. Consequently, patients with fractures of the zygoma, orbit, or frontal bone are at greater risk for such injuries.

It is essential that ocular assessment be done at the initial evaluation of the facial bone fracture patient. Often edema may develop rather quickly, which would prevent a complete ocular examination at a later date.

The initial ocular assessment should involve five parameters: (1) visual acuity, (2) pupillary reactions to light, (3) eyelid or globe lacerations, (4) funduscopic examination, and (5) ocular motility. The visual acuity

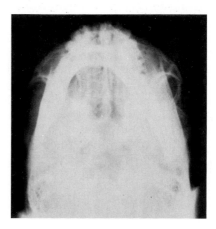

**Fig. 17–11.**
A markedly depressed left zygomatic arch fracture is demonstrated by a submental-vertex view.

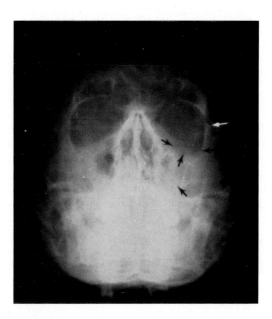

**Fig. 17–12.**
A comminuted left tripod malar fracture is visualized on a Waters' view. A step deformity of the orbital rim can be anticipated on physical examination (arrows). Note the opacity of the left maxillary sinus.

can be grossly evaluated by assessing the patient's ability to read material, count fingers, or merely perceive light. The pupillary reactions to light should be assessed by direct stimulation of the pupil in comparison to an alternating light testing procedure. Direct stimulation of the pupil should elicit a constrictive reaction. The alternating light testing procedure requires moving a light from the normal eye to the injured eye. Initially a dilatation will occur before the constriction. The eyelids and globe should be evaluated for any lacerations. Funduscopic examination should check for both the red reflex and for visualization of the retina. Ocular movement should be evaluated by having the patient's eyes follow the examiner's finger throughout the full range of motion. After evaluation is completed, any concern should require an immediate ophthalmology consultation for further evaluation.

After resolution of the edema, the clinician may be able to identify depression over the zygomatic arch, step-off deformities of the orbital rim, flattening of the malar eminence, or inferior displacement of the lateral canthus. Oral excursion may be limited to less than 2 cm. (Limitation of oral excursion can occur if the zygomatic arch is depressed 1 cm and impedes the movement of the coronoid process of the mandible.) Diplopia with superior gaze may be present if the inferior rectus muscle is trapped by an orbital floor fracture. Enophthalmos may occur if a significant orbital floor defect is present.

The best roentgenographic studies obtainable from the emergency room are the Waters' view of the facial bones and the submental-vertex view of the zygomatic arches. Displacement of the malar fragment and/or opacity in the maxillary sinus is readily visible on a Waters' view. A CT scan of the orbits must be obtained to further delineate the extent of the fractures (Fig. 17-13).

Surgical reduction of the isolated zygomatic arch fracture can be done either intraorally or extraorally on an outpatient basis. After reduction of the bony fragments, stabilization is secured by placement of plates across the fracture lines at two or three sites to achieve solid fixation to resist the pull of the masseter muscle postoperatively (Fig. 17-14). Many fractures can be fixated at two points with plates placed at the frontal zygomatic suture line and the zygomatic maxillary buttress. Fractures of the zygoma should be reduced within 3 weeks of injury.

Postoperatively, antibiotic coverage is continued for a week. A light dressing may be applied over the ipsilateral eye, but it is removed on the first postoperative day. Weekly, the patient's muscular symmetry and extraocular muscle function are monitored.

Complications secondary to zygoma fractures are unusual, but may include infection, malunion, and nonunion. Infection usually occurs in those cases requiring orbital floor reconstruction with an implant, especially if the maxillary sinus has also been packed. The infection may develop early or late with respect to the repair of the fracture, and requires removal of the

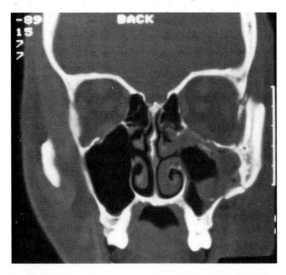

**Fig. 17–13.**
A coronal CT scan demonstrates a displaced left malar fracture. Opacification of the left maxillary sinus is clearly evident. Also note the ability for the CT scan to demonstrate the extraocular muscles.

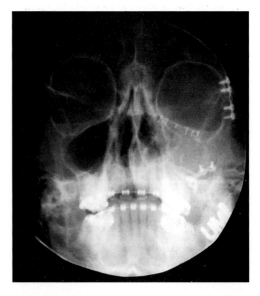

**Fig. 17–14.**
Postreduction view of zygoma complex fractures stabilized by plates across three sites. Sometimes the plate at the zygoma/maxillary buttress is not needed.

implant as well as antibiotics administered for systemic effect. Malunion of the zygoma may cause facial asymmetry and interference with mandibular function. Correction can be achieved by osteotomies at the zygomaticofrontal and zygomaticomaxillary suture line, elevation of the zygoma, bone grafting, and fixation. Nonunions will necessitate bone grafting and rigid fixation. Any residual contour deformity may be corrected at a later date with the use of onlay bone, cartilage, or synthetic grafts.

## BLOW-OUT FRACTURES

Strictly speaking, the term *blow-out fracture* should be restricted to fractures of the orbital floor without involvement of the orbital rim. Blow-out fractures result from the transmission of a sudden increased intraocular pressure through the weakest point of the orbital floor, most commonly near the infraorbital nerve canal. A second common site of fracture is the medial orbital wall.

The most common cause of blow-out fractures is the automobile accident. One third of the cases usually result from blunt trauma secondary to fist blows, ball injuries, falls, and other forms of assault. Although the orbital rim protects the eyeball itself against direct injury from objects larger than 5 cm, ocular injury must be ruled out in all blow-out fractures. The incidence of ocular injury with orbital fractures varies widely, but the incidence of hyphema and retinal hemorrhage appears to be the greatest. However, more severe injuries such as decreased vision or blindness may also occur. Direct ocular injury is more common in low-velocity injuries (14%) than in auto accidents (0.6%).

During examination, the patient may volunteer the presence of diplopia, infraorbital nerve numbness, and, possibly, decreased vision. Clinically, periorbital edema and ecchymosis may handicap the initial examination. However, the eyelids can usually be pried open to allow a gross examination of vision and light perception. Diplopia may occur as a result of limitation of superior gaze (Fig. 17-15). As the periorbital edema resolves, diplopia may lessen in severity. If the periorbital edema is minimal, enophthalmos may be present.

The most common causes of diplopia in blow-out fractures are entrapment of either the inferior rectus muscle or inferior oblique muscle; or a periorbital fat herniation. Other causes of immediate diplopia include injury to cranial nerves III, IV, and VI; direct injury or hemorrhage into the extraocular muscles; or displacement of the eyeball into the maxillary sinus. The "traction test" will simplify the differential diagnosis. Topical anesthesia is applied to the conjunctiva. The eyeball is pinched with a fine forceps at the insertion of the inferior rectus muscle and rotated. If rotation of the eyeball cannot be accomplished, entrapment of the inferior rectus muscle is demonstrated. If rotation of the eyeball is achieved, then the diplopia is a result of one of the other causes.

Enophthalmos may be evident on the initial examination or it may be masked by the periorbital edema. With subsequent resolution of the edema, enophthalmos will become more apparent. The mechanism of enophthalmos includes herniation of the orbital fat into the maxillary sinus, posterior position of the ocular globe as a result of entrapment of the inferior rectus muscle, or the downward displacement of the ocular globe through a large orbital floor fracture. Additionally, enophthalmos may develop as a result of orbital fat necrosis secondary to the injury, to pressure from an orbital hematoma, or to a low-grade inflammatory process.

The most pertinent roentgenographic studies are a Waters' view initially, followed by a CT scan. A coronal CT scan is the most accurate in diagnosing this defect. However, its use may be limited by the positioning requirements of the patient or by the presence of multiple dental fillings. Abnormal findings would include lowering of the orbital floor, orbital fat entrapment in the maxillary sinus (Fig. 17-16), or massive orbital contents displacement into the maxillary sinus.

Treatment of blow-out fracture is twofold. If definite ocular injury is demonstrated on initial examination, an ophthalmologic consultation must be obtained immediately for evaluation. If no ocular injury is present, surgical considerations are postponed until the resolution of periorbital edema. The two primary indications for

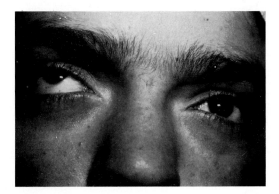

**Fig. 17–15.**
Impairment of superior gaze occurring after a blow to the left eye. A traction test confirmed entrapment of the inferior rectus muscle.

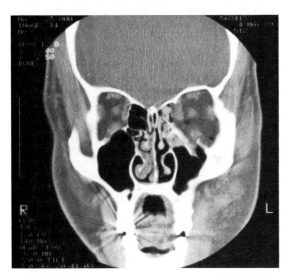

**Fig. 17–16.**
A coronal CT scan demonstrating a left blow-out fracture. Soft-tissue entrapment can be seen. Note the artifacts created by the dental fillings on the right side.

surgical correction of a blow-out fracture include diplopia, confirmed by a positive traction test; or enophthalmos. Usually, roentgenographic evidence will support the diagnosis of a blow-out fracture, but a normal study should not postpone surgery if there is a positive traction test or enophthalmos present.

The surgical procedure should be performed within 2 weeks after injury, because the incarcerated contents become more difficult to release after this period. If surgery is postponed more than 2 or 3 weeks, motility problems and enophthalmos may appear as late complications. The surgical procedure consists of exploration of the orbital floor through a lower eyelid incision, release of the entrapped inferior rectus muscle, retrieval of the herniated orbital contents, and reconstruction of the orbital floor with either a synthetic implant or a cranial bone graft.

Antibiotics are recommended both preoperatively and postoperatively because of the involvement with the maxillary sinus. An eye patch is usually applied at the completion of the operation and removed on the first postoperative day. The patient is followed as an outpatient for persistence of either diplopia or enophthalmos.

Useful binocular vision commonly occurs at the end of 3 months. However, if diplopia is not improved by that time, an ophthalmology consultation will be required for further evaluation and possible prescription of glass prisms to allow useful vision. After 6 months, extraocular muscle surgery may be necessary to correct the persistent diplopia.

The persistence of enophthalmos presents a difficult problem. Enophthalmos may be corrected by osteotomies and reconstruction with a cranial bone graft. However, this surgical procedure is a major effort to correct a deformity that might have been prevented at the initial surgical repair.

## NASAL FRACTURES

Fractures of the nasal bones are the most common of all facial bone fractures. Early treatment will allow easy reduction with satisfactory postoperative results. Neglect of treatment may produce both physiologic and cosmetic deformities much more difficult to correct.

The type of nasal fracture may vary from a simple displacement of the nasal pyramid from a lateral blow to a more complex comminuted fracture with a resultant "smashed-nose" appearance from a frontal force. Associated injuries include fractures extending through the cribriform plate, medial canthal ligament displacement, or lacrimal gland or duct injuries. Sequelae of the comminuted nasal fracture include traumatic telecanthus, dacryocystitis, and epiphora.

Clinical evaluation plays the most important role in making an accurate diagnosis. The presence of preexisting disease, nasal deformity, or a previous nasal operation should be investigated at the time of the initial examination. On physical examination, nasal and periorbital edema is common. Nasal obstruction may be present secondary to edema, clots, or displaced nasal bone fractures. Movement of the nasal bone fragments

may be elicited by palpation. Subcutaneous emphysema may be present. The possibility of a telescoping-type injury should be considered if the nasolabial angle is greater than 100 degrees (especially in a man) or if a step deformity is noted dorsally at the junction of the nasal bone with the septum.

The importance of identifying a hematoma of the septum at the time of the initial examination cannot be stressed too strongly. If overlooked, a septal hematoma can progress either to a partial nasal obstruction or to a septal perforation. Topical application of 10% cocaine will shrink the nasal mucosa and allow examination of the nasal passageways by a speculum. The presence of a septal hematoma should be treated immediately by incision and drainage.

Often, the posteroanterior and lateral roentgenographic views of the nasal bones are not helpful in supporting the clinical impression of a nasal fracture. A Waters' view may better demonstrate fractures of either the nasal septum or the bony pyramid. However, the clinical impression is much more meaningful in diagnosing this fracture.

Ideally, nasal fractures should be treated when they are initially diagnosed. Usually, however, the presence of nasal edema does not permit immediate reduction. At the end of 3 to 5 days, the edema will resolve sufficiently to allow satisfactory reduction of the nasal fracture. Most simple fractures are treated by closed reduction. However, complicated fractures that result from a frontal impact are more likely to be treated by an open reduction. The fragments are reduced under direct vision and wired together. Medial canthal ligament injuries are repaired. Bone grafting may be done.

Although closed reduction can be performed with the patient under either general anesthesia or a combination of local and topical anesthesia, general anesthesia is recommended to protect the airway from posterior nasal bleeding. After satisfactory reduction, a nasal speculum should be used to demonstrate the patency of the airways and to evaluate the position of the nasal septum. A displaced septum should be returned to its position in the vomerine groove. Nasal packing is inserted to maintain the nasal bone reduction. A nasal splint is applied for further stabilization.

Postoperatively, the nasal packing will be left in place for approximately 5 days and the nasal splint for 7 days. Usually, the nasal splint is worn only at night during the second week. Any activity that would endanger the nasal reduction (e.g., contact sports) should be avoided for 6 weeks. During the interval of packing, nasal decongestants and antibiotics are used.

Late complications of nasal fracture include nasal deformity and airway obstruction. The nasal deformity may be secondary to malunion of the nasal bones or to a septal injury. Malunion usually occurs as a result of the patient's failure to seek early medical attention. Correcting a nasal fracture more than 14 days past the injury is rarely successful and will require rhinoplasty to correct the deformity. Persistent nasal deformity or airway obstruction may be the result of a septal injury and will also require rhinoplasty and possible submucous cartilage resection for correction. In the pediatric age group, rhinoplasties are normally postponed until the age of 15 years to avoid any possible growth disturbances with the development of the nose. In the adult, rhinoplasty can be performed after satisfactory wound healing has occurred, usually about 3 months after the injury.

## FRONTAL SINUS FRACTURES

Frontal sinus fractures are not common, but they do warrant special considerations. Such injuries are usually accompanied by fractures of other facial bones and may be associated with an intracranial injury.

On clinical examination, anesthesia of the forehead and scalp may be present as a result of soft-tissue injury to the supratrochlear and supraorbital nerves. If a depressed supraorbital ridge fracture is present, diplopia will be demonstrated as a result of dysfunction of the superior rectus and superior oblique muscles. Periorbital ecchymosis and edema will be present, which may mask the frontal depression secondary to the fracture. Tenderness and crepitation to palpation may be elicited. Rhinorrhea may also be noted.

Roentgenographic studies should include a skull series and Caldwell and lateral views of the facial bones. If air fluid levels or cloudiness is seen in the sinus, or if a pneumocephalus is present, a CT scan in both axial and coronal views should be obtained. The presence of an intracranial aerocele is pathognomonic for a dural

tear and would implicate a fracture of the posterior wall of the frontal sinus.

The treatment of frontal sinus fractures depends on the extent of the fracture, the amount of fragmentation present, nasal frontal duct involvement, and the presence of a dural tear with CSF leak. Antibiotic coverage should begin on the day of injury. Surgical correction of a depressed or compound anterior wall fracture requires elevation and wiring or microplating of the bony fragments. Treatment of posterior wall fractures is controversial and involves open exploration with sinus obliteration by a variety of means. In the presence of a dural tear, a transfrontal craniotomy with repair of the dura should be done in conjunction with reduction of the fracture or cranialization of the sinus.

The potential complications of frontal sinus fractures can be life-threatening. A posterior wall fracture with a dural tear may develop either a retrograde meningitis or brain abscess. Frontal sinus infections may also extend into the orbital cavities. The frontal sinus duct may be obstructed, with the subsequent development of a mucocele.

## FACIAL FRACTURES IN THE PEDIATRIC PATIENT

The incidence of facial fractures in the pediatric age group varies widely, partly because plain x-rays are unreliable in the diagnosis of such injuries in children.

There are not many large series of pediatric facial fractures reported in the literature. Consequently, controversy regarding the incidence, the effect of injury on growth, and the actual treatment of such injuries has been unresolved.

Everyone does agree that the facial skeleton is constantly changing from birth to the age of 18 years. Facial bones initially are resilient, but brittleness begins to increase significantly after the age of 2 to 3. The paranasal sinus development changes the vulnerability of the facial bones to injury. The maxillary sinus aeration begins at birth and continues until the age of 12. The frontal sinus aeration begins at approximately 5 years of age and continues to late puberty. The role of dentition, as well as the mixed dentition present in pediatric patients, limit one's ability to adequately stabilize either the maxillary or mandibular fractures.

Certain generalized patterns of pediatric facial bone fractures can be apparent, however. Skull fractures are more common than facial bone fractures in the age group under 12 years. Mid-facial fractures are extremely rare before the eighth birthday. Mandibular fractures that occur in the pediatric population under 10 years of age will involve the condyle 66% of the time. After the age of 15 the adult pattern of mandibular fracture prevails. Forty percent of all patients with facial bone fractures will have skull fractures. In the earlier pediatric age group most fractures probably are greenstick because of the resiliency of the facial bones.

The diagnosis of facial bone fractures in the pediatric patient is difficult both clinically and radiographically. The child may not understand or ask questions about the injury. Cooperation in the physical examination may be difficult to obtain, but tenderness to palpation usually can be elicited. The key factor in identifying facial bone fractures in the pediatric age group is maintaining a high level of suspicion. Because plain x-rays are notoriously unreliable in the diagnosis, axial and coronal CT scans must be obtained in children when facial fractures are suspected.

In general, the treatment plan for facial fractures of pediatric patients may not be guided by the principles of adult treatment described in earlier pages. Three types of injuries may be present. First, the minimally displaced fracture in the pediatric age group may do best if left alone and simply observed. Second, severely displaced fractures require anatomic reduction and stabilization, especially in the older child. Third, fractures that fall between the first two groups in patients with a high degree of facial growth potential may not require aggressive surgical treatment.

Several questions have been raised when trying to apply the principles of wide exposure and rigid fixation to the pediatric patient. Although wide exposure to the craniofacial abnormalities of the upper third of the face and skull is well tolerated, some have questioned whether scarred soft tissue of the midface may inhibit growth.

Many have also advocated that rigid fixation is not as necessary in the pediatric patient as in the adult. Certainly, severely displaced fractures will need stabilization. However, wire fixation or single point fixation may be all that is necessary for adequate treatment. In fact, mild displacement of facial fractures may only need reduction to be stable. The stiffness of rigid fixation and screw fixation may cause secondary growth disturbances. Wire fixation or microplate fixation may be a better choice in the younger patient. If rigid plates are used, they should be removed after bone healing has been achieved. Additionally, acute bone grafting continues to be controversial and should be used sparingly.

Treatment of mandibular fractures should be as simple as possible. Open reduction and internal fixation is avoided unless severe or unfavorable angle fractures are present. Fractures involving the condyle are treated in a conservative manner if the head is still in the glenoid fossa. If the child has good occlusion on physical examination after the swelling has resolved, then observation, early motion, and a liquid diet are appropriate treatment. If occlusion cannot be demonstrated, then immobilization with acrylic splints or arch bars with IMF for 3 weeks is indicated. However, if the condyle head is displaced outside of the glenoid fossa, open reduction and internal fixation followed with immobilization for 3 weeks is recommended.

A facial deformity may result from abnormal development secondary to growth center disturbance after a facial bone fracture. Therefore the importance of making the diagnosis cannot be overemphasized. Even if the facial fractures are minimally displaced and require no surgical treatment, the long-term effect on growth must be monitored. The effect of condylar fractures on the development of the mandible is unpredictable. Some patients have compensatory overgrowth on the injured side, whereas others may have less growth. The parents of the patient should be alerted to the possibility of growth abnormality and the child should be observed throughout adolescence. Any abnormality that may develop would then require further evaluation and possible surgical intervention.

## SOFT-TISSUE INJURY MANAGEMENT

Soft-tissue injuries are seen on a daily basis in any emergency room. The appropriate management includes not only evaluation of the wound itself but also evaluation for any deeper injury and repair by the appropriate methods. Complicated wounds require the expertise of a surgical specialist. However, many wounds are simple and can be treated by either the emergency room or primary care physician.

The general principles of wound repair apply to injuries occurring in any region of the body. However, for the purpose of discussion, most of the examples will be confined to the head and neck area. Before any local anesthesia is administered, evaluation of facial nerve function can be done simply by asking the patient to raise the eyebrows, close the eyes, and smile. If any weakness is present, then a nerve injury should be considered. Vertically oriented lacerations across the cheek have a potential for underlying parotid duct injury, especially if the laceration appears to extend into the parotid gland. Cannulating Stensen's duct opposite the second maxillary molar can often be done in the emergency room. Injection of methylene blue solution will allow the diagnosis to be made. If either a parotid duct or facial nerve injury is identified, the patient should be referred to a surgical specialist for management in the operating room.

Commonly, most soft-tissue injuries are isolated and can be managed in the emergency room. Such wounds range in severity from simple lacerations to dog bite injuries to more complicated soft-tissue wounds. For those lacerations that do not require the expertise of a surgical specialist, simple general principles may guide the emergency room or primary care physician in a prompt and satisfactory repair.

## Surgical Technique

Local infiltration, either with plain xylocaine or xylocaine with epinephrine, is the most common choice of anesthesia. In facial wounds, 1% xylocaine with epinephrine, 1:200,000, is the more appropriate choice because the head and neck area is extremely vascular. The use of epinephrine decreases the amount of bleeding; prolongs the duration of anesthesia; and allows for greater volume of infiltration, if necessary. However, epinephrine may cause cardiac irritability. Large amounts should be avoided in patients with cardiac disease, arrhythmias, or hypertension. Epinephrine should not be injected in wounds that have a high risk for infection or in wounds with marginally viable tissue.

Proper administration of local anesthesia may avoid some patient discomfort. Direct wound infiltration through the wound margin by using a 25- or 27-gauge needle is better tolerated than injection through the intact skin. The injection should be done as a slow, steady application of anesthesia in contrast to the sudden, painful injection of a bolus of the local solution.

After the wound is anesthetized, it should be treated with an appropriate solution such as povidone-iodine (Betadine) and draped. If any foreign material is still present, or if suspicion of bacteria seeding is high, local irrigation of the wound is performed. Such irrigation provides mechanical cleansing of the wound. The choice of the solution for irrigation is not as important as the actual cleansing of the wound. The simplest technique for irrigation is the use of a 25-cc syringe with a 22-gauge needle. The amount of irrigation necessary to clean the wound depends, of course, on the contamination and tissue injury of the wound. The irrigation may also be supplemented by using a toothbrush or scrub brush to remove any embedded particles.

Any bleeding point should be coagulated. Most emergency rooms now have battery-operated, disposable cauteries that can be used. This coagulation will help minimize the chance of postclosure bleeding and the subsequent increased risk of infection or development of hematomas.

Most simple lacerations do not require much surgical manipulation. Occasionally, there may be an area of questionable tissue on the wound margin that will require debridement. Conservation should be the primary goal whenever debriding edges of such wounds. However, the nonviable tissue should be removed to provide optimal results for wound healing. If the extent of the debridement is of concern to the physician, then surgical consultation should be obtained.

Lacerations that extend through the dermis into the subcutaneous tissue will require a two-layer closure. Closure of the dermal subcutaneous junction with an absorbable suture is the first step and provides the strength in wound repair. The choice of absorbable suture can be either 5-0 Dexon or Vicryl. The sutures are placed in such a manner that the knot is inverted. The needle is first passed through the subcutaneous tissue into the dermis on one side of the wound and passed through the dermis into the subcutaneous tissue on the other side of the wound where it is tied. Such a technique allows the knot to be covered by the full layer of the skin and thus minimizes the chances for "spitting" of the suture.

In small lacerations, the physician can proceed from one end of the wound to the other. However, for longer wounds, it is easier to divide the wound into quarters with placement of the first three sutures. This approach allows for more accurate closure and avoids the appearance of "dog ears."

After the dermal layer is approximated, closure of the skin layer should be completed. The use of small, interrupted sutures of 6-0 nylon placed at short intervals is an acceptable technique. (Slightly more demanding is the subcuticular suture, which may present a better outcome by avoiding the chances of crosshatching seen occasionally with interrupted suture repair.) The interrupted skin sutures should not strangulate the skin. Sutures should be removed before the sixth day to avoid crosshatching, or "railroad tracks." The application of sterile strips can be done at the time of suture removal.

Wounds to the lower eyelids are usually closed with 6-0 silk to minimize the possible irritation of sutures on the ocular globe. Nylon sutures are stiff and can cause corneal abrasions.

## Anatomic Considerations

The technique described will allow the emergency room or primary-care physician to handle all wounds with confidence that optimal wound healing can occur. However, wounds at various anatomic sites require special attention. These are discussed briefly.

Many physicians do not consider scalp wounds to be significant and simply close them with staples or large sutures. However, in men, male-pattern baldness may develop, and thus the scar may become visible at some future time. Closure of such wounds should therefore be done with care. If possible, one should close the galea with a 4-0 absorbable suture (Dexon or Vicryl) or one of the newer, longer-lasting sutures (such as Maxon). Interrupted sutures with 4-0 nylon can then be used to complete the skin closure.

Eyelid wounds that are superficial and that do not involve the underlying tarsal plate or levator musculature can be closed with simple sutures. Normally, lacerations to the upper eyelid are closed with 6-0 nylon, whereas 6-0 silk is used for lower eyelid wounds.

Repair of small through-and-through lacerations of either the nose or ear can be accomplished in the emergency room. Sometimes infiltration of local anesthesia is not well tolerated for nasal wounds, but repair of wounds at either site is done in a similar manner. In nasal wounds, repair is done by placing 5-0 absorbable sutures for the nasal mucosa repair and a 6-0 nylon suture in the skin layer. For ear lacerations, 6-0 nylon sutures are used for both the preauricular and postauricular skin closure. Sutures are not placed in the cartilage of either the ear or the nose.

Lip lacerations are common and may completely split either the upper or lower lip. Such injuries will require layer closure for optimal results. The labial mucosa closure can be accomplished with a 5-0 absorbable suture. The orbicularis oris muscle should be approximated with a 4-0 absorbable suture such as Dexon. The dermis is closed with the 5-0 absorbable suture and the skin with a 6-0 nylon suture. For the vermilion portion of the wound, 6-0 silk sutures would be appropriate. If the laceration violates the vermilion cutaneous border, careful approximation of the border should be done to avoid a notching defect. The closure can be accomplished by placing a stitch either just above or below the vermilion cutaneous junction and approximating this point first. Subsequent interrupted sutures can then be placed for final closure.

Postoperative care for the wounds is important for optimal results. Antibiotics are prescribed for dog bites and wounds that extend into the oral cavity. No dairy products are allowed for 2 days in wounds involving the oral cavity. Because most wounds will develop some edema after closure, a light compression dressing should be applied and maintained for several days postrepair.

On the second or third day after injury, the dressing is removed and the wound examined for any sign of inflammation that may suggest an early infection. For wounds that are close to the eye or on the lip, an antibiotic ointment is usually applied for the first several days after repair. The patient is advised to clean the wound with a 50% mixture of peroxide and water and to reapply a light coating of the antibiotic ointment.

The sutures of facial wounds should be removed by the fourth to sixth day, depending on the type of wound and type of closure. Steri-Strips can be applied after suture removal.

After the sutures are removed, the patient should be seen in 3 weeks for follow-up. The patient is instructed in the general principles of wound healing, and followed every 3 months for the first year after injury until the maturation of the wound is complete. If the physician or the patient is unhappy with the final results of the scarring, then the patient should be referred to a surgical specialist for possible revision.

## BIBLIOGRAPHY

Bartlett SP, De Luzier III JB: Controversies in the management of pediatric facial fractures, *Clin Plast Surg* 1:245, 1992.

Converse JM, Smith B, Wood-Smith D: Orbital and naso-orbital fractures. In Converse JM, editor: *Reconstructive plastic surgery*, ed 2, Philadelphia, 1977, WB Saunders.

De Marino DP et al: Three-dimensional computed tomography in maxillofacial trauma, *Arch Otolaryngol Head Neck Surg* 112:146, 1986.

Dingman RO, Converse JM: Clinical management of facial injuries and fractures of facial bones. In Converse JM, editor: *Reconstructive plastic surgery*, ed 2, Philadelphia, 1977, WB Saunders.

Dingman RO, Natvig P: *Surgery of facial fractures*, Philadelphia, 1964, WB Saunders.

Finkle DR et al: Comparison of the diagnostic methods used in maxillofacial trauma, *Plast Reconstr Surg* 73:32, 1985.

Gruss JS: Naso-orbital-ethmoid fractures: classification and the rule of primary bone grafting, *Plast Reconstr Surg* 75:3, 1985.

Gruss JS: Discussion: orbital roof fractures in the pediatric population, *Plast Reconstr Surg* 84:217, 1989.

Gruss JS: Complex craniomaxillofacial trauma: evolving concepts in management: a trauma unit's experience, 1989 Fraser R. Gurd lecture, *J Trauma* 30(4):377, 1990.

Gussack GS et al: Pediatric maxillofacial trauma: unique features in diagnosis and treatment, *Laryngoscope* 94:925, 1987.

Hoopes JE, Wolforte FG, Jabaley ME: Operative treatment of fractures of the mandibular condyle in children, *Plast Reconstr Surg* 46:357, 1970.

Kawamoto HK Jr: Late post-traumatic enophthalmos: a correctable deformity? *Plast Reconstr Surg* 69:423, 1982.

LaFort R: Fractures de la mâchoire superieur, *Cong Int Med*, C.R. (Paris), p. 275, 1900.

Lineweaver W et al: Post traumatic condylar hyperplasia, *Ann Plast Surg* 22:163, 1989.

Luce EA, Tubb TD, Moore AM: Review of 1,000 major fractures and associated injuries, *Plast Reconstr Surg* 63:26, 1979.

Maniglia AJ, Kline SN: Maxillofacial trauma in the pediatric age group, *Otolaryngol Clin North Am* 16:717, 1983.

Manson PN et al: Midface fracture: advantages of immediate extended open reduction and bone grafting, *Plast Reconstr Surg* 76:1, 1985.

Manson PN: Management of facial fractures, *Perspect Plast Surg* 2:1, 1988.

Mong AJ, Grossman MD: A prospective analysis of the incidence of ocular injury in 283 consecutive facial fracture patients. Paper presented during Residents Day at U. of Louisville Dept. of Ophthalmology, Louisville, Ky, June 18, 1990.

Nohum AM: The biomechanics of maxillofacial trauma, *Clin Plast Surg* 2:59, 1975.

McCoy FJ et al: An analysis of facial fractures and their complications, *Plast Reconstr Surg* 29:381, 1962.

Milaukas AT, Fueger GF: Serious ocular complications associated with blow-out fractures of the orbit, *Am J Ophthalmol* 62:670, 1966.

Morgan BDG et al: Fractures of the middle third of the face: a review of 300 cases, *Br J Plast Surg* 25:147, 1972.

Mulliken JD et al: Management of facial fractures in children, *Clin Plast Surg* 4:491, 1977.

Murray JAM et al: Open vs. closed reduction of the fractured nose, *Arch Otolaryngol* 110:797, 1984.

Ousterhout DK, Vargervik K: Maxillary hypoplasia secondary to midfacial trauma in childhood, *Plast Reconsr Surg* 30:491, 1987.

Parker MG, Lehman J Jr: Management of facial fractures in children, *Perspect Plast Surg* 3:1, 1989.

Reynolds JR: Late complications vs. methods of treatment in a large series of mid-facial fractures, *Plast Reconstr Surg* 61:871, 1978.

Rock WD, Brian DJ: The effects of nasal trauma during childhood upon growth of the nose and midface, *Br J Orthod* 10:38, 1983.

Sataloff RT et al: Surgical management of the frontal sinus, *Neurosurgery* 15:593, 1984.

Schaefer SD, Diehl JT, Briggs WH: The diagnosis of cerebrospinal fluid rhinorrhea by metrizamide CT scanning, *Laryngoscope* 90:871, 1980.

Schultz RC: Facial injuries from automobile accidents: a study of 400 consecutive cases, *Plast Reconstr Surg* 40:45, 1967.

Schultz RC: Supraorbital and glabellar fractures, *Plast Reconstr Surg* 45:227, 1970.

Spiessl B: Rigid internal fixation of fractures of the lower jaw, *Trauma Reconstr Surg* 13:124, 1972.

Steidler NE et al: Incidence and management of major middle third facial fractures at the Royal Melbourne Hospital: a retrospective study, *Int J Oral Surg* 9:92, 1980.

Steidler NE et al: Residual complications in patients with major middle third facial fractures, *Int J Oral Surg* 9:259, 1980.

Stranc MF, Robertson GA: A classification of injuries of the nasal skeleton, *Ann Plast Surg* 2:468, 1979.

Tessier P: Definitive surgical treatment of the severe facial deformities of craniofacial dysosteses: Crouzon's and Apert's disease, *Plast Reconstr Surg* 48:419, 1971.

Wolfe SA: Application of craniofacial surgical precepts in orbital reconstructive following trauma and tumor removal, *J Maxillofac Surg* 10:212, 1981.

Zin KY et al: The effect of rigid fixation on the developing craniofacial skeleton: an experimental study, *Plast Reconstr Surg* 87:229, 1991.

# CHAPTER 18

# Special Topics

## REFLEX SYMPATHETIC DYSTROPHY

Reflex sympathetic dystrophy is a syndrome of unknown cause that often follows a relatively minor injury. It has been called by several names: Sudeck's atrophy, causalgia, shoulder-hand syndrome, posttraumatic dystrophy, and others. The pathogenesis of the disorder is unclear, but a disturbance in the sympathetic nervous system apparently develops and leads to the characteristic symptoms and signs of intense pain (allodynia) and vasomotor disturbances. The condition usually affects the extremity rather than the torso. Early recognition is difficult.

### Clinical Features

Clinical manifestations can be variable, but persistent burning pain that develops after an injury is the characteristic feature. Three stages (acute, dystrophic, and atrophic) are often described. The acute stage lasts up to 6 to 12 weeks and is characterized by the development of persistent, burning pain. The injury is often trivial but the pain is often severe and out of proportion to the amount of trauma. Initially, the pain is localized to the area of the injury, but gradually it spreads throughout the extremity. Hypersensitivity to light touch is also a common symptom. The extremity appears swollen and warm, and excessive perspiration may be present. In the later dystrophic and atrophic stages, motion in the affected joints becomes restricted, and the involved area becomes cool. Skin and muscle atrophy develop and the skin appears dry, shiny, and glossy. Stiffness and intractable pain may persist for several weeks or months.

The roentgenogram often reveals patchy osteoporosis (Fig. 18-1). The bone scan is often positive showing regional uptake, which is diagnostic and reflects increased blood flow.

### Treatment

Reflex sympathetic dystrophy is best treated by prevention. All injuries should have immediate attention, and pain and swelling should be controlled. Early use of the extremity is also important. Once reflex sympathetic dystrophy develops, it is difficult to treat. The most important aspect of therapy is restoration of motion by exercise. Active use of the extremity should be encouraged in spite of the pain. The edema may be controlled by elevation. Physical therapy in the form of passive range-of-motion exercises may be helpful but should not replace active home exercise by the patient. Smoking should be discouraged. Repeated sympathetic blocks are sometimes helpful. The treatment is often prolonged, but most patients eventually improve.

## ROTATIONAL DEFORMITIES OF THE LEGS IN CHILDREN

Developmental abnormalities of the lower extremities are common and are often a source of concern to parents. The cause of these deformities is unknown, but hereditary and persistent postnatal malpositioning play important roles. Most correct themselves spontaneously.

### In-toeing

The in-toeing gait pattern seen in young children is the most common rotational deformity and is usually secondary to one or more of the following causes: (1) internal rotation deformity of the hip secondary to contracture or excessive femoral anteversion, (2) internal (medial) torsion of the tibia, or (3) metatarsus varus (adductus) of the foot.

All three of these deformities are aggravated by positions or postures that are often assumed by the child or infant. Lying in the prone position with the legs extended and the feet internally rotated is often associated with in-toeing deformity. Sitting in the "reverse-tailor" position with the feet internally rotated beneath the buttocks is directly related to persistent tibial rotation and adduction of the forefoot (Fig. 18-2). Children may assume these positions for extended periods while sleeping, playing, or watching television.

Children with internal rotation deformities have a high incidence of bowing of the lower extremities. This is often more apparent than actual, because the lower limb is never visualized in the true anteroposterior plane but rather in the oblique plane. The gait is occasionally clumsy, and the appearance may be unsightly.

### Internal Femoral Torsion

The diagnosis is made by clinical examination. It is helpful to mark the patellae and observe their position as the child walks. If the child toes in and the patellae face medially, excessive femoral anteversion or an internal rotation contracture of the hips should be suspected. If the child toes in and the patellae face straight forward, then the deformity is distal to the knee, either internal tibial torsion or metatarsus varus. Internal femoral torsion can also be measured with the patient prone, the hips extended, and the knees flexed 90 degrees (Fig. 18-3). External and internal measurements of hip motion are then made, with the tibia acting as a

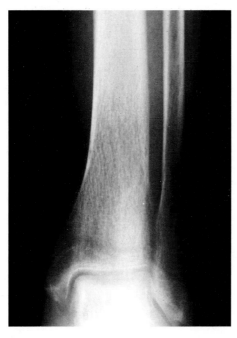

**Fig. 18–1.**
Roentgenogram of the ankle several weeks after a relatively minor sprain. Severe osteoporosis (Sudeck's bone atrophy) of the lower portions of the tibia and fibula are present.

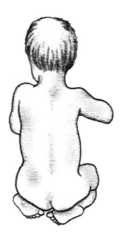

**Fig. 18–2.**
The reverse-tailor position.

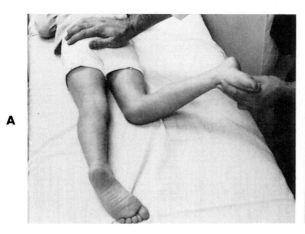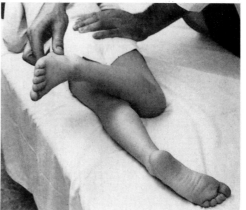

A      B

**Fig. 18–3.**
Measuring femoral torsion. The tibia can act as a pointer. Internal femoral torsion is present when internal rotation (**A**) is 30 degrees greater than external rotation (**B**). External femoral torsion exists when external rotation exceeds internal rotation by the same amount.

pointer. An internal rotation deformity exists at the hip when internal rotation exceeds external rotation by more than 30 degrees.

### Internal Tibial Torsion

An approximate measurement of tibial torsion can be obtained by having the patient sit on the examining table with the knees flexed 90 degrees over the side. The tibial tubercle is palpated and directed straight forward. The malleoli are then grasped with the thumb and index finger, and the position of the axis of the ankle joint is determined (Fig. 18-4). Normally, 20 to 30 degrees of external tibial torsion is present in adults, and the lateral malleolus will be slightly posterior to the medial malleolus. In children with internal tibial torsion, the lateral malleolus will be anterior to the medial malleolus.

### Metatarsus Varus

With the child in the same sitting position, the foot is examined for deformity. If metatarsus varus is present, the lateral border of the foot is convex, and the medial border is concave (Fig. 18-5).

### Treatment

There is no evidence that in-toeing causes any significant adult problems, even if mild deformity persists. Thus treatment of femoral torsion is minimal and is first directed at simply avoiding abnormal sitting postures. The child is encouraged to sleep on the side rather than in the prone position. The reverse-tailor position should be avoided. A stool or chair, rather than the floor, should be used for sitting. Passive stretching exercise of the hips may be performed and the family is reassured that internal rotation deformity of the hips usually corrects itself spontaneously by the age of 6 years. Roller-skating is an excellent exercise for these children. The rare severe case that does not correct itself by the age of 8 years may require surgery although some mild deformities persist into adulthood.

Tibial torsion is best treated by observation and reassurance. Spontaneous correction usually occurs with growth. Improper sitting and sleeping habits should be corrected. Stretching exercises are of no value. Shoes with corrective wedges or torque heels appear to be of no benefit in the treatment of any of these problems.

The treatment of metatarsus varus will depend on whether the deformity is fixed or not. If the foot is flexible, and the deformity easily overcorrectable, passive stretching exercises and a straight or reverse-last shoe are sometimes tried, although their effectiveness is unknown (Fig. 18-6). If passive correction of the forefoot is not possible, early treatment with corrective casts may be indicated. The correction should begin shortly after birth. When the disorder is seen after the age of 1 or 2 years, operative intervention is occasionally necessary. Early diagnosis is therefore important.

## Out-toeing

External rotation deformity of the lower extremities is usually caused by the following: (1) external rotation of the hip secondary to soft-tissue contracture or femoral retroversion (external femoral torsion); (2) external tibial torsion; or (3) calcaneovalgus, or flatfeet. Out-toeing is often associated with a genu valgum deformity and may be aggravated by sleeping in the prone position (Fig. 18-7). The use of wide diapers or of a child's "walker" with a wide pad may potentiate an externally rotated gait.

If femoral retroversion is the cause, examination will reveal that external rotation of the hips is significantly greater than internal rotation. External tibial torsion is diagnosed by the marked posterior position of the lat-

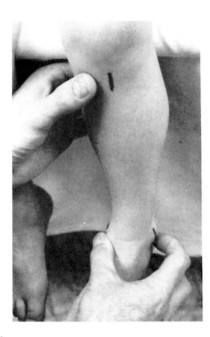

**Fig. 18–4.**
Measuring tibial torsion.

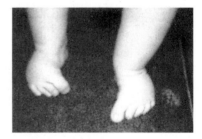

**Fig. 18–5.**
Metatarsus varus (adductus). The lateral border of the foot is convex.

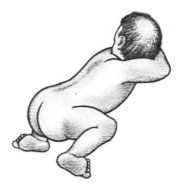

**Fig. 18–7.**
The prone sleeping position, which often potentiates external rotation deformities.

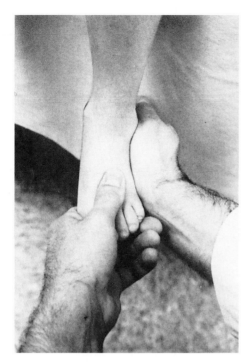

**Fig. 18–6.**
Stretching exercises for metatarsus varus. The heel is firmly grasped. The forefoot is then passively manipulated into the corrected position and held for 10 seconds. The exercise is repeated two or three times at regular intervals during the day.

eral malleolus as compared with the medial. The flatfoot deformity is often associated with eversion of the heels (see Chapter 12).

### Treatment

Observation and reassurance are all that is indicated. Improper postural habits should be corrected. Wide diapers and walkers with wide canvas slings are avoided. Stretching exercises are begun for any hip deformity. Any additional treatment is not helpful and surgery is rarely necessary.

## ANGULAR DEFORMITIES OF THE LEGS IN CHILDREN

### Genu Varum (Bowed Legs)

Genu varum with mild internal tibial torsion is a common, almost normal finding in early childhood. This developmental bowing spontaneously corrects itself with growth and weight bearing in more than 95% of patients. In many cases there is even a normal physiologic "swing" to a knock-knee deformity between the ages of 18 months and 3 years. The knock-knee deformity will then usually correct itself between the ages of 4 and 7 years.

The child is commonly brought to the doctor because of the wide space between the knees and the mild in-toeing gait. Other possible causes of bowing (such as rickets and Blount's disease) can generally be ruled out by the child's history. Roentgenograms may be necessary. There is usually no evidence of any intrinsic bone disease. The amount of genu varum can be determined by measuring the distance between the medial femoral condyles with the child standing and the medial malleoli touching.

Developmental genu varum is usually not severe and rarely requires any treatment. The family can be reassured that spontaneous correction will usually occur by the age of 3 years. Any associated metatarsus varus should be ap-

propriately treated, however. Severe cases should be referred at a young age to rule out Blount's disease.

### Blount's Disease

This is a pathologic, developmental bowing that results from altered growth of the upper medial tibial epiphysis (Fig. 18-8). The cause is unknown, but abnormal pressure may play a role. Blount's disease is more common in obese early walkers. It may be unilateral, in contrast to physiologic bowing, which is almost always bilateral. Two forms of Blount's disease are described: an *infantile* type, which begins before age 3; and an *adolescent* form, which starts after age 8. Before the age of 2, the infantile form may be difficult to differentiate from physiologic bowing, especially if it is bilateral. Although physiologic bowing resolves with growth, Blount's disease progressively worsens. A strong family history and severe bowing are indications for roentgenographic evaluation.

Early recognition (before age 2) and differentiation from physiologic bowing are important. Bracing before age 3 may be effective. Otherwise, surgical correction is usually necessary.

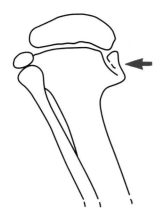

**Fig. 18–8.**
Diagram of Blount's disease, showing disturbance of the growth of the medial tibial epiphysis.

### Genu Valgum (Knock-Knee)

Knock-knee may be the result of a variety of disorders, including injury and metabolic disease. However, most genu valgum is present as one stage in the normal physiologic "swing" between developmental genu varum and normal alignment. It is usually bilateral and is most common between the ages of 2 and 4 years.

The severity of the deformity can be determined by measuring between the medial malleoli or Achilles tendons with the child standing, the medial femoral condyles touching, and the patellae facing forward (Fig. 18-9). If reassurance is needed, similar measurements

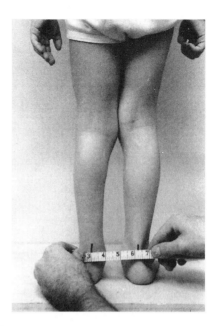

**Fig. 18–9.**
Measuring genu valgum.

can be taken on return visits to confirm spontaneous correction.

Most patients need only reassurance and follow-up. The rare case that persists beyond the age of 7 years may require brace correction. If the deformity is excessive or unequal, a thorough search should be made for the underlying abnormality.

## LEG LENGTH INEQUALITY

Limb length discrepancies in the lower extremities may result from several causes. The most common are fractures, osteomyelitis, neuromuscular disease, and vascular anomalies. Usually the affected limb is shorter, but occasionally the inequality is the result of overgrowth as a result of epiphyseal stimulation by inflammation or injury. Often, no cause is found. The inequality may cause a mild limp and compensatory scoliosis.

In children, a thorough search should be made to determine the cause. If any is found, the appropriate treatment is instituted. If no cause is noted and the difference is less than 1 cm, the child is followed by repeated careful measurements until mature to determine whether the inequality is static or increasing. Both types of inequality require

specialized care, and surgical correction of the asymmetry may be indicated. In children with growth remaining, equalization of the discrepancy may be accomplished either by lengthening the shortened extremity or by partially stopping epiphyseal growth on the longer extremity.

In the adult, the amount of leg length discrepancy that is clinically significant is controversial, but it would appear that up to 2.0 cm of shortening is well tolerated. However, chronic low back pain that may be accompanied by a leg length discrepancy should probably be treated with a shoe lift to compensate for the difference. It is not known whether the leg length discrepancy actually causes the low back pain, but occasionally the pain will be relieved by the lift.

## SPINAL BRACES

Braces are appliances that allow partial movement of a joint. They perform several functions, including protection and stabilization. They are most commonly used to temporarily support and restrict motion in the

treatment of painful disorders of the spine. There is no evidence that wearing a brace "weakens" the back, but the patient should always be encouraged to exercise and maintain proper muscular tone if the brace is be-

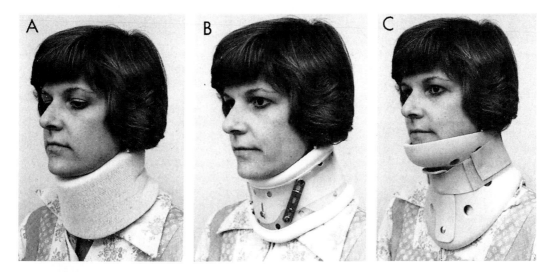

**Fig. 18–10.**
Cervical collars. **A,** The soft foam collar. **B,** The adjustable collar. **C,** The Philadelphia collar.

ing used for pain management only and not for fracture stabilization.

## Cervical Collars

Cervical collars extend from the head to the thorax and are usually soft, although semirigid collars are also available (Fig. 18-10). The soft collar is usually more comfortable but restricts motion less than the other collars. These appliances are all used in the treatment of degenerative disc disease and minor ligamentous or muscular injuries of the cervical spine.

## Taylor Brace

This is a fundamental back brace useful in dorsal and lumbar spine disease (Fig. 18-11). It is a high, semirigid brace that may be modified. Degenerative disc disease and minor fractures may be treated with this brace or one of its modifications (long Taylor, modified Taylor, and short Taylor).

## Jewett (Hyperextension) Brace

This three-point brace provides pressure over the lumbar spine, sternum, and symphysis pubis. It is used in minor fractures of the dorsal spine when extension is desired. It is also useful in the treatment of epiphysitis.

## Knight Spinal Brace (Chairback)

This is a rigid lumbar orthosis that is useful in treating chronic low back pain when more support is required than a light lumbar support can provide. It is also used in the treatment of disc disease and spondylolisthesis.

## Light Lumbar Supports

These supports are usually made of canvas and may be reinforced with metal stays. They are commonly used in the treatment of lumbar disc disease and chronic low back pain syndromes. They may also function to increase the intraabdominal pressure that aids in the support of the lower portion of the back. They are more comfortable than the Knight spinal brace but provide less support.

## DISABILITY RATING

The physician is often called upon to determine the amount of disability that is present as the result of musculoskeletal disease or injury. This determination is often used as the basis for settlement in workmen's compensation cases as well as in personal injury litigation. However, it is usually the "physical impairment rating" expressed as a percentage rather than "disability" that must be determined. It is not the duty of the physician to determine how this impairment affects the patient so-

cially or economically. Often, however, it is the impairment rating that is used as the sole basis for the determination of disability by those administrators responsible for these rulings.

Disability may be defined in various ways and is not a medical term but rather an administrative one. It does not simply mean pain that has persisted for several months. (Pain without objectively validated limitations in daily activities has no impairment.) Medically, it is physical

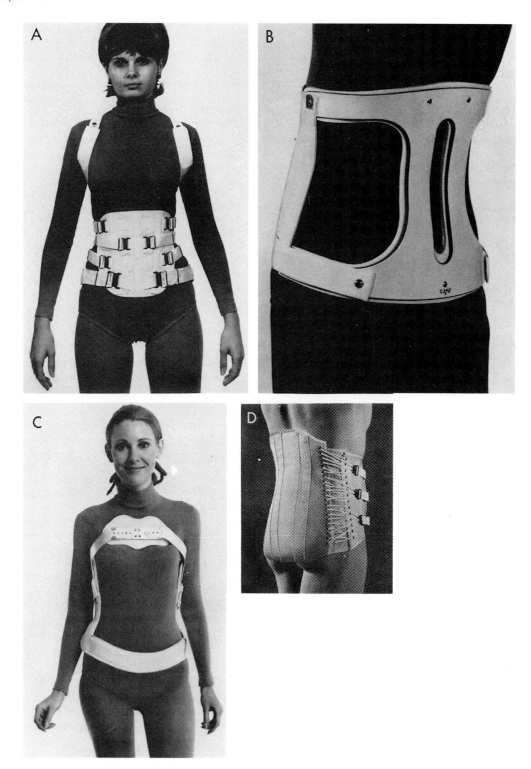

**Fig. 18–11.**
Spinal braces. **A**, The Taylor brace. **B**, The Knight spinal (chairback) brace. **C**, The Jewett hyperextension brace. **D**, The lumbosacral support. (From Camp International, Inc, Jackson, Mich. Used by permission.)

impairment that prohibits the performance of normal physical function. Under Social Security, *disability* means the inability to do any work for at least 12 months because of a physical impairment. Legally, it means permanent bodily injury for which restitution may be judged necessary. Under workmen's compensation statutes, disability is often divided into: (1) temporary total disability, during which time the patient is under care and unable to work; (2) temporary partial disability, during which time recovery is sufficient that some employment may be begun; and (3) permanent disability, which is permanent loss of function after maximum recovery.

Physical impairment can usually be measured accurately on the basis of the loss of physical function. A careful clinical history and physical examination are mandatory. Laboratory and roentgenographic analysis may also be necessary.

For the determination of specific ratings for each impairment, the following manuals are excellent: *Guides to the Evaluation of Permanent Impairment* (AMA), and *Disability Evaluation Under Social Security*. Remember, a disability rating follows a patient for life. It can adversely affect future employability.

## JOINT REPLACEMENT SURGERY

Great advances have been made in the past 25 years in the surgical treatment of degenerative and rheumatoid arthritis. These advances have been due primarily to improvements in the techniques of joint arthroplasty. This procedure is most commonly used for conditions of the hip and knee, but devices have been developed for use in almost every joint (Fig. 18-12). The indications for surgery are the presence of arthritis and failed medical management.

The basic purpose of these techniques is to implant a device into the joint that replaces the degenerated articular surfaces. Most of the procedures utilize a hard plastic, high-density polyethylene for the socket (Fig. 18-13). This articulates with a metallic component, both components usually being fixed to the bone by a cementing compound, methylmethacrylate, or by an ingrowth system.

The goal of joint replacement surgery is to eliminate the disability that results from pain, loss of motion, and malalignment. It is suitable in patients with bilateral disease, and advanced age is not a contraindication. It has been used successfully in almost every age group, and 90% of patients over 65 years of age can expect a 15-year implant survival. Rehabilitation after a joint replacement is usually rapid.

Mechanical problems after total knee replacement are slightly more common than after total hip replacement, but the results are uniformly good in both procedures. More than 90% of patients undergoing arthroplasty have excellent relief of pain and improvement in motion. Short-term problems are those related to infection and venous thrombosis, both of which are treated prophylactically. Long-term concerns include aseptic loosening and also osteolysis, a term used to describe an inflammatory response to particulate debris that can lead to bone loss and implant failure.

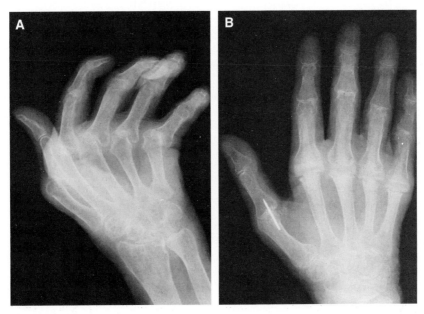

**Fig. 18–12.**
**A**, Severe rheumatoid arthritis of the hand with dislocations of the metacarpophalangeal joints. **B**, Postoperative roentgenogram after metacarpophalangeal replacement. The alignment and function are markedly improved. The thumb has also been fused.

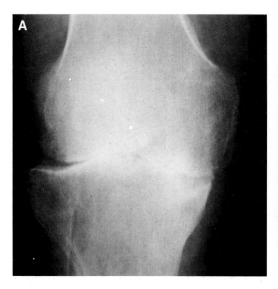
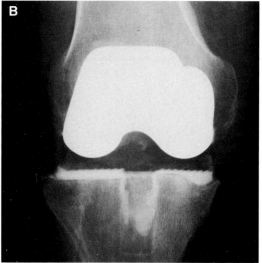

**Fig. 18–13.**
**A,** Degenerative arthritis of the knee. **B,** Postoperative roentgenogram after total knee replacement. Because of the occasional problem of loosening, newer procedures have been developed for use in the knee and hip that do not require the bonding cement.

## COMPARTMENT SYNDROMES OF THE LOWER LEG

Compartment syndromes are disorders of the extremities in which increased tissue pressure compromises the circulation to the muscles and nerves within the space (see Chapter 15). These conditions are most common in the lower part of the leg, where four natural compartments exist (anterior, lateral, deep posterior, and superficial posterior). The anterior compartment is most commonly involved.

The disorder may be acute or chronic. Chronic cases may be confused with stress fractures, tendinitis, and other forms of "shin splints." The acute case is associated with significantly greater morbidity.

### Clinical Features

The acute form may follow fractures, burns, trauma, or vascular injury. Excessive pain, numbness, and weakness are the most common complaints. The pain is often severe because of muscle and nerve ischemia. The chronic case is usually related to exercise, and symptoms are generally mild. Weakness, hypoesthesia, and pain on passive stretch of the involved muscle are usually present. The affected area may also be swollen and tense. The peripheral pulse is often diminished. There is usually an increase in intracompartmental tissue pressure that can be measured directly.

Roentgenographic findings are usually normal (except in fractures), but should be obtained in the chronic case to rule out stress fracture.

### Treatment

The chronic case usually subsides with rest, but fasciotomy is occasionally performed to prevent recurrence. The acute form requires immediate surgical decompression. Without treatment, necrosis of muscle and nerve may occur and result in permanent weakness, contracture, and nerve dysfunction similar to Volkmann's ischemic contracture in the upper extremity.

## INJECTION AND ASPIRATION THERAPY

Locally injected analgesics and steroids are often used in the treatment of musculoskeletal diseases. Their use in many specific disorders has been described in previous chapters. This section will deal with their usage in other common conditions.

In general, these compounds are used to relieve pain and improve the function of inflamed joints, tendons, and bursae. The exact mechanism by which this is accomplished is unknown. An increase in local blood flow and improvement in local tissue metabolism are common explanations. A placebo effect is undoubtedly present in some cases. Systemic absorption is less after local injection than it is with oral administration. However, some absorption does occur, and plasma cortisol

**TABLE 18–1.**

Guidelines for Common Steroid Injections

| Site | Diagnosis | Needle Size (gauge, inches) | Anesthetic Volume (ml) |
|---|---|---|---|
| Subacromial bursa | Rotator cuff tendinitis | 22, 1½ | 4-5 |
| Bicipital groove | Biceps tendinitis | 22, 1½ | 2-3 |
| A-C joint | Arthritis | 25, 1½ | 1-2 |
| L,M epicondyle | Epicondylitis | 25, ⅝ | 1.5 |
| First extensor sheath | DeQuervain's disease | 25, ⅝ | 1.5 |
| Trochanteric bursa | Tendinitis | 22, spinal | 4-5 |
| Knee joint | Arthritis | 22, 1½ | 5-10 |
| Knee, soft tissue | Tendinitis | 25, 1½ | 3-4 |
| Plantar fascia | Fasciitis | 25, 1½ | 1 |
| Toe MPJ | Arthritis | 25, ⅝ | 1.5 |

**Note:** Using 1 ml of the appropriate steroid, the volume is increased by the addition of local anesthetic. Injecting a "space" should not cause pain during the injection while the medicine is going in. If it does, the needle tip may be in the synovium, capsule, or fat pad, and the needle should be redirected or the shot may not be as effective. Injecting soft tissue should be performed slowly so as not to cause pain from the sudden volume pressure.

levels can be suppressed for up to 1 week after injection. Markers of bone formation such as osteocalcin can also be depressed transiently but return to normal in 2 weeks after intraarticular use of a corticosteroid. However, markers for bone resorption do not change, suggesting that there is no effect on bone resorption and only a temporary effect on bone formation. Greater systemic absorption occurs when a given dose is divided equally and instilled into two joints than when administered into one joint. Although not well documented, subtle adverse effects of cortisone use may also be seen. (Joint injections may temporarily help other conditions such as hay fever and allegies, for example.) It is known that absorption causes insomnia in some patients the first night after injection. The control of the diabetic patient may also be temporarily altered by the use of intraarticular cortisone. Because of the systemic absorption, 3 to 4 weeks should pass before reinjecting large joints.

There is little to be gained by a "series" of shots or by repeating an injection to relieve a small amount of residual pain after a successful first shot. There is also nothing gained by giving a shot too early, and nothing lost by trying other treatments first.

A variety of materials are available, but the most commonly used is 1% plain lidocaine, usually mixed with 1 ml of one of the various corticosteroids, either short acting or long acting. Many of these steroids are offered in different strengths, although the more concentrated solutions may offer no advantage over the less concentrated ones. The duration of action varies inversely with the degree of solubility. The stronger, less soluble forms should be avoided in superficial injections because they are more likely to cause *subcutaneous atrophy* and *depigmentation. (Dark skin depigmentation effects may be more apparent.)* The more water-soluble compounds may cause less lipoatrophy but have a shorter duration of action. (Atrophy may reverse occasionally when the steroid is absorbed.) The lidocaine and steroid may be injected separately but are usually mixed together. The use of a small amount of lidocaine alone for skin and soft-tissue infiltration may be necessary in the apprehensive patient. If a joint is to be entered that has a thick capsule, it may also need to be infiltrated because passing a larger needle through the capsule may be uncomfortable for the patient. Do not use the steroid mixture to anesthetize the site, use only the anesthetic. Otherwise, atrophy may occur. The anesthetic is best injected with a 25-gauge needle (⅝-inch or 1½-inch). This needle size may also be used to inject the steroid/lidocaine mixture, especially if the injection is superficial. A 22-gauge, 1½-inch needle is sometimes necessary in deeper injections. A "giving" sensation usually occurs as the needle penetrates the tough, fibrous capsule, especially in the knee. To avoid joint trauma, the needle should not be advanced once the joint has been entered. Aspirating the syringe while withdrawing the needle may prevent residual drops of the mixture from contaminating the skin and subcutaneous tissue.

The dose of cortisone is usually based on volume, with 1 to 2 ml used for larger joints and lesser amounts for smaller joints (Table 18-1). Tendons, except the quadriceps and elbow epicondyles, are not usually directly injected. Instead, it is usually a *space* (joint, tendon sheath, or subacromial space) that is injected. There should be little resistance when injecting a space. If resistance occurs, the needle tip is probably incorrectly placed in soft tissue, and its position should be changed. The volume of fluid injected will depend on the size of the joint or soft-tissue area.

If aspiration is necessary, which it sometimes is in the knee, an 18-gauge needle works best. It is less apt to be occluded by joint debris or synovium. As much fluid as possible is removed by expressing the fluid toward the needle. The pain of aspirating with the large bore needle may be prevented by infiltrating the injection site first with lidocaine using a 25-gauge needle. Aspiration of some fluid also ensures proper needle placement for the injection of large joints such as the knee. If aspiration is performed, the needle may simply be left in position, and the syringe exchanged for one containing the medication.

A mild *postinjection inflammation* ("flare") occurs in 5% of patients following the injection and may last 12 to 24 hours. It is characterized by increased local pain and begins several hours after the injection. It may be caused by poor technique or the steroid vehicle. It usually responds to ice, rest, and analgesics.

*Facial flushing* is an occasional side effect of intrasynovial steroid use. It begins within a few hours of injection and subsides in 1 to 2 days. It is more common with triamcinolone. (Triamcinolone may have the most side effects but it also acts the longest.) It is benign and self-limited.

Rarely, allergic or anaphylactic reaction to intraarticular steroids can occur, a situation that, paradoxically, may require the same drug for its treatment.

If the diagnosis is correct, treatment failures are usually the result of an inaccurate injection. If there is no response to the first injection, it may be repeated in 2 to 3 weeks.

When employing these compounds, it is important not to rely solely on their use in the treatment of any disorder. They are used only as an adjunct to the appropriate treatment of the underlying abnormality. Sufficient knowledge of the relevant regional anatomy is also essential, and no more than four to six injections should be given over a 6-month period.

**Note:** It has not been proven that there are any serious long-term systemic adverse effects to the occasional steroid injection, and the investigations into whether or not any local cartilage or soft tissue damage can occur are conflicted. Threshold doses among individuals regarding side effects seem to differ, but even short courses of treatment at high doses appear to have low risk. Any recommended limits to the yearly number of injections a patient may have seem arbitrary, although some reasonable restrictions are obviously sensible and appropriate.

## General Principles

1. Maintain strict sterile technique.
2. Avoid injection and aspiration in the presence of local infection. A needle passed into a joint through an area of cellulitis may spread the infection into the joint.
3. Avoid the injection of major weight-bearing tendons (e.g., patellar tendon, Achilles tendon) and joints. Such injections may mask the normal symp-

toms and allow a level of activity that could be locally harmful. An exception is for temporary relief of the degenerated joint.
4. Avoid injecting previously infected joints.
5. Avoid injecting markedly unstable joints.
6. Do not inject prosthetic joints.
7. Avoid injecting the skeletally immature patient (except those with known arthritis).
8. Inject slowly to avoid pain caused by the volume effect.
9. Less absorption occurs if the area is rested for 48 hours.
10. Avoid reverse tracking of the steroid.
11. A "safe" dose of steroid cannot be determined because of individual patient variability.
12. There does not appear to be any added risk in giving injections to patients taking warfarin or other anticoagulants.

## Soft-Tissue Injection

Painful disorders of the soft tissue include such conditions as bursitis, tendinitis, tenosynovitis, trigger points, and so-called fibrositis. Most of these conditions have been previously described. Trigger points, fibrositis, and other similar syndromes are poorly understood disorders that present with pain and localized tenderness. A common site for the development of these tender areas is the spine, especially the interscapular and lumbosacral areas. Injecting these tender points is a common practice, but symptomatic relief is hard to analyze.

The depth of the injection varies from 1.25 to 5 cm, and it may be necessary to inject several areas. The best relief is obtained when the area is well defined. If the area to be infiltrated lies directly over bone, it is usually safe to insert the needle until it touches bone. Fluid may be injected at this point, and the needle is then retracted for further infiltration (Fig. 18-14). However, particular care should be exercised when the injected area does not lie over bone but rather over soft structures such as viscera.

## Joint Injection

There are occasional instances where intraarticular aspiration and injection are helpful. These are more easily performed when an effusion is present. Except for the shoulder and hip, most joints are entered on their extensor aspect (Fig. 18-15). The major neurovascular bundle is usually found on the flexor side. Fluid will also usually distend the joint most in the direction of the extensor side, which makes entrance easier.

The knee is the joint most commonly entered. If fluid is present in the suprapatellar pouch, the joint may be

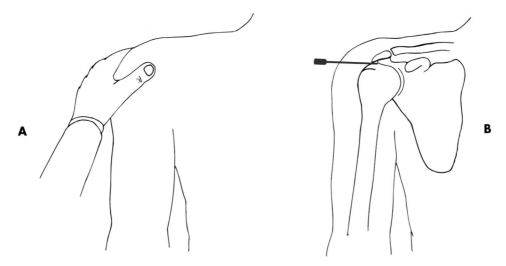

**Fig. 18–14.**
Injecting the subacromial space and rotator cuff. **A,** The sulcus between the acromion and humeral head is palpated. The finger may be kept in position and used as a guide for the needle, or the site may be marked with the fingernail. **B,** The needle is passed into the space, and fluid is injected. Fluid should flow freely. The tendon is not directly injected. The bicipital groove anteriorly and the acromioclavicular joint may also require injection.

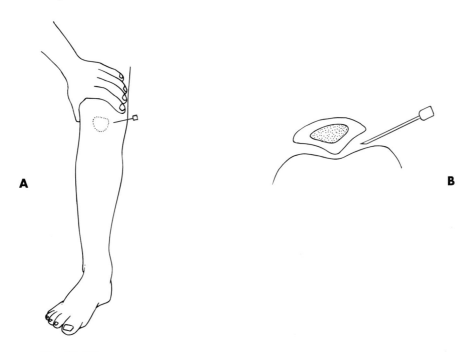

**Fig. 18–15.**
Knee joint injection. The knee should be placed in extension. **A,** The knee is injected in the groove between the patella and femur medially. The finger is used to establish the line of needle placement. **B,** The patellofemoral space is usually wider medially because of a slight tilt to the patella. The knee can also be injected with the patient sitting and the knee bent or straight. The needle can be inserted beside the patellar tendon if the knee is bent and directed to the notch of the femur.

entered through the area of maximum swelling. Otherwise, the medial or lateral surface is used so that the needle passes between the patella and femur with the knee extended. Relaxation of the extensor mechanism is necessary. Other joints, including the smaller joints, are entered in a similar manner. Distracting (traction) distally on a small joint often makes needle entry easier by slightly opening the joint.

# FROSTBITE

The severity of injury produced by exposure to cold depends upon many factors. The most important are the duration of exposure and the degree of temperature. High humidity and wind also increase the amount of damage. Surface moisture also has a negative effect, because it allows for more rapid cooling of the involved part. In addition, previous cold injury and preexisting peripheral vascular disease increase the susceptibility to future injury. Frostbite will usually require several hours of exposure to cold unless the exposure is at high altitudes, where frostbite occurs more rapidly.

Although any area can be affected, the nose, ears, hands, and feet are the most common sites of involvement. The signs and symptoms will depend upon the amount of damage. Mild injury may cause only hyperemia and edema. Soft flesh is usually palpable beneath the frozen, stiff skin. Upon recovering from this degree of involvement, the part often becomes bright red and very painful. Vesicles may appear later.

With more severe injury, the part never recovers, and necrosis of varying degrees begins to appear after thawing. A sign that gangrene may develop is the appearance of heat, edema, and pain in the surrounding tissues. Even after recovery, the part often remains sensitive to cold, and permanent paresthesias and discomfort are often the end result.

## Treatment

Cold injury can be prevented by avoiding tight-fitting clothing and by wearing several layers of loosely fitted clothing that is relatively windproof but not completely impervious to moisture. Long periods of immobility should be avoided, and socks and gloves should be kept dry.

Treatment depends on the severity of involvement. Mild exposure is treated by removing all wet and constricting clothing in a sheltered area. The part is warmed by applying gentle pressure or, as in the case of the hands and feet, by placing the part under an armpit or on the abdomen beneath the clothing of another individual. The part should never be rubbed or massaged.

More severe degrees of acute injury are treated by rapid warming. Smoking is not permitted because vasoconstriction impedes healing. Constriction is also avoided by keeping the patient well hydrated with oral or even IV fluids. Use of the part should always be avoided, and after transfer to the appropriate facility, the extremity is placed in warm water that is kept at 40° to 42° C (104° to 108° F) for 20 to 30 minutes. Higher temperatures or prolonged warming time are unnecessary and may even be harmful. The extremity should be temporarily removed whenever more warm water is being added. Touching the sides or bottom of the vessel should be avoided. The affected part should never be exposed to an open fire, excessive dry heat, or hot water. The extremity is insensitive and may be burned. Exercise should be avoided. Rewarming is often painful, and the patient may require narcotics. Injuries more than 24 hours old are not rewarmed.

Following rewarming, the extremity is elevated to control the edema, and the area is exposed to the air. Refreezing should be prevented. Blisters should be left intact. Daily whirlpool baths with an antibacterial solution at body temperature are begun, and the injured part is observed for tissue demarcation that may take several weeks. Early debridement should be avoided because actual tissue loss is usually much less than initially estimated. Only the onset of infection with wet gangrene requires immediate surgery with removal of the site of sepsis. Antibiotics and tetanus prophylaxis are given as necessary.

Postfrostbite sequelae such as sensitivity, paresthesias, and edema may benefit from sympathectomy.

**Note:** The feet may swell after the shoes are removed, and will not fit again if the patient has to be moved.

# RHABDOMYOLYSIS

This is a condition in which disintegration or dissolution of muscle tissue occurs leading to membrane lysis and leakage of muscle constituents. Myoglobin is eventually excreted in the urine.

The disorder can develop with muscle damage from trauma, exertional heat stroke, simple strenuous overexertion, prolonged seizure activity, electrical injury, pressure from lying without moving for a prolonged time, infectious and inflammatory myositis, and some metabolic myopathies. It may also be a complication of a disorder called neuroleptic malignant syndrome. This is a potentially fatal idiosyncratic reaction to certain neuroleptic drugs (particularly haloperidol) characterized by fever, muscular rigidity, and altered consciousness.

## Clinical Features

The primary problem is myoglobin, which may cause renal failure when released in large amounts. Symptoms may range in severity. Muscle tenderness, fever, altered consciousness, painful muscle cramps, and acute weakness are often presenting features. Ischemic compartment syndromes may even result from plasma leakage into damaged muscle.

Laboratory testing usually reveals myoglobinuria, elevated CPK and aldolase levels, hyperkalemia and hyperphosphatemia. Screening for myoglobinuria may be performed with a simple urine dipstick test using orthotolidine or benzidine.

Treatment involves aggressive IV fluid replacement to prevent acute renal failure and to correct electrolyte imbalance. Early recognition can help prevent renal consequences, which occur in 30% of cases.

## DISORDERS OF TREATMENT

Several musculoskeletal problems develop with some frequency during treatment for other conditions. They often occur during hospitalization and can usually be prevented by simple means.

### Ulnar Neuritis

This condition may develop in the hospitalized patient and usually results from sleeping in the supine position with the elbows slightly flexed and resting on the bed. It also often results when the elbows are used to push up from the bed. Pain and numbness along the ulnar nerve distribution are typical symptoms, and the nerve is tender to palpation at the elbow. The condition is often bilateral. It sometimes develops from the patient lying in supine position during surgery.

The disorder is prevented by having the patient wear soft pads strapped to the elbow to prevent pressure. The patient is not allowed to lie with the elbows in slight flexion, and a trapeze should always be available so that the patient will not have to use the elbows for propping up. Once the symptoms occur, surgical treatment is occasionally necessary.

### Crutch Palsy

The improper use of crutches may occasionally result in crutch palsy. The patient often supports the weight of the body with the axillary portion of the crutch. Variable degrees of pain and paresthesias may develop in the arm with prolonged usage. The symptoms are most often caused by pressure on the lower portion of the brachial plexus, and the ring and small fingers are typically affected.

The condition is easily prevented by instructing the patient to apply pressure on the hand portion of the crutch and not on the axillary portion.

### Trochanteric Bursitis

Bursitis over the greater trochanter is occasionally seen in the hospitalized patient as a result of prolonged recumbency in the lateral position. Pressure over the trochanter results in inflammation of the bursa. Ultrasound, hot packs, antiinflammatory medication, and a local steroid injection are usually curative.

### Frozen Shoulder

Inactivity of the shoulder, often in association with cardiac or pulmonary disorders, may lead to stiffness in the shoulder and reflex sympathetic changes in the upper extremity. The etiology of this condition, sometimes called shoulder-hand syndrome or adhesive capsulitis, is unclear. The stiffness, similar to that seen in frozen shoulder from other causes, is progressive, but fortunately, full, pain-free motion is the eventual outcome. The sympathetic component is manifested as pain, edema, osteoporosis, and dystrophic skin changes.

The most important aspect of treatment is prevention. The patient is encouraged to move the shoulders as often as possible, and passive range of motion is also performed.

## RICKETS

This is a systemic disease of infancy and childhood in which mineralization of growing bone is deficient as a result of abnormal calcium, phosphorus, or vitamin D metabolism. (Osteomalacia is the same condition in the adult.) Renal osteodystrophy is a term used to describe a similar condition in patients with chronic kidney disease. Certain forms of the disorder may respond only to very high doses of vitamin D and are referred to as vitamin D–resistant rickets (VDRR).

### Physiology

Normal serum levels of calcium are critical for healthy nerve and muscle function. Homeostasis is maintained by the following: (1) calcium absorption through the small bowel, (2) removal of calcium from the bone reservoir, and (3) renal reabsorption. All three mechanisms are controlled to varying degrees by a metabolite of vitamin D, 1,25-dihydroxyvitamin D; and parathyroid hormone (PTH). Phosphate levels are bound to those of calcium in a great part in that when hydroxyapatite bone crystals are resorbed for calcium, phosphate is released as well. Phosphate levels are also under renal regulation. Tubular resorption is regulated by PTH, which can cause phosphate diuresis. Therefore any disorder that raises parathyroid hormone levels increases renal excretion of phosphate.

Vitamin D is a fat-soluble vitamin present in high concentrations in fatty fish (e.g., tuna and salmon), eggs, butterfat, and cod liver oil. Most milk products are fortified with vitamin D. The vitamin is absorbed from the GI tract with dietary lipids and stored in the liver. The daily requirement is 400 to 800 I.U. Vitamin D requires sunlight to be converted to its active metabolites in the liver. Vitamin D enhances absorption of calcium from the small bowel, transfer of calcium from bone crystal, and proximal tubular resorption of calcium.

Parathyroid hormone mobilizes calcium and phosphorus from bone in response to low serum calcium levels; and enhances calcium transfer in the small bowel and reabsorption by the renal tubules. When serum calcium levels are diminished, parathyroid activity is increased. Osteoclastic activity is enhanced (reflected by increased serum alkaline phosphatase levels) and normal serum calcium levels are restored. Ongoing resorption leaves soft osteoid behind (osteomalacia). In children, enchondral ossification is affected as well, leading to a decrease in longitudinal growth and deformity, especially at the knee. In severe cases of rickets, parathyroid enlargement may occur and excess bone resorption may result in osteitis fibrosa.

### Etiology

True, classic vitamin D deficient rickets is rare today in Western society. Absorption of vitamin D, however, may be blocked in several gastrointestinal disorders. Similar conditions may also prevent absorption of calcium and phosphorus, but in the absence of these diseases, deficiencies of calcium and phosphorus are also rare.

A number of acquired or inherited renal tubular abnormalities may cause resorptive defects and result in rickets and osteomalacia. A number of separate syndromes have been identified including classic vitamin D resistant rickets, which is probably the most common form of rickets in general medicine.

Chronic renal failure can produce the condition sometimes referred to as renal rickets or renal osteodystrophy. The renal abnormalities result in retention of phosphate.

### Clinical Features

The child with classic rickets usually develops a number of specific abnormalities. Softening of the skull bones (craniotabes) may be present early in the disorder. Enlargement of the ribs at the costochondral junctions produces the "rachitic rosary." Limb deformities and epiphyseal swelling are often present. The height of the child with rickets is often below the normal range. Children are often irritable and fatigue easily. Pigeon breast deformity is common, and there is often an indentation of the lower ribcage, at the insertion of the diaphragm, that is sometimes referred to as Harrison's grooves. Thoracic volume may actually be decreased, resulting in diminished pulmonary ventilation.

Physical findings in the adult with osteomalacia are more subtle. Malaise and bone pain may be present. Many patients are presumed to have osteoporosis.

### Special Studies

In rickets, characteristic radiographic changes occur at the ends of growing bones and lead to widening and irregularity of the epiphyseal plate.

Roentgenographic abnormalities in the adult with osteomalacia are often confused with osteoporosis. Pseudofractures (Looser's zones) may develop where major arteries cross bone. Insufficiency compression fractures are common in vertebral bodies.

The laboratory assessment of the various disorders of bone metabolism requires a high degree of interest. Many of the conditions are so similar that only a complicated laboratory evaluation may establish the diagnosis. BUN, creatinine, alkaline phosphatase, calcium, and phosphorus levels should be determined in any patient suspected of having metabolic bone disease.

### Treatment

Because of the complex nature of many of these disorders, a qualified endocrinologist and nephrologist should be consulted for treatment.

The need for orthopedic intervention is rare. Surgical care is indicated for slipped capital femoral epiphysis, which occurs commonly in renal rickets. Deformity may require bracing.

## PAGET'S DISEASE (OSTEITIS DEFORMANS)

Paget's disease is a nonmetabolic bone disorder of unknown origin that causes excessive bone destruction (osteolysis) and excessive attempts at repair, which results in weakened bone of increased mass. Monostotic and polyostotic disease are both described. Males are affected twice as often as females.

The disorder is unusual before the age of 40, and up to 3% of patients over the age of 50 years may show localized lesions. Clinically important disease is much less common.

### Clinical Features

Bone pain is usually the first symptom, but many lesions are asymptomatic. The onset of the disease is variable, and symptoms result mainly from the effects of complications. Painful bowing of the long bones develops, sometimes leading to pathologic fractures. Half of the patients have hip or pelvic involvement and hip pain is a common complaint. Secondary osteoarthritis may develop. Increased blood shunting in the extremity may cause warmth in the limb and occasionally lead to heart failure.

Characteristic bone hypertrophy leads to skull enlargement and bony overgrowth of the spine. This can produce neurologic complications (e.g., vision and hearing loss, radicular pain, and cord compression). Serum calcium and phosphate levels are normal, and the alkaline phosphatase level is elevated. There is increased urinary excretion of pyridinoline cross-links, although this test is expensive and not usually needed in routine cases. Roentgenograms show dense, expanded bones with characteristic radiolucency and opacity (Fig. 18-16). Bone scanning will reflect the extent and activity of the disease.

### Treatment and Prognosis

NSAIDs are usually helpful in controlling the bone pain. For progressive disease with symptomatology, calcitonin and biphosphonates are among the drugs that have some effectiveness.

Many monostotic lesions probably remain asymptomatic and the prognosis of the mild form is good. Progression of the disease is common. Malignant degeneration occurs in less than 1% of patients and should be considered when there is a sudden increase in pain. Bone biopsy may be needed in uncertain cases. Sarcomatous change carries a grave prognosis.

Surgical intervention may be required for neurologic complications or joint symptoms. Surgery is often associated with profuse blood loss. Elective cases benefit from preoperative treatment to suppress bone activity and vascularity.

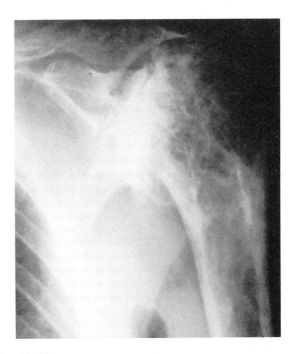

**Fig. 18–16.**
Paget's disease of the humerus. Osteoarthritis of the glenohumeral joint is also present.

## MISCELLANEOUS NEUROMUSCULAR DISORDERS

A variety of neuromuscular problems may present as "orthopedic" conditions with weakness, numbness, and/or pain. The following section describes some of the more common neuromuscular disorders that fit this category.

### Peripheral Nerve Compression Syndromes

Localized injury and compression of peripheral nerves are both common problems. The more common disorders have been previously discussed. Other syndromes are similarly caused by trauma or inflammation (Table 18-2). Early recognition is the key to effective treatment. Often, only the distal sensory portion of the nerve is involved. If superficial, Tinel's sign is usually positive. Minor sensory deficits are commonly present.

### Postpolio Sequelae

Many victims of polio were left with varying degrees of weakness and deformity. Most of these patients are now more than 50 years of age. In recent years, some of them have begun to experience new symptoms, mainly increased fatigue, difficulty swallowing, cognitive defects, weakness, and joint pain. Most of the time, their musculoskeletal complaints can be attributed to arthritic changes (wrist and knee especially) or other expected disorders such as carpal tunnel syndrome. Sometimes, the symptoms have no clear etiology, and

**TABLE 18–2.**

Miscellaneous Peripheral Nerve Syndromes

| Nerve | Common Cause | Symptoms | Treatment/Prognosis |
|---|---|---|---|
| Proximal radial (Saturday night palsy) | Pressure from arm over chair (or person) Fracture midhumerus | Wrist drop Sensory loss on dorsum of wrist or first dorsal web space | Cock-up splint Spontaneous recovery likely in 6-12 wk Surgical exploration occasionally required if as a result of fracture |
| Superficial radial nerve at wrist | Tight watchband or glove Swelling a result of de Quervain's disease | Sensory loss in first web space, thumb, index finger | Remove, treat cause Spontaneous recovery is usual |
| Femoral nerve | Hemorrhage in groin as a result of anticoagulation Iatrogenic as a result of stretching from retractor during abdominal surgery | Weakness of knee extension, stair walking Anterior thigh atrophy, numbness | Exercise to maintain strength Spontaneous recovery is likely |
| Peroneal nerve at fibular head | Cast rubbing, keeping leg crossed Fracture of fibular neck | Foot drop or weak great toe Numbness on dorsum of foot, first web space | Remove cause. Drop foot brace if needed Recovery usual but sometimes incomplete if as a result of fracture |
| Infrapatellar branch of saphenous nerve (crosses patellar tendon from medial to lateral) | Kneeling, surgical incision, prepatellar bursitis | Numbness, lateral to patellar tendon. Pain over nerve at patellar tendon | Remove cause. Recovery likely. Permanent if as a result of surgical incision |
| Spinal accessory nerve | Iatrogenic loss as a result of biopsy of node in posterior triangle Trauma (contusion) | Trapezius paralysis and atrophy | Occasional recovery if as a result of closed trauma Permanent if iatrogenic |
| Long thoracic nerve | Direct trauma, traction? Backpacking, weightlifting | Scapular winging (serratus anterior paralysis) | Recovery is common but variable. No effective treatment |
| Superficial peroneal nerve on dorsum of foot | Tight laces on shoes Swelling as a result of extensor tenosynovitis | Variable numbness on dorsum of foot, first web space | Remove cause. Treat inflammation. Recovery is usual |

the weakness and fatigue may even follow the same pattern as the original infection.

This "syndrome" has received a great deal of media attention, sometimes alarming many patients. Among the possible causes for these symptoms are: (1) "burnout" or overuse of a few surviving motor units; (2) progressive anterior horn cell loss; (3) age-related muscle and ligament weakness, which further compromises marginal muscle function; (4) improper or inappropriate braces and orthotics; (5) reactivated polio virus; (6) an ALS-like syndrome; and (7) decompensation of the balance between denervation and reinervation. The most likely factors involved are overuse, age-related progression, and the use of poor or outdated prosthetic devices.

### Management

Reassurance and understanding are the most important tactics in treatment. Few patients who have had polio have any serious progression of their weakness. The role of exercise has not been clearly established, but ex-

cessive physical strain should be avoided, and these patients will probably benefit from a careful, *nonfatiguing*, resistive exercise program. Braces, orthotics, and other assistive devices should be evaluated and updated or modified as necessary.

## Charcot-Marie-Tooth Disease

This is a heterogeneous group of noninflammatory inherited peripheral neuropathies, sometimes called peroneal muscular atrophy, hereditary motor and sensory neuropathy (HMSN), or idiopathic dominantly inherited hypertrophic polyneuropathy. The etiology is chronic segmental demyelination of peripheral nerves with hypertrophic changes caused by remyelination.

### Clinical Features

The onset is usually between 10 and 20 years of age but can be delayed to age 50. The familial nature of the disease helps to establish the diagnosis. The presentation is variable from family to family, but affected individuals in a family tend to have similar symptomatology. The male/female ratio is 3:1.

The onset is usually gradual and the condition typically runs a slowly progressive course. The lower extremities are primarily involved. A high arch (cavus) and hammered toes are characteristic developments. Atrophy of the lower legs often produces a storklike appearance. Muscle wasting does not involve the upper legs. Hypertrophic changes may develop in some peripheral nerves. Sensory loss, painful paresthesias, or other neurologic signs may occur, although the sensory loss is usually mild. Deep tendon reflexes (DTRs) are absent in many cases, and decreased proprioception often interferes with balance and gait. Poorly healing foot ulcers develop in some cases. Late in the disorder, the hands may become involved.

Electrophysiologic studies are often diagnostic and may also be helpful in defining various subtypes of this group of neuropathies. Occasionally, muscle and nerve biopsies are required but the early onset, slow progression, and familial nature of the condition is usually sufficient to establish the diagnosis.

### Treatment and Prognosis

Genetic counseling is needed. Occupational and physical therapy are helpful to preserve function. Bracing and surgery are indicated to add stability and restore a plantigrade foot.

Disability is usually mild and compatible with a long life. Ten percent to 20% of patients are asymptomatic. A small number of cases are nonambulators by the sixth or seventh decade.

## Syringomyelia

This disease of the spine is characterized by the formation of fluid-filled cavities within the spinal cord, sometimes extending into the brain stem. The cause is unknown but the condition is thought to be the result of obstruction of the fourth ventricle (often associated with a Chiari I malformation) that causes fluid to be diverted down the central cord. Later in life, syrinxes may be a result of trauma or of an intramedullary tumor.

### Clinical Features

The onset is usually insidious and symptoms may not develop until the third or fourth decade. The cervical spine is the area most commonly affected. Intrinsic hand atrophy, weakness, and sensory loss may develop. The latter may lead to unnoticed burns or other injuries in the hand. Neck involvement may cause the development of a Charcot joint in the shoulder or elbow. Reflexes are absent in the upper extremity and hyperactive in the legs. Trophic skin changes eventually occur.

Plain roentgenograms usually reveal widening of the bony canal in the region of involvement. Myelography and other imaging studies are recommended.

The condition is slowly progressive in most cases but the course may be quite variable, ranging from death in a few months to slow incapacitation over several years. Surgical intervention often halts progression but often does not lead to improvement in neurologic findings.

## Herpes Zoster

This is a common condition also known as "shingles." It develops from the reactivation of a varicella (chickenpox) virus, which often resides asymptomatically in dorsal root ganglia. As a result, the affected nerve root becomes painful and a typical skin eruption develops along the distribution of the root. The thoracic region is more commonly involved and the disorder often develops when there is a weakening of the immune system.

The skin rash may not develop for several days, which makes an early diagnosis difficult. The pain is usually quite severe. The skin later becomes reddened, and eventually clusters of vesicles appear. These, too, are painful and last for 1 to 2 weeks.

Treatment includes pain relief and oral antiviral agents.

## Multiple Sclerosis

Multiple sclerosis (MS) is a chronic demyelinating neurologic disorder of unknown etiology that presents with recurrent episodes of neurologic dysfunction. (Patients with pain in the legs will often worry that their symptoms are from MS.) The early diagnosis is difficult because of the variability of presenting symptoms. The hallmark of MS is relapsing and remitting neurologic deficits. Pathologically, the lesions of MS are those of patchy loss of myelin in the white matter. Inflammation and edema may be present in the acute stage, and scarring occurs in the chronic phase.

The disease usually presents in the third decade, and females are more commonly affected than males. Pain is rare. Paresthesias, disturbances in sensation and gait, and visual and bladder dysfunction are the most common initial symptoms. Many of these mimic other disorders, which makes a diagnosis difficult to establish. Although the diagnosis is ultimately based on clinical evidence (objective neurologic findings such as ataxia, incoordination, hyperactive reflexes, positive Babinski sign, visual loss, and Lhermitte's sign—tingling paresthesias with neck flexion), a number of laboratory and imaging tests are helpful.

### Special Studies

Magnetic resonance imaging (MRI) is the preferred imaging modality. Typical abnormalities (periventricular plaques) are found in the majority of cases and, when combined with a positive history and neurologic examination, usually establish the diagnosis without further testing. The cerebrospinal fluid (CSF) usually has elevated protein and leukocyte levels. The gamma globulin level is often increased (70% of cases), and agar gel electrophoresis of concentrated CSF often shows migration in a typical pattern called oligoclonal bands.

Evoked potentials (electrical responses to sensory stimulation recorded by surface electrodes) are often abnormal although, like most other tests, they are not specific for MS.

### Prognosis

The long-term outcome is variable, although many (one third of all) patients have a relatively benign course. Predicting the prognosis for an individual patient is difficult.

## EXERCISE AND GOOD HEALTH

Regular exercise is the key to good health. People who are physically fit have more energy, sleep better, and are less depressed. They suffer fewer illnesses and pains than average and enjoy a more positive sense of well-being. Exercise is just as important for the person who does heavy labor all day as it is for those who do desk work. Doing hard work does burn some calories and strengthen muscles, but it does little to make patients fit and may even cause chronic pain to muscles and back. Most patients need some kind of regular exercise, and the best is known as *aerobic* (literally, "with air"). Before starting, a general physical examination may be needed if there is any indication of chronic illness.

### Aerobic Exercise

For the exercise to be considered aerobic, it must be fast enough to improve cardiovascular fitness. The heart rate is usually used to determine whether the exercise is sufficient to develop the aerobic effect. To be effective, the activity simply needs to raise the pulse to what is known as the "target heart rate" (THR) and *sustain* the THR for at least 15 to 20 minutes during the exercise.

The individual's THR is determined by first subtracting the patients age from 220 to obtain that individual's maximum heart rate (MHR). That figure is then multiplied by 0.60 to 0.80 to determine the target heart rate zone (Table 18-3). Exercise performed in this zone improves aerobic conditioning.

### Walking and Jogging

These are certainly the simplest of aerobic exercises. Because it is "low impact" (no excessive jumping or pounding), brisk walking is easier on the back and legs and provides about the same benefits as jogging. Walking is also the least risky exercise for those individuals with chronic medical problems. In addition to improving cardiovascular function, walking may also: (1) help slow bone loss, especially in women, (2) extend life (walking 12 to 20 miles per week will decrease the annual death risk by about 27%), (3) help control cholesterol levels, and (4) help control weight.

As with all exercise, the activity should be begun slowly. Eventually the patient should walk at least four times per week for about 45 to 60 minutes while pausing from time to time to check the heart rate. Usually, walking at a rate of 120 steps per minute is adequate. For walking, warming up is not necessary, but a "cool-down period" after running is better than stopping abruptly.

Once the patient is comfortable walking, jogging may be tried. A slow pace is more than adequate.

**TABLE 18–3.**

Target Heart Rates (Measured at 60% to 80%)*

| Age (yr) | 25 | 30 | 35 | 40 | 45 | 50 | 55 | 60 | 65 |
|---|---|---|---|---|---|---|---|---|---|
| **Target heart rate range** | 117-156 | 114-152 | 111-148 | 108-144 | 105-140 | 102-136 | 99-132 | 96-128 | 93-124 |

* Notes:
1. The level of exertion required to exercise in the THR zone correlates well with the individual's maximum oxygen capacity ($VO_2$ max), which is the best measurement of aerobic fitness.
2. Brisk walking or similar activity that burns 2,000 calories per week can protect against heart disease.
3. Patients should be encouraged to climb stairs rather than ride elevators. Even short bursts of exercise such as this are helpful.
4. If knee pain occurs, patients may have to avoid climbing hilly areas or stairs, activities that place the extensor mechanism under flexion load.
5. It should take about 2 months of gradually increasing exercise for the patient to reach the THR.
6. Walking burns about 80 calories per mile.
7. After jogging or other vigorous exercise, patients should "cool down" by walking slowly for 5 to 10 minutes.
8. Hand-held or ankle weights may be used when walking but are not necessary.
9. With regular exercise, the resting pulse decreases, a sign of more effective cardiovascular function.

### Other Exercises

Swimming, cycling, rowing, cross-country skiing, and jumping rope are also excellent aerobic activities. Swimming removes the body weight and may be better in patients with painful joints. Swimmers should avoid any stroke that requires the neck to be extended and the chin raised because this can irritate cervical disc disease. Goggles and snorkel help prevent excessive neck motions and subsequent pain. Swimming at a THR for 20 to 30 minutes three times per week is sufficient. If cycling is tried, the bike needs to fit properly so that the lower portion of the back will not become strained.

Stretching exercises may be good before any vigorous exercise. Stretching should be done after warming up for 5 minutes by walking (see Chapter 15). Cold muscles should not be stretched.

## LOCAL SOFT-TISSUE TREATMENT

All musculoskeletal problems involve the soft parts at least to some degree. For purposes of discussion, these problems are divided into acute and chronic disorders.

### Treatment of Acute Injuries

These injuries are generally those of muscle strains of varying degree, contusions, and ligamentous sprains. They are all accompanied by hemorrhage and swelling. For the first 24 to 72 hours, ice is applied for 30 minutes every hour. Rest, ice, soft compression, and elevation (*RICE*) are also used. Crushed ice in a plastic bag is preferred to the chemical cold packs, which can cause blistering and severe chemical burns. After 3 days, gentle range-of-motion and stretching exercises are begun several times a day while cold is applied. Cold is maintained for about 5 minutes after the exercise.

Protected use of the part is allowed as tolerated. Heat in any form, vigorous stretching, massage, and exercise are avoided to prevent further injury. Hematomas that may form usually do not require aspiration. In the majority of cases, these absorb spontaneously over the course of several weeks.

(**Note:** Ice is also helpful in cases of chronic "overuse" problems such as tendinitis. It is usually applied for 5 minutes after the offending activity.)

### Treatment of Chronic Disorders

Among the forms of "therapy" available for patient care are occupational and physical therapy and other rehabilitation services. In referring patients for these services, consultation with the therapist or physiatrist may be helpful. The diagnosis should be included, as well as specific instructions regarding the treatments and their frequency. In addition, a maximum time limit (usually 2 to 4 weeks) should be set to determine whether or not the treatments are truly effective. If the patient is hospitalized, the prescribed treatments are often given twice a day. For an outpatient, they are usually given once a day or every other day. For the therapy to be continued, the patient should show more than just temporary improvement. If not, the treatment should be stopped and the patient reevaluated.

Most therapeutic modalities have developed over the years on a purely empiric basis, and various treatments have been in vogue at various times. All of these treatments are expensive, and patient improvement is often anecdotal and short-lived. Modalities do not speed healing. A placebo effect caused by the "hands-on" aspect of the care undoubtedly plays a considerable role. Among the more commonly used treatments available at this time are the following: (1) heat therapy for pain relief, (2) massage, (3) therapeutic exercises, and (4) traction.

### Heat Therapy

Whether to use ice or heat therapeutically in the treatment of pain is an arbitrary judgment. Heat remains the most popular. Heat treatment is either superficial or deep. The theories behind thermotherapy are that it increases blood flow, helps resolve edema and inflammatory products, and increases the extensibility of collagen, thus producing pain relief and diminishing stiffness.

Superficial heat (1 to 5 mm) can be delivered at home as well as in a therapy office. Paraffin baths (usually for hands), infrared lamps, hot packs (such as hot water bottles and heating pads), and various forms of whirlpool "hydrotherapy" are available. Perhaps the simplest, least expensive is "moist heat" at home. A small towel is dampened and any excess moisture removed (many heat pads come with soft pads designed for this purpose). A plastic sheet is placed between the towel and heat source. Heat is then applied to the affected area for 1 to 2 hours one or two times a day (or more, as needed). Care should be taken not to raise the temperature level too high and cause a skin burn.

Deep heat is usually available as shortwave diathermy, microwaves, and ultrasound. Diathermy and ultrasound are more commonly used. The type must be specified.

The following points should be remembered when using any form of heat:

1. Patients should not fall asleep with their heating pad.
2. Heat before exercise (especially stretching) often enhances the effect of the exercise.
3. Heat should not be used in areas of cancer, near the gonads, or near a developing fetus.
4. Heat should be avoided in tissues without pain sensation or adequate circulation. The increased temperature increases the metabolic demand but the tissues are unable to respond with increased vascular supply. Necrosis may then occur.

### Massage

A number of various massage techniques are used for "spasm" or "nodules." They are usually types of kneading and stroking and are most commonly used for spine pain.

### Therapeutic Exercise

In general, if stiffness is present (e.g., a frozen shoulder), stretching or gentle manipulation (sometimes preceded by deep heat) are recommended. If weakness is present, resistive exercises are taught to the patient so that these can be performed at home.

New trends in the management of most soft-tissue injuries emphasize progressive exercise and restoration of function over passive modalities. After a short period, during which modalities and medicine may be needed for pain control, further rest is no longer justified in most cases and may even be counterproductive, leading to more atrophy and weakness. Exercises are taught and, for the most part, the completion of the rehabilitation is up to the patient. It is costly and unnecessary to have the patient return to therapy for exercise.

### Traction

Various forms of spinal "stretching" are used, generally in the treatment of chronic spine pain. There is no evidence that any real distraction of disc or facet joints ever occurs, although patients sometimes report improvement with cervical traction.

### Others

Trigger point injections, phonophoresis (ultrasound with cortisone cream), dimethyl sulfoxide (DMSO, investigational), acupuncture, biofeedback, electrotherapy, ice massage, and manipulation are all available. Transcutaneous electrical nerve stimulation (TENS) seems to be helpful in some chronic pain problems with localized pain, although its effect seems to decline over time. TENS may alter pain perception by stimulation of certain afferent fibers to inhibit spinal cord transmission of painful stimuli. Phonophoresis is the process of attempting to "drive" molecules of hydrocortisone (in the cream form) into the soft tissue with the use of ul-

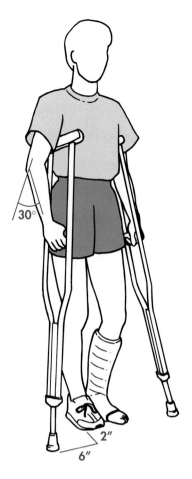

**Fig. 18–17.**
Proper crutch fit. The length of the crutch should be such that with the crutch slightly ahead (4 cm) and to the side (10 cm), there should be three fingerbreadths between the axilla and the axillary pad. The underarm area should be fitted first. Then the hand grip is placed so that the grip is at the level of the wrist with the elbow bent 30 degrees. The hand grip of other devices (walker, cane) should be adjusted in the same manner. To go up stairs, the good foot goes first, the affected foot second, and the crutches last. To go down stairs, the crutches go first, the affected foot second, and the good foot last. Pressure goes on the hands. The patient should not hang on the axillary pad, but should pinch it against the chest.

trasonic waves. It became popular with physical therapists because it gave them a means of administering medication in conjunction with physical therapy. Some studies have shown that cortisone does penetrate into the soft tissue with ultrasound, but the studies are few and the results are somewhat conflicting. More complete discussions of occupational therapy and other rehabilitation services may be found in some of the works cited in the bibliography.

### Canes, Crutches, and Walkers

Assistive devices are a tremendous benefit in both short- and long-term patient care. They can improve stability and relieve pain. However, the fitting of these devices and presentation of instructions regarding them are often insufficient and occasionally left to nonmedical personnel.

Use of the cane has long been advocated for pain relief in the treatment of arthritis of the lower extremity. Such arthritis often causes a painful and unsightly limp, which is usually fatiguing and may even cause low back pain. As advances have been made in orthopedic surgery, and demands made by patients, both the patient and physician may too quickly opt for a high-tech joint replacement rather than succumb to the "indignity" of trying the most time-honored device for relieving pain and limp. Suggesting the use of a cane in an arthritic patient almost always requires some sensitive coaxing, and better education of the general public regarding the benefits of a cane would be helpful in this regard. It is usually the patient's pride or a psychologic aversion to using the cane that needs to be overcome. The positive aspects of cane use should be presented. Patients need to understand that they would probably look better using a cane that could eliminate their pain and limp than they would walking with the limp itself. An attractive cane used to be a symbol of elegance and not a stigma of the aging process. If those attitudes could be encouraged, perhaps more patients could be treated nonsurgically.

Although it can be used on either side, the cane is almost always used in the hand opposite the leg with weakness or pathologic joint disease. If used on the same side, it can produce excessive trunk sway. The length of the cane should be such that the handle is at wrist level with the elbow flexed 30 degrees. It has been shown that for every pound of pressure applied to the cane, 8 pounds of pressure are reduced on the affected hip.

Crutches, walkers, and four-poster canes are used for stability as well as for pain relief and protection from weight bearing. They provide a broad base that increases the base of support and decreases the precision of coordination necessary during ambulation. Four-poster canes can only be used to push in the downward direction. Crutches need to be accurately adjusted (Fig. 18-17). Crutches that are too long may cause pressure on the axillary structures and result in crutch palsy. The hand piece of the crutch or walker should be at the same height as the cane so that it lies at wrist level with the elbow flexed 30 degrees.

## CONTROVERSIES IN ORTHOPEDIC SURGERY

The referring physician may be required to help make certain decisions regarding musculoskeletal patient care that involve problematic issues. Eventually this activity may even be mandated as more physicians and patients take part in managed care. The following areas are some that seem to be the most contentious.

### Lumbar Fusion for Disc Degeneration

Fusion (arthrodesis) for arthritic conditions involving peripheral joints has been and remains an excellent procedure for the relief of pain and the correction of deformity. It has been supplanted by total arthroplasty in some joints, but it remains the procedure of choice in others. Because of the great success with peripheral joint fusion, attempts have been made over the years to transfer that knowledge and technique to degenerative conditions of the lumbar spine in an attempt to cure low back pain. In years past, fusion was actually used by some surgeons each time a lumbar discectomy was performed. Because of the high failure rate in curing low back pain, arthrodesis of the spine for disc degeneration lost popularity. Recently, technical advances in roentgenographic imaging techniques and internal fixation devices have rekindled interest in the procedure. However, some recent studies have questioned the appropriateness of these procedures and their cost. Lumbar fusion is clearly indicated for trauma, scoliosis, and spondylolisthesis, but considerable uncertainty remains regarding its efficacy for the relief of the common low back pain resulting from disc degeneration.

### Arthroscopy

With the advent of intraarticular endoscopic evaluation and surgery, tremendous advances have been made in patient care. Now, procedures such as meniscectomy, which used to require arthrotomy and hospitalization, can be routinely performed in the outpatient setting. As the role of arthroscopy evolved, the indications for the procedure were naturally broadened (partially because of tremendous public pressure). As with other rapidly advancing technical procedures, there remains some dispute regarding the indications for its use, especially in two areas, the arthritic knee and the knee with anterior pain ("chondromalacia").

In the treatment of osteoarthritis of the knee, the most difficult patient case is the middle-aged, active person with minimal roentgenographic and clinical arthritis, whose mild disease and young age would make total replacement inappropriate but who lacks evidence of meniscal injury. In years past, this patient may have had open debridement (the "house cleaning" procedure of Magnuson), in which osteophytes and degenerative cartilage are removed and exposed bone is drilled to encourage the formation of new cartilage. The success of this operation was somewhat limited; but because the same procedure can be performed by the arthroscopic route, it has again attracted interest. The indications for the surgery are difficult to define. Young patients with mild disease do best. Patients with previous meniscectomy, extensive disease, or deformity do less well. Results may be equivocal and tend to deteriorate with time. It is uncertain how much the role of lavage and rest may play in the relief of pain. In some studies, joint lavage by itself was as effective as arthroscopic debridement after 1 year.

The second area of controversial arthroscopic use involves the disorder called *anterior knee pain* (Chapter 11). This "syndrome" typically occurs in many adolescents and may continue for years. Some of these patients may be found to have chondromalacia arthroscopically. They sometimes respond poorly to physical therapy and there is a great tendency to try to find some surgical cure by shaving the articular cartilage in the back of the patella. Anterior knee pain and the pathologic changes of chondromalacia are probably unrelated, and even though conservative management has a high failure rate, arthroscopic investigation of the knee in such cases (with or without debridement of cartilage lesions) does not seem to be beneficial. Conservative care usually remains the treatment of choice.

## The Role of Physical Medicine

Soft-tissue injuries make up the majority of musculoskeletal disorders that present to most orthopedic offices. On a cost basis, they account for a great part of workers' compensation injuries, especially those to the low back. Traditionally, most soft-tissue injuries were treated with a long initial period of rest, sometimes followed by therapeutic modalities such as ultrasound and massage. In the case of low back pain, the use of modalities was sometimes continued for weeks and months in an effort to control pain. If therapeutic exercises were ever initiated, it was often as a last resort—late in the program, after deconditioning had occurred. Patient compliance was often low.

It appears that there is little scientific support for the use of modalities, certainly not beyond the initial few days of pain control, ice, and rest. As healing occurs, a careful, gradual, progressive exercise program must be initiated and maintained by the patient at home, and progress must be assessed. It should be supervised by a physician and/or therapist. Patient rehabilitation cannot be accomplished by passive treatments, especially in the absence of an exercise program to restore function. Immobilization and inactivity after the initial period of rest only prolong recovery. Heat and liniments (usually consisting of menthol, camphor, or red pepper extract) act mainly as counterirritants to try to control

pain, and by themselves are inappropriate and should not be continued for more than a short time. The main reason for therapy is for the patient to function better.

## Thoracic Outlet Syndrome

Everything about this disorder seems clouded in uncertainty. In spite of a number of anatomic studies suggesting its etiology, the exact cause of the condition remains obscure. Some authors consider the disorder to be quite common, whereas others dispute its existence. Except for those rare cases of documented vascular involvement, the diagnosis is difficult to establish with any assurance because the symptoms, in most cases, are only related to pain (possibly neural). The available electrical tests are also of debatable benefit, and even MRI is not helpful. The standard clinical tests (such as Adson's) are not specific, and the results of both surgical and medical management are also variable and difficult to measure. Most patients with neural symptoms consistent with thoracic outlet syndrome deserve an extended trial of conservative treatment. Surgery should probably be reserved for those with obvious vascular involvement or those emotionally stable patients whose symptoms cannot be explained on the basis of other causes of arm pain. The variety of surgical approaches also attests to the uncertainty, and a complication rate as high as 30% to 40% has been reported in many series.

## Muscle Spasm

There appears to be little evidence that true "spasm" of skeletal muscle actually occurs very often, and the term has purposely been avoided in this book so as not to confuse it with pain. (The exceptions might include leg cramps and muscle guarding associated with fractures.) However, the phrase is commonly used by both patients and physicians in describing the signs and symptoms of painful disorders, usually involving the *spine*. Most studies suggest instead that sustained involuntary muscular contraction does not occur commonly. Spinal discomfort, especially, would not seem to be related to muscle spasm: in most cases (except for spondylolisthesis or acute soft-tissue strains and sprains) the cause lies at the level of the disc, either through degeneration and/or nerve root compression and not at the site of the referred pain.

The proliferation of "muscle relaxants" has occurred partly because of these misconceptions. (It has also occurred because of some reluctance by physicians to use narcotics for pain control, probably the result of concern over potential abuse problems.) The use of muscle relaxants is not based on any solid scientific evidence, however. Even the package inserts of most of these drugs contain the same disclaimer: "The mode of action of this drug has not been clearly identified but may be related to its sedative properties." If sedatives are used for pain control, there is always the additional problem of drowsiness common to most muscle relaxants.

Pain of unknown cause should not be treated with muscle relaxants. For acute muscular or ligamentous injury at any site, the treatment remains ice, compression, protection, and pain medication, if indicated. For spinal pain of bone, disc, or nerve origin, the patient may require narcotics. Rehabilitative exercises eventually may also be necessary. The use of muscle relaxants for pain management in any clinical setting does not seem to be indicated.

## COMMON MYTHS AND MISCONCEPTIONS

The issue of misinformation is one that physicians face and deal with on a regular basis. Patients routinely have questions based on misconceptions. These questions must be answered, although no clear easy explanation may be available in some cases. Sometimes, the health care provider may lack the time to address the question adequately, or it may simply be easier to fall back on some time-honored response that may be totally unscientific in nature.

Some of this misinformation is even passed on in scientific writing, and after a time it may even become "factual." The issue of muscle "spasm" discussed earlier in this chapter is an example.

Lastly, we need to appreciate the impact that some emotion-laden words used to explain conditions have on the patient, and not use these words indiscriminately. For example, "arthritis" may seem like a fairly innocent term to describe a painful joint, but many patients will interpret the word to mean a sentence to a life filled with chronic pain.

Some of the more common examples of these are listed below and most are controversial:

1. Are spurs painful? The college dictionary defines a spur as a sharp, pointed instrument, and medical dictionaries define it as a bony projection. The term osteophyte is probably better. These bony outgrowths are usually the result, rather than the cause, of disorders. An exception may be the spinal osteophyte, which can occasionally cause symptoms by crowding of adjacent neural tissue. Removal of the bony tissue is not indicated in most cases.
2. Do changes in weather affect joint symptoms? There is no clear evidence of any link between joint pain and any of the parameters (such as humidity or barometric pressure) used to describe weather. Arthritis pain typically waxes and wanes but there is no correlation with weather.
3. Does favoring one leg cause opposite leg problems? The forces applied to the unaffected leg are no greater than those in normal individuals, even though the force transmitted to the affected leg may be less (as a result of amputation, polio or other causes). Even leg length differences up to two centimeters seem to be well tolerated.
4. Is joint noise pathologic? The etiology of crepitus or grating is often unclear. The late stages of osteoarthritis may be associated with audible and palpable crepitus, probably as a result of abnormal motion of rough surfaces. Crepitus at the patellofemoral joint is common but usually benign and not a sign of joint pathology, especially in the young.

   The loud noise reproducible when the MCP or other joints are manipulated also appears to be innocent and there is no evidence that it leads to arthritis. Mild swelling and loss of strength have been reported in rare cases, however. The etiology of such noise is uncertain, but it may be a result of sudden pressure change that causes the release of vibratory energy.
5. Disruption or tear? When applied to musculotendinous problems, the term "tear" is probably a misnomer. By definition, tear means to separate or pull apart by force. Most of the time, the term is used to describe a terminal event in tendons that have aged and chronically weakened. "Tear" also suggests pain. "Disruption" may be a better description. A healthy tendon is difficult to pull apart, whereas a degenerated one is easily disrupted, often with minor force.

## BIBLIOGRAPHY

Armstrong RD et al: Serum methylprednisolone levels following intraarticular injection of methylprednisolone acetate, *Ann Rheum Dis* 40:571-574, 1981.

Bennett RL, Knowlton GC: Overwork weakness in partially denervated skeletal muscle, *Clin Orthop* 12:22, 1958.

Bloomberg MH: *Orthopedic braces*, Philadelphia, 1964, JB Lippincott.

Blount WP: Don't throw away the cane, *J Bone Joint Surg Am* 38:695-708, 1956.

Buckwalter JA, Lohmander S: Operative treatment of osteoarthrosis, *J Bone Joint Surg Am* 76:1405-1417, 1994.

Chan PS, Steinberg DR, Bozentka DJ: Consequences of knuckle cracking: a report of two acute injuries, *Am J Orthop* 28:113-114, 1999.

Chang RW et al: A randomized, controlled trial of arthroscopic surgery versus closed needle joint lavage for patients with osteoarthritis of the knee, *Arthritis Rheum* 31:289-296, 1993.

Charnley J: The long-term results of low-friction arthroplasty of the hip performed as a primary intervention, *J Bone Joint Surg Br* 54:61, 1972.

Colwell CW et al: Osteonecrosis of the femoral head in patients with inflammatory arthritis or asthma receiving corticosteroid therapy, *Orthopedics* 19:941-946, 1996.

DiBenedette V: Keeping pace with many forms of walking, *Phys Sports Med* 16:145, 1988.

*Disability evaluation under Social Security*, Chicago, 1979, American Medical Association.

Doege TC, editor: *Guides to the evaluation of permanent impairment*, ed 4, Chicago, 1993, AMA.

Ekelund LG et al: Physical fitness as a predictor of cardiovascular mortality in asymptomatic North American men: the lipid research clinics mortality follow-up study, *N Engl J Med* 319:1379, 1988.

Emkey RD et al: The systemic effect of intraarticular administration of corticosteroid on markers of bone formation and bone resorption in patients with rheumatoid arthritis, *Arthritis Rheum* 39:277-282, 1996.

England JD, Garcia CA: Electrophysiological studies in the different genotypes of Charcot-Marie-Tooth disease, *Curr Opin Neurol* 9:338-342, 1996.

Epperson LW: The late effects of poliomyelitis, *Ala J Med Sci* 25:173, 1988.

Fadale PD, Wiggins MC: Corticosteroid injections: their use and abuse, *J Am Acad Orthop Surg* 2:133-140, 1994.

Feldman MD, Schoenecker PL: Use of the metaphyseal-diaphyseal angle in the evaluation of bowed legs, *J Bone Joint Surg Am* 75:1602-1609, 1993.

Gibson JN et al: Arthroscopic lavage and debridement for osteoarthritis of the knee, *J Bone Joint Surg Br* 74:534-537, 1992.

Gray RG, Gottlieb NL: Intraarticular corticosteroids: an updated assessment, *Clin Orth* 177:235-263, 1983.

Greene WB: Infantile tibia vara, *J Bone Joint Surg Am* 1:130-143, 1993.

Griffin JE et al: Patients treated with ultrasonic driven hydrocortisone and with ultrasound alone, *Phys Ther* 47:594-601, 1967.

Gross RH: Leg length discrepancy: how much is too much, *Orthopedics* 1:307, 1978.

Halstead LS: Assessment and differential diagnosis for post-polio syndrome, *Orthopedics* 14:1209-1223, 1991.

Hanley EN: Lumbar spine fusions: matching expectations and outcomes, *AAOS Bulletin* 6-7, 1993.

Harding AE: From the syndrome of Charcot, Marie and Tooth to disorders of peripheral myelin proteins, *Brain* 118:809-818,1995.

Heinrich SD, Sharps CH: Lower extremity torsional deformities in children. A prospective comparison of two treatment modalities, *Orthopedics* 14:655-661, 1991.

Ionasescu VV: Charcot-Marie-Tooth neuropathies: from clinical description to molecular genetics, *Muscle Nerve* 18:267-275, 1995.

Johnson RM et al: Cervical orthoses: a study comparing their effectiveness in restricting cervical motion in normal subjects, *J Bone Joint Surg Am* 59:332, 1977.

Kaplan FS, Singer FR: Paget's disease of bone, *J Am Acad Orthop Surg* 3:336-344, 1995.

Key LL, Bell NH: Osteomalacia and disorders of vitamin D metabolism. In Stein JH, editor: *Internal medicine*, ed 4, St Louis, 1994, Mosby.

Knight R: Developmental deformities of the lower extremity, *J Bone Joint Surg Am* 36:521, 1954.

Kramer KM, Levine AM: Posttraumatic syringomyelia, *Clin Orthop* 334:190-199, 1997.

Koehler BE, Urowitz MB, Killinger DW: The systemic effects of intraarticular corticosteroid, *J Rheumatol* 1:117-125, 1974.

Kottke FJ, Stillwell GK, Lehmann JF: *Krusen's handbook of physical medicine and rehabilitation*, ed 3, Philadelphia, 1982, WB Saunders.

Ladd AL et al: Reflex sympathetic imbalance: response to epidural blockage, *Am J Sports Med* 17:660, 1989.

Leon AS et al: Leisure-time physical activity levels and risk of coronary heart disease and death: the multiple risk factor interventional trial, *JAMA* 258:2388, 1987.

Levenson JL: Neuroleptic malignant syndrome, *Am J Psychiatry* 142:1137-1144, 1985.

Line RL, Rust GS: Acute exertional rhabdomyolysis, *Am Fam Physician* 52:502-506,1995.

Magnuson PB: Technique of debridement of the knee for arthritis, *S Clin North Am* 26:249-255, 1946.

Mankin HJ: Rickets, osteomalacia and renal osteodystrophy: an update, *Orthop Clin North Am* 21:81-96, 1990.

Matsen FA, Clawson DK: The deep posterior compartmental syndrome of the leg, *J Bone Joint Surg Am* 57:34, 1975.

Matsen FA, Winquist RA, Krugmire RB: Diagnosis and management of compartment syndromes, *J Bone Joint Surg Am* 62:286, 1980.

Maynard FM: Post-polio sequelae. Differential diagnosis and management, *Orthopedics* 8:857, 1985.

McAdams TR, Swenson DR, Miller RA: Frostbite: an orthopedic perspective, *Am J Orthop* 28:21-26, 1999.

McCauley RL et al: Frostbite injuries: a rational approach based on pathophysiology, *J Trauma* 23:143, 1983.

McGinty JB et al: Uses and abuses of arthroscopy: a symposium, *J Bone Joint Surg Am* 74:1563-1577, 1992.

Merkow RL, Lane JM: Paget's disease of bone, *Orthop Clin North Am* 21:171-189, 1990.

Morley AJM: Knock-knee in children, *Br Med J* 2:976, 1957.

Nickel VL: *Orthopedic rehabilitation*, New York, 1982, Churchill Livingstone.

Ochoa JL, Verdugo RJ: Reflex sympathetic dystrophy: a common clinical avenue for somatoform expression, *Neurol Clin* 13:351-363, 1995.

Owen RR, Jones D: Polio residual clinic: conditioning exercise program, *Orthopedics* 8:882, 1983.

Payne R: Neuropathic pain syndromes with special reference to causalgia and reflex sympathetic dystrophy, *Clin J Pain* 2:59, 1986.

Peach PE, Olejnik S: Effect of treatment and noncompliance on post-polio sequelae, *Orthopedics* 14:1199-1209, 1991.

Poplawski WB, Wiley AM, Murray JT: Posttraumatic dystrophy of the extremities: a clinical review and trial of treatment, *J Bone Joint Surg Am* 65:642, 1983.

Roos DB: Thoracic outlet syndromes: update 1987, *Am J Surg* 154:568-573, 1987.

Rusk HA: *Rehabilitation medicine*, ed 4, St Louis, 1977, CV Mosby Co.

Salenius P, Vankka E: The development of the tibiofemoral angle in children, *J Bone Joint Surg Am* 57:259, 1975.

Schutzer SF, Gossling HR: The treatment of reflex sympathetic dystrophy syndrome, *J Bone Joint Surg Am* 66:625, 1984.

Sheridan GW, Matsen FA: Fasciotomy in the treatment of the acute compartment syndrome, *J Bone Joint Surg Am* 58:112, 1976.

Sherman M: Physiologic bowing of the legs, *South Med J* 53:830, 1960.

Slattery MR, Jacobs DR, Nichaman MZ: Leisure time physical activity and coronary heart disease death: the railroad study, *Circulation* 79:304, 1989.

Staheli LT: Rotational problems in children, *J Bone Joint Surg Am* 75:939-950, 1993.

Stanton-Hicks M et al: Reflex sympathetic dystrophy: changing concepts and taxonomy, *Pain* 63:127-133, 1995.

Stanton RP et al: Reflex sympathetic dystrophy in children: an orthopedic perspective, *Orthopedics* 16:773-782, 1993.

Swanson AB: Flexible implant arthroplasty for arthritic finger joints, *J Bone Joint Surg Am* 54:435, 1972.

Swanson JW: Multiple sclerosis: update in diagnosis and review of prognostic factors, *Mayo Clin Proc* 64:577, 1989.

Tachdjian MO: *Pediatric orthopedics*, Philadelphia, 1972, WB Saunders.

Thorsteinsson G: Management of postpolio syndrome, *Mayo Clin Proc* 72:627-638, 1997.

Williams B: Orthopedic features in the presentation of syringomyelia, *J Bone Joint Surg Br* 61:314-322, 1979.

Wuir WS et al: Comparison of ultrasonically applied vs intra-articular injected hydrocortisone levels in canine knees, *Orthop Rev* 19:351-356, 1990.

Young GR: Energy conservation, occupational and the treatment of post-polio sequelae, *Orthopedics* 14:1233-1242, 1991.

# Anterior Dermatome

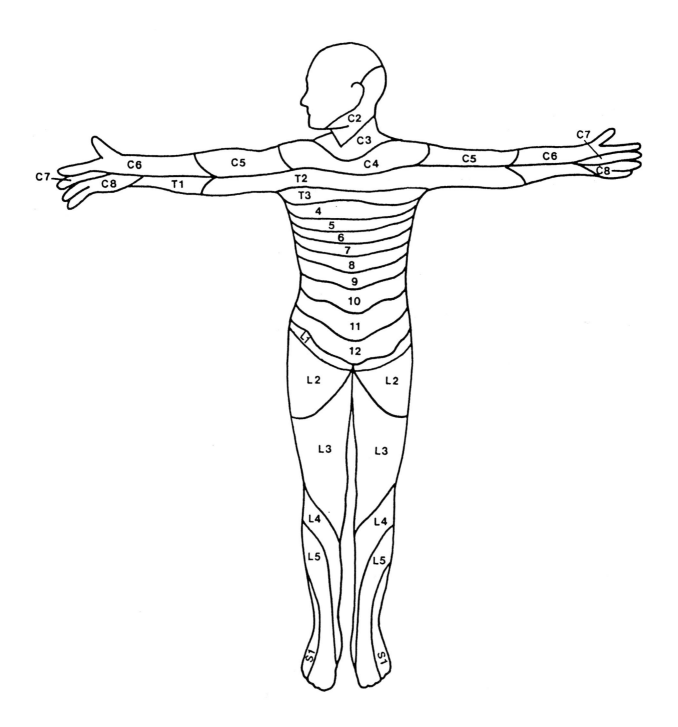

# Posterior Dermatome

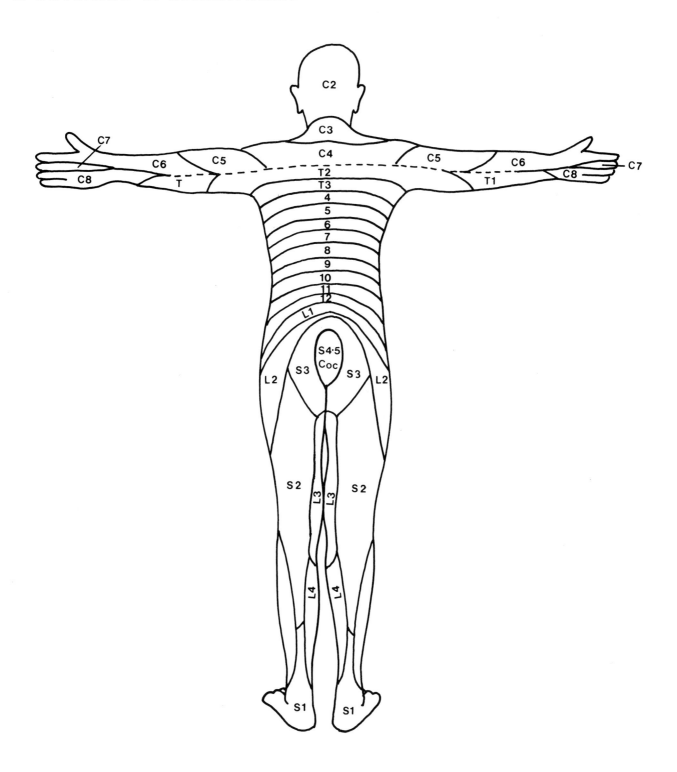

# Patient Teaching Guides

## ANKLE FRACTURE

### ABOUT YOUR DIAGNOSIS

An ankle fracture is a break of any of the bones of the ankle joint. Its causes include a blow to the ankle, a fall landing on the feet, or most commonly, a twisting injury to the ankle. A physical examination and an x-ray will diagnose the injury. Most of the time an ankle fracture will heal, but it is possible to have some long-term pain and disability depending on the circumstances of the injury.

### LIVING WITH YOUR DIAGNOSIS

The symptoms of an ankle fracture are pain in the ankle, particularly when bearing weight or moving the ankle. The signs include swelling, bruising, and possibly a deformity of the joint. Depending on the severity, an ankle fracture may not be more than a severe sprain in which the ligament attachment has been pulled off the bone. On the other hand, a fracture can result in a major disruption of the joint. This may include a dislocation of the ankle.

### TREATMENT

Treatment will depend on the severity and location of the fracture. It can range from treatment similar to a sprain (with rest, ice, compression, and bracing for protected mobility) to surgery (with placement of screws and plates to hold the bones together while they heal). A cast or a removable splint that will hold the bones in a stable position until they heal is the most common treatment. This will take 4 to 6 weeks in most cases. If a cast is used, there will be some weakness of the lower leg muscles after removal. This is probably the most common side effect and will resolve with physical therapy. Potential complications include failure of the fracture to heal (called a nonunion). Other complications include restriction of blood flow to the foot or toes if the cast is too tight or if there is swelling in the cast. Infection or bleeding related to surgery can also occur.

### DO:

- Take medications for pain control as prescribed.
- Eat a diet containing adequate supplies of calcium to help with bone healing.
- Keep your foot elevated for the first few days to minimize swelling. You may have crutches to use for walking.
- Apply cold to your ankle the first day or so to minimize swelling.
- You will probably not receive any exercises to do until removal of the cast. Following those exercises or participating in physical therapy will hasten your recovery.

### DON'T:

- Spend too much time on your feet or with your foot hanging down, since this will increase swelling. You should not place heat on the ankle for the same reason. Swelling may result in restriction of circulation to the foot.
- Get a plaster cast wet; even a fiberglass cast takes a long time to dry, so avoid getting it wet.
- Stick objects such as coat hangers, pencils, or knitting needles down the cast to scratch. If you break the skin, you may get an infection.
- Damage the cast because this will make it less effective. Although a cast is designed to protect the ankle, it is not indestructible.
- Remove your cast too soon. This may result in reinjury and significantly prolong the time to recovery.
- Remove your plastic or metal splint unless instructed to. It cannot keep your bones in position for healing unless it is in place.

### CALL YOUR DOCTOR WHEN:

- You notice any numbness, tingling, coldness, or duskiness of your toes. This could indicate that the cast is too tight or that there has been swelling of the ankle, resulting in restriction of circulation to your foot.

- You have damaged your splint or cast so that it is loose, or is allowing your ankle to move more than it should.
- You had surgery and fever develops, or if redness, swelling, or pus are present at the incision; these signs suggest that an infection is present.
- You have increasing pain or are unable to use your ankle at some time after surgery; this could be an

indication that plates or screws have broken or shifted.

## FOR MORE INFORMATION:

For a description of the injury, x-rays, and surgical treatment, visit the website at http://www.medmedia.com/00a1/29.htm

# ANKLE SPRAIN

## ABOUT YOUR DIAGNOSIS

Ankle sprains are the result of stretching or of partially or completely tearing one or several of the ligaments that hold the ankle joint together. Ankle sprains occur when the ankle joint is forced to bend farther than normal. The most common type of sprain occurs when the foot is turned inward and the full weight comes down on the ankle. This causes a sprain on the outside of the ankle. Almost everyone has a sprain sometime in his or her life. Almost all heal completely without further problems.

## LIVING WITH YOUR DIAGNOSIS

The symptoms of a sprain include a popping or tearing sensation at the time of injury. This results in pain whenever the ankle bears weight. Usually there is fairly quick swelling at the site of injury. Bruising will often develop during the next 24 hours.

## TREATMENT

Treatment will help prevent swelling, protect the joint until it heals, and prevent unnecessary muscle weakness. Treatment also helps remove any swelling, enabling you to get moving again as quickly as possible. The initial treatment helps to prevent swelling and consists of four components. First, apply ice to the injury immediately because the swelling can start in a few minutes. The less swelling you have, the quicker you will be back to normal activity. Second, rest the joint for 1 or 2 days. This may include using crutches to rest the ankle if you have to be up and around during the first day or two. Third, compress the injured area with a compression wrap or air splint. Fourth, elevate the ankle above the level of the hip. You can remember these treatment components with the acronym RICE (*R*est, *I*ce, *C*ompression, and *E*levation).

The next treatment is protected motion that allows the ankle to move without moving too far and further injuring the joint. This may be something as simple as using a compression wrap or a splint or brace. Your doctor may prescribe physical therapy. This will keep muscles from weakening and help remove any swelling that has taken place. Sometimes your doctor may suggest heat or alternating cold and heat to try to remove swelling. Do not use heat until at least 72 hours after the injury; to use it earlier will almost always cause more swelling, and this will slow recovery. Lastly, your doctor may recommend exercises or physical therapy after you have recovered to try to prevent future injuries. Severe injuries may require casting of the foot or even surgery. This is usually necessary when the ligaments are completely torn or if there are multiple ligaments injured.

## DO:

- Take any medicines prescribed by your doctor. Prescription pain medicines may be used for severe sprains. Over-the-counter medications may be used for less severe sprains.
- Follow your instructions for RICE immediately after your injury. Your doctor may prescribe physical therapy.
- Use your crutches as directed. If you are an athlete, your trainer may be able to help speed your recovery. After you have recovered, you may want to consider exercises to increase the strength of the lower leg muscles. There are also exercises that may improve "proprioception" (the ability to recognize the position of your foot without looking at it). Both types of exercises may help prevent future injury.

## DON'T:

- Perform activities that will increase swelling; this will slow your return to complete activity. Therefore avoid early application of heat, excessive activity, and standing or sitting with the ankle hanging. If you keep a shoe on or apply a splint, brace, or compression wrap, you should watch for signs that it is getting too tight and cutting off circulation to the toes. Symptoms would include numbness or tingling in the foot or toes, blueness or duskiness of the toes, or coldness in the toes. If any one of these occurs, loosen whatever is tight or contact your doctor.
- Stop all movement of the joint. Although it is desirable to keep the joint moving, you must avoid a second injury before the first one heals.

## CALL YOUR DOCTOR WHEN:

- Swelling is increasing or if you notice any of the above symptoms of decreased circulation to the foot.

- You are not noticing significant improvement within 7 to 10 days after the sprain.
- You notice any popping, catching, or giving way of the ankle after the swelling has gone away. These may be signs of a more severe injury than was originally apparent.

## FOR MORE INFORMATION:

A description of the injury, the ligaments involved, and treatments for severe sprains are available at the website: http://www.medmedia.com/00a1/25.htm

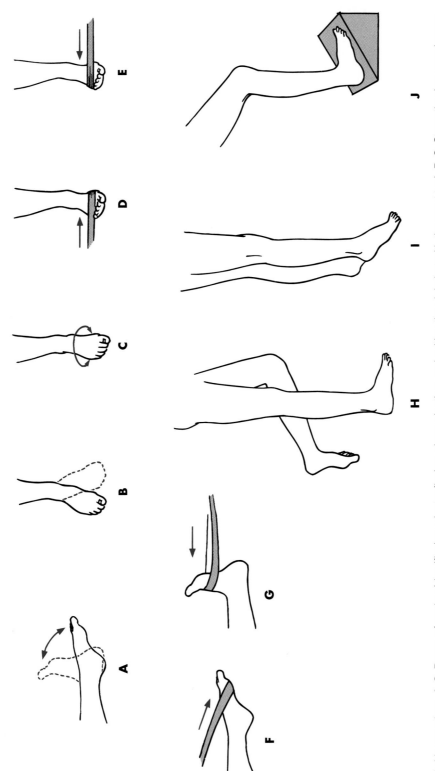

Ankle exercises. **A-C,** Range of motion (dorsiflexion, plantar flexion, circumduction, and writing the alphabet with the great toe). **D-G,** Strengthening exercises using a rubber strap (invertors, evertors, plantar flexors, dorsiflexors). **H,** Static one-leg standing with eyes closed. **I,** Toe raises. **J,** Heel cord stretches. Each exercise is performed 10 to 15 times. Ice is applied for a few minutes before and after each exercise period, and the exercises are performed three times a day. (From Mercier LR: *Practical orthopedics,* ed 5, St Louis, 2000, Mosby.)

This section may be photocopied and distributed to families.
From Mercier LR: *Practical orthopedics,* ed 5. Copyright © 2000, Mosby, St Louis.
Reproduced from Ferri FF, editor: *Ferri's Clinical Advisor 2000 CD-ROM,* St Louis, 2000, Mosby. In Ferri FF, editor: Ferri's Patient Teaching Guides.

# ANKYLOSING SPONDYLITIS

## ABOUT YOUR DIAGNOSIS

Ankylosing spondylitis is a form of arthritis that primarily affects the entire spine, although it may involve the hips and shoulders. It usually affects young men, and there seems to be a genetic link. Back pain is the most common symptom, and it may be quite difficult to make the correct diagnosis in the early stages of the condition. Most of the usual blood tests for arthritis are normal. In the later stages of the condition, radiographic (x-ray) findings can be quite dramatic, showing complete fusion of the spine. This may cause the patient to walk in a stooped posture. Ankylosing spondylitis can have features such as eye irritation, heart problems, and spinal cord compression. A decreased ability to expand the chest can be another early finding.

## LIVING WITH YOUR DIAGNOSIS

Ankylosing spondylitis is a gradually progressive disease, and it can result in serious impairments. Precautions include sleeping without pillows to prevent the neck from fusing in an abnormally flexed position. If this happens, it becomes difficult to see straight ahead when walking or driving. Physical therapy, including water therapy, is combined with use of medications such as aspirin and antiinflammatory drugs to minimize deformity and pain.

## TREATMENT

Nonsurgical treatment is geared toward preventing fusion in undesirable positions. Physical therapy is important but possibly not cost effective. Analgesics and antiinflammatory drugs can be effective in managing the pain. Surgical treatment involves cutting the bones in the spine to realign the body into a functional position. This is a complex surgical procedure with considerable risk, and patient and surgeon should choose this option with care. The hips are sometimes involved, and replacement arthroplasty may be needed.

## DO:

- Maintain as much motion as possible to prevent fusion in an awkward position.
- Perform regular non–weight-bearing exercise.

## DON'T:

- Spend long periods in a poor posture, particularly with the head hanging forward.

## CALL YOUR DOCTOR WHEN:

- You fall and notice a sudden change in the alignment of your neck or back, whether or not you are feeling pain.

## FOR MORE INFORMATION:

Visit these websites:
http://www.spondylitis.org/symptoms.htm
http://www.medmedia.com/oa4/46.htm

# ARTHRITIS, JUVENILE RHEUMATOID

## ABOUT YOUR DIAGNOSIS

Juvenile rheumatoid arthritis (JRA) refers to a form of arthritis occurring in children that is different from adult rheumatoid arthritis. Juvenile rheumatoid arthritis will develop in 1 of every 1000 children. The arthritis is caused by inflammation (changes in the immune system) in the joint. These changes can cause stiffness, warmth, swelling, and pain. Although there is no cure for this type of arthritis, there are many very good treatments, and a substantial number of children will have a complete remission of their condition. There are three types of JRA, and these can be associated with different types of problems.

Pauciarticular JRA affects only a few joints (usually less than four) and occurs in half of the children with JRA. This type most commonly starts in the preschool years and is more likely to occur in girls. Knees, elbows, and ankles are usual spots for the arthritis to occur. Inflammation in the eyes develops in about half of children with pauciarticular JRA. The eye disease can develop at any point during the course of JRA; thus all children with JRA must be regularly seen by an eye doctor. The inflammation is usually detected by the eye doctor by examining the eyes with a special light (called a slit lamp). Untreated, the eye inflammation can lead to vision loss and scarring, so it is important to continue regular eye examinations.

Polyarticular JRA affects many joints and occurs in about 40% of children who have JRA. Often the arthritis involves the small joints of the hands and fingers. Joints commonly affected include the neck, knees, ankles, feet, wrists, and hands. Again, girls are more likely to develop this condition. Some children have a positive blood test called a rheumatoid factor, and their arthritis can be very similar to adult rheumatoid arthritis. Children with polyarticular JRA can also have eye inflammation develop, but this does not occur as often as in the children with pauciarticular JRA.

Systemic JRA occurs in about 10% of children with JRA, with boys and girls both affected equally. Often this condition starts with fever, rash, changes in the blood cells, and joint pain. The inflammation of the joints may not develop for many weeks to months, so this type of JRA can be very hard to diagnose at first. Rarely, systemic JRA can involve the heart, lymph nodes, liver, and lungs.

Approximately 70,000 children in the United States have some form of JRA. Although certain hereditary and environmental factors may increase an individual's risk of developing JRA, the exact cause is unknown. Juvenile rheumatoid arthritis is not an infectious illness. In other words, you cannot "catch" it from another individual.

To diagnose JRA in a child, a physician obtains a medical history, performs an examination of the joints, and orders laboratory tests and possibly x-rays of the joints. Laboratory tests may include an erythrocyte sedimentation rate (ESR), which measures inflammation in the body, a complete blood cell count (CBC), a rheumatoid factor (RF), and an antinuclear antibody (ANA). The RF and ANA are specific proteins found in the blood and may aid a physician in the diagnosis of JRA. However, there is no single blood test that will prove or disprove whether a child has JRA.

Juvenile rheumatoid arthritis is a chronic disease that may last for many months or years. However, about 75% of children eventually outgrow this disease. Although there is no cure for JRA, earlier detection, improved medications, and comprehensive treatment greatly improve the chances for a full and active life.

## LIVING WITH YOUR DIAGNOSIS

Juvenile rheumatoid arthritis causes joint pain and stiffness that can affect a child's ability to do daily activities. Stiffness and discomfort are usually worse in the morning, then get better toward the end of the day. The child may hold the affected joint close to the body because of the pain. Arthritis affecting the hands and wrists can affect the ability to write, dress, and carry items. Arthritis affecting the hips, knees, or feet can decrease the ability to walk, play, or stand. If arthritis affects the neck, it can decrease the ability to look around. A child may not want to participate in play activities because of the pain and fatigue. The pain of JRA may also keep the child awake at night, which may increase the fatigue.

## TREATMENT

The best way to manage JRA is through a combination of medication, therapies, exercise, education, and "pacing" of activities to prevent fatigue. Treatment should be from a physician experienced in the treatment of arthritis. Medications help to decrease the inflammation that causes pain and swelling. Nonsteroidal antiinflammatory drugs (NSAIDs) are often the first line of therapy. Possible side effects of NSAIDs include stomach upset, ulcers, diarrhea, constipation, headache, dizziness, difficulty hearing, and a rash. If these medications do not adequately control the pain, a physician may prescribe "disease modifying" medications that often are effective in slowing the progression of the disease. These medications include gold shots, hydroxychloroquine, and methotrexate. Gold shots and methotrexate may affect the blood, liver, or kidneys and possibly cause a rash. Hydroxychloroquine may affect the eyes and cause a rash. Prednisone, a potent antiinflammatory drug, is used if the disease cannot be managed by other medications or if the child has serious systemic JRA. Prednisone may cause acne, high blood sugar, increased blood pressure, difficulty sleeping, and weight gain. When used for a long time, prednisone may also slow down a child's growth rate and cause thinning of the bones. The eye disease is treated with prednisone eye drops; if severe, more potent oral medications may be required.

Learning about JRA is essential because your child may have the disease for a long time, and careful management is important to prevent problems. Exercise is important to maintain joint movement and muscle strength. The pacing of activities helps manage fatigue. The use of splints can help by resting painful, swollen joints.

## DO:

- Have your child take medications as prescribed.
- Call the doctor if your child experiences any side effects from medications.
- Learn as much as you can about this condition and its treatments.
- Encourage your child to exercise.
- Encourage your child to participate in the same activities as other children of similar age; however, your child should alternate periods of activity with rest.

- Speak to your child's teachers and school nurse. Ask them what services are available in the school system to help your child manage pain and fatigue.

## DON'T:

- Wait to see whether a medication's side effect will go away. Always call your doctor if you have any questions.
- Give up. If one medication doesn't work for your child, discuss it with your physician until you find a medicine that helps decrease the pain and stiffness.
- Have your child continue with an exercise program that causes increased pain. This may mean that the program needs to be modified.
- Forget to have regular eye examinations. Children with JRA can have eye inflammation develop. Also, some of the drugs used to treat JRA can cause side effects in the eyes.

## CALL YOUR DOCTOR WHEN:

- Your child has any side effects listed above from any of the medications.
- The medication is not helping the joint pain, stiffness, swelling, or fatigue.
- Your child needs a referral to a physical or occupational therapist for exercise, joint protection, or splinting.

## FOR MORE INFORMATION:

Contact the Arthritis Foundation in your area. If you do not know the location of the nearest office, call the national office at 1-800-283-7800 or access the website at www.arthritis.org. Children with JRA will benefit from contact with other children, and the Internet can be a good way to find a pen pal. Many cities have support groups for children with JRA and their parents.

## ARTHRITIS, PSORIATIC

### ABOUT YOUR DIAGNOSIS

Psoriatic arthritis causes inflammation leading to pain, swelling, and warmth in certain joints and also a rash. The joints most commonly affected are the fingers, neck, and lower back. Although the psoriasis rash usually occurs before the joint pain, some individuals are unaware of this rash. Psoriasis may affect the nails, scalp, umbilicus (belly button), and genital areas. Fatigue may also occur in this disease. Less commonly, psoriatic arthritis may also cause inflammation of the eyes, nails, and heart.

Although certain hereditary and environmental factors may increase an individual's risk of developing psoriatic arthritis, the exact cause of this disease is unknown. Psoriatic arthritis is not an infectious illness: in other words, you cannot "catch" it from another individual.

Psoriatic arthritis usually begins between the ages of 30 and 50 years. It occurs equally in men and women. To diagnose psoriatic arthritis, a physician obtains a medical history, performs an examination of the joints, skin, and nails, and orders laboratory tests and possibly x-rays of the joints, neck, and lower back. Laboratory tests may include an erythrocyte sedimentation rate (ESR), which measures inflammation in the body; and a complete blood cell count (CBC).

### LIVING WITH YOUR DIAGNOSIS

The joints most commonly affected are the fingers, neck, and lower back. Psoriatic arthritis of the fingers can decrease your ability to write, open jars, and lift and carry items. If the back is affected, it can decrease your ability to bend or stand. If the neck is affected, it may affect your ability to look around. For some individuals, the rash of psoriasis causes embarrassment in social situations. There is no cure for psoriatic arthritis. However, with earlier detection, improved medications, and comprehensive treatment, individuals with psoriatic arthritis can lead a full life.

### TREATMENT

The best way to manage psoriatic arthritis is through a combination of medication, therapy, exercise, and education. Medications help to decrease the inflammation that causes pain and swelling. Nonsteroidal antiinflammatory drugs (NSAIDs) are often the first line of therapy. Potential side effects of NSAIDs include stomach upset,

diarrhea, constipation, ulcers, headache, dizziness, difficulty hearing, and a rash. If these medications do not adequately control the pain and swelling, a physician may prescribe "disease modifying" medications that may slow down the disease process. These medications include hydroxychloroquine, sulfasalazine, and methotrexate. Hydroxychloroquine may cause nausea, diarrhea, and a rash, and rarely may affect the eyes. Sulfasalazine and methotrexate may affect the blood and liver, and may cause a rash. A dermatologist (skin doctor) may prescribe medications to manage the psoriasis.

Learning about your arthritis is essential because you may have psoriatic arthritis for the rest of your life. Exercise is important to maintain joint movement and muscle strength. Alternating periods of rest and activity can help to manage fatigue.

### DO:

- Take your medication as prescribed.
- Call your doctor if you are experiencing side effects from medications.
- Ask you doctor what over-the-counter pain medications and skin products you may take along with the prescription medications.
- Exercise, because this can help maintain joint range of motion and muscle strength.

### DON'T:

- Wait and see if a medication's side effect will go away. Always call your doctor if you have any questions.
- Give up. If one medication does not work for you, discuss this with your physician until you find a medicine that helps decrease joint pain, stiffness, and the skin disorder.
- Go on a specific diet without the consent of your physician.
- Continue an exercise program that causes pain. If pain after exercise continues, it usually means the exercise needs to be modified specifically for you.

### CALL YOUR DOCTOR WHEN:

- You experience any of the side effects listed above from any of the medications.

- The medication is not helping the joint pain, stiffness, or swelling, or the skin disorder.
- You need a referral to a physical or occupational therapist for exercise or joint protection.

## FOR MORE INFORMATION:

Contact the Arthritis Foundation in your area. If you do not know the location of the nearest office, call the national office at 1-800-283-7800 or access the website at www.arthritis.org.

Call the National Psoriasis Foundation at (503) 297-1545.

# ARTHRITIS, RHEUMATOID

## ABOUT YOUR DIAGNOSIS

Rheumatoid arthritis (RA) causes inflammation leading to pain, stiffness, and swelling in joints. The joints most commonly affected are the hands, wrists, feet, and knees. Fatigue can also be severe in RA. Less commonly, RA can cause inflammation in other parts of the body including the lungs, eyes, heart, blood vessels, skin, and nerves. Rheumatoid arthritis used to be called "crippling arthritis" because of the potential joint damage. Now, because of better treatment, less joint damage may occur.

Although certain hereditary and environmental factors may increase an individual's risk of developing RA, the exact cause of RA is unknown. Rheumatoid arthritis is not an infectious illness: in other words, you cannot "catch" it from another individual.

Rheumatoid arthritis affects 1% to 5% of the adult population throughout the world. It occurs two to three times more often in women than in men, and occurs more commonly during a woman's childbearing years. To diagnose RA, a physician obtains a medical history, performs an examination of the joints, and orders laboratory tests and possibly x-rays of the joints. Laboratory tests may include an erythrocyte sedimentation rate (ESR), which measures inflammation in the body; a complete blood cell count (CBC); and a test called a rheumatoid factor (RF). Because only 75% of individuals with RA have a "positive" RF and other individuals without RA may also have a positive test, this blood test does not confirm a diagnosis of RA with 100% accuracy.

## LIVING WITH YOUR DIAGNOSIS

Rheumatoid arthritis causes joint pain and stiffness that can affect your ability to do daily activities. Rheumatoid arthritis of the hands, wrists, or shoulders can decrease your ability to write, open jars, dress, and carry items. Arthritis affecting hips, knees, or feet can decrease your ability to walk, bend, or stand. If arthritis affects your neck, it may limit your ability to look around. There is no cure for RA. However, with earlier detection, improved medications, and comprehensive treatment, individuals with RA can lead a full life.

## TREATMENT

The best way to manage RA is with a combination of medications, therapies, exercise, education, and "pacing" of activities to prevent fatigue. Medications help decrease the inflammation that causes pain and swelling. Nonsteroidal antiinflammatory drugs (NSAIDs) are often the first line of therapy. If these medications do not adequately control the pain and swelling, a physician may prescribe "disease modifying" medications that may slow down the RA disease process. These medicines include hydroxychloroquine, methotrexate, and gold shots. Because these medications may take up to a few months to be effective, the doctor may prescribe prednisone. Prednisone is a strong antiinflammatory medication that works quickly.

All medications can cause side effects. The NSAIDs may cause stomach upset, diarrhea, constipation, ulcers, headache, dizziness, difficulty hearing, or a rash. Hydroxychloroquine may cause nausea, diarrhea, and a rash, and it rarely may affect the eyes. Methotrexate and gold shots may affect your blood, liver, or kidneys and may cause a rash. Prednisone may cause skin bruising, high blood sugar, increased blood pressure, difficulty sleeping, cataracts, weight gain, and thinning of the bones.

Learning about your arthritis is essential because you may have RA for a long time, maybe for the rest of your life. Exercise is important to maintain joint movement and muscle strength. Alternating periods of rest and activity can help to manage fatigue.

## DO:

- Take your medication as prescribed.
- Call your doctor if you are experiencing side effects from medications.
- Ask your doctor which over-the-counter pain medications you may take with your prescription medications.
- Exercise to maintain joint range of motion and muscle strength.

## DON'T:

- Wait to see whether a possible medication side effect will go away on its own.
- Give up. If one medication doesn't work, discuss with your physician other medicines that might help decrease your pain and stiffness.
- Go on a special diet without the consent of your physician.

- Continue an exercise program that causes pain. If pain after exercise continues, it usually means the exercise program needs to be modified specifically for you.

## CALL YOUR DOCTOR WHEN:

- You experience side effects that you believe are caused by your medications.
- The medication and other treatments are not helping the pain, swelling, or fatigue.

- You believe you may need a referral to a physical or occupational therapist for exercise or joint protection.

## FOR MORE INFORMATION:

Contact the Arthritis Foundation in your area. If you do not know the location of the nearest office, call the national office at 1-800-283-7800 or access the website at www.arthritis.org.

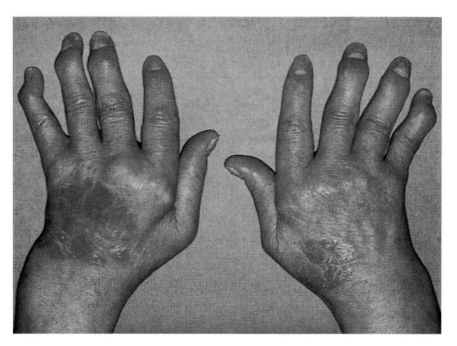

Rheumatoid arthritis can involve various organs and be associated with several medical disorders. (From Ferri FF, editor: Ferri's Patient Teaching Guides. In Ferri FF, editor: *Ferri's Clinical Advisor 2000 CD-ROM*, St Louis, 2000, Mosby.)

# CARPAL TUNNEL SYNDROME

## ABOUT YOUR DIAGNOSIS

Carpal tunnel syndrome (CTS) may cause pain or "tingling/numbness" in the hand, the wrist, and sometimes the arm. It is seen four times more often in women than in men, and it occurs most often in middle-aged patients. More than 50% of patients with CTS have it in both hands.

Several nerves travel from the spine, down the arm and into the hand, and help make possible fine movements of the fingers and hand (e.g., handwriting, buttoning, and fine coordination). The nerve affected in CTS is the "median nerve." It travels under the transverse carpal ligament along with the flexor tendons of the wrist and hand through the carpal tunnel, a very small space in the wrist.

## LIVING WITH YOUR DIAGNOSIS

Carpal tunnel syndrome may be caused by repetitive motion of the hand or fingers, resulting in inflammation or mild injury of the median nerve. Other medical conditions (obesity, diabetes, hypothyroidism, pregnancy, or tuberculosis) may cause or contribute to CTS. The most common symptoms of CTS are numbness or burning/aching pain (some have no pain) of the hand and/or fingers, which may awaken an individual from sleep or occur while bending the wrist (e.g., when driving or holding a telephone receiver). Also, some patients may have a weak grip and/or wasting of the palm muscles.

## TREATMENT

Several treatment options are available for CTS. Nonsurgical treatments are usually tried first, depending on the stage of the syndrome. Your physician may suggest wearing a wrist splint to keep your wrist in a neutral position to reduce further irritation of the nerve. Fifty percent of patients improve when treated in early stages of CTS, although relapse is common. A wrist splint may be especially helpful if worn when sleeping. Steroid medication injections into the carpal tunnel may help to reduce the inflammation. Oral antiinflammatory medications such as aspirin or ibuprofen may be prescribed to help reduce inflammation and relieve symptoms.

Surgery may be considered if conservative treatments have failed to provide adequate long-term symptom relief. A minor surgical procedure may be done through a small incision in the palm and wrist to release the compression of the median nerve. In some cases, a special endoscope may be used to release the nerve. In either case, it is usually done in outpatient surgery. The patient usually goes home the same day with the wound bandaged and wearing a sling and/or wrist splint.

## DO:

- Make sure —if your work requires repetitive wrist or hand action—that your wrists and arms have adequate support. Try using a wrist support at the keyboard if you type often. If you begin having symptoms of CTS, rest or divide your work if possible to minimize repetitive wrist or hand action.
- If you are diabetic, try to keep your blood sugar under adequate control.
- Follow your physician's instructions about activity and medication.

## DON'T:

- Strike things with the butt of your palm. This may injure your median nerve and cause CTS.
- Allow your weight to remain above the normal limits for your age and height. This may worsen the symptoms of CTS.
- Delay in getting treatment. Once muscle wasting has occurred, the chances of full recovery are significantly reduced.
- Use vibrating hand tools.
- Use awkward positions of the hand or wrist.
- Perform repetitive movements of the hand or wrist (especially forceful grasping or pinching).
- Apply direct pressure over the palm and wrist.

## CALL YOUR DOCTOR WHEN:

- The conservative measures prescribed by your doctor have not provided any relief of your symptoms.
- The pain, numbness, or tingling worsens significantly.
- Your grip becomes weaker.
- You have any problems associated with your medications.

## FOR MORE INFORMATION:

Contact:
The Neuropathy Association
PO Box 2055
Lenox Hill Station
New York, NY 10021
1-800-247-6968
E-mail: info@neuropathy.org
Website: http://www.neuropathy.org

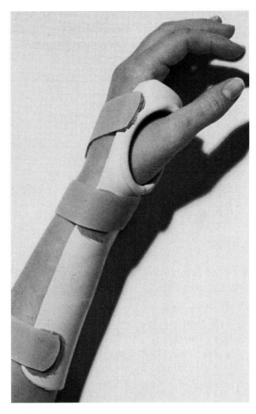

Polypropylene occupational wrist splint. (From Mercier LR: *Practical orthopedics*, ed 5, St Louis, 2000, Mosby.)

# CERVICAL DISC DISEASE

## ABOUT YOUR DIAGNOSIS

The neck (cervical) portion of your spinal column is made of seven vertebrae separated by cartilaginous discs. These discs are the "shock absorbers" of the head and neck. They act as a cushion between the bones and allow some of the bending movements of the head and neck. Degenerative changes or trauma may rupture the annulus fibrosus, the tough band of cartilage surrounding each disc, and disc material may bulge or herniate into the spinal canal or nerve root canal. The herniated or bulging piece of the disc or degenerative bone spur may compress the spinal cord or nerve root, causing pain in the neck or a tingling and numbness that may radiate to the shoulder, upper back, arm, or hand. Some patients also have weakness, clumsiness, and difficulty walking.

## LIVING WITH YOUR DIAGNOSIS

The pain from a bulging or herniated disc is worse on movement and may be aggravated by coughing, laughing, or straining when having a bowel movement.

Degenerative changes in the discs are a normal process as we age. Tobacco abuse, poor posture, and strenuous work with poor lifting technique may accelerate the degenerative changes. The discs gradually become worn, less plump, and eventually flatten. When the disc space becomes narrow enough that the vertebrae rub one another, then wear and tear changes develop at the edges of the vertebrae. This wear and tear causes bone spurs to develop that may begin to press on the spinal cord or nerve root. As the nerve becomes irritated, it may cause pain, tingling, numbness, or weakness.

## TREATMENT

If your physician suspects that you have a cervical disc that is causing a problem, one or more of the following tests may be ordered: computed tomography (CT) scan (special x-ray pictures of the neck); magnetic resonance imaging (MRI, special non–x-ray pictures of the neck); myelogram/CT (x-ray of the spinal canal and nerve roots); or an electromyogram/nerve conduction velocity test (EMG/NCV, an electrical test of the nerves and muscles). Conservative treatments such as physical therapy, localized heat, cervical traction, and special exercises are usually performed by a trained physical therapist. Injection of steroids and an anesthetic medication into the cervical spinal canal is usually performed by anesthesiologists with special training in pain control. Generally, surgery is the final option if conservative treatments have failed to relieve the symptoms. Your surgeon will discuss the risks and benefits of surgery.

## DO:

- Perform gentle stretching and bending of your neck.
- Maintain good posture while sitting and walking.
- Always wear a seat belt when traveling in a motor vehicle.
- Place a pillow under your head and neck when lying in bed.
- Participate in a daily exercise program approved by your physician.

## DON'T:

- Use tobacco. Tobacco causes cumulative injury to your spine by damaging the normal repair process in the discs and vertebrae.
- Make a habit of "popping" your neck.
- Slouch in a chair or bed.
- Return to work without clearance from your physician.
- Engage in any strenuous activities until cleared with your physician.
- Resume driving until pain free without pain medication.

## CALL YOUR DOCTOR WHEN:

- You have any problems associated with your medications.
- Your symptoms become much worse or if you have new weakness.
- You have difficulty walking, have weakness or inability to move your limbs, or have loss of control of your bowels or bladder.

## FOR MORE INFORMATION:

Contact:
North American Spine Society
6300 North River Road, Suite 500
Rosemont, IL 60018-4231
(847) 698-1630
E-mail: nassman@aol.com
Website: http://www.webd.alink.net/nass/

# CERVICAL SPONDYLOSIS

## ABOUT YOUR DIAGNOSIS

Cervical spondylosis is a term used to describe one of the causes of neck pain. It usually involves arthritis at the level of the vertebral bodies in the neck and may cause pressure on the nerves or spinal cord. This can make the condition difficult to differentiate from disc herniation or rupture. Pain may be present in the neck and may radiate to the shoulder blades, arm, and hand and fingers. Weakness in the arms may develop gradually and only be discovered during a physical examination.

## LIVING WITH YOUR DIAGNOSIS

Cervical spondylosis can begin as an intermittent problem or become apparent with severe pain on awakening. Numbness and tingling may develop in the arm and fingers. There is usually no history of injury. The acute neck pain usually responds to rest and use of medication. Partial paralysis sometimes develops and necessitates surgical decompression.

## TREATMENT

Limitation of neck motion with a collar or neck brace generally helps to decrease the pain. Most patients dislike the collar at first; some, however, actually become dependent on the collar and do not want to go without it. Acute painful episodes are treated with rest and medications such as analgesics and antiinflammatory drugs. Muscle relaxants are used sparingly and only for short periods of time. When the acute pain subsides, neck exercises are started and are performed with the collar. Traction may be an option for some patients, although others may not be able to tolerate it, and a few become worse with it. Exercises in which patients actively move their necks are recommended for increasing motion and strength. Spinal manipulation is not recommended for this diagnosis. In rare instances an operation is necessary to relieve pressure on the nerves or spinal cord. This is usually recommended after nonsurgical treatment has not provided relief.

## DO:

- Treat acute, painful episodes with rest. Immobilize the neck and take medications such as analgesics and antiinflammatory drugs as directed.
- Perform as directed exercises that focus on active neck motion and strengthening.

## DON'T:

- Undergo spinal manipulations if you are experiencing acute pain.

## CALL YOUR DOCTOR WHEN:

- Pain has not responded to rest and medication. Sudden muscle weakness or paralysis should also be dealt with immediately.

## FOR MORE INFORMATION:

Read the *Mayo Clinic Health Letter* of August 1993 at this website:
http://www.mayo.ivi.com/mayo/9308/htm/neck_qa.htm

# CHARCOT'S JOINT

## ABOUT YOUR DIAGNOSIS

Charcot's joint is a destructive process that primarily affects joints in the weight-bearing extremities such as the feet, ankles, knees, and possibly hips. Many times Charcot's joint can be confused with an infection involving these areas, and it may be difficult for your physician to differentiate between these two conditions. By definition, a patient with a Charcot's joint has decreased sensation in the affected area and peripheral neuropathy, which is most commonly due to diabetes. There are other causes of peripheral neuropathy, but they are much less common than diabetes. As a result, it is common for persons with diabetes to experience peripheral neuropathy first, which is followed by Charcot's joint. A high index of suspicion is generally required to make the diagnosis early in the disease process.

A person with Charcot's joint experiences swelling, pain, and increased skin temperature over the affected joint or joints. These are the same signs and symptoms that occur with infections, so this cause has to be considered as well. The use of weight-bearing or standing roentgenograms (x-rays) is essential not only to establish the diagnosis but also to determine the degree of destruction of the joints. Most patients with Charcot's joint have acute inflammation without a history of trauma or of a cut or break in the skin, which would suggest an infection. Charcot's joint is generally considered treatable but not curable.

## LIVING WITH YOUR DIAGNOSIS

Prevention is the key to minimizing the deformities that can occur. Contact your doctor at the earliest sign of swelling, redness, or increased skin temperature directly over an affected joint or joints. Ignoring the warning signs may lead to destruction of the joints with disintegration of the bones and collapse. Many times Charcot's joint is an extremely painful condition, even though it occurs in areas affected by peripheral neuropathy. Persons with this severe pain usually seek treatment sooner than persons with little pain, who often do not seek treatment until the deformity becomes severe.

## TREATMENT

There are no medications available specifically to treat Charcot's joint. The acute inflammatory phase is managed with immobilization of the extremity and use of crutches or a walker to decrease or eliminate weight bearing through the extremity. It can take as long as 6 weeks for the acute inflammation to subside. After the inflammation subsides, the joint or joints are braced and likely require bracing or other support to prevent further flare-ups and destruction of the joints.

## DO:

- Control your diabetes with proper medication, diet, and exercise.
- Modify, should a Charcot's joint develop, the exercise program to eliminate weight bearing. Substitute non–weight-bearing forms of exercise such as cycling or water exercises.

## DON'T:

- Begin an aggressive walking or running program immediately after being fitted with braces or splints.

## CALL YOUR DOCTOR WHEN:

- You notice the recurrence of swelling, heat, or redness around any weight-bearing joint, particularly if it recurs in a joint that was treated.

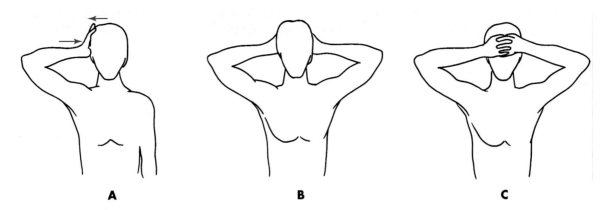

Isometric neck exercises. **A**, The hand is placed against the side of the head slightly above the ear, and pressure is gradually increased while resisting with the neck muscles and keeping the head in the same position. The position is held 5 seconds, relaxed, and repeated five times. **B**, The exercise is performed on the other side and then **C**, from the back and front. The exercise should be performed three or four times daily. (From Mercier LR: *Practical orthopedics,* ed 5, St Louis, 2000, Mosby.)

# DISC HERNIATION

## ABOUT YOUR DIAGNOSIS

Disc herniation usually refers to protrusion of the soft, rubbery material that lies between the vertebral bodies in the spinal column and acts as shock absorbers. When they begin to bulge or protrude, the discs can apply pressure to the nerves as they exit the spinal cord. This can produce pain, numbness, and possibly weakness, extending down the arms and into the hands and fingers or down the leg and into the feet and toes. The causes of disc herniation are varied but most commonly are related to a degenerative, arthritis-like process. Improper bending and lifting techniques, particularly in the lifting of heavy objects, can lead to disc herniation. This is a relatively common condition and usually can be managed.

## LIVING WITH YOUR DIAGNOSIS

The signs and symptoms of disc herniation include pain somewhere along the spinal column, whether it be in the neck or back, with radiation of the pain into either the arms or legs. The pressure of the disc on the nerve can actually cause weakness or paralysis in some muscles.

## TREATMENT

Most disc protrusions can be treated with rest, medication, and time. Sometimes, however, disc herniation does not respond to conservative measures, and surgical intervention may be needed. Medications typically used for the new onset of back pain and pain radiating down into the arms or legs include nonsteroidal antiinflammatory drugs (NSAIDs) and pain relievers.

A concern with back pain that does not respond quickly to medical therapy is the potential for addiction to narcotics and other medications. These medications are to be used for short periods of time and are generally not recommended for long-term use. The side effects of conservative treatment are generally related to the use of medications. Possible complications of surgical treatment include permanent damage to the nerve and wound infection.

Rest is recommended until the pain begins to subside; this may take 2 weeks or more. Should the pain symptoms subside, treatment is directed at rehabilitation and reeducation on proper lifting techniques. Many cities now have back centers that focus on rehabilitation and retraining in proper lifting techniques. For low back difficulties, including herniation, elastic low back supports may be of benefit.

## DO:

- Rest and take your medications as prescribed.
- Use proper lifting techniques.

## DON'T:

- Lift heavy objects, particularly using inappropriate lifting techniques.

## CALL YOUR DOCTOR WHEN:

- You notice partial paralysis of muscles or loss of bowel or bladder control; this may represent a surgical emergency.

## FOR MORE INFORMATION:

Visit the website at http://www.medfacts.com/d_disk.htm

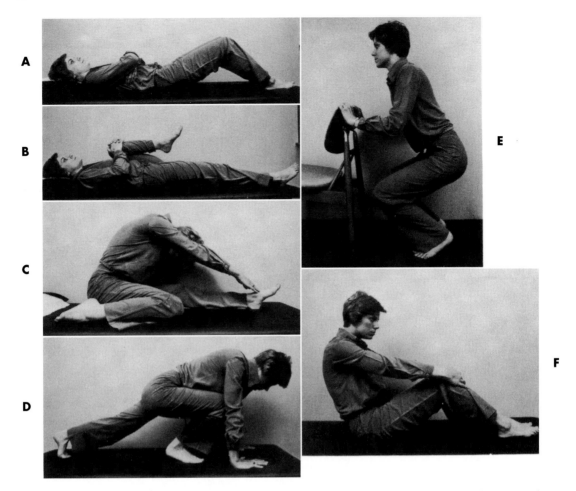

Low back exercises. **A**, Pelvic tilt performed to decrease the lumbar lordosis and raise the anterior aspect of the pelvis. The small of the back is pressed to the floor and the abdominal and buttock muscles are tightened. **B**, Hip flexion, performed to stretch the tight posterior spinal musculature and unload the posterior disc. Each knee is drawn up and pulled firmly to the chest several times and held for 10 to 20 seconds. The exercise is then repeated with both knees. After the acute pain has subsided, the remainder of the exercises are performed: **C**, Hamstring stretching exercises; **D**, hip flexor stretching exercises; **E**, quadriceps strengthening and heel cord stretching exercise; and **F**, abdominal strengthening exercise (sit-ups, which may be partial). All exercises are performed on a carpeted floor and should be repeated in sets of five to ten at least three times daily. (From Mercier LR: *Practical orthopedics*, ed 5, St Louis, 2000, Mosby.)

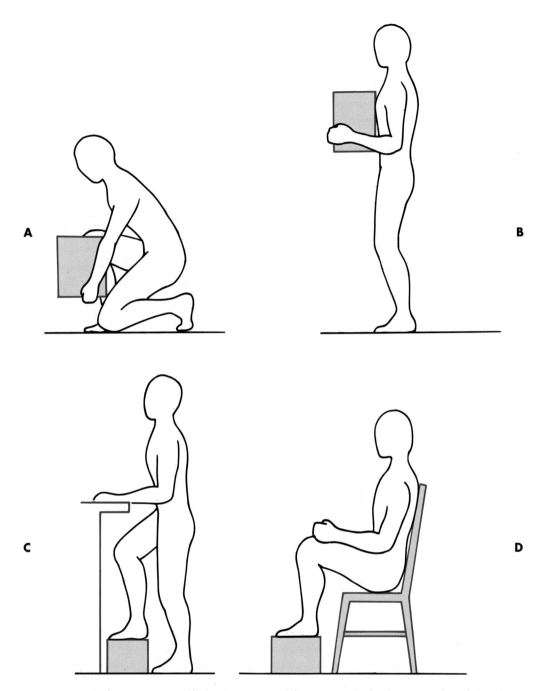

General postural instructions. Patients should be instructed to do the following: **A**, Bend the knees and hips and keep the back straight when lifting. **B**, Hold objects close to the body when carrying. **C**, Place one foot on a stool when standing. **D**, Keep the knees higher than the hips when sitting, and keep the back straight when standing by "tucking in" the abdomen and tightening the buttocks to decrease swayback. In addition, they should avoid high-heeled shoes and sleeping on the abdomen, activities that increase lordosis. (From Mercier LR: *Practical orthopedics*, ed 5, St Louis, 2000, Mosby.)

# FEMORAL NECK FRACTURE

## ABOUT YOUR DIAGNOSIS

A femoral neck fracture is a break of the thigh bone at the hip. In younger individuals this may be caused by a severe fall or an auto accident, but it is much more commonly seen in older individuals, particularly women. A femoral neck fracture usually results from osteoporosis or thinning of the bone associated with increasing age. If the bone of the hip is thin enough, even twisting can result in a break. Indeed, in many elderly individuals, a twist while standing causes the break, and then they fall. As many as one fourth of all women older than 75 years may have osteoporosis severe enough to experience a hip fracture. Hip fractures are diagnosed by physical examination and an x-ray. Many individuals have a complete recovery after surgery.

## LIVING WITH YOUR DIAGNOSIS

The symptoms of a hip fracture are pain in the hip, buttock, or pubic area, especially with movement of the hip or leg. A sign commonly seen is shortening of the affected leg in comparison with the other leg. In addition, the foot of the affected leg will often turn in. A later sign may be bruising on the hip, especially in thin individuals.

## TREATMENT

Treatment is nearly always surgical. There are a variety of surgical options depending on where the hip fracture is located and on the condition of the bone. These options range from placing pins across the fracture to using metal plates and screws to hold the bone fragments together. Other choices include replacing the ball of the hip joint with a metal one, or replacing the socket as well as the ball. At times, if the patient is in very poor health and cannot tolerate surgery, the treatment may be bed rest to try to allow the fracture to heal. This has a very poor success rate, with many complications, and is reserved for individuals who simply cannot tolerate surgery. The main side effects of surgery are those seen with any surgery: namely, infection and bleeding. Sometimes, the surgery fails to stabilize the joint, usually because the remaining bone is too thin for the artificial joint or the screws or pins to hold.

## DO:

- Take the medication your doctor will prescribe for pain. After most surgeries, a physical therapy program is started and will have the patient out of bed within a few days after surgery. This is important to prevent weakening of the muscles. Pain medicines will make this more comfortable and should be used appropriately to speed recovery.
- Eat an adequate diet to provide protein and calcium that will speed healing of the bone.
- Perform the exercises that form your physical therapy, a crucial part of recovery from surgery. Most individuals will achieve a total recovery if they are diligent in the physical therapy regimen.
- Prevent further hip fractures. It is possible to slow or even reverse osteoporosis with appropriate diet, exercise, and medical therapy, including hormone replacement therapy (estrogen) for women who have gone through menopause. The stronger the bone, the less likely you are to sustain a hip fracture. If osteoporosis is present, there are medicines that may help reverse the process. You should discuss this with your doctor. In addition, there are things to do in the home that will decrease the chance of falls. These include adequate lighting and avoiding tripping hazards such as loose rugs and poorly fitted shoes. Many home health agencies can offer help in making the home safer.

## DON'T:

- Take medications that have side effects of dizziness or drowsiness. These may increase the risk of falls.
- Take medicines such as steroids, thyroid medicines, and diuretics that may increase osteoporosis. These should be used only if the benefits outweigh the risks of osteoporosis.
- Use alcohol and tobacco. These increase the risk of osteoporosis, as does a lack of weight-bearing exercise.
- Eat a diet low in calcium and excessive in protein. This increases the risk of osteoporosis.
- Provide a living environment with poor light and lots of tripping hazards. This will increase the risk of a fall.
- Fail to comply with physical therapy, or experience prolonged bed rest. The most significant long-term

adverse effects of hip fractures have been pneumonia or blood clots to the lungs because of prolonged bed rest. Indeed, this is largely why the outcome of nonsurgical treatment is poor. With advances in surgical techniques that allow ambulation to start within a few days after surgery, these adverse effects have decreased. However, failure to comply with a physical therapy program, as well as prolonged bed rest, will increase these risks.

## CALL YOUR DOCTOR WHEN:

- You have any increasing pain in your hip after surgery. This could be a sign of infection, bleeding, or loosening of the hip replacement or screws.
- You are having increasing difficulty walking. This also can be a sign of loosening of the hip replacement.

- Signs of infection are present, such as fever, or swelling or redness of the incision line.
- You experience any shortness of breath and coughing. These could be signs of pneumonia or a blood clot to the lungs, which can be complications of a hip fracture.

## FOR MORE INFORMATION:

For a description of fractures and of surgical repairs, visit the website at http://www.medmedia.com/oo4/156.htm

For a description of surgery and recovery, visit the website at http://www.depuy.com/PatientEd/Hip/Hip.htm

For information on osteoporosis, visit the website at http://www.oznet.ksu.edu/dp_fnut/NUTLINK/pages/bones.htm

Or call the Osteoporosis and Related Bone Diseases National Resource Center at 1-800-624-BONE.

# FIBROMYALGIA

## ABOUT YOUR DIAGNOSIS

Fibromyalgia (FM) means pain in the muscles, tendons, and ligaments. In FM, there are specific areas of pain in the body called tender points. We do not know the cause of FM. However, research has looked at sleep, levels of chemicals called serotonin and substance P, as well as muscle and growth hormone as possible important factors in the cause of FM.

It is estimated that FM may occur in up to 2% of the population. It is about eight times more common in women than men. Fibromyalgia usually occurs in individuals between the ages of 20 and 50 years, although it is also common in women older than 60 years. Although we do not know the cause of FM, it is not an infectious illness. A physician is able to diagnose FM by obtaining a medical history and performing an examination of the joints and muscles. Most blood tests and x-rays show no abnormalities. However, your doctor may perform blood tests to determine whether your pain and fatigue result from other diseases that may cause similar symptoms, and x-rays may be done to look for any bone or joint abnormalities.

## LIVING WITH YOUR DIAGNOSIS

Individuals with FM experience pain and fatigue. Pain is usually worse in the areas of the upper back and neck and the lower back and hips, although pain can occur around any of the tender points. The fatigue can be severe. Individuals with FM may also have headaches, numbness or tingling in the hands or feet, abdominal bloating, diarrhea or constipation, and forgetfulness. Fibromyalgia may affect your activities at work and at home because of the pain and fatigue. Although there is no cure for FM, individuals with this diagnosis can feel better with appropriate therapies. Treatment focuses on managing the symptoms with medications, exercise, stress management, and fatigue management.

## TREATMENT

The best way to manage FM is through a combination of sleep improvement, exercise, stress management, and medications. Medications can improve the amount and quality of sleep. Individuals with FM often awaken frequently throughout the night and wake up feeling tired. This interrupted sleep pattern prevents them from reaching the deepest form of sleep. A physician may prescribe a medicine to reach this deeper stage of sleep. By improving sleep, the pain will also decrease. The most common medications include amitriptyline, nortriptyline, and cyclobenzaprine. These medications are used in large doses to treat depression, and in small doses to manage pain and sleep. The most common side effects from these medications are grogginess upon awakening, dry mouth, constipation, weight gain, and rash.

Appropriate exercises are very helpful in decreasing pain. Stretching and posture exercises should be done every day to maintain good body alignment and prevent pain. Endurance exercises should be done three or four times a week and can include walking, biking, or water therapy. This type of exercise will improve your ability to do activities for a longer length of time. It is important to *begin exercise slowly and to increase gradually.*

Although stress does not cause FM, it is more difficult to manage daily life when you hurt and are tired. Often individuals with FM have forgotten how to "relax." You should look at your life realistically and explore whether family or financial problems or depression is interfering with your ability to feel better. A counselor can offer services that range from relaxation therapy to family counseling.

## DO:

- Call your doctor if you are experiencing side effects from medications.
- Ask your doctor what over-the-counter pain medications you may take with your prescribed medicines.
- Work with your health professionals. Management of FM may be difficult but it is not impossible. Communication and follow-up are key factors in feeling better.

## DON'T:

- Expect medications alone to decrease your pain and fatigue from FM. Feeling better involves improved sleep, exercise, and stress management.
- Take any diet supplement without discussing it first with your physician.
- Stop exercising.

## CALL YOUR DOCTOR WHEN:

- You experience side effects from your medications.
- You continue to wake frequently throughout the night.
- You need a counselor to help with family or financial problems.
- You need additional exercise instruction.
- You need an occupational therapist to help you manage your fatigue.

## FOR MORE INFORMATION:

Contact the Arthritis Foundation in your area. If you do not know the location of the nearest office, call the national office at 1-800-283-7800 or access the website at www.arthritis.org.

You may also contact the Fibromyalgia Network at 1-800-853-2929.

# FROSTBITE

## ABOUT YOUR DIAGNOSIS

Frostbite is the result of freezing of living human tissues. It can be a very serious injury. It is commonly caused by exposure of bare or poorly protected skin, hands, and feet to subfreezing temperatures. Increasing wind speed, known as "wind chill," is often a factor. Alcohol consumption, fatigue, and dehydration increase the risk of frostbite. Once frostbite occurs, it is irreversible. Recovery can take weeks, and the loss of skin, fingers, and toes, as well as deformity and discoloration, are possible. The best treatment, therefore, is prevention.

## LIVING WITH YOUR DIAGNOSIS

The signs of impending frostbite are pain, a decreasing ability to sense touch, and redness upon exposure to cold. If recognized and treated at this stage, mild swelling and peeling of the skin may be the only effects. As the process progresses, the affected area becomes pale and firm. As the area is rewarmed, large blisters, blood blisters, and an obvious appearance of dead tissue (black, blue, or dark gray) can occur.

## TREATMENT

The best treatment is prevention! Dress adequately for conditions. Protect and monitor small children closely! Drink plenty of nonalcoholic and noncaffeinated fluids. Plan ahead. Limit exposure when possible. If injury is suspected, immediately seek shelter and warmth. The best treatment is immersing the injured area in warm water (optimally 104° F). Do not use hot water because this may cause more injury. If possible, rewarm the entire body, encourage fluid intake, and elevate the affected area after rewarming. If blistering occurs, do not rupture the blisters. Wrap the area in dry, clean bandages and seek emergency care.

## DO:

- Anticipate weather conditions and dress accordingly.
- Drink plenty of nonalcoholic fluids.
- Seek shelter at the first sign of symptoms.
- Protect and monitor small children closely in adverse weather.
- Elevate the injured area after rewarming.
- Warm the entire body when able.
- Remove all wet clothing as soon as possible.
- Seek emergency care immediately if blisters or dead tissue appear.

## DON'T:

- Rub the injured area with snow! This worsens the injury.
- Consume alcohol before exposure to subfreezing cold.
- Become fatigued or dehydrated in subfreezing cold.
- Ignore frostbite's early symptoms: pain, numbness, and redness.
- Rupture any blisters that form, if at all possible.
- Allow frostbitten areas to refreeze.

## CALL YOUR DOCTOR WHEN:

- You suspect frostbite injury.

## FOR MORE INFORMATION:

About a book on First Aid, access the website at
http://www.medaccess.com/first_aid/FA_TOC.htm
About cold injuries, access the website at
http://www.nols.edu/School/Pubs/FirstAid/EX9Cold#HYPO
Or contact your local chapter of the American Red Cross

# FROZEN SHOULDER

## ABOUT YOUR DIAGNOSIS

Frozen shoulder, also known as adhesive capsulitis, usually develops without any identifiable cause. It is a painful condition that almost universally results in decreased range of motion of the shoulder joint. It may develop gradually, preventing one from realizing the magnitude of the problem. On the other hand, the symptoms can be quite sudden and severe with nearly complete loss of shoulder motion. Adults in their 40s and 50s are most at risk; however, anyone with a previous shoulder injury may be affected. Persons with a history of diabetes are at greater risk for adhesive capsulitis than are persons who do not have diabetes. The condition can often be present in both shoulders and may resist all forms of treatment.

Roentgenograms (x-rays) usually are needed to rule out other possible causes of shoulder stiffness, such as degenerative arthritis, tumors, and shoulder dislocation.

## LIVING WITH YOUR DIAGNOSIS

Frozen shoulder has been termed a "benign" process because it tends to improve over the course of 1 to 3 years. Unfortunately, many patients cannot endure the pain or the limitation of motion while they wait for the symptoms to resolve. As a result, physical therapy plays an important role in the conservative management of this condition.

## TREATMENT

When frozen shoulder develops spontaneously, without a prior shoulder injury or operation, conservative management with physical therapy is preferred. However, when this condition develops after an operation on the shoulder, a more aggressive treatment plan, including possible further surgical intervention, may be necessary. Analgesics and antiinflammatory drugs may help to reduce pain, but use of these drugs has to be combined with a supervised therapy program for maximum relief. Injection of steroid-type medications into the joint itself often is helpful.

## DO:

- Take your medications as prescribed.
- Undertake a supervised therapy program that combines range-of-motion exercises with strengthening exercises.

## DON'T:

- Discontinue your physical therapy without consulting your doctor.

## CALL YOUR DOCTOR WHEN:

- You notice shoulder pain that is not responding to rest and is associated with a decrease in the overall range of motion of the shoulder joint.

## FOR MORE INFORMATION:

Contact the website at http://www.vir.com/frankenstein/faq/shoulder/frozen.faq.html

# GOUT

## ABOUT YOUR DIAGNOSIS

Gout is an abrupt and very painful form of arthritis. It usually affects only one joint at a time, typically the great toe, foot, ankle, knee, wrist, or elbow. Gout usually affects men older than 40 years. It is unusual in women until they have passed through menopause (the change of life).

Gout "attacks" are caused by the release of "crystals" into a joint, resulting in inflammation, pain, and swelling. These crystals are made of a substance in the blood called uric acid. In individuals with gout, either too much uric acid is made or not enough uric acid is eliminated by the kidneys. Alcohol, aspirin, certain medicines, and rarely certain foods (e.g., liver and other organ meats, sardines, and anchovies) may cause levels of uric acid to rise in individuals, making them more prone to developing gout. The only way to diagnose gout with certainty is to place a needle into the affected joint, remove the joint fluid, and look for the gout crystals under a microscope.

## LIVING WITH YOUR DIAGNOSIS

Individuals who have an attack of gout notice rapidly developing pain, swelling, warmth, and redness in the affected joint. The pain can be so intense that even lightly touching the joint will cause severe pain. The pain is usually continuous and more painful if the joint is moved. Everyday activities such as walking, dressing, and lifting may be difficult.

Attacks may occur at any time; however, attacks can be triggered by certain events such as injuries, surgery, an acute illness, or ingestion of alcoholic beverages. Once the attacks are treated, the symptoms usually resolve within hours to a few days. If attacks are not treated, they may last several days. In between attacks the symptoms resolve completely. Individuals with higher uric acid levels in their blood are more prone to recurring attacks. Persistently elevated uric acid levels for many years can cause deposits of uric acid in nodules under the skin. These are called "tophi." Some individuals with gout are also prone to developing kidney stones.

## TREATMENT

There are two ways to approach the therapy for gout: (1) treatment of attacks and (2) prevention of attacks.

Preventive treatment is necessary in individuals with tophi, kidney stones, and frequent attacks.

Attacks of gout are usually treated with nonsteroidal antiinflammatory drugs (NSAIDs) such as indomethacin. Potential side effects of NSAIDs include stomach upset, ulcers, constipation, diarrhea, headaches, dizziness, difficulty hearing, and skin rash. Colchicine is another type of antiinflammatory drug that is particularly effective early in the attack. Potential side effects of colchicine include stomach cramps, nausea, vomiting, and diarrhea. Occasionally, a more potent antiinflammatory medicine such as prednisone, a cortisone-like medicine, is necessary. Potential side effects of cortisone-like medicines are increased appetite, weight gain, difficulty sleeping, easy bruising, and stomach upset. Removal of the joint fluid from the affected joint, followed by a cortisone injection, is another common treatment for gout. Cortisone injections usually provide the most rapid and complete relief of pain and swelling. Aside from the discomfort of the injection, there are very few side effects from cortisone injections.

Prevention of gouty attacks is accomplished by lowering uric acid levels. Two common medicines that lower uric acid levels are allopurinol and probenecid. The specific medicine your doctor chooses will depend on other medicines you are taking and other medical conditions you have. The most common side effects of allopurinol and probenecid are skin rash and upset stomach.

## DO:

- Rest the affected joint until the symptoms begin to improve.
- Take your medicines as prescribed.
- Ask your doctor which over-the-counter medications you may take with your prescription medications.
- Follow your doctor's advice by limiting your use of alcoholic beverages and avoiding certain foods or medications.

## DON'T:

- Wait to see if side effects from the medications will go away.

## CALL YOUR DOCTOR WHEN:

- You experience any medication side effects.
- The treatment is not decreasing your symptoms in a reasonable amount of time.
- You begin to lose more movement in the affected joint.
- You experience worsening warmth, redness, or pain after a cortisone injection.

## FOR MORE INFORMATION:

Contact the Arthritis Foundation in your area. If you do not know the location of the nearest office, call the national office at 1-800-283-7800 or access the website at www.arthritis.org.

# INFLAMMATORY MYOPATHY (MYOSITIS)

## ABOUT YOUR DIAGNOSIS

Myositis is a condition that causes inflammation in muscles. Two types of myositis are polymyositis and dermatomyositis. They are uncommon conditions that cause muscle weakness in children and adults. Although muscle inflammation is the most common feature of these types of myositis, other organs in the body can be affected such as the skin, lungs, esophagus (food pipe), and joints. No one knows what causes these types of myositis, but it is not an infectious illness (like colds); therefore, you cannot "catch" it from another individual.

Myositis is diagnosed by a medical history, physical examination, and blood tests that detect muscle inflammation. In individuals who appear to have myositis, further studies of the nerve and muscle, as well as a muscle biopsy specimen, are used to confirm the diagnosis. Treatment of myositis usually improves the symptoms, but most individuals need to stay on therapy for several years.

## LIVING WITH YOUR DIAGNOSIS

Myositis causes weakness, especially in muscles around the shoulder and hip. Individuals therefore have difficulty carrying heavy objects, combing their hair, reaching overhead, getting out of bed or chairs, walking up stairs, and standing for long periods. Some individuals have muscle pain. Fatigue, fever, and poor appetite are common. Arthritis causing pain, swelling, and stiffness in joints can make day-to-day activities difficult. Occasionally, individuals with myositis have an associated lung condition that causes a cough or difficulty breathing. Because the esophagus is made of muscle, some individuals with myositis have difficulty swallowing or have problems with heartburn. Dermatomyositis differs from polymyositis by its typical skin rash, which appears on the chest, shoulders, face, and hands. Many of the symptoms of myositis improve with treatment.

## TREATMENT

Myositis is most commonly treated with corticosteroids (cortisone-like medicines such as prednisone). Potential side effects of corticosteroids are increased appetite, weight gain, difficulty sleeping, easy bruising, and stomach upset. Longer-term use of corticosteroids can lower your resistance to infection, as well as cause stomach ulcers, muscle weakness, and bone thinning (osteoporosis). Corticosteroids should always be taken with food to prevent stomach upset. In addition, patients should receive adequate amounts of calcium and vitamin D to help prevent osteoporosis.

Despite corticosteroid therapy, some individuals continue to have symptoms and require more potent medications such as methotrexate or azathioprine (Imuran). Methotrexate can cause poor appetite, nausea, headaches, mouth sores, and diarrhea. Imuran can cause nausea, vomiting, and diarrhea. Routine blood cell counts and liver function tests are necessary to monitor for abnormalities with both methotrexate and azathioprine.

Treatment may continue for several years. All individuals with myositis should rest their muscles during the early part of the treatment. After the muscle inflammation is improved, special exercises to strengthen muscles should be started.

## DO:

- Rest your muscles until the muscle inflammation improves.
- Take your medicines as prescribed.
- Ask your doctor which over-the-counter medications you may take with your prescription medications.
- Eat a well-balanced diet low in carbohydrates and fat to prevent excessive weight gain.

## DON'T:

- Wait to see if side effects from medications will go away.
- Begin a rigorous exercise program without your doctor's advice.
- Stop taking the corticosteroid medicine unless your physician instructs you to do so.
- Forget to inform your doctor and dentist that you are taking a corticosteroid (prednisone).
- Overeat, because corticosteroids may increase your appetite.

## CALL YOUR DOCTOR WHEN:

- You experience any medication side effects.
- The treatment is not decreasing your symptoms in a reasonable amount of time.
- You begin to notice the return of muscle weakness.

## FOR MORE INFORMATION:

Contact the Arthritis Foundation in your area. If you do not know the location of the nearest office, call the national office at 1-800-283-7800 or access the website at www.arthritis.org.

The Myositis Association of America, Inc. will also provide information about these conditions. Call (540) 433-7686; or write the Myositis Association of America, 1420 Huron Court, Harrisonburg, VA 22801.

From Mercier LR: *Practical orthopedics*, ed 5. Copyright © 2000, Mosby, St Louis.
Reproduced from Ferri FF, editor: Ferri's Patient Teaching Guides. In Ferri FF, editor: *Ferri's Clinical Advisor 2000 CD-ROM*, St Louis, 2000, Mosby.

# KNEE PAIN

## ABOUT YOUR DIAGNOSIS

Knee pain is a relatively vague diagnosis. If you are referred to an orthopedic surgeon, he or she attempts to define whether the pain is located in the anterior (front) part of the knee just beneath the kneecap or is deep within the knee joint itself. The many causes of knee pain include a sprained or torn ligament, torn cartilage, or arthritis of the kneecap or entire joint. Inflammatory conditions such as rheumatoid arthritis or osteoarthritis also may manifest themselves with knee pain. Knee pain is extremely common and is usually self-limiting. In other words, when the offending activity is discovered and discontinued, the knee pain usually resolves. Depending on the particular cause of knee pain, it is often curable.

## LIVING WITH YOUR DIAGNOSIS

Knee pain is usually accompanied by swelling and sometimes by a clicking or popping sensation. Sometimes the knee can actually catch and lock. In that situation, a torn piece of cartilage has become trapped within the joint and is preventing bending or straightening of the knee.

## TREATMENT

Initially, the most important aspect is to determine the cause of knee pain, particularly if an activity such as aggressive walking or jogging has been recently started. Many persons who participate in court sports that require lateral movement experience knee symptoms, and when these activities are eliminated for 2 to 6 weeks, the symptoms gradually subside.

The use of nonsteroidal antiinflammatory drugs (NSAIDs) such as ibuprofen or naproxen, which can be obtained over the counter, helps to decrease inflammation and pain. These medications should be used with caution; they can cause stomach problems and should be taken with meals. Patients with a history of ulcers or bleeding ulcers should consult their physician before starting to use these medications.

Kneecap pain usually can be managed with physical therapy to aggressively strengthen the quadriceps muscles in the front of the thigh and stretch the hamstring and calf muscles on the back of the thigh and lower leg. Sprained ligaments often heal with rest and time. However, torn ligaments around the knee sometimes require immobilization followed by aggressive physical therapy for rehabilitation. A surgeon may recommend surgical reconstruction. As with any surgical procedure, there can be risks and complications, which are usually discussed with you before the actual surgical procedure.

Once the symptoms have subsided, activities can be gradually resumed, beginning with straight-ahead activities such as walking or cycling. Working back into the preferred activity can be attempted with caution.

## DO:

- Take your medications as prescribed.
- Consult your primary care physician when beginning a new medication if you take other prescription medications.
- Eliminate the activity that causes the pain.
- Resume activity gradually; resume the offending activity with extreme caution.

## DON'T:

- Use nonsteroidal antiinflammatory medications if you have a history of bleeding ulcers.
- Continue the offending activity, such as running, in the belief that you can "run it off." This can cause additional injury to the knee, which may worsen or damage the joint itself.

## CALL YOUR DOCTOR WHEN:

- You have attempted conservative measures on your own and the symptoms persist.
- You are undergoing a prescribed physical therapy or rehabilitation program and your symptoms worsen. Physical therapists usually offer to contact the physician, but do not hesitate to ask if you notice that the therapy seems to be worsening the symptoms.
- You have side effects from the medication.

## FOR MORE INFORMATION:

Visit the website at http://www.mayo.ivi.com/mayo/9312/htm/kneepain.htm

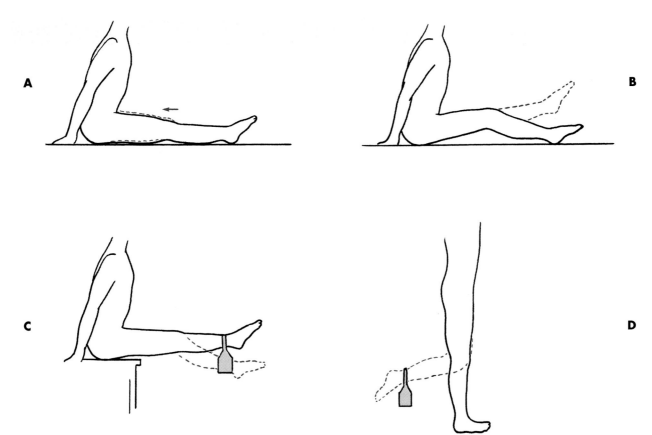

Knee exercises. **A**, Isometric quadsetting. The muscle is tightened and the knee stiffened and relaxed several times. **B** and **C**, Isotonic short-arc knee extension. The knee is straightened through the last 30 degrees (to prevent peripatellar pain). Weights are gradually added beginning with 2 kg and progressing to 10 kg. **D**, Isotonic knee curls for hamstring strengthening. Weight is increased as with quad strengthening. All exercises are performed as five sets of ten lifts each, three times a day. Exercises should not cause pain or swelling. (From Mercier LR: *Practical orthopedics*, ed 5, St Louis, 2000, Mosby.)

# LOW BACK PAIN

## ABOUT YOUR DIAGNOSIS

*Acute* back pain usually results from an injury or an accident and lasts 1 to 7 days. *Chronic* low back pain may last for more than 3 months. Management of low back pain depends on the cause and duration of pain.

The back is made up of vertebrae; discs between the vertebrae; the spinal cord, which contains the nerves; and surrounding structures, such as muscles and ligaments. The muscles in the back and abdomen help support the spine. If the muscles, nerves, or vertebrae are injured, pain can result.

Approximately 80% of persons in the United States experience some type of low back pain during their lifetimes. Some persons have low back pain after sitting for a prolonged length of time or after reaching for an object that is out of reach. Many low back injuries are caused by twisting or other sudden movement. Some persons experience low back pain after an accident or fall. Obesity, poor posture, and weak back and abdominal muscles all contribute to low back pain. Low back pain may occur in association with diseases such as osteoarthritis, ankylosing spondylitis, Reiter's syndrome, or fibromyalgia.

A physician diagnoses low back pain by taking a medical history, performing a physical examination, and possibly ordering roentgenograms (x-rays). The doctor may order blood tests to determine whether the low back pain is caused by another disorder that may cause similar symptoms. Computed tomography (CT), magnetic resonance imaging (MRI), or a bone scan may be performed if the doctor needs a clearer picture of the bones or nerves, the discs between the vertebrae, and other soft tissue. Sometimes an electromyogram (EMG), which helps identify muscle and nerve problems, may be obtained if the physician believes the back is causing numbness or tingling in the legs because of pressure on the nerves. Most of the time roentgenograms are not needed.

## LIVING WITH YOUR DIAGNOSIS

You may experience difficulty bending at the waist, lifting, walking, and standing. Sometimes the pain may keep you awake at night. If the low back pain lasts for months, it may affect your ability to do your job.

## TREATMENT

Management of low back pain depends on the cause of the pain. If the pain is due to an injury, the physician may recommend a short period of bed rest and application of heat or cold to the affected area. Sometimes the physician may prescribe acetaminophen or nonsteroidal antiinflammatory drugs (NSAIDs) to decrease the pain. If the pain is particularly severe, stronger narcotic-containing pain medicines may be needed for a short time. If you are having muscle spasms, a doctor may prescribe a muscle relaxant. All medications have side effects. The NSAIDs may cause stomach upset, diarrhea, ulcers, headache, dizziness, difficulty hearing, or a rash. Side effects of muscle relaxants include drowsiness, dizziness, and a rash.

Physical therapy may be helpful to decrease low back pain. If you are experiencing chronic low back pain, low back and abdominal exercises are helpful.

## DO:

- Take your medications as prescribed.
- Call your doctor if you are experiencing side effects from medications.
- Develop, if you are overweight, a weight loss plan with your physician.
- Participate in daily back-stretching and strengthening exercises.
- Practice good posture when sitting, standing, or lifting.

## DON'T:

- Wait for a possible medication side effect to go away on its own.
- Give up. If your back pain does not decrease, ask your physician about participating in a multidisciplinary low back management program.
- Stop exercising.

## CALL YOUR DOCTOR WHEN:

- You have side effects of medications.
- You continue to have low back pain.
- You need a referral to a physical therapist or counselor.
- You have new pain that runs down the side of your legs.

- You have new numbness or tingling in your legs.
- You have difficulty urinating or have loss of control of your bowels or bladder.

## FOR MORE INFORMATION:

Contact the Arthritis Foundation in your area. If you do not know the location of the nearest office, call the national office at 1-800-283-7800 or access the website at www.arthritis.org.

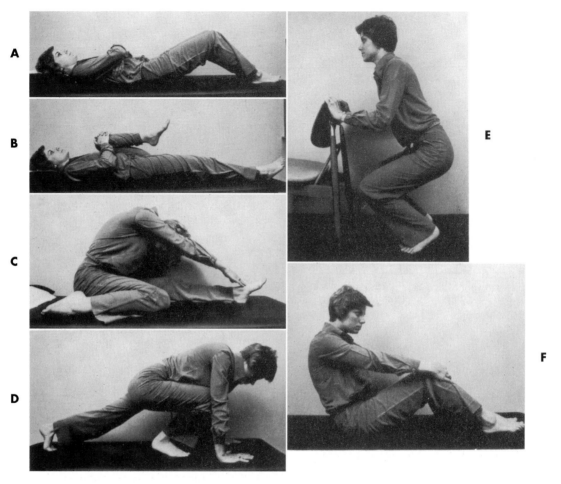

Low back exercises. **A**, Pelvic tilt performed to decrease the lumbar lordosis and raise the anterior aspect of the pelvis. The small of the back is pressed to the floor and the abdominal and buttock muscles are tightened. **B**, Hip flexion, performed to stretch the tight posterior spinal musculature and unload the posterior disc. Each knee is drawn up and pulled firmly to the chest several times and held for 10 to 20 seconds. The exercise is then repeated with both knees. After the acute pain has subsided, the remainder of the exercises are performed: **C**, Hamstring stretching exercises; **D**, hip flexor stretching exercises; **E**, quadriceps strengthening and heel cord stretching exercise; and **F**, abdominal strengthening exercise (sit-ups, which may be partial). All exercises are performed on a carpeted floor and should be repeated in sets of five to ten at least three times daily. (From Mercier LR: *Practical orthopedics*, ed 5, St Louis, 2000, Mosby.)

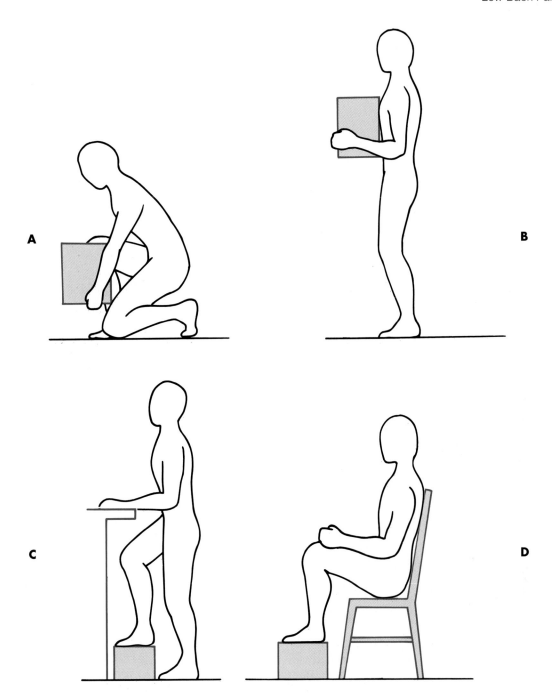

General postural instructions. Patients should be instructed to do the following: **A**, Bend the knees and hips and keep the back straight when lifting. **B**, Hold objects close to the body when carrying. **C**, Place one foot on a stool when standing. **D**, Keep the knees higher than the hips when sitting, and keep the back straight when standing by "tucking in" the abdomen and tightening the buttocks to decrease swayback. In addition, they should avoid high-heeled shoes and sleeping on the abdomen, activities that increase lordosis. (From Mercier LR: *Practical orthopedics*, ed 5, St Louis, 2000, Mosby.)

## LUMBAR DISC DISEASE

### ABOUT YOUR DIAGNOSIS

Your lumbar spine (low back) is made of five vertebrae separated by cartilaginous discs that serve as the "shock absorbers" of the spine. They act as a cushion between the bones and allow some flexibility of the lower back. Degenerative changes or trauma may rupture the annulus fibrosus, the tough band of cartilage surrounding each disc, and disc material may bulge or herniate into the spinal canal or nerve root canal. The herniated or bulging piece of the disc or degenerative bone spur may compress the spinal cord or nerve root, causing pain in the back or tingling and numbness that may radiate to the buttocks, hips, groin, or legs. The pain from a bulging or herniated disc is worse on movement and may be worsened by coughing, laughing, or straining while having a bowel movement. Some patients also have weakness, clumsiness, drop foot, or walking intolerance.

### LIVING WITH YOUR DIAGNOSIS

Degenerative changes in the discs are a normal process as we age. Tobacco abuse, poor posture, and strenuous work with poor lifting technique may accelerate the degenerative changes. The discs gradually become worn, less plump, and eventually flattened. When the disc space becomes narrow enough that the vertebrae rub one another, wear and tear changes develop at the edges of the vertebrae. This wear and tear causes bone spurs to develop that may begin to press on the end of the spinal cord and/or one of its nerve roots. As the nerve becomes irritated, it may cause back and leg pain, tingling and numbness, or weakness in the legs or feet. Rarely, with extremely large, acute disc herniations, a loss of bladder and bowel control may occur.

### TREATMENT

If your physician suspects that you have a lumbar disc that is causing a problem, one or more of the following tests may be ordered: computed tomography (CT) scan (special x-ray pictures of the neck); magnetic resonance imaging (MRI, special non–x-ray pictures of the neck); myelogram/CT (x-ray of the spinal canal and nerve roots); or an electromyogram/nerve conduction velocity test (EMG/NCV, an electrical test of the nerves and muscles). Conservative treatments such as physical therapy, ultrasound, localized heat, and special exercises are usu-

ally performed by a trained physical therapist. Injection of steroids and an anesthetic medication into the spinal canal may provide some relief in patients with chronic pain. Generally, surgery is the final option if conservative treatments have failed to relieve the symptoms. Your surgeon will discuss the risks and benefits of surgery.

### DO:

- Maintain good posture while sitting and walking.
- Always wear a seat belt when traveling in a motor vehicle.
- Make, if you must sit for long periods, a lumbar support by placing a small pillow or rolled towel between your low back and the seat. Stand and walk about frequently (about every hour) to reduce low back fatigue and strain.
- Always lift heavy objects with proper straight spine posture. Hold the object close to your body and use your thigh and leg muscles to lift.
- Participate in a regular exercise program approved by your physician.

### DON'T:

- Sit for long periods. If you must sit or drive for long periods, stop in a safe place and walk for 10 minutes.
- Lift or twist, push or pull heavy objects; always use your leg muscles to lift.
- Use tobacco. It causes cumulative injury to your spine by damaging the normal repair process in the discs and vertebrae.
- Return to work without clearance from your physician.
- Engage in any strenuous activities until cleared with your physician.
- Resume driving until you are pain free or your pain is tolerable without pain medications.

### CALL YOUR DOCTOR WHEN:

- You have any problems associated with your medications.
- Your symptoms become much worse or if you have new signs of weakness.
- You have difficulty walking, develop weakness or inability to move your limbs, or have loss of control of your bowels or bladder.

# FOR MORE INFORMATION:

Contact:
North American Spine Society
6300 North River Road, Suite 500
Rosemont, IL 60018-4231
(847) 698-1630
E-mail: nassman@aol.com
Or visit the website at http://www.webd.alink.net/nass/

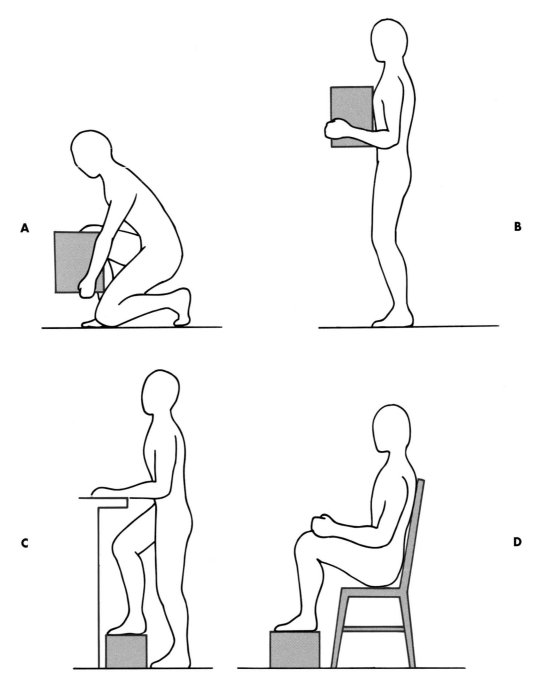

General postural instructions. Patients should be instructed to do the following: **A**, Bend the knees and hips and keep the back straight when lifting. **B**, Hold objects close to the body when carrying. **C**, Place one foot on a stool when standing. **D**, Keep the knees higher than the hips when sitting, and keep the back straight when standing by "tucking in" the abdomen and tightening the buttocks to decrease swayback. In addition, they should avoid high-heeled shoes and sleeping on the abdomen, activities that increase lordosis. (From Mercier LR: *Practical orthopedics*, ed 5, St Louis, 2000, Mosby.)

## LYME DISEASE

### ABOUT YOUR DIAGNOSIS

Lyme disease (LD) can affect many parts of the body including the skin, nerves, brain, heart, and joints.

Lyme disease is a curable infection caused by a microorganism called *Borrelia burgdorferi*. This organism is carried and spread to individuals by certain types of ticks. However, only half of the individuals who have LD actually remember being bitten by a tick. Lyme disease is mainly present in certain regions of the United States including the Northeast, the Midwest (mainly in Wisconsin and Minnesota), and along the West Coast. Although LD is an infection, you cannot catch it from an individual who already has it.

Lyme disease is usually diagnosed by the types of symptoms it causes. A blood test may help confirm the diagnosis, but it is not 100% accurate. Therefore, Lyme tests should not be relied upon to make the diagnosis unless you have symptoms that are very likely caused by LD.

### LIVING WITH YOUR DIAGNOSIS

Lyme disease often occurs in stages, and individuals may only have one or a few of the symptoms before it is diagnosed and treated. Treatment of LD cures the infection and prevents progression of the disease. Some of the earliest symptoms of LD are a rash and flulike symptoms such as fever, chills, muscle and joint aches, fatigue, headache, and enlarged lymph glands. The rash occurs at the site of the tick bite (often on the armpit, groin, or thigh) and is usually raised or flat, and red with a white area in the center. A later stage of LD affects the brain, nerves, and heart. The infection can cause meningitis; headache; weakness in the face, arm, and legs; or nerve pain in the arms and legs. Infections in the heart can cause inflammation and heart rhythm changes, causing fluttering in the chest, chest pain, shortness of breath, lightheadedness, or fainting. The last stage of LD occurs months after the infection. In this stage arthritis develops, causing attacks of pain, swelling, and stiffness in joints, especially the knee. Fatigue may persist throughout the stages of LD.

### TREATMENT

Because LD is an infection, it is treated with antibiotics. Depending on the stage of the disease or the types of symptoms being treated, the antibiotics may be given by mouth or by vein. Unfortunately, despite treatment, some individuals with LD have persistent fatigue, headaches, muscle aches, and joint pain. These symptoms are not caused by an ongoing infection and do not improve with further antibiotic therapy. While the infection is being treated with antibiotics, symptoms such as pain can be treated with acetaminophen or nonsteroidal antiinflammatory drugs (NSAIDs). Potential side effects of NSAIDs include stomach upset, ulcers, constipation, diarrhea, headaches, dizziness, difficulty hearing, and rash.

Prevention of LD can be accomplished by reducing your risk of exposure to ticks when you are in areas where LD is known to occur. Precautions include using good insect repellents (containing "DEET"), wearing long sleeves and pants, tucking pant legs into socks, wearing closed shoes rather than sandals or loafers, brushing off clothes, and inspecting for ticks. If a tick becomes attached, it should be removed with a pair of tweezers by grasping the tick close to the skin and gently pulling it out.

### DO:

- Take your medicines as prescribed.
- Ask your doctor which over-the-counter medications you may take with your prescription medications.
- Take preventive measures to avoid tick exposure.

### DON'T:

- Wait to see whether side effects from medications will go away.

### CALL YOUR DOCTOR WHEN:

- You experience any medication side effects.
- The treatment does not decrease your symptoms in a reasonable amount of time.
- You have new or unexplained symptoms.

### FOR MORE INFORMATION:

Contact the Arthritis Foundation in your area. If you do not know the location of the nearest office, call the national office at 1-800-283-7800 or access the website at www.arthritis.org.

# METATARSALGIA

## ABOUT YOUR DIAGNOSIS

*Metatarsalgia* is a term used to describe pain in the ball of the foot. This type of forefoot pain can be confused with many other causes of forefoot pain, so it is important to ensure the diagnosis is correct. Specifically, metatarsalgia refers to inflammation or pain of the metatarsal heads (or, in other words, "bone pain"). This pain usually is due to increased forces through the forefoot, such as those caused when wearing high heels or when the normal fat pad has shrunk. Increased pressure through the ball of the foot results in inflammation of one or more of the metatarsal bones. Diagnoses that can be confused with metatarsalgia include Morton's neuroma (nerve pain), sesamoiditis, and synovitis.

## LIVING WITH YOUR DIAGNOSIS

Metatarsalgia usually can be managed without surgical intervention, but it may persist for several months or even years. Only after all nonsurgical treatments have failed should you consider surgical intervention. Many times a simple pad or soft shoe insert makes a dramatic difference. To prevent a recurrence, you must stop wearing the offending shoes. Appropriate shoes are necessary to provide adequate cushioning for the painful foot.

## TREATMENT

Metatarsalgia is managed with appropriate footwear such as running shoes, soft shoe inserts, and sometimes custom soft orthotic devices. All are designed to reduce friction and pressure through the forefoot. The soles of shoes can be modified to further reduce pressure by means of placement of a metatarsal bar or rigid rocker on the sole. When calluses are present, regular trimming may provide dramatic relief. Medications and diet are not as effective as local care and do not seem to alter the course of this painful condition. Surgical intervention before adequate attempts at conservative therapy may result in unpredictable results and actually worsen the condition.

## DO:

- Eliminate as much pressure and friction as possible by changing the type and style of shoes you wear.
- Switch to non–weight-bearing forms of exercise such as cycling or swimming.

## DON'T:

- Wear fashionable but impractical shoes.

## CALL YOUR DOCTOR WHEN:

- The pain becomes constant or does not respond to conservative therapy.

## FOR MORE INFORMATION:

Visit the website at
    http://www.countryliving.com/rb/health/07acheb9.htm

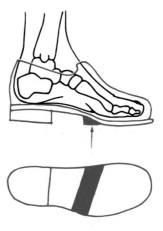

The anterior metatarsal bar *(arrow)*. It is placed behind the metatarsal heads so that weight is transferred to the metatarsal necks. (From Mercier LR: *Practical orthopedics*, ed 5, St Louis, 2000, Mosby.)

# NECK PAIN

## ABOUT YOUR DIAGNOSIS

The neck is made up of the vertebrae (neck bones), spinal cord (which contains the nerves), discs between the vertebrae, and the surrounding soft tissue such as the muscles and ligaments. The vertebrae, or bony parts of the spine, protect the spinal cord. Neck pain may be caused by an injury or disease that affects this area.

Neck pain commonly occurs after one lies in an uncomfortable position for a prolonged period, or sometimes occurs as the result of poor posture. It may occur in association with diseases such as osteoarthritis, rheumatoid arthritis, ankylosing spondylitis, and fibromyalgia. Neck pain may result from an injury to the neck. Stress that causes increased muscle tension may worsen neck pain.

A physician diagnoses neck pain by taking a medical history, performing a physical examination, and possibly by ordering roentgenograms (x-rays). The physician may order blood tests to determine whether the neck pain is due to diseases that may cause similar symptoms. Computed tomography (CT), magnetic resonance imaging (MRI), or a bone scan may be performed if the physician needs a clearer picture of the bones, nerves, discs between the vertebrae, and other soft tissue. Sometimes an electromyogram (EMG), which helps identify muscle and nerve problems, may be obtained if the doctor believes the neck problem may be causing numbness or tingling in the arms due to pressure on the nerves.

## LIVING WITH YOUR DIAGNOSIS

You may experience difficulty looking from side to side, driving, and reading. Sometimes the pain may keep you awake at night. Neck pain can cause headaches. If the neck pain lasts for months, it may affect your ability to do your job.

## TREATMENT

Management of neck pain depends on the cause of the pain. If the pain is due to an injury, your physician may recommend the use of heat or ice on the affected area. Sometimes the physician may prescribe acetaminophen or nonsteroidal antiinflammatory drugs (NSAIDs) to decrease the pain. If the pain is particularly severe, stronger narcotic-containing pain medicines may be needed for a short time. If you experience muscle spasms, your doctor may prescribe a muscle relaxant. Physical therapy may be helpful to decrease the neck pain by means of deep heat treatments, traction, or exercise.

All medications have side effects. NSAIDs may cause stomach upset, diarrhea, ulcers, headache, dizziness, difficulty hearing, or a rash. Some side effects of muscle relaxants are drowsiness, dizziness, and a rash.

## DO:

- Take your medications as prescribed.
- Call your doctor if you are experiencing side effects from medications.
- Practice good posture when sitting and standing.
- Ask your doctor about the use of a cervical pillow.
- Perform neck exercises every day.

## DON'T:

- Wait to see whether a possible side effect of medication goes away on its own.

## CALL YOUR DOCTOR WHEN:

- You experience side effects of medications.
- You continue to have neck pain or headaches.
- You have numbness or tingling in your arms.
- You need a referral to a physical therapist.

## FOR MORE INFORMATION:

Contact the Arthritis Foundation in your area. If you do not know the location of the nearest office, call the national office at 1-800-283-7800 or access the website at www.arthritis.org.

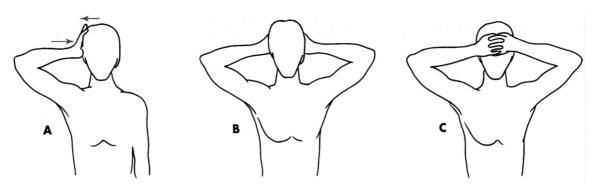

Isometric neck exercises. **A**, The hand is placed against the side of the head slightly above the ear, and pressure is gradually increased while resisting with the neck muscles and keeping the head in the same position. The position is held 5 seconds, relaxed, and repeated five times. **B**, The exercise is performed on the other side and then **C**, from the back and front. The exercise should be performed three or four times daily. (From Mercier LR: *Practical orthopedics*, ed 5, St Louis, 2000, Mosby.)

## OSTEOARTHRITIS

### ABOUT YOUR DIAGNOSIS

Osteoarthritis (OA) is also called "wear and tear arthritis" or degenerative joint disease. Osteoarthritis commonly affects the weight-bearing joints of the body such as the hips, knees, and spine, but it may also affect the hands. In OA, the cushion on the end of the bone, the cartilage, begins to wear down, resulting in pain.

Although the exact cause of OA is unknown, a variety of factors may increase an individual's risk of developing OA. In the past, it was believed that OA developed as an individual got older because the joints "just wore out." However, age is just one cause of OA. Obesity, repetitive movements, and a prior severe injury to a joint can lead to OA. Osteoarthritis of the fingers develops more often in women than in men. Osteoarthritis occurs more often in some families.

Osteoarthritis is not an infectious illness. In other words, you cannot "catch" OA from another individual. A physician can diagnose OA by obtaining a medical history, performing an examination of the joints, and ordering x-rays. An x-ray will show that the joint space (where the cartilage separates the two bones) is narrowed or absent. The x-ray may also show bone spurs that can be responsible for some of the pain. Blood tests are usually normal in osteoarthritis.

### LIVING WITH YOUR DIAGNOSIS

Most individuals begin to notice OA as gradual joint pain and stiffness, most commonly in the hands, knees, hips, and back. Pain and stiffness usually worsen with activity and toward the end of the day. Osteoarthritis may also affect the neck and feet. Pain and stiffness may make it more difficult to perform some daily activities such as bending at the waist, grasping or reaching for objects, turning the neck, and walking or climbing stairs. There is no cure for OA; however, medications, exercises, and assistive devices can decrease the pain and improve one's quality of life.

### TREATMENT

The best management of OA is a combination of different treatments. Acetaminophen or nonsteroidal antiinflammatory drugs (NSAIDs) are used to decrease the pain and stiffness. Potential side effects of NSAIDs include stomach upset, ulcers, constipation, diarrhea,

headaches, dizziness, difficulty hearing, and a rash. The NSAIDs should be taken with food. Cortisone injections into the joint can be helpful. A physical therapist can provide exercises to strengthen muscles that provide stability to the joints, which may help decrease pain. Water exercise programs may be particularly beneficial because the water decreases the stress on the joints. An occupational therapist provides hand exercises and may discuss ways to do certain activities differently or suggest an assistive device to avoid pain. Joint surgery such as a hip or knee replacement may be recommended if the pain is particularly severe and if an x-ray shows there is no space between the two bones of a joint.

### DO:

- Take your medication as prescribed.
- Ask your doctor what over-the-counter pain medications you may take with your prescription medications.
- Eat a well-balanced diet and lose those extra pounds if you are overweight.
- Perform a physician-prescribed exercise program, because exercise can decrease the pain of osteoarthritis.

### DON'T:

- Wait to see whether a side effect from the medication will go away.
- Overeat and assume a gain of 2 or 3 pounds a year will not affect the pain of OA.
- Continue an exercise program that causes pain. If pain after exercise continues, it usually means the exercise needs to be modified specifically for you.

### CALL YOUR DOCTOR WHEN:

- You experience any medication side effects.
- The medication and other treatments are not decreasing the pain.
- You believe you may need a referral to a physical therapist or an occupational therapist.

### FOR MORE INFORMATION:

Contact the Arthritis Foundation in your area. If you do not know the location of the nearest office, call the national office at 1-800-283-7800 or access the website at www.arthritis.org.

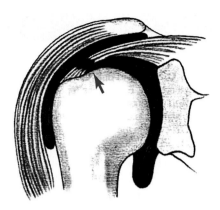

Rupture of the rotator cuff *(arrow).* Full thickness rupture allows joint fluid to escape from the glenohumeral joint into the subacromial region. This is often an MRI clue to a full thickness tear. (From Mercier LR: *Practical orthopedics,* ed 5, St Louis, 2000, Mosby.)

# OSTEOPOROSIS

## ABOUT YOUR DIAGNOSIS

Osteoporosis is a metabolic bone disease in which bones become brittle, predisposing them to fractures.

Decreased estrogen levels in postmenopausal women is one of the most common causes of osteoporosis. Oral steroids taken for asthma or arthritis may also cause osteoporosis.

Osteoporosis may be caused by poor nutritional intake of vitamins and minerals, such as vitamin D and calcium. Cigarette smoking, alcohol consumption, and a sedentary lifestyle predispose individuals to osteoporosis. Petite white women with a positive family history of osteoporosis are at high risk. Hyperthyroidism, hyperparathyroidism, or Cushing's syndrome can also lead to osteoporosis.

Osteoporosis has been diagnosed in 4 million to 6 million individuals in the United States. It is four times more common in women than men. Risk increases with age. There are at least 275,000 osteoporotic fractures of the hip every year.

Osteoporosis may be detected on an x-ray of a bone. The osteoporosis must be advanced to be noticeable on x-ray. Dual energy x-ray absorptiometry (DEXA) is a more sensitive measure of bone density and can be used to follow bone density over time. Osteoporosis is defined as a bone density of 2.5 standard deviations below the peak mean bone density of the general population. Patients with bone densities below this level are at high risk for having fractures. Patients with intermediate bone densities and a previous history of fracture also have osteoporosis.

Osteoporosis may be prevented or cured with proper medical therapy.

## LIVING WITH YOUR DIAGNOSIS

Many individuals with osteoporosis have no symptoms. Some have a loss of height and curvature of the spine. Others may have pain from a hip, spine, or wrist fracture.

## TREATMENT

A regular weight-bearing exercise such as walking is an excellent preventive therapy. Dietary calcium intake should be between 1000 and 1500 mg of elemental calcium a day. Vitamin D is necessary for the absorption of calcium from the diet; 400–800 international units (IU) of vitamin D are recommended daily. Postmenopausal women should also consider estrogen replacement therapy with 0.625 mg of conjugated equine estrogen per day. Alendronate, an oral bisphosphonate, in a dosage of 5 to 10 mg once a day has been approved for the prevention of osteoporosis. All of these preventive therapies may also be used in patients with established osteoporosis. In addition, calcitonin, available as a nasal spray or as an injection, is indicated for women who cannot take estrogen and who are postmenopausal by more than 5 years. Surgery is often required to repair fractured bones.

Side effects of treatment may include kidney stones caused by excess calcium replacement, vitamin D toxicity, or esophageal ulcers caused by alendronate therapy. Estrogen therapy has been associated in some studies with a mild increase in the risk for breast cancer, and a marked increase in endometrial uterine cancers. Women who have not had a hysterectomy must take estrogen in combination with a progestin to minimize the risk of endometrial cancer. Estrogen may also lead to breast tenderness and resumption of menses in postmenopausal women. Benefits of estrogen therapy include a markedly decreased risk of coronary artery disease and increased vaginal lubrication. Each woman with osteoporosis should discuss individual concerns about estrogen replacement therapy with a knowledgeable physician before beginning this therapy. Raloxifene (Evista) is a newer product recently approved for the prevention of osteoporosis. It shares some of the benefits of estrogens such as increased bone density and lowering of lipids and is without significant adverse effects on the endometrium and breasts. It can, however, cause hot flashes and increase the risk of thrombosis.

## DO:

- Minimize any risk factors for osteoporosis by quitting cigarette smoking, decreasing alcohol or caffeine intake, increasing exercise, and taking adequate calcium and vitamin D.
- Have a vitamin D level measured in your blood, especially if you live in a northern climate and have low sun exposure.
- Have regular breast examinations and mammograms if you take estrogen.

## DON'T:

- Take alendronate with food; it will not be absorbed.
- Take alendronate when you lay down; it may cause esophageal ulcers. Instead, stand up and take it with a full glass of water.
- Take calcium without consulting your doctor if you have a history of kidney stones or hyperparathyroidism.
- Take more vitamin D than recommended by your physician.
- Take estrogen alone if you are postmenopausal and you have a uterus. Instead, take estrogen with a progestin.

## CALL YOUR DOCTOR WHEN:

- You wish to have a bone density measurement.
- You would like an assessment of your current calcium intake.
- You notice any new hip, back, wrist, or rib pain, especially if it occurs after falling, coughing, or sneezing.

- You wish to discuss the risks and benefits of estrogen replacement.
- You notice a new lump on your breast.
- You have heartburn while taking alendronate.

## FOR MORE INFORMATION:

Contact:
National Osteoporosis Foundation
1150 17th Street NW, Suite 500
Washington, DC 20036-4603
(202) 223-2226
Website at http://www.nof.org/osteoporosis

The Endocrine Society
4350 East West Highway, Suite 500
Bethesda, MD 20814-4410
1-888-ENDOCRINE
Website: http://www.endo-society.org.

The NIH Consensus Development Conference Statement is online at the website http://text.nom.nih.gov/nih/cdc/www/43txt.html.

# POLYMYALGIA RHEUMATICA

## ABOUT YOUR DIAGNOSIS

Polymyalgia rheumatica (PMR) is a type of inflammation that produces pain and stiffness in the muscles around the neck, shoulders, buttocks, hips, and thighs. It seldom occurs in individuals younger than 50 years. No one knows what causes the inflammation in PMR, but it is not an infectious illness (like colds). Therefore you cannot "catch" it from another individual.

Polymyalgia rheumatica is diagnosed mostly by its symptoms. However, most individuals with PMR have evidence of inflammation as indicated by the results of two blood tests: the erythrocyte sedimentation rate (ESR) and the C-reactive protein (CRP). Because there are other diseases that can cause symptoms similar to those of PMR, your doctor will probably order other blood tests to be sure you do not have another problem.

## LIVING WITH YOUR DIAGNOSIS

Individuals with PMR commonly notice pain and stiffness (a feeling of restricted motion) in the muscles around the neck, shoulders, buttocks, hips, and thighs. The pain and stiffness are most noticeable in the morning and may improve with activity during the course of the day. Occasionally, PMR may also cause pain and swelling in the joints. In addition, PMR can also cause fatigue, poor appetite, fever, and sweats. Approximately 20% of individuals with PMR also have another condition called "temporal arteritis," which may cause headaches and sudden vision changes. Your doctor will determine whether you also have this condition. Fortunately, the treatment of PMR results in considerable improvement in nearly all of these symptoms within a few days. Although PMR responds to therapy, some patients may require treatment for more than 2 or 3 years.

## TREATMENT

The most common treatment for PMR is corticosteroids (cortisone-like medicines such as prednisone). Nonsteroidal antiinflammatory drugs (NSAIDs) such as ibuprofen are sometimes also used. Potential side effects of corticosteroids are increased appetite, weight gain, difficulty sleeping, easy bruising, and stomach upset. Longer-term use of corticosteroids can lower your resistance to infection, and cause stomach ulcers and bone thinning (osteoporosis).

Corticosteroids should always be taken with food to prevent stomach upset. In addition, patients should receive adequate amounts of calcium and vitamin D to help prevent osteoporosis.

## DO:

- Take your medicines as prescribed.
- Ask your doctor which over-the-counter medications you may take with your prescription medications.
- Inform your doctor and dentist that you are taking a corticosteroid (prednisone).
- Eat a well-balanced diet low in carbohydrates and fat to prevent excessive weight gain.
- Perform a physician-prescribed weight-bearing exercise program.

## DON'T:

- Wait to see whether side effects from the medicines will go away.
- Stop taking the corticosteroid medicine unless your physician instructs you to do so.
- Overeat, because corticosteroids may increase your appetite.
- Continue an exercise program that causes pain.

## CALL YOUR DOCTOR WHEN:

- You have any medication side effects.
- Your pain and/or stiffness return during treatment.
- You have new headaches, cramping in your tongue or jaw, or sudden changes in your vision.
- You run out of prednisone (cortisone).

## FOR MORE INFORMATION:

Contact the Arthritis Foundation in your area. If you do not know the location of the nearest office, call the national office at 1-800-283-7800 or access the website at www.arthritis.org.

# PSEUDOGOUT

## ABOUT YOUR DIAGNOSIS

Pseudogout is an abrupt and often very painful form of arthritis generally affecting individuals older than 60 years. It usually affects only one joint at a time such as a knee, ankle, wrist, elbow, or shoulder. Because it resembles gout but has a different cause, it is called pseudogout, meaning "false gout."

Pseudogout "attacks" are caused by the release of "crystals," made of calcium and phosphorus, into a joint. These crystals cause inflammation in the joint, leading to pain and swelling. No one knows why some individuals get pseudogout and others do not. It is not caused by an infection. In other words you cannot "catch" it. The only way to be certain of the diagnosis of pseudogout is to place a needle into the affected joint, remove joint fluid, and look for the pseudogout crystals under a microscope.

## LIVING WITH YOUR DIAGNOSIS

Individuals with pseudogout commonly have pain, swelling, warmth, and redness develop rapidly in the affected joint. The pain is often constant and it gets worse if the joint is moved a lot. Everyday activities such as walking, dressing, and lifting may be difficult. In some cases more than one joint may be affected. Some individuals experience fever and fatigue with the arthritis.

There is no way to know when or how many attacks an individual will have once the first attack occurs. Attacks may occur at any time; however, certain events, such as surgery or an acute illness, can trigger attacks. Once the attacks are treated, the symptoms generally resolve within days; untreated they may last for several weeks or more. Between attacks the symptoms resolve completely for most individuals.

## TREATMENT

Nonsteroidal antiinflammatory drugs (NSAIDs) such as ibuprofen, naproxen, or indomethacin are commonly used to treat pseudogout. Potential side effects of NSAIDs include stomach upset, ulcers, constipation, diarrhea, headaches, dizziness, difficulty hearing, and skin rash. Occasionally, a more potent antiinflammatory medicine such as prednisone, a cortisone-like medicine, is necessary. Potential side effects of cortisone-like medicines are increased appetite, weight gain, difficulty sleeping, easy bruising, and stomach upset. Colchicine is another type of antiinflammatory medication used to treat pseudogout. Colchicine's potential side effects include stomach cramps, nausea, vomiting, and diarrhea. Removal of the joint fluid from the affected joint followed by a cortisone injection into the joint is another common treatment for pseudogout. Cortisone injections usually provide the most rapid and complete relief of pain and swelling. Aside from the discomfort of the injection, there are very few side effects with cortisone injections. Regardless of the specific treatment used, it is important to rest the affected joint until the symptoms begin to subside.

## DO:

- Rest the affected joint until the symptoms begin to improve.
- Take your medicines as prescribed.
- Ask your doctor which over-the-counter medications you may take with your prescription medications.

## DON'T:

- Wait to see whether side effects from medications will go away.
- Give up; ask your doctor about other treatment options if your symptoms are not going away on their own.

## CALL YOUR DOCTOR WHEN:

- You experience any medication side effects.
- The treatment is not decreasing your symptoms in a reasonable amount of time.
- You begin to lose full motion in the affected joint.
- You experience worsening warmth, redness, or pain after a cortisone injection.

## FOR MORE INFORMATION:

Contact the Arthritis Foundation in your area. If you do not know the location of the nearest office, call the national office at 1-800-283-7800 or access the website at www.arthritis.org.

# RAYNAUD'S PHENOMENON

## ABOUT YOUR DIAGNOSIS

Raynaud's phenomenon causes temporary decreased blood flow to the fingers, toes, and ears; and, less often, to the tip of the nose. Raynaud's phenomenon usually occurs with exposure to cold temperatures when blood flow decreases in the fingers and toes. The skin in the area involved will first turn white because there is no blood in that area. Next, the skin may turn blue, and once the blood flows back into the skin, become purple or red. If Raynaud's is not treated, sores or ulcers may develop in the areas with the decreased blood flow. If the blood flow is decreased for a long time, the skin in the affected areas could turn black and die. Rarely, Raynaud's phenomenon affects organs inside the body.

Raynaud's phenomenon may occur at any age but usually occurs between the ages of 20 and 40 years. It occurs more often in women than in men. Although we do not know the cause of Raynaud's, it is not an uncommon illness. To diagnose Raynaud's, a physician obtains a medical history and performs a physical examination. There are no specific blood tests to diagnose Raynaud's, but a physician may perform certain blood tests to determine whether Raynaud's phenomenon is associated with other conditions.

## LIVING WITH YOUR DIAGNOSIS

Raynaud's phenomenon may cause pain and numbness when the affected areas turn white. Some individuals have swelling, warmth, or a throbbing pain when the affected areas turn purple or red. To prevent these problems, you should keep the body warm and avoid any unnecessary exposure to cold. If you have a job that involves working outside or that exposes your body to cold temperatures indoors, you should see whether your job can be modified or explore other employment options.

## TREATMENT

The best way to manage Raynaud's phenomenon is through a combination of therapies and preventive measures. To keep the body warm you should dress in layers, wear lined mittens rather than gloves, wear a hat and scarf, and always carry a sweater with you to adjust to the room temperature. To avoid exposure to cold, have someone warm up your car in the winter, use an oven mitt to get items out of the refrigerator/freezer, and warm up the bathroom by letting the warm water run for a while before you take a shower or bath. Smoking causes the blood vessels to close down, leading to less blood flow in the affected areas and a greater chance of sores or an infection developing in those areas. Therefore individuals with Raynaud's must stop smoking. If emotional stress seems to cause a Raynaud's attack, relaxation and biofeedback may be helpful to increase the circulation in certain areas of the body. If the Raynaud's is severe, a physician may prescribe a medication such as nifedipine that can improve the blood flow. The most common side effects of this medication may include swelling in the hands and feet, lightheadedness or dizziness, and a rash. If these medications do not help and if your symptoms are severe, your physician may suggest a type of surgery called a sympathectomy. This surgery involves cutting the nerves that cause the blood vessels to close down, thereby increasing blood flow.

## DO:

- Call your doctor if you are experiencing side effects from medications.
- Ask your doctor what over-the-counter medications you may take or should avoid.
- Stop smoking.
- Examine your fingers, toes, nose, and ears daily for any new sores or infections.
- Moisturize your affected areas with ointments at least daily.

## DON'T:

- Wait to see whether a possible medication side effect will go away on its own.
- Continue smoking.
- Expose yourself unnecessarily to cold.

## CALL YOUR DOCTOR WHEN:

- You experience side effects that you believe may be caused by your medications.

- The medication and other treatments are not helping to improve your symptoms.
- You are concerned about a sore in an affected area.
- You need a referral to a stop smoking program.
- You believe you need a referral to a vocational rehabilitation specialist to explore other job options.

## FOR MORE INFORMATION:

Contact the Arthritis Foundation in your area. If you do not know the location of the nearest office, call the national office at 1-800-283-7800 or access the website at www.arthritis.org.

# ROTATOR CUFF TENDINITIS/TEAR

## ABOUT YOUR DIAGNOSIS

Rotator cuff diseases include inflammation (tendinitis) and possibly a partial- or full-thickness tear of the tendon (see figure). This causes marked pain in the shoulder region. This pain may worsen at night or with activities in which the arms are held over the head. Rotator cuff problems are caused by cumulative trauma throughout one's lifetime. It is believed to be partially caused by impingement of the tendon on a bone spur within the shoulder. Rotator cuff tendinitis or tear is fairly common. It is usually detected by means of placing the shoulder through ranges of motion that reproduce the pain. The diagnosis is generally made by means of history and physical examination. Magnetic resonance imaging (MRI) is helpful when a tear is suspected. Rotator cuff tendinitis or tear can be managed to the point that pain can usually be completely alleviated.

## LIVING WITH YOUR DIAGNOSIS

Signs and symptoms of rotator cuff tendinitis and possible tear include pain in the shoulder that worsens with activities such as lying down to sleep at night or working with one's arms over one's head. The tendinitis not only causes pain in the shoulder region but also can eventually lead to a tear in the rotator cuff tendon itself. When that happens, the shoulder becomes much weaker, and it becomes quite difficult to perform any activities above your head.

## TREATMENT

Rotator cuff tendinitis generally can be managed successfully with nonsurgical methods. Nonsteroidal anti-inflammatory drugs (NSAIDs) can help not only to control inflammation but also to relieve pain. Cortisone injections may also be effective. Exercise, specifically physical therapy focused on rotator cuff rehabilitation to strengthen the internal and external rotator tendons of the shoulder, can make a difference in the overall pain (see figure). Surgical decompression or possible repair of the torn tendon is considered when physical therapy does not make a difference or when the tendon actually sustains a tear. Surgical treatment may have complications, and you should discuss them thoroughly with your physician before you undergo this form of treatment.

## DO:

- Take your medications as prescribed.
- Perform your exercises as directed.

## DON'T:

- Take addictive pain medications as long-term therapy for rotator cuff tendinitis or tear.
- Perform activities that necessitate using your hands above your head.
- Attempt to strengthen the shoulder with push-ups. This has not been found to make a difference and may worsen the pain.

## CALL YOUR DOCTOR WHEN:

- The pain is severe enough to prevent you from sleeping satisfactorily at night and is not controlled with over-the-counter medications.

## FOR MORE INFORMATION:

Visit the website at http://www.sechrest.com/mmg/shoulder/cufftear.html

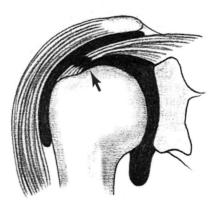

Rupture of the rotator cuff *(arrow)*. Full thickness rupture allows joint fluid to escape from the glenohumeral joint into the subacromial region. This is often an MRI clue to a full thickness tear. (From Mercier LR: *Practical orthopedics,* ed 5, St Louis, 2000, Mosby.)

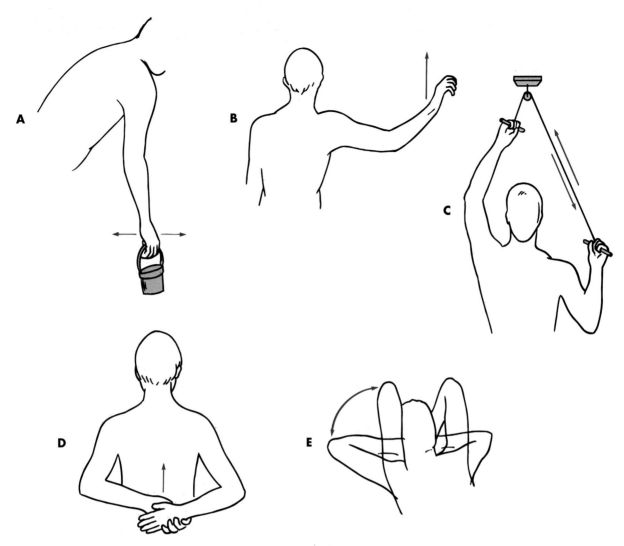

Shoulder strengthening exercises. **A,** Pendulum exercises. **B,** Wall-climbing exercise. **C,** Rope and pulley exercises. The normal arm assists in the elevation of the stiffened arm. **D,** Exercise for restoring internal rotation. **E,** Exercise for restoring external rotation. Each exercise should be performed hourly or at least four times a day. Applying moist heat before the exercise may be helpful. In addition, activities that aggravate the pain, such as overhead work, should be avoided. For sitting work, a chair that supports the arms and shoulders should be used, and the patient should sit as close to the working surface as possible. (From Mercier LR: *Practical orthopedics,* ed 5, St Louis, 2000, Mosby.)

# SCOLIOSIS

## ABOUT YOUR DIAGNOSIS

Scoliosis is defined as a lateral (or sideways) curvature of the spine that measures more than 10 degrees. It usually begins during childhood or adolescence and may continue to slowly worsen into adulthood. Typically, the greater the angle of the curvature, the greater is the risk that it will progress. Curves less than 30 degrees at the end of growth rarely progress and do not usually necessitate close observation. Curves greater than 50 to 75 degrees are at a high risk for progression and may necessitate aggressive therapy.

Pain is the most common reason that adults seek treatment of scoliosis. Although the pain is believed to be caused by muscle fatigue along the outside of the curve, the true source of the pain remains unclear. Some patients may notice a loss of height, an increase in the prominence of a rib, or changes in their waistline, which can signal a progression of the curve.

A series of roentgenograms (x-rays) taken over several years is the most accurate method for monitoring the curve. A slowly progressive curve may remain nonpainful and as a result not require formal treatment. However, a rapidly progressive curve that produces pain and deformity may require more aggressive management.

## LIVING WITH YOUR DIAGNOSIS

The diagnosis of scoliosis includes a wide range of deformities from mild to painful and severe. Although the deformity may not be noticeable until late in the course of the progression of the curve, the emotional aspects of this disease may be quite severe, particularly for adolescents. Breathing difficulties may develop with large curves but are usually preceded by pain and fatigue.

## TREATMENT

Analgesics and antiinflammatory drugs may reduce the pain of scoliosis. There are no medications, injections, diets, or exercises that affect the curve itself. The nonoperative management of scoliosis includes routine roentgenograms taken at regular intervals to monitor for progression. Bracing can be effective in preventing progression but does not correct a curve that has already developed. Exercises have not proved to be of benefit in this diagnosis, nor has electrical stimulation of muscles. An operation is indicated when the curve progresses or results in severe pain. When the curve is not progressive, you have to decide whether the pain warrants a complex surgical procedure. The surgeon must be sure that there is not some other cause for the back pain that may be unrelated to the scoliosis.

## DO:

- Take your medications as prescribed.
- Wear your brace as directed, but be aware that many curves can progress despite bracing.

## DON'T:

- Stop wearing your brace without your doctor's recommendation.

## CALL YOUR DOCTOR WHEN:

- You notice a change in the deformity, such as an increased rib prominence, change in leg length, or new onset of pain.

## FOR MORE INFORMATION:

Visit the website at http://www.yahoo.com/Health/Diseases_and_Conditions/Scoliosis

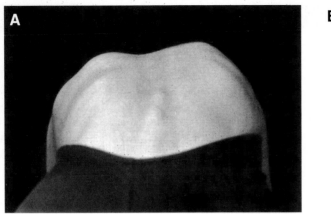
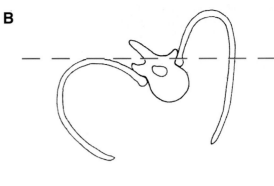

**A,** Scoliosis with rib prominence resulting from vertebral rotation is best exhibited on forward bending (the Adams position). **B,** Cross section of the chest showing rib distortion as a result of vertebral rotation. (From Mercier LR: *Practical orthopedics,* ed 5, St Louis, 2000, Mosby.)

# WARTS, PLANTAR

## ABOUT YOUR DIAGNOSIS

All warts, including plantar warts, are caused by the family of viruses called the human papillomavirus (HPV) group. Certain HPV viruses are more likely to infect one area of the body than the other. In the case of plantar warts, the HPV virus infects the bottom of the foot.

Anyone can get warts; they are very common in the United States. The group of individuals most likely to get warts is those people between the ages of 10 and 20 years. Plantar warts are often obtained by walking barefoot in public locker rooms, showers, and pool areas. Individuals with plantar warts leave the virus behind on the moist floor, and it is then picked up by bare feet.

Plantar warts can be a big problem because they are on the bottom of the foot. When we stand on them, the warts are like a big lump in our shoe and it hurts. The pain can become so severe that simply standing becomes difficult.

## LIVING WITH YOUR DIAGNOSIS

A plantar wart begins as a thickening of the skin on the bottom of the foot. At first this may seem like a small callus or bunion, but over time the plantar wart becomes larger, hurts, and takes on a very sharp border. It is flat and usually flesh colored, but it can bleed and become brown or blackish.

The plantar wart will often grow and make walking, running, and even standing very painful. A large number of plantar warts will go away on their own; more than 65% of all warts will go away in 2 years with no treatment.

## TREATMENT

Because the plantar wart forms on the sole of the foot, it is often covered by thick skin. After soaking in a shower or bath, gentle abrasion with a coarse cloth or pumice rock will remove some of this thick skin. This will help the medication to get to the wart but not go too deeply and cause soreness or bleeding. The usual medication placed on a plantar wart is 40% salicylic acid in plaster form (Duoplast). Salicylic acid ointment can also be applied and then covered with an occlusive tape. The pre-made plaster (Duoplast) is easier to use.

The plaster is cut to the size of the plantar wart and applied once a week. The acid will kill the wart and the skin around it. Each time the plaster is taken off, the underlying whitish dead skin must be removed. Sometimes the plaster will cause inflammation and tenderness. If this occurs you should stop the treatment for 2 or 3 days. Treatment should be continued until the wart is gone. This may take several weeks.

If the plantar wart does not go away, or if it becomes very sore with treatment, you need to call your doctor. Your doctor has other treatments that may be more successful. Warts can come back even after a cure. You must remember to avoid reinfection if at all possible.

## DO:

- Treat plantar warts early; waiting makes treatment more difficult.
- Wear protective footwear (flip-flops, sandals) in public showers, locker rooms, and pool areas.
- Gently remove dead skin overlying the wart.
- Use salicylic acid plasters or ointment on plantar warts.
- Wash hands after touching your plantar warts.

## DON'T:

- Cut, dig, or pick at your plantar warts.
- Put your feet in contact with warts on other parts of the body.
- Cause your warts to bleed.
- Continue treatment of your plantar warts if they become painful or sore.

## CALL YOUR DOCTOR WHEN:

- Your wart does not go away with salicylic acid treatment, or if it becomes worse.

## FOR MORE INFORMATION:

Contact:
The American Academy of Dermatology
930 N. Meachum Road
Schaumburg, IL 60173
(847) 330-0230

# Index

**A**

Abdomen, shoulder pain referred from, 69
Abduction
    definition of, 4
    shoulder, 49*f*
Abscess
    Brodie's, 231, 325
    sonography of, 332-333
    subungual, 102*f*
Abuse, fractures associated with, 22, 23*f*
Acetabulum
    fractures of, 157*f*, 310-311, 311*f*
    protrusio acetabuli, 171
Acetic acids, 247*t*
Achilles tendon
    bursae, 210
    "pump bump," 259, 259*f*
    roentgenography of, 324
    rupture of, 211, 211*f*
    tendinitis of, 210
Acromioclavicular joint
    anatomy of, 49*f*
    dislocation, 64, 262
    osteoarthritis of, 65
    roentgenography of, 297
    sports-related injuries, 262
Acute cartilage necrosis, 166
Acute compartment syndrome, 17
Acute rheumatic fever, 228, 228*t*
Adduction, 4
Adhesive capsulitis. *see* Frozen shoulder
Adson's test, 40*f*
Alendronate, for osteoporosis, 145
Alignment, 6
Alkaptonuria, 243
Allen's test, 116, 116*f*
Allis' sign, 161*f*
Allopurinol, 239
Anaerobic infections, 231
Anesthesia
    metacarpal block, 97*f*
    for soft-tissue management, 371
    for treating fractures, 12-13
Aneurysm, aortic, 147

Page references with *"t"* denote tables;
those with *"f"* denote figures

Aneurysmal bone cyst
    of knee, 319-320
    of thoracic spine, 289-290
Angiography, 334, 334*f*
Angular deformities, of lower extremities
    Blount's disease, 323, 377, 378*f*
    genu valgum, 378, 378*f*
    genu varum, 377
Animal bites, 233
Ankle
    anatomy of, 200, 201*f*
    developmental variants of, 324-325
    exercises, 206*f*
    fractures of, 218-220
    instability tests, 205*f*
    magnetic resonance imaging of, 349,
        351*f*-352*f*
    pathology of, 324-325
    roentgenography of
        anatomy, 324-325
        anteroposterior view, 323, 323*f*
        examination, 323-324
        lateral view, 323
        oblique view, 323, 323*f*
    running injuries, 259-260
    sports-related injuries
        sprain, 269
        wrapping and taping techniques for
            preventing, 269, 270*f*-271*f*
    sprain
        clinical features of, 204-205, 205*f*, 269
        description of, 204
        sports-related, 269
        treatment of, 205, 207, 269
    wrapping and taping techniques for, 269,
        270*f*-271*f*
Ankylosing spondylitis
    clinical features of, 138, 314
    definition of, 138
    diagnosis of, 138
    differential diagnosis of, 139
    extraskeletal manifestations of, 138-139
    gender predilection, 138
    laboratory findings of, 138
    prognosis, 139-140
    roentgenographic findings of, 138, 139*f*
    treatment of, 139
Ankylosis, 4

Ansaid. *see* Flurbiprofen
Anserine bursa, 193, 194*f*
Anserine bursitis, 257
Antalgic gait, 4
Anterior capsular insufficiency, 262
Anterior cruciate ligament
    anatomy of, 177, 178*f*
    injury
        chronic knee instability secondary to,
            186-187, 187*f*
        clinical features of, 183-185
        description of, 183
        Lachman test, 185, 185*f*
        treatment, 185-186
Anterior inferior tibiofibular, 204
Anterior knee pain syndrome, 257-258, 396
Anterior talofibular ligament, 204, 204*f*
Antibiotics, 233
Antiinflammatory medications
    description of, 246
    nonsteroidal anti-inflammatory medica-
        tions. *see* Nonsteroidal anti-inflam-
        matory medications
    side effects of, 246-248
Anulus fibrosus, 26
Apophysis, 276-277
Apposition, 6, 7*f*
"Apprehension" test, 189*f*
Arnold-Chiari malformation, 339
Arthritis
    glenohumeral joint, 65
    gouty
        clinical features of, 238, 238*t*
        definition of, 238
        diagnostic studies
            crystal analysis, 236
            synovial fluid analysis, 236*t*
        roentgenographic findings of, 238,
            239*f*
        treatment of, 238-239
    Lyme, 245-246
    osteoarthritis
        of glenohumeral joint, 65
        of hand, 92, 96*t*
        of hip, 168-169
        of knee, 192-193
        of sacroiliac joint, 154
        of wrist, 92, 96*t*